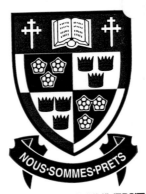

NOUS·SOMMES·PRETS

SIMON FRASER UNIVERSITY
W.A.C. BENNETT LIBRARY

Obesity and
Mental Disorders

Medical Psychiatry

Series Editor Emeritus

William A. Frosch, M.D.
Weill Medical College of Cornell University
New York, New York, U.S.A.

Advisory Board

Jonathan E. Alpert, M.D., Ph.D.
Massachusetts General Hospital and
Harvard University School of Medicine
Boston, Massachusetts, U.S.A.

Bennett Leventhal, M.D.
University of Chicago School of Medicine
Chicago, Illinois, U.S.A.

Siegfried Kasper, M.D.
Medical University of Vienna
Vienna, Austria

Mark H. Rapaport, M.D.
Cedars-Sinai Medical Center
Los Angeles, California, U.S.A.

Obesity and Mental Disorders

edited by

Susan L. McElroy
University of Cincinnati
Cincinnati, Ohio, U.S.A.

David B. Allison
University of Alabama at Birmingham
Birmingham, Alabama, U.S.A.

George A. Bray
Louisiana State University System
Baton Rouge, Louisiana, U.S.A.

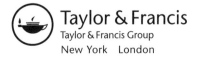

Taylor & Francis
Taylor & Francis Group
New York   London

Published in 2006 by
Taylor & Francis Group
270 Madison Avenue
New York, NY 10016

No claim to original U.S. Government works
Printed in the United States of America on acid-free paper
10 9 8 7 6 5 4 3 2 1

International Standard Book Number-10: 0-8247-2944-7 (Hardcover)
International Standard Book Number-13: 978-0-8247-2944-8 (Hardcover)

This book contains information obtained from authentic and highly regarded sources. Reprinted material is quoted with permission, and sources are indicated. A wide variety of references are listed. Reasonable efforts have been made to publish reliable data and information, but the author and the publisher cannot assume responsibility for the validity of all materials or for the consequences of their use.

Library of Congress Cataloging-in-Publication Data

Catalog record is available from the Library of Congress

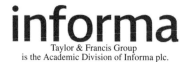

Taylor & Francis Group
is the Academic Division of Informa plc.

Visit the Taylor & Francis Web site at
http://www.taylorandfrancis.com

Preface

Obesity and mental disorders are major public health problems that co-occur to a significant, but unknown, degree. Indeed, whether or not these conditions are related has been a focus of scientific debate for over 50 years. However, the evaluation and treatment of the patient with obesity and a comorbid mental disorder have received extremely little empirical study, and presently there are very few treatment guidelines to help clinicians manage such individuals.

Many emerging lines of evidence suggest that reexamination of the relationship between obesity and mental disorders is in order, particularly for mental health professionals. In this regard, the significant overlap between obesity and psychopathology in clinical populations may be the most important. Weight gain, overweight, and obesity frequently complicate the treatment of patients with mental disorders, especially those with psychotic disorders, mood disorders, and eating disorders. Conversely, mood and eating symptoms and disorders are common in persons of all ages seeking treatment for obesity, as well as some of the general medical conditions associated with obesity, such as type 3 diabetes and cardiovascular disease.

However, the reasons for the overlap between obesity and mental disorders in clinical populations are not understood. First, iatrogenic factors likely play a role. Many of the drugs used to treat psychotic and mood disorders are associated with weight gain. Conversely, some of the drugs used to treat the general medical conditions that co-occur with obesity may induce psychological systems. Second, both obesity and many mental disorders are increasingly severe public health problems. Substantial epidemiological evidence indicates that obesity has increased in prevalence in the general population from the late 1970s to the present. Birth cohort data suggest that mood and eating disorders are becoming more prevalent in younger populations. Thus, obesity and mental disorders may be co-occurring to a greater degree simply by chance alone. On the other hand, since smoking cessation is often associated with weight gain, some have hypothesized that the current obesity epidemic is due in part to decreasing rates of smoking. Third, mounting family history, twin, and genetic data suggest that obesity and many mental disorders, including psychotic, mood, and eating disorders, are polygenic, heterogeneous conditions. In light of recent epidemiologic studies showing that obesity co-occurs with certain types of psychopathology in certain populations, including major depression in females and binge eating disorder in males and females, it might be possible that certain forms of obesity and certain types of mental disorders share common inherited pathogenic factors.

In short, it is unknown how much of the clinical overlap between obesity and mental disorders is due to iatrogenic factors, because of the chance co-occurrence of two common conditions, due to shared inherited pathogenic factors, or to various combinations of these possibilities. A better understanding of this overlap would likely lead to improved treatment of obesity and mental disorders when they co-occur, and possibly of the individual conditions.

This book provides an accessible and expert summary of obesity, its relationship to mental disorders, and its management (including when associated with psychopathology) for the mental health professional. The first chapter of the book defines obesity and provides an overview of its epidemiology, causes, and natural history. The next eight chapters provide a state-of-the-art update on the relationship between obesity and mental disorders. Specifically, chapters two through seven summarize the relationship between obesity and schizophrenia, depressive and bipolar disorders, eating disorders, substance use disorders, smoking, and impulsive-compulsive spectrum disorders. Chapters eight and nine review two important and common syndromes often associated with both obesity and psychopathology, namely the metabolic syndrome and polycystic ovary syndrome.

The third part of the book summarizes behavioral treatments of obesity. Chapter 10 provides a comprehensive update of dietary therapy for obesity without psychopathology. Chapter 11 reviews research on the use of dietary therapy, exercise, behavioral weight management, and specialized psychotherapies in the treatment of obese patients with psychotic, mood, and eating disorders.

The last part of the book focuses on the medical treatments of obesity with and without associated mental disorders. Chapters 12, 13, and 14 in this section provide overviews of pharmacologic agents used in the treatment of three separate but related conditions: obesity without psychopathology (or "uncomplicated obesity"), binge eating and binge eating disorder, and medication-induced weight gain. Chapters 15, 16 and 17 summarize the most up-to-date literatures regarding the medical treatment of three important "subtypes" of obesity: uncomplicated obesity, obesity with mood disorders, and obesity with eating disorders. The last two chapters (Chapters 18 and 19) discuss the crucial role of bariatric surgery in the treatment of severe obesity, including in the obese patient with psychopathology.

It is our hope that this volume will serve as a reference source for physicians, researchers and other health care professionals seeking answers to the many questions related to understanding and treating obesity and mental disorders.

Susan L. McElroy M.D.
David B. Allison Ph.D.
George A. Bray M.D.

Contents

Contributors

Robert M. Anthenelli   Department of Psychiatry and Neuroscience, Tri-State Tobacco and Alcohol Research Center and Addiction Sciences Division, University of Cincinnati College of Medicine and Cincinnati Veterans Affairs Medical Center, Cincinnati, Ohio, U.S.A.

Jose C. Appolinario   Obesity and Eating Disorders Group, Institute of Psychiatry of the Federal University of Rio de Janeiro and Institute of Endocrinology and Diabetes of Rio de Janeiro, Rio de Janeiro, Brazil

Louis J. Aronne   Department of Medicine, Weill-Cornell University Medical College, New York, New York, U.S.A.

Josué Bacaltchuk   Eating Disorders Program (PROATA), Federal University of São Paulo and Janssen-Cilag Farmaceutica, São Paulo, Brazil

Bryann R. Baker   Compulsive, Impulsive and Anxiety Disorders Program, Mount Sinai School of Medicine, New York, New York, U.S.A.

Richard A. Bermudes   Department of Psychiatry and Behavioral Sciences, University of California Davis Medical Center, Sacramento, California, U.S.A.

Reena Bhargava   Division of GI and Endocrine Surgery, Department of Bariatric Surgery, University of Cincinnati School of Medicine, Cincinnati, Ohio, U.S.A.

George A. Bray   Pennington Biomedical Research Center, Louisiana State University System, Baton Rouge, Louisiana, U.S.A.

Scott Crow Department of Psychiatry, University of Minnesota, Minneapolis, Minnesota, U.S.A.

Martina de Zwaan Department of Psychosomatic Medicine, University of Erlangen, Erlangen, Germany

Bethany Doerfler Department of Medicine, Northwestern University Feinberg School of Medicine and Wellness Institute, Northwestern Memorial Hospital, Chicago, Illinois, U.S.A.

Kimberly Frost-Pineda Department of Psychiatry, Neuroscience, Anesthesiology, and Community Health and Family Medicine, University of Florida, Gainesville, Florida, U.S.A.

Keith S. Gersin Division of GI and Endocrine Surgery, Department of Bariatric Surgery, University of Cincinnati School of Medicine, Cincinnati, Ohio, U.S.A.

Mark S. Gold Department of Psychiatry, Neuroscience, Anesthesiology, and Community Health and Family Medicine, University of Florida, Gainesville, Florida, U.S.A.

Anna Guerdjikova Department of Psychiatry, University of Cincinnati College of Medicine, Cincinnati, Ohio, U.S.A.

Jaimee L. Heffner Mental Health Care Line, Cincinnati Veterans Affairs Medical Center, Cincinnati, Ohio, U.S.A., and Department of Psychology, Ohio University, Athens, Ohio, U.S.A.

Eric Hollander Department of Psychiatry, Clinical Psychopharmacology, and Compulsive, Impulsive and Anxiety Disorders Program, Seaver and New York Autism Center of Excellence, Mount Sinai School of Medicine, New York, New York, U.S.A.

L. K. George Hsu Department of Psychiatry, Tufts-New England Medical Center, Boston, Massachusetts, U.S.A.

Paul E. Keck Jr. Psychopharmacology Research Program, Department of Psychiatry, University of Cincinnati College of Medicine; General Clinical Research Center and Mental Health Care Line, Cincinnati Veterans Affairs Medical Center, Cincinnati, Ohio, U.S.A.

Jakub Z. Konarski Mood Disorder Psychopharmacology Unit, Institute of Medical Science, Toronto, Ontario, Canada

Renu Kotwal Psychopharmacology Research Program, Department of Psychiatry, University of Cincinnati College of Medicine, Cincinnati, Ohio, U.S.A.

Robert F. Kushner Department of Medicine, Northwestern University Feinberg School of Medicine and Wellness Institute, Northwestern Memorial Hospital, Chicago, Illinois, U.S.A.

Shishuka Malhotra Private Practice and President of Neuro Behavioral Clinical Research, Inc., United Health Network, Canton, Ohio, U.S.A.

Susan L. McElroy Psychopharmacology Research Program, Department of Psychiatry, University of Cincinnati College of Medicine, Cincinnati, Ohio, U.S.A.

Roger S. McIntyre Department of Psychiatry, University of Toronto, Toronto, Ontario, Canada

James E. Mitchell Neuropsychiatric Research Institute, University of North Dakota School of Medicine and Health Sciences Department of Clinical Neuroscience, University of Erlangen, Erlangen, Germany

Tricia Cook Myers Neuropsychiatric Research Institute, University of North Dakota School of Medicine and Health Sciences Department of Clinical Neuroscience, University of Erlangen, Erlangen, Germany

Erik B. Nelson Psychopharmacology Research Program, Department of Psychiatry, University of Cincinnati College of Medicine, Cincinnati, Ohio, U.S.A.

Charles B. Nemeroff Emory University School of Medicine, Department of Psychiatry, Atlanta, Georgia, U.S.A.

Helen C. Oppenheim Department of Psychiatry, Neuroscience, Anesthesiology, and Community Health and Family Medicine, University of Florida, Gainesville, Florida, U.S.A.

Natalie L. Rasgon Department of Psychiatry and Behavioral Science, Department of Obstetrics and Gynecology, Stanford University School of Medicine, Stanford, California, U.S.A.

Margaret F. Reynolds Behavioral Neuroendocrinology Program, Stanford University School of Medicine, Stanford, California, U.S.A.

Donna H. Ryan   Pennington Biomedical Research Center, Louisiana State University, Baton Rouge, Louisiana, U.S.A.

Calvin Selwyn   Division of GI and Endocrine Surgery, Department of Bariatric Surgery, University of Cincinnati School of Medicine, Cincinnati, Ohio, U.S.A.

Lisa Sharma   Compulsive, Impulsive and Anxiety Disorders Program, Mount Sinai School of Medicine, New York, New York, U.S.A.

Latha V. Soorya   Department of Psychiatry, Seaver and New York Autism Center of Excellence, Mount Sinai School of Medicine, New York, New York, U.S.A.

Leona Spelman   Neuroscience Centre, St. Vincent's Hospital, Fairview, Dublin, Ireland

Lorraine Swan-Kremeier   Neuropsychiatric Research Institute, University of North Dakota School of Medicine and Health Sciences Department of Clinical Neuroscience, University of Erlangen, Erlangen, Germany

Jogin H. Thakore   Neuroscience Centre, St. Vincent's Hospital, Fairview, Dublin, Ireland

Jonathan A. Waitman   Department of Medicine, Weill-Cornell University Medical College, New York, New York, U.S.A.

Kerry Wangen   Department of Psychiatry, University of California–Irvine, Orange, California, U.S.A.

Suzan Winders-Barrett   Mental Health Care Line, Cincinnati Veterans Affairs Medical Center, and Department of Psychology and Psychiatry, University of Cincinnati College of Medicine, Cincinnati, Ohio, U.S.A.

1

Obesity Is a Major Health Problem: Causes and Natural History

George A. Bray

Pennington Biomedical Research Center, Louisiana State University System, Baton Rouge, Louisiana, U.S.A.

OVERVIEW OF OBESITY

How fat are we? Before we can answer this question and discuss its implications, we need a definition of what we mean by fatness or obesity. Obesity means too much body fat, but because body fat is affected by age and sex, it has proven more effective to use a surrogate relating height and weight called the body mass index (BMI). This is measured as the weight in kilograms (kg) divided by the stature in meters (m) squared (kg/m^2). The BMI is largely independent of height and provides a reasonable assessment of fatness. The normal range of BMI is 18.5 to $24.9\,kg/m^2$. Overweight is defined as a BMI between 25 and $29.9\,kg/m^2$, and obesity as a BMI $>30\,kg/m^2$ (1,2).

Using the BMI, the prevalence of obesity can be assessed around the world. In the United States, 60.4% of the adult population aged 20 to 74 is overweight and 30.5% are obese in the most recent survey of the American population by the National Center of Health Statistics (3,4). The epidemic is worldwide and is affecting children as well as adults (1,5). It is against this background of a rising prevalence of obesity that strategies to prevent and treat obesity need to be developed.

A careful analysis of the shifting distribution curves for body weight shows that most of the increase is in the upper half of the distribution curve, which skews body weight to the heavy side. This would suggest that the people at risk for obesity in the current epidemic are people in the upper part of the body weight distribution curve who have a genetic susceptibility to store fat in our society of nutritional abundance. These people probably begin to gain weight in childhood and then continue into adult life (6,7). This environmental response of genetically susceptible people to nutritional abundance has been labeled as a "toxic environment" (8).

In this overview of obesity, it is important to start with a number of realities for obesity that underlie the problem. These are briefly summarized below:

- Obesity is a chronic, relapsing, stigmatized disease that is increasing in prevalence.
- It is due to an imbalance between energy intake and energy expenditure.
- Treatments rarely cure obesity.
- The therapeutic armamentarium of physicians is limited and labors under the negative halo of treatment mishaps.
- Drugs do not work when they are not taken.
- Weight loss plateaus on any treatment when compensatory mechanisms come into play.
- Frustration with plateaued weight that often averages less than 10% leads to discontinuing therapy, then to weight regain and labeling the weight loss program as a failure.

The current epidemic of obesity is a time bomb for future development of diabetes and its many complications. As such, it deserves efforts at prevention and, where needed, treatment. The disease of obesity has its pathology rooted in the enlargement of fat cells. Secretory products of these enlarged fat cells produce most of the pathogenetic changes that result in the complications associated with obesity. Physicians and the health care system have two strategies to deal with this problem. The first is to prevent the development of obesity, or to reverse it before the complications develop. Alternatively, the health care system can wait until the complications develop and then institute appropriate therapy. With the current high quality therapies available to treat hypertension, diabetes mellitus, and hypercholesterolemia, many physicians would prefer this latter strategy. However, if treatment for obesity were effective, the former approach would clearly be preferable. In one long-term trial, the incidence of new cases of diabetes was reduced to zero over two years in patients who lost and maintained a weight loss of 12% or more compared to an incidence of 8.5% for new cases of diabetes in those who did not lose weight. Thus, effective treatment can have a major impact in reducing the risk of developing serious diseases in the future.

One reason that most physicians are reluctant to treat obese patients is that their treatments are limited in number and effectiveness. At this writing, there are only two drugs approved by the United States Food and Drug Administration for long-term use in obesity. As monotherapy, both agents can produce a weight loss of 8% to 10%. However, to achieve the reduction in the rate of new cases of diabetes noted above, the weight loss needs to exceed 12%, a goal that cannot be easily achieved with current monotherapy. Thus, there is a great need for new treatment to be used when prevention fails.

Obesity is a stigmatized disease. One commonly held view is that obese people are lazy and weak-willed. If fat people just had willpower, they would push themselves away from the table and not be obese. This widely held view is shared by the public and by health professionals alike. The clamoring of women to be lean and well proportioned supports this view. The declining relative weight of centerfold models in Playboy and of women who are winners of the Miss America contest also supports this view. Many physicians just do not like to see obese patients come into their offices. Dealing with this problem will pose a major challenge to any efforts to improve the lot of people who are obese.

Two other issues aggravate the problem of treating obesity. The first is the "negative halo" that surrounds the use of appetite suppressants because amphetamine is addictive. There was never any evidence that dexfenfluramine was addictive. Nonetheless, the drug was scheduled by the United States Drug Enforcement Agency as a Schedule IV drug because on paper it had chemical similarities to amphetamine.

The second issue is the concern about the plateau of body weight that is reached when homeostatic mechanisms in the body come into play and stop further weight loss. There is an analogy with treatment of hypertension. When an antihypertensive drug is given, blood pressure drops and then stops falling within a few weeks to reach a "plateau" at a new lower level. The antihypertensive drug has not lost its effect when the plateau occurs, but its effect is being counteracted by physiological mechanisms designed to maintain blood pressure. In the treatment of obesity, a similar plateau in body weight is often viewed as a therapeutic failure for the weight loss drug. This is particularly so when weight is regained when the drug is stopped. These attitudes and biases need to change before any effective new therapy will become widely accepted.

The final issue is the disaster that recently befell many patients who took the combination of fenfluramine and phentermine. Aortic regurgitation occurred in up to 25% of the patients treated with this combination of drugs and led many physicians to say "I told you so" and "I'm certainly glad I did not use those drugs." Much of this will subside with time, but there will remain a residue of concern among some physicians and among regulators about the potential problems that might surface when new treatments for obesity are made available to the public.

THE CAUSES OF OBESITY

Etiologic Classification

A number of specific etiologies that cause obesity are described further.

Psychological and Social Factors

Psychological factors in the development of obesity are widely recognized, although attempts to define a specific personality type that causes obesity have been unsuccessful. One condition linked to weight gain is seasonal affective disorder, which refers to the depression that occurs during the winter season in some people living in the north, where days are short. These patients tend to increase body weight in winter. This can be effectively treated by providing higher-intensity artificial lighting in the winter (9).

Behavioral Patterns of Eating

Restrained eating: A pattern of conscious limitation of food intake is called "restrained" eating (10). It is common in many, if not most, middle-age women of "normal weight." It may also account for the inverse relationship of body weight to social class; women of upper socioeconomic status often use restrained eating to maintain their weight. In a weight-loss clinic, higher restraint scores were associated with lower body weights (11). Weight loss was associated with a significant increase in restraint, indicating that higher levels of conscious control maintain lower weight. Greater increases in restraint correlate with greater weight loss, but also with higher risk of "lapse" or loss of control and overeating.

Binge eating disorder: Binge eating disorder is a psychiatric illness characterized by uncontrolled episodes of overeating, usually in the evening (12). The patient may respond to treatment with drugs that modulate serotonin.

Night eating syndrome: Night eating syndrome is the consumption of at least 25% (and usually more than 50%) of energy between the evening meal and the next morning (13,14). It is one pattern of disturbed eating in the obese. It is related to sleep disturbances and may be a component of sleep apnea, in which day-time somnolence and nocturnal wakefulness are often found.

Socioeconomic and Ethnic Factors

Obesity is more prevalent in lower socioeconomic groups in the United States and elsewhere. The inverse relationship of socioeconomic status (SES) and overweight is found both in adults and children. In the Minnesota Heart Study, for example, the SES and BMI were inversely related. People of higher SES were more concerned with healthy weight-control practices, including exercise, and tended to eat less fat (15). In the National Heart,

Lung and Blood Institute Growth and Health Study, SES and overweight were strongly associated in Caucasian 9- and 10-year-old girls and their mothers, but not in African American girls (16). The association of SES and overweight is much stronger in Caucasian women than in African American women. African American women of all ages are more obese than are Caucasian women. African American men are less obese than white men, and socioeconomic factors are much less evident in men. The prevalence of obesity in Hispanic men and women is higher than in Caucasians. The basis for these ethnic differences is unclear. In men, the socioeconomic effects of obesity are weak or absent. This gender difference, and the higher prevalence of overweight in women, suggests important interactions of gender with many factors that influence body fat and fat distribution. The reason for this association is not known.

Neuroendocrine Obesity

Hypothalamic obesity: Hypothalamic obesity is rare in humans, but it can be regularly produced in animals by injuring the ventromedial or paraventricular region of the hypothalamus or the amygdala (17,18). These brain regions are responsible for integrating metabolic information on nutrient stores provided by leptin with afferent sensory information on food availability. When the ventromedial hypothalamus is damaged, hyperphagia develops, the response to leptin is eliminated, and obesity follows. Hypothalamic obesity in humans may be caused by trauma, tumor, inflammatory disease, surgery in the posterior fossa, or increased intracranial pressure (17). The symptoms are usually present in one or more of the three patterns: (i) headache, vomiting, and diminished vision due to increased intracranial pressure, (ii) impaired endocrine function affecting the reproductive system with amenorrhea or impotence, diabetes insipidus, and thyroid or adrenal insufficiency or, (iii) neurologic and physiologic derangements, including convulsions, coma, somnolence, and hypothermia or hyperthermia.

Cushing's syndrome: Obesity is one of the cardinal features of Cushing's syndrome (19). Thus, the differential diagnosis of obesity from Cushing's syndrome and pseudo-Cushing's syndrome is clinically important for therapeutic decisions (19,20). Pseudo-Cushing's is a name used for a variety of conditions that distort the dynamics of the hypothalamic–pituitary–adrenal axis and can confuse the interpretations of biochemical tests for Cushing's syndrome. Pseudo-Cushing's includes depression, anxiety disorders such as obsessive-compulsive disorder, poorly controlled diabetes mellitus, and alcoholism.

Hypothyroidism: Patients with hypothyroidism frequently gain weight because of a generalized slowing of metabolic activity. Some of this weight gain is fat. However, the weight gain is usually modest, and marked obesity is uncommon. Hypothyroidism is common, however, particularly in older women.

Polycystic ovary syndrome: The definition of the polycystic ovary syndrome (PCOS) is based on a conference held at the National Institutes of Health in April 1990 and includes menstrual irregularity plus hyperandrogenism, excluding other pathology such as congenital adrenal hyperplasia and androgen secreting tumors (21). Obesity, particularly central obesity, is common in this syndrome. Similarly, insulin resistance is often present, even when obesity is minimal. The basis for the association of the hypothalamic–adrenal–gonadal problem and the obesity is unclear. Luteinizing hormone is usually increased and the ovary is the source for the increased amounts of testosterone, possibly through stimulation by insulin-like growth factor-1. Metformin has been effective in reducing insulin resistance and restoring fertility in PCOS.

Growth hormone deficiency: Lean body mass is decreased and fat mass is increased in adults and children who are deficient in growth hormone, compared with those who have normal growth hormone secretion. However, the increase in fat does not produce clinically significant obesity. Growth hormone replacement reduces body fat generally and visceral fat selectively (22). Acromegaly produces the opposite effects with reduced body fat, particularly visceral fat. Treatment of acromegaly, which lowers growth hormone, increases body fat and visceral fat. Since growth hormone selectively decreases visceral fat, the gradual decline in growth hormone with age may be one reason for the increase in visceral fat with age.

Drug-Induced Weight Gain

Several drugs can cause weight gain, including a variety of psychoactive agents and hormones (Table 1) (23). The degree of weight gain is generally not sufficient to cause true obesity, except occasionally in patients treated with high-dose corticosteroids, some psychoactive drugs, or valproate.

Cessation of Smoking

Weight gain is very common when people stop smoking and is at least partly mediated by nicotine withdrawal. Weight gain of 1 to 2 kg in the first few weeks is often followed by an additional 2 to 3 kg weight gain over the next four to six months. Average weight gain is 4 to 5 kg, but can be much greater (24). Researchers have estimated that smoking cessation increases the odds ratio of obesity 2.4-fold in men and 2.0-fold in women, compared with nonsmokers.

Sedentary Lifestyle

A sedentary lifestyle lowers energy expenditure and promotes weight gain in both animals and humans. Restriction of physical activity in rats causes weight gain, and animals in zoos tend to be heavier than those in the wild.

Table 1 Drugs that Produce Weight Gain and Alternatives

Category	Drugs that cause weight gain	Possible alternatives
Neuroleptics	Thioridazine	Molindone
	Olanzepine	Haloperidol
	Quetiapine	Ziprasodone
	Resperidone	
	Clozapine	
Antidepressants	Amitriptyiine	Protriptyline
Tricyclics	Nortriptyline	Bupropion
Monoamine oxidase inhibitors	Imipramine	Nefazadone
Selective serotonin reuptake	Mitrazapine	Fluoxetine
inhibitors	Paroxetine	Sertraline
Anticonvulsants	Valproate	Topiramate
	Carbamazepine	Lamotrigine
	Gabapentin	Zonisamide
Antidiabetic drugs	Insulin	Acarbose; Miglitol;
	Sulfonylureas	Metfbrmin; Orlistat;
	Thiazolidinediones	Sibutramine
AntiSerotonin	Pizotifen	
Antihistamines	Cyproheptidine	Inhalers; deconqestants
β-Adrenergic blockers	Propranolol	ACE Inhibitors;
α-Adrenergic blockers	Terazosin	Calcium channel blockers
Steroid Hormones	Contraceptives	Barrier methods
	Glucocorticoids	Non-steroidal
	Progestational	anti-inflammatory
	steroids	agents

Source: From George A. Bray, 2001.

In an affluent society, energy-sparing devices in the workplace and at home reduce energy expenditure and may enhance the tendency to gain weight (25). In children, there is a graded increase in BMI as the number of hours of television watching increases (26).

A number of additional observations illustrate the importance of decreased energy expenditure in the pathogenesis of weight gain. The highest frequency of overweight occurs in men in sedentary occupations. Estimates of energy intake and energy expenditure in Great Britain suggest that reduced energy expenditure is more important than increased food intake in causing obesity (25). A study of middle-aged men in the Netherlands found that the decline in energy expenditure accounted for almost all the weight gain (27). According to the Surgeon General's Report on Physical Activity, the percentage of adult Americans participating in physical activity decreases steadily with age, and reduced energy expenditure in adults and children predicts weight gain (28). In the United States, and possibly in other countries, the amount of time spent watching television is related to the degree of obesity in children; and the number of automobiles is related to the degree of obesity in adults (26). Finally, the fatness of men in several affluent countries (The Seven Countries Study) was inversely related to levels of physical activity (29).

Diet

The amount of energy intake relative to energy expenditure is the central reason for the development of obesity. However, diet composition also may be variably important in its pathogenesis. Dietary factors become important in a variety of settings.

Breast feeding: Several recent papers have suggested that breast feeding may reduce the prevalence of obesity in later life. In a large German study of more than 11,000 children, von Kries et al. (30) showed that the duration of breast feeding as the sole source of nutrition was inversely related to the incidence of obesity, defined as a weight above the 95th percentile, when children entered the first grade. In this study, the incidence was 4.8% in children with no breast feeding, falling in a graded fashion to 0.8% in children who were solely breast fed for 12 months or more. A second large report also showed that breast feeding reduced the incidence of overweight, but not obese adolescents (31). The third report with fewer subjects and more ethnic heterogeneity failed to show this effect (32). However, the potential that breast feeding can reduce the future risk of obesity is another reason to recommend breast feeding for at least 6 to 12 months.

Overeating: Voluntary overeating (repeated ingestion of energy exceeding daily energy needs) can increase body weight in normal-weight men and women. When these subjects stop overeating, they invariably lose most or all of the excess weight. The use of overeating protocols to study the consequences of food ingestion has shown the importance of genetic factors in the pattern of weight gain (33).

Progressive hyperphagic obesity is one clinical form of overeating (34). A small number of patients begin to be overweight in childhood and then have unrelenting weight gain, usually surpassing 140 kg (300 lb) by 30 years of age. The recent death of a 13-year-old weighing 310 kg (680 lb) illustrates a nearly maximal rate of weight gain of 25 kg/yr. These patients gain about the same amount of weight year after year. Because approximately 22 kcal/kg is required to maintain an extra kilogram of body weight in an obese individual, the energy requirements in these patients must increase year by year, with the weight gain being driven by excess energy intake.

Japanese sumo wrestlers who eat large quantities of food twice a day for many years, and who have a very active training schedule, have low visceral fat relative to total weight during training. When their active career ends, however, the wrestlers tend to remain overweight and have a high probability of developing diabetes mellitus (35).

Dietary Fat Intake

Epidemiologic data suggest that a high-fat diet is associated with obesity. The relative weight in several populations, for example, is directly related to the percentage of dietary fat in the diet (36–38). A high-fat diet introduces palatable foods into the diet, with a corresponding increase in energy density (i.e., lesser weight of food for the same number of calories). This makes over-consumption more likely. Differences in the storage capacity for various macronutrients also may be involved. The capacity to store glucose as glycogen in liver and muscle is limited and needs to be replenished frequently. This contrasts with fat stores, which are more than 100 times the daily intake of fat. This difference in storage capacity makes eating carbohydrates a more important physiologic need that may lead to overeating when dietary carbohydrate is limited and carbohydrate oxidation cannot be reduced sufficiently.

Dietary carbohydrate and fiber: When the consumption of sugar and body weight are examined there is usually an inverse relationship. However, there are recent data to suggest that the consumption of sugar-sweetened beverages in children may enhance the risk of more rapid weight gain. Both the baseline consumption and the change in consumption over two years were positively related to the increase in BMI over two years. That is, children who drank more sugar-sweetened beverages gained more weight and those who increased their beverage consumption had an even greater increase (39).

A second relationship between obesity and carbohydrate intake may be through the glycemic index. The glycemic index is a way of describing the ease with which starches are digested in the intestine with the release of glucose, which can be readily absorbed. A high glycemic index food is one that is readily digested and produces a large and rapid rise in plasma glucose. A low glycemic index food, on the other hand, is more slowly digested and associated with a slower and lower rise in glucose. Comparative studies show that feeding high glycemic index food suppresses food intake less than low glycemic index foods. The low glycemic index foods are the fruits and vegetables that tend to have fiber. Potatoes, white rice, and white bread are high glycemic index foods. Legumes and whole wheat are low glycemic index foods.

In a review of six studies, Roberts documented that consumption of higher glycemic index foods was associated with higher energy intake compared with consumption of lower glycemic index foods. Thus, higher fiber foods that release carbohydrate more slowly appear to stimulate less food intake than foods that release glucose more rapidly (40).

In addition to the relation of energy intake and glycemic index, there are recent data to support the idea that diets with higher fiber intake are associated with lower weight. The Seven Countries Study initiated by Keys et al. (29) more than 20 years ago has been a fertile source for epidemiologic data. A recent reexamination of data from this group has shown that the fiber intake within each of the participating countries was inversely related to body weight. Men eating more fiber had lower body weight. Epidemiological data also suggest that countries with higher fiber consumption have lower prevalences of obesity (29). In addition, fiber intake may be related to the development of heart disease and diabetes (41,42).

Dietary calcium: Nearly 20 years ago, McCarron et al. (43) reported that there was a negative relationship between BMI and dietary calcium intake in the data collected by the National Center for Health Statistics (NCHS). More recently, Zemel et al. (44) found that there was a strong inverse relationship between calcium intake and the risk of being in the highest quartile of BMI. These studies have prompted a reevaluation of studies measuring calcium intake or administration of oral calcium. In the prospective trials, subjects receiving calcium had a greater weight loss than those who were receiving placebo. Increasing calcium from 0 to nearly 2000 g/d was associated with a reduction in BMI of about 5 BMI units (45). Taken together, these data suggest that low calcium intake may be playing a role in the current epidemic of obesity.

Frequency of eating: The relationship between the frequency of meals and the development of obesity is unsettled. Many anecdotal reports argue that overweight persons eat less often than normal-weight persons, but documentation is scanty. However, frequency of eating does change lipid and glucose metabolism. When normal subjects eat several small meals a day, serum cholesterol concentrations are lower than when they eat a few large meals a day. Similarly, mean blood glucose concentrations are lower when meals are frequent (46). One explanation for the effects of frequent small meals compared with a few large meals could be the greater insulin secretion associated with larger meals.

Genetic and Congenital Disorders

Discovery of the basis for the 5 single-gene defects that produce obesity in animals was followed by the recognition that these same defects, though rare, also produce human obesity.

The rare humans with leptin deficiency correspond to the obese (ob/ob) mouse animal model (47–49). Leptin is a 167 amino acid protein produced in adipose tissue and the placenta and possibly other tissues that signals the brain through leptin receptors about the size of adipose stores. In three families, consanguineous marriages led to expression of the recessive leptin deficient state. These very fat children are hypogonadal, but are not hypothermic or endocrine deficient They lose weight when treated with leptin.

A defect in the leptin receptor has also been described, and these patients are very fat, just as are the leptin-deficient children (50). They do not respond to leptin because they lack the leptin receptor.

A third defect results from mutations in the melanocortin receptor (51–53). Several forms of this receptor transmit signals for activation of the adrenal gland by ACTH (melanocortin 1-receptor), activation of the melanocyte (melanocortin 2-receptor), and suppression of food intake by α-MSH (melanocortin 3-receptor and melanocortin 4-receptor). Genetic engineering to eliminate the MC4R in the mouse brain produces massive obesity. Several reports claim a genetic defect in this receptor is the culprit in some humans with obesity. These individuals are of either sex and are massively obese. A much rarer form of human obesity has been reported when production of proopiomelanocortin (POMC), the precursor for peptides that act on the melanocortin receptors, is defective (54). These people have red hair, endocrine defects and are moderately obese.

The peroxisome proliferator-activated receptor-γ (PPAR-γ) is important in the control of fat cell differentiation (55). Defects in the PPAR-γ receptor in humans have been reported to produce modest degrees of obesity that begin later in life. The activation of this receptor by thiazolidinediones, a class of anti-diabetic drugs, is also a cause for an increase in body fat.

The final human defect that has been described is in prohormone convertase 1 (56,57). In one family, a defect in this gene and in a second gene were associated with obesity. Members of the family with only the PC-1 defect were not obese, suggesting that it was the interaction of two genes that lead to obesity.

Several congenital forms of obesity exist, which are more abundant than most of the single-gene defects. The Prader–Willi syndrome results from an abnormality on chromosome 15q11.2 that is usually transmitted paternally (58). This chromosomal defect produces a "floppy" baby who usually has trouble feeding. Obesity in these children begins at about age two and is associated with overeating, hypogonadism, and mental retardation (58).

The Bardet–Biedl syndrome (BBS) (59,60) is a rare variety of congenital obesity. It is named after the two physicians who described it in separate publications in the 1920s. It is a recessively inherited disorder that can be diagnosed when four of the six cardinal features are present. These six cardinal features are: (i) Progressive tapetoretinal degeneration, (ii) distal limb abnormalities, (iii) obesity, (iv) renal involvement, (v) hypogenitalism in men and, (vi) mental retardation (61). The genetic defect in one form of the BBS has been identified on chromosome 20q12 as a "chaperonin-like" protein that is involved in folding proteins (62). It is allelic with the McKusick–Kaplan syndrome (MKKS). This latter syndrome is characterized by polydactyly, hydrometrocolpus and heart problems, but without obesity.

Natural History of Obesity

Individuals can become overweight at any age, but this is more common at certain ages. At birth, those who will and those who will not become obese later in life can rarely be distinguished by weight, except for the infants of diabetic mothers, for whom the likelihood of obesity later in life is increased. Thus, at birth, a large pool of individuals will eventually become overweight, and a smaller group will never become overweight. I have labeled these pools "preoverweight" (Fig. 1) and "never overweight," using the NCHS data for prevalence of BMI $> 25\,\mathrm{kg/m^2}$ as the solid line. Several surveys suggest that one-third of overweight adults become overweight before age 20, and two-thirds do so after that (34). Thus, 75% to 80% of adults will become overweight at some time in their lives. Between 20% and 25% of the population will display their overweight before age 20, and 50% will do so after age 20. Some of these overweight individuals will develop clinically significant problems such as diabetes, hypertension, gallbladder disease, or the metabolic syndrome. These are the overweight people that I call "clinically overweight."

Because most preoverweight people will become overweight, it is important to have as much insight as possible into the risk factors. These predictors fall into two broad groups: demographic and metabolic. When an individual becomes overweight (i.e., BMI $> 25\,\mathrm{kg/m^2}$) without clinically significant problems, they manifest "overweight" or "preclinical overweight." With the passage of time or a further increase in weight, they may show clinical signs of diabetes, hypertension, gallbladder disease, or

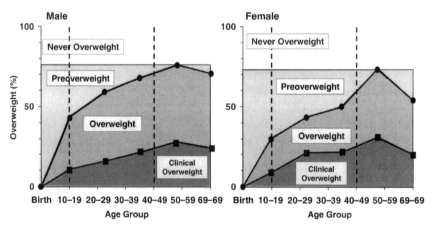

Figure 1 Natural history of overweight. Because many non-overweight babies become overweight, this group is labeled preoverweight. About one-third of those who become overweight do so before age 20, and two-thirds do so after. The remainder are not overweight.

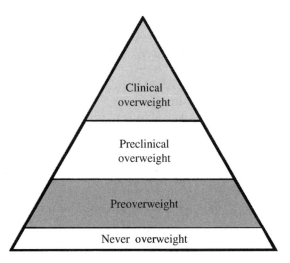

Figure 2 Pyramid of overweight. Many individuals who become overweight do not have diabetes, hypertension, or other diseases. These are called preclinical overweight. Those who develop clinical disease are clinically overweight.

dyslipidemia. I call this group "clinically overweight." The relationship of one to the other may be depicted as a pyramid (Fig. 2).

At the base is the reservoir of never overweight and preoverweight individuals, many of whom will become overweight in their adult life. Some of these will in turn show signs of clinical disease and become clinically overweight.

Overweight Developing Before Age 10

Prenatal Factors

Caloric intake by the mother may influence body size, shape, and later body composition. Birth weights of identical and fraternal twins have the same correlation ($r = 0.63$), indicating that birth weight is a poor predictor of future obesity. In the first years of life, the correlation of body weight among identical twins begins to converge, rapidly becoming much closer together ($r = 0.9$), whereas that of dizygotic twins diverges during this same period ($r = 0.5$). Infants born to diabetic mothers have a higher risk of being overweight as children and adults (63). Infants who are small-for-dates, short, or have a small head circumference are at higher risk of developing abdominal fatness and other comorbidities associated with obesity later in life (63).

Infancy Through Age 3

Body weight triples and body fat normally doubles in the first year of life. This increase in body fat and how long the infant was breast fed in the first year of life are important predictors of overweight later in life. In infants and young children with overweight parents, an infant above the 85th percentile at age one to three has a fourfold increased risk of adult overweight if either parent is overweight, compared with non-overweight infants. If neither parent is overweight, this infantile overweight does not predict overweight in early adult life (64). These observations are similar to the older observations suggesting that the risk for adult obesity was 80% for children with two overweight parents, 40% for those with one overweight parent, and less than 10% if neither parent was overweight (34).

Childhood Obesity from Ages 3 to 10

Ages 3 to 10 are high-risk years for developing obesity. Adiposity rebound describes the inflection point between a declining BMI and an increasing BMI that occurs between age 5 and 7 years. The earlier this rebound occurs, the greater the risk of overweight later in life. About half of the overweight grade school children remain overweight as adults. Moreover, the risk of overweight in adulthood was at least twice as great for overweight children as for non-overweight children. The risk is 3 to 10 times higher if the child's weight is above the 95th percentile for their age. Parental overweight plays a strong role in this group as well. Nearly 75% of overweight children age 3 to 10 remained overweight in early adulthood if they had one or more overweight parent, compared with 25% to 50% if neither parent was overweight. Overweight 3- to 10-year-old with an overweight parent thus constitutes an ideal group for behavioral therapy. When body weight progressively deviates from the upper limits of normal in this age group, it is labeled "progressive obesity" (34); this is usually severe and lifelong, and is associated with an increase in the number of fat cells.

Overweight Developing in Adolescence and Adult Life

Adolescence

Weight in adolescence becomes a progressively better predictor of adult weight status. In a 55-year follow-up of adolescents, the weight status in adolescence predicted later adverse health events (65). Adolescents above the 95th percentile had a 5- to 20-fold greater likelihood of overweight in adulthood. In contrast with younger ages, parental overweight is less important, or has already had its effect. While 70% to 80% of overweight adolescents with an overweight parent were overweight as young adults, the numbers were only modestly lower (54–60%) for overweight adolescents without overweight parents. Despite the importance of childhood and adolescent weight status, however, it remains clear that most overweight individuals develop their problem in adult life (34).

Adult Women

Most overweight women gain their excess weight after puberty. This weight gain may be precipitated by a number of events, including pregnancy, oral contraceptive therapy, and menopause.

Pregnancy: Weight gain during pregnancy and the effect of pregnancy on subsequent weight gain are important events in the weight gain history of women (66). A few women gain considerable weight during pregnancy, occasionally more than 50 kg. The pregnancy itself may leave a legacy of increased weight, as suggested by one study that evaluated women prospectively between the ages of 18 and 30 years (67). Women who remained nulliparous ($n = 925$) were compared with women who had a single pregnancy of 28 weeks' duration during that period and who were at least 12 months postpartum. The primiparas gained 2 to 3 kg more weight and had a greater increase in waist circumference divided by hip circumference (WHR) compared with the nulliparous women during this period. The overall risk of weight gain associated with child-bearing after age 25, however, is quite modest for most American women (66).

Oral contraceptives: Oral contraceptive use may initiate weight gain in some women, although this effect is diminished with the low-dose estrogen pills. One study evaluated 49 healthy women initiating treatment with a low-dose oral contraceptive (30 mg ethinyl estradiol plus 75 mg gestodene). Anthropometric measurements before and after the initiation of this formulation were used to compare 31 age- and weight-matched women (68). Baseline BMI, percent fat, percent water, and WHR did not change significantly after six cycles in the birth control pill users. A similar number of women gained weight in both groups (30.6% of users, and 35.4% of controls). The typical weight gain in the pill user group was only 0.5 kg, but the small weight gain in these women was attributable to the accumulation of fat, not body water. Approximately 20% of women in both groups lost weight.

Menopause: Weight gain and changes in fat distribution occur after menopause. The decline in estrogen and progesterone secretion alters fat cell biology so that central fat deposition increases. Estrogen replacement therapy does not prevent weight gain, although it may minimize fat redistribution (69). A prospective study of 63 early postmenopausal women compared 34 who initiated continuous estrogen and progesterone therapy to the remaining women who refused it. Body weight and fat mass increased significantly in both the treatments (73.2–75.6 kg) and the control groups (71.5–73.5 kg). However, WHR increased significantly only in the control group (0.80–0.85). Caloric and macro nutrient intake did not change in either group. A two-year trial with estrogen in postmenopausal women also showed an increase in body fat (70).

Adult Men

The transition from an active lifestyle during the teens and early 20s to a more sedentary lifestyle thereafter is associated with weight gain in many men. The rise in body weight continues through the adult years until the sixth decade. After ages 55 to 64, relative weight remains stable and then begins to decline. Evidence from the Framingham Study and studies of men in the armed services suggests that men have become progressively heavier for height during this century.

Weight Stability and Weight Cycling

Weight cycling associated with dieting is popularly known as yo–yo dieting (71). Weight cycling refers to the downs and ups in weight that often happen to people who diet, lose weight, stop dieting, and regain the weight they lost and sometimes more. The possibility that loss and regain is more detrimental than staying heavy has been hotly debated. In a review of the literature between 1964 and 1994, a group of experts concluded that most studies did not support any adverse effects on metabolism associated with weight cycling. Also, little or no data supported the contention that it is more difficult to lose weight a second time after regaining weight from a previous therapeutic approach. Most researchers agree that weight cycling neither necessarily increases body fat, nor adversely affects blood pressure, glucose metabolism, or lipid concentrations.

REFERENCES

1. Obesity: preventing and managing the global epidemic. Report of a WHO consultation. World Health Organ Tech Rep Ser2000; 894:i–xii, 1–253.
2. Clinical Guidelines on the Identification, Evaluation, and Treatment of Overweight and Obesity in Adults—The Evidence Report. National Institutes of Health. Obes Res 1998; 6 Suppl 2:51S–209S.
3. Flegal KM, Carroll MD, Ogden CL, Johnson CL. Prevalence and trends in obesity among US adults, 1999–2000. JAMA 2002; 288:1723–1777.
4. Mokdad AH, Ford ES, Bowman BA, et al. Prevalence of obesity, diabetes, and obesity-related health risk factors, 2001. JAMA 2003; 289:76–79.
5. Ogden CL, Flegal KM, Carroll MD, Johnson CL. Prevalence and trends in overweight among US children and adolescents, 1999–2000. JAMA 2002; 288:1728–1732.
6. Bhargava SK, Sachdev HS, Fall CH, et al. Relation of serial changes in childhood body-mass index to impaired glucose tolerance in young adulthood. N Engl J Med 2004; 350:865–875.
7. Whitaker RC, Pepe MS, Wright JA, Seidel KD, Dietz WH. Early adiposity rebound and the risk of adult obesity. Pediatrics 1998; 101:E5.
8. Brownell K, Horgen K. Food Fight. New York: McGraw-Hill, 2004.
9. Partonen T, Lonnqvist J. Seasonal affective disorder. Lancet 1998; 352: 1369–1374.

10. Lawson OJ, Williamson DA, Champagne CM, et al. The association of body weight, dietary intake, and energy expenditure with dietary restraint and disinhibition. Obes Res 1995; 3:153–161.
11. Williamson DA, Lawson OJ, Brooks ER, et al. Association of body mass with dietary restraint and disinhibition. Appetite 1995; 25:31–41.
12. Yanovski SZ. Binge eating disorder affects outcome of comprehensive very-low- calorie diet treatment. Obes Res 1994; 2:205–212.
13. Stunkard AJ. The night eating syndrome: a pattern of food intake among certain obese patients. Am J Med 1955; 19:78–86.
14. Stunkard A. Two eating disorders: binge eating disorder and the night eating syndrome. Appetite 2000; 34:333–334.
15. Jeffery RW, Forster JL, Folsom AR, Luepker RV, Jacobs DR Jr, Blackburn H. The relationship between social status and body mass index in the Minnesota Heart Health Program. Int J Obes 1989; 13:59–67.
16. Obarzanek E, Schreiber GB, Crawford PB, et al. Energy intake and physical activity in relation to indexes of body fat: the National Heart, Lung, and Blood Institute Growth and Health Study. Am J Clin Nutr 1994; 60:15–22.
17. Bray GA, Gallagher TF Jr. Manifestations of hypothalamic obesity in man: a comprehensive investigation of eight patients and a reveiw of the literature. Medicine (Baltimore) 1975; 54:301–330.
18. Bray GA, York DA. The MONA LISA hypothesis in the time of leptin. Recent Prog Horm Res 1998; 53:95–117; discussion 117–118.
19. Plotz CM, Knowlton Al, Ragan C. The natural history of Cushing's syndrome. Am J Med 1952; 13:597–614.
20. Orth DN. Cushing's syndrome. N Engl J Med 1995; 332:791–803.
21. Dunaif A. Polycystic ovary syndrome. Polycystic ovary syndrome. Health News 1998; 4:4.
22. Lonn L, Johansson G, Sjostrom L, Kvist H, Oden A, Bengtsson BA. Body composition and tissue distributions in growth hormone deficient adults before and after growth hormone treatment. Obes Res 1996; 4:45–54.
23. Allison DB, Mentore JL, Heo M, et al. Antipsychotic-induced weight gain: a comprehensive research synthesis. Am J Psychiatry 1999; 156:1686–1696.
24. Flegal KM, Troiano RP, Pamuk ER, Kuczmarski RJ, Campbell SM. The influence of smoking cessation on the prevalence of overweight in the United States. N Engl J Med 1995; 333:1165–1170.
25. Prentice AM, Jebb SA. Obesity in Britain: gluttony or sloth? BMJ 1995; 311:437–439.
26. Crespo CJ, Smit E, Troiano RP, Bartlett SJ, Macera CA, Andersen RE. Television watching, energy intake, and obesity in US children: results from the third National Health and Nutrition Examination Survey, 1988–1994. Arch Pediatr Adolesc Med 2001; 155:360–365.
27. Kromhout D. Changes in energy and macro nutrients in 871 middle-aged men during 10 years of follow-up (the Zutphen study). Am J Clin Nutr 1983; 37:287–294.
28. Surgeon General's report on physical activity and health. From the Centers for Disease Control and Prevention. JAMA 1996; 276:522.

29. Kromhout D, Bloemberg B, Seidell JC, Nissinen A, Menotti A. Physical activity and dietary fiber determine population body fat levels: the Seven Countries Study. Int J Obes Relat Metab Disord 2001; 25:301–306.
30. von Kries R, Koletzko B, Sauerwald T, et al. Breastfeeding and obesity: cross sectional study. BMJ 1999; 319:147–150.
31. Gillman MW, Rifas-Shiman SL, Camargo CA Jr, et al. Risk of overweight among adolescents who were breastfed as infants. JAMA 2001; 285:2461–2467.
32. Hediger ML, Overpeck MD, Kuczmarski RJ, Ruan WJ. Association between infant breastfeeding and overweight in young children. JAMA 2001; 285:2453–2460.
33. Bouchard C, Tremblay A, Despres JP, et al. The response to long-term overfeeding in identical twins. N Engl J Med 1990; 322:1477–1482.
34. Bray GA. The Obese Patient: Major Problems in Internal Medicine. Philadelphia: W.B. Saunders, 1976.
35. Nishizawa T, Akaoka I, Nishida Y, Kawaguchi Y, Hayashi E. Some factors related to obesity in the Japanese sumo wrestler. Am J Clin Nutr 1976; 29:1167–1174.
36. Bray GA, Popkin BM. Dietary fat intake does affect obesity! Am J Clin Nutr 1998; 68:1157–1173.
37. Yu-Poth S, Zhao G, Etherton T, Naglak M, Jonnalagadda S, Kris-Etherton PM. Effects of the National Cholesterol Education Program's Step I and Step II dietary intervention programs on cardiovascular disease risk factors: a meta-analysis. Am J Clin Nutr 1999; 69:632–646.
38. Astrup A, Ryan L, Grunwald GK, et al. The role of dietary fat in body fatness: evidence from a preliminary meta-analysis of ad libitum low-fat dietary intervention studies. Br J Nutr 2000; 83 Suppl 1:S25–S32.
39. Ludwig DS, Peterson KE, Gortmaker SL. Relation between consumption of sugar-sweetened drinks and childhood obesity: a prospective, observational analysis. Lancet 2001; 357:505–508.
40. Roberts SB, Pi-Sunyer FX, Dreher M, et al. Physiology of fat replacement and fat reduction: effects of dietary fat and fat substitutes on energy regulation. Nutr Rev 1998; 56:S29–41; discussion S41–S49.
41. Woik A, Manson JE, Stampfer MJ, et al. Long-term intake of dietary fiber and decreased risk of coronary heart disease among women. JAMA 1999; 281: 1998–2004.
42. Salmeron J, Manson JE, Stampfer MJ, Coiditz GA, Wing AL, Willett WC. Dietary fiber, glycemic load, and risk of non-insulin-dependent diabetes mellitus in women. JAMA 1997; 277:472–477.
43. McCarron DA, Morris CD, Henry HJ, Stanton JL. Blood pressure and nutrient intake in the United States. Science 1984; 224:1392–1398.
44. Zemel MB, Shi H, Greer B, Dirienzo D, Zemel PC. Regulation of adiposity by dietary calcium. Faseb J 2000; 14:1132–1138.
45. Davies KM, Heaney RP, Recker RR, et al. Calcium intake and body weight. J Clin Endocrinol Metab 2000; 85:4635–4638.
46. Jenkins DJ, Wolever TM, Vuksan V, et al. Nibbling versus gorging: metabolic advantages of increased meal frequency. N Engl J Med 1989; 321:929–934.

47. Montague CT, Farooqi IS, Whitehead JP, et al. Congenital leptin deficiency is associated with severe early-onset obesity in humans. Nature 1997; 387:903–908.
48. Strobel A, Issad T, Camoin L, Ozata M, Strosberg AD. A leptin missense mutation associated with hypogonadism and morbid obesity. Nat Genet 1998; 18:213–215.
49. Ozata M, Ozdemir IC, Licinio J. Human leptin deficiency caused by a missense mutation: multiple endocrine defects, decreased sympathetic tone, and immune system dysfunction indicate new targets for leptin action, greater central than peripheral resistance to the effects of leptin, and spontaneous correction of ieptin-mediated defects. J Clin Endocrinol Metab 1999; 84:3686–3695.
50. Clement K, Vaisse C, Lahlou N, et al. A mutation in the human leptin receptor gene causes obesity and pituitary dysfunction. Nature 1998; 392:398–401.
51. Farooqi IS, Keogh JM, Yeo GS, Lank EJ, Cheetham T, O'Rahilly S. Clinical spectrum of obesity and mutations in the melanocortin 4 receptor gene. N Engl J Med 2003; 348(12):1085–1095.
52. Vaisse C, Clement K, Guy-Grand B, Froguel P. A frameshift mutation in human MC4R is associated with a dominant form of obesity. Nat Genet 1998; 20:113–114.
53. HinneyA, Schmidt A, Nottebom K, et al. Several mutations in the melanocortin-4 receptor gene including a nonsense and a frameshift mutation associated with dominantly inherited obesity in humans. J Clin Endocrinol Metab 1999; 84:1483–1486.
54. Krude H, Biebermann H, Luck W, Horn R, Brabant G, Gruters A. Severe early- onset obesity, adrenal insufficiency and red hair pigmentation caused by POMC mutations in humans. Nat Genet 1998; 19:155–157.
55. Ristow M, Muller-Wieland D, Pfeiffer A, Krone W, Kahn CR. Obesity associated with a mutation in a genetic regulator of adipocyte differentiation. N Engl J Med 1998; 339:953–959.
56. Jackson RS, Creemers JW, Ohagi S, et al. Obesity and impaired prohormone processing associated with mutations in the human prohormone convertase 1 gene. Nat Genet 1997; 16:303–306.
57. Perusse L, Rankinen T, Zuberi A, et al. The human obesity gene map: the 2004 update. Obes Res 2005; 13(3):381–490.
58. Gunay-Aygun M, Cassidy SB, Nicholls RD. Prader-Willi and other syndromes associated with obesity and mental retardation. Behav Genet 1997; 27:307–324.
59. Green JS, Parfrey PS, Harriett JD, et al. The cardinal manifestations of Bardet-Biedl syndrome, a form of Laurence-Moon-Biedl syndrome. N Engl J Med 1989; 321:1002–1009.
60. Grace C, Beales P, Summerbell C, Kopelman P. The effect of Bardet-Biedl syndrome in the components on energy balance. Int J Obes Relat Metab Disord 2001; 25(Suppl 2):S42.
61. O'Dea D, Parfrey PS, Harnett JD, Hefferton D, Cramer BC, Green J. The importance of renal impairment in the natural history of Bardet-Biedl syndrome. Am J Kidney Dis 1996; 27:776–783.

62. Katsanis N, Beales PL, Woods MO, et al. Mutations in MKKS cause obesity, retinal dystrophy and renal malformations associated with Bardet-Biedl syndrome. Nat Genet 2000; 26:67–70.

63. Barker DJ, Hales CN, Fall CH, Osmond C, Phipps K, Clark PM. Type 2 (non- insulin-dependent) diabetes mellitus, hypertension and hyperlipidaemia (syndrome X): relation to reduced fetal growth. Diabetologia 1993; 36:62–67.

64. Whitaker RC, Wright JA, Pepe MS, Seidel KD, Dietz WH. Predicting obesity in young adulthood from childhood and parental obesity. N Engl J Med 1997; 337:869–873.

65. Must A, Jacques PF, Dallal GE, Bajema CJ, Dietz WH. Long-term morbidity and mortality of overweight adolescents. A follow-up of the Harvard Growth Study of 1922 to 1935. N Engl J Med 1992; 327:1350–1355.

66. Williamson DF, Madans J, Pamuk E, Flegal KM, Kendrick JS, Serdula MK. A prospective study of childbearing and 10-year weight gain in US white women 25 to 45 years of age. Int J Obes Relat Metab Disord 1994; 18:561–569.

67. Smith DE, Lewis CE, Caveny JL, Perkins LL, Burke GL, Bild DE. Longitudinal changes in adiposity associated with pregnancy. The CARDIA Study. Coronary Artery Risk Development in Young Adults Study. JAMA 1994; 271:1747–1751.

68. Reubinoff BE, Grubstein A, Meirow D, Berry E, Schenker JG, Brzezinski A. Effects of low-dose estrogen oral contraceptives on weight, body composition, and fat distribution in young women. Fertil Steril 1995; 63:516–521.

69. Aloia JF, Vaswani A, Russo L, Sheehan M, Flaster E. The influence of menopause and hormonal replacement therapy on body cell mass and body fat mass. Am J Obstet Gynecol 1995; 172:896–900.

70. Haarbo J, Christiansen C. Treatment-induced cyclic variations in serum lipids, lipoproteins, and apolipoproteins after 2 years of combined hormone replacement therapy: exaggerated cyclic variations in smokers. Obstet Gynecol 1992; 80:639–644.

71. Weight cycling. National Task Force on the Prevention and Treatment of Obesity. JAMA 1994; 272:1196–202.

2

Obesity and Psychotic Disorders

Jogin H. Thakore and Leona Spelman
*Neuroscience Centre, St. Vincent's Hospital, Fairview,
Dublin, Ireland*

INTRODUCTION

Schizophrenia is associated with increased death rates and a reduced life span. Accidents and suicide do not account for the vast majority of such deaths. Evidence suggests that many illnesses, including cardiovascular disease, contribute to this excess mortality. Obesity is a physiological characteristic associated with the development of cardiovascular illness and it is clear that our patients with schizophrenia are frequently overweight, and at times, obese. This may simply mirror the worldwide epidemic of obesity, though it is unclear whether the distribution of body fat (i.e., android or gynoid) differs between those with schizophrenia and their well counterparts as most studies to date have reported body weight changes only as a function of body mass index (BMI). Antipsychotic agents and the unhealthy lifestyle of those with schizophrenia have been the culprits most cited as causing this weight gain. Yet, the increase in cardiovascular-associated mortality in schizophrenia was observed prior to the introduction of antipsychotic medication, posing a problem for this commonly held belief. Increases in visceral obesity, which are not accurately measured using BMI and which may occur independently of medication exposure, are a potential explanation. One means to address such issues is to study those experiencing their first-episode of schizophrenia and who have not been exposed to any psychotropic medication. Though important, the role of antipsychotic medication (conventional and atypical) will not be discussed, as this is addressed elsewhere (discussed in chap. 10). With all these issues in mind, this chapter will focus on relationships among obesity, obesity-related illnesses, and first-episode, drug-naive schizophrenia.

MORTALITY STUDIES IN SCHIZOPHRENIA

As early as 1841, it was reported that mentally ill people, institutionalized in asylums in Britain, had a risk of death 6 to 7 times than that of the general population (1). Studies performed in the early decades of the 20th century from the United States and Europe also reported increased mortality among psychiatric patients treated in a hospital (2,3). These studies highlighted the causes of death due to infections secondary to overcrowding and poor hygiene (4). However, studies performed after the introduction of antipsychotic medication in 1952 and those reflecting the community-based treatment of schizophrenia are perhaps more relevant to us today than the older studies based on institutionalized subjects. Additionally, in tandem with the changing face of contemporary psychiatry, mortality studies have become more sophisticated demonstrating that psychiatric patients have higher death rates than the general population (5,6). This information leads us to ask the obvious question as to what contributes to this excess mortality. Natural and unnatural causes (including suicide) contribute in some way to early death among individuals with schizophrenia.

The impact of suicide on the increased mortality in schizophrenia is substantial (6–10). In fact, suicide is the largest single cause of the excess mortality of schizophrenia (7). In acknowledging this fact it is also important to consider that although the incidence of suicide is increased throughout the course of schizophrenia, compared to the general population, it is highest in the year following diagnosis (11). With this in mind, the lifetime risk of suicide for schizophrenia has been recently revised (12). In this chapter, the authors used computerized curve modeling to review 29 contemporary mortality reports for schizophrenia and consequently calculated a lifetime risk of suicide at 4% instead of the previously reported 10% risk (12,13). Therefore, suicide, although the single most important cause of premature mortality in schizophrenia, is far outweighed by the proportion of the excess deaths caused by accumulated natural causes (7).

The first meta-analysis of the excess mortality of schizophrenia found a significantly increased mortality from natural and unnatural (suicide, accidents, and homicide) causes (7). Brown reported that 28% and 12% of the excess mortality is attributable to suicide and accidents, respectively. Thus, 60% of the excess mortality is attributable to physical disease (7). A later study by the same author examined specific causes of the excess mortality of schizophrenia using the standardized mortality ratio (SMR) (8). SMR is derived from the number of deaths observed in a population divided by the number of expected deaths and multiplied by 100. The study concluded that the SMRs for natural and unnatural causes were significantly higher in a group of schizophrenia patients and were mostly accounted for by cardiovascular disease, diabetes, and epilepsy (8). Earlier studies from the United Kingdom and Sweden also found that cardiovascular disease contributed significantly to the increased mortality in schizophrenia, though these findings were not universally accepted (14–18).

More recent studies, however, have confirmed the findings of Brown et al. and others (7,8,14–16). A Swedish research group reported appreciable increases in deaths from cardiovascular causes among patients with a diagnosis of schizophrenia over the time period of 1976–1995 (19). Norway is in a unique position as Ødegard, the creator of the first nationwide psychiatric case register, published mortality statistics for psychiatric patients from 1916–1974, thereby allowing observation of trends over many decades (3,20–22). A recent Norwegian study confirmed the changing trends and reported an increase in SMRs for cardiovascular death and suicide in psychiatric patients from 1980–1992 (9). A medical examiner case study conducted in the United States confirmed this observation by concluding that the majority of deaths among schizophrenia patients were the result of natural diseases, mostly atherosclerotic cardiovascular disease (23). Therefore, the findings within schizophrenia mirror the increasing impact of cardiovascular disease as a cause of mortality within the general population as the 20th century has progressed and in projections of mortality to the year 2020 (24,25). In addition, the mortality from undetermined causes in schizophrenia is high (15). Although suicidal acts contribute to this statistic, another contributing factor may be sudden death due to cardiac arrhythmias (26–29). As patients with pre-existing cardiac disease are at an increased risk, this may further impact the effect of cardiovascular events on the mortality in schizophrenia (30).

MORBIDITY FROM GENERAL MEDICAL
DISEASE IN SCHIZOPHRENIA

In considering mortality statistics, it is also useful to specifically examine the literature on general medical morbidity associated with schizophrenia as it has been posited that nearly 50% of patients with schizophrenia have a co-occurring general medical condition (31–33). Despite the high percentage of comorbidity, this statistic is a conservative estimate as it has been suggested that the extent and consequences of general medical comorbidity in patients with schizophrenia are generally under-recognized (32). In epidemiological studies higher than expected rates of cardiovascular disease, infectious diseases, type 2 diabetes mellitus, respiratory disease, certain forms of cancer, and a variety of other illnesses have been found in patients with schizophrenia (16,34–36). However, it must be stated that early

studies failed to meet methodological standards necessary to provide conclusive evidence (34). More recent evidence has shed light on this topic. In
a study by Dixon et al. (37) among 719 people with a diagnosis of schizophrenia, the majority of patients reported at least one medical problem.
The prevalence of diabetes exceeded those expected in the general population and the rates of hypertension and heart disease resembled those found
in an older cohort in the general population, as measured in the national
health interview survey (38). Thus, patients with schizophrenia would
appear to develop cardiovascular disease at a younger age than the general
population (37).

However, the finding of a lower prevalence of general medical illnesses
in older schizophrenia patients, mean age of 68.4 years, as compared to
patients with mood disorders and Alzheimer's disease lead us to postulate
about the existence of a survivor cohort (39). Thus, people with schizophrenia may develop physical illnesses earlier in life than other groups and
have died before reaching middle or old age when one would expect
morbidity and mortality to increase (25). In fact, numerous investigators
have concluded that the excess mortality of schizophrenia is highest in
the young and generally decreases with age (14,16,40). In addition to
becoming physically sick at younger ages, patients with schizophrenia are
rarely treated for their physical illness in the early, less severe phases and
appear for medical attention only when cardiovascular and pulmonary diseases are severe and potentially life-threatening (41). This problem is further
compounded by reduced detection of comorbid physical illness in schizophrenia by the medical profession despite the fact that general medical
comorbidity has been linked with more severe psychiatric symptoms
(37,42,43). With these facts in mind it is timely to examine the phenomenon
of medical illness, and in particular cardiovascular disease, in association
with schizophrenia.

CARDIOVASCULAR RISK FACTORS AND SCHIZOPHRENIA

Lifestyle factors including unhealthy diet and lack of exercise, alcohol use,
tobacco smoking, and poverty are all considered to be important etiological
factors for the development of cardiovascular disease (7,11,44). The pattern
of excess smoking in schizophrenia populations may contribute to the
increased mortality from cardiovascular and respiratory diseases reported
in this group, as is mirrored in global projections of mortality (25,44). In
addition, a reluctance to seek medical attention and poor compliance with
recommended treatments may have an impact on the less favorable outcomes of patients with schizophrenia (7).

These lifestyle issues, often acting in concert, have been identified as
substantial risk factors for developing cardiovascular illness and are often
referred to as modifiable risk factors (45,46). Risk factors which are

independently related to the development of cardiovascular disease but which are considered nonmodifiable are personal characteristics such as age, gender, family history of premature heart disease, and other genetic factors (47,48). Other risk factors that are considered modifiable include obesity, diabetes, insulin resistance, hypertension, dyslipidemias, and hyper-triglyceridemia. These biochemical parameters together form the metabolic syndrome (49). This syndrome, which appears to occur 2 to 4 times more often in those with schizophrenia than in an appropriately matched population, and obesity are believed to play a critical role in the development of cardiovascular illness (50).

OBESITY AND SCHIZOPHRENIA

The debate concerning obesity and schizophrenia has thus far centered on the role of medication (51). There is little doubt that both conventional and atypical antipsychotic medications can induce weight gain (52). However, the potential to do so varies among the different compounds as exemplified by a meta-analysis by Allison et al. (53) (discussed in chap. 10). Moreover, the epidemiologic situation may be more complex than is appreciated. For example, Homel et al. (54) examined the rates of change in BMI for individuals with and without schizophrenia between 1987 and 1996, a period in which atypical antipsychotic drug usage increased. The BMI in the general population rose steadily during the period in question, taking into account age and gender. The average BMI in those with schizophrenia was significantly higher than man in the general population. Even though females between 18 and 30 years of age showed a dramatic increase in BMI, there was no specific trend over time in the total schizophrenic population indicating that the often quoted linear relationship between obesity, as measured by BMI, and atypical antipsychotic drug usage may be too simple. Furthermore, a population-based record linkage study from Western Australia spanning from 1980 to 1998 observed that ischemic heart disease (IHD) was the major cause of death in psychiatric patients including those with schizophrenia (55). Indeed, the rates of death due to IHD remained high in schziophrenia whereas a diminution was observed in the general population. Curiously, the higher IHD-associated mortality rates applied to male patients with schizophrenia and not females. However, Homel et al. (54) showed that the increase in schizophrenia-related obesity in their study was seen mostly in females. Thus, we are left with two excellent studies, which seem to indicate that the rates of obesity have increased in females without the expected increase in IHD which begs the following questions: Are we measuring the best predictive indicator of cardiovascular disease? Is schizophrenia associated with cardiovascular disease independently of medication exposure?

VISCERAL FAT DISTRIBUTION AND SCHIZOPHRENIA

In terms of the first question, large-scale epidemiological studies indicate that there is a clear association between morbid obesity (BMI $>40 \, \text{kg/m}^2$), type 2 diabetes, and cardiovascular disease (56). However, the location of the fat is more critical in lesser forms of obesity such as those generally seen in schizophrenia (57). Significant increases in visceral or intra-abdominal fat (IAF), termed "android obesity," are linked to the development of dyslipidemias, atherosclerosis, hypertension, and diabetes (58). Though Vague (59) was the first to emphasize that obesity was not homogenous and that certain patterns of obesity (namely, android or abdominal) were linked to glucose intolerance and lipid abnormalities, he was not the first to describe this association. This distinction must pass to JB Morgagni who, using anatomical dissection, made the link between excessive visceral fat, hypertension, and atherosclerosis some 250 years ago (60). This sort of quantification of visceral fat is only possible at postmortem examination. Suitable "in vivo" alternative means of measurement are classified as indirect, with waist-to-hip ratio (WHR) and waist circumference, and direct with imaging techniques such as magnetic resonance imaging (MRI) and CT scanning (61).

In both WHR and waist circumference, the waist refers to the midpoint between the iliac crest (measured standing) and the hip refers to the most rotund part across the buttocks. In terms of WHR and waist circumference, cut-off values are >0.85 for women and >0.90 for men and $>88 \, \text{cm}$ for women and $>100 \, \text{cm}$ for men, respectively, as these values are associated with greater metabolic disturbance. CT is still probably the gold standard in terms of measuring visceral fat distribution and the L4–L5 junction is the best site for examination if a single scan is being used to estimate this area. The advantage of MRI is the lack of exposure to ionizing radiation though error rates in comparison to CT in terms of estimating subcutaneous fat and visceral fat can approach 8% to 22%, respectively.

Most studies reporting patterns of obesity in schizophrenia have recruited subjects who are receiving or who have been exposed to psychotropic medication. Few have used the methods described earlier to evaluate fat distribution. First-episode, drug-naïve patients with schizophrenia offer a unique opportunity to study the interrelationship between illness and regional fat distribution, without the confounding variable of prior antipsychotic drug exposure. To date, three studies have been published which sought to specifically determine visceral fat distribution in first-episode schizophrenia. The first was by our group and used CT scans to determine visceral fat area in 15 subjects with first-episode, drug-free schizophrenia ($n = 8$ drug-free and $n = 7$ drug-naïve) and an appropriate healthy control group (62). We found that patients had a higher BMI and WHR, higher plasma levels of cortisol, and over 3 times as much IAF than did normal age- and sex-matched controls. However, this study had two limitations. First, patients were not matched with controls in terms of BMI. Since the BMI of patients was higher than that of controls, our results may have been explicable in terms of a simple mass effect, namely, that IAF levels were increased in proportion to BMI. Second, although all patients had been free of intramuscular antipsychotics for six months and oral antipsychotics for six weeks, not all were atypical-antipsychotic naïve, which is of importance as these agents can induce weight gain (63,64).

Therefore, we conducted a separate study in which we aimed to determine whether first-episode, drug-naïve patients ($n = 19$) with schizophrenia had increased amounts of visceral fat in comparison to a control group who were matched with patients in terms of age, sex, diet, exercise, smoking status, alcohol intake, and most importantly, BMI (controls = 23.0 ± 0.43; patients = $24.6 \pm 0.73 \, kg/m^2$) (65). In addition, we were interested in estimating the effects of risperidone and olanzapine on the visceral fat distribution in the patient group.

We found that patients with schizophrenia consumed less fiber but more saturated fat, had higher WHRs, and had just over 3 times as much IAF ($116.8 \pm 20.2 \, cm^2$) as did the BMI-matched group of control subjects ($38.0 \pm 4.8 \, cm^2$). Pharmacological intervention with risperidone and olanzapine over a six-month period did not improve the quality of their diet as patients continued to consume less fiber and more saturated fat than did controls. However, following treatment, patients took more vigorous exercise. BMI, a measure of total body fatness, increased equally and significantly with both risperidone and olanzapine ($29.4 \pm 0.82 \, kg/m$). Intra-abdominal fat also increased equally with both risperidone ($26.9 \pm 12.1 \, cm^2$) and olanzapine ($18.2 \pm 11.4 \, cm^2$), but these increases were not statistically different from pretreatment values ($116.8 \pm 20.2 \, cm^2$ vs. $131.7 \pm 20.9 \, cm^2$). Our results in this study indicated that usage of the atypical antipsychotics, risperidone and olanzapine, did not significantly increase IAF stores, but was consistent with our previous findings of conventional neuroleptics.

In contrast, in the third study, Zhang et al. (66) found no difference between first-episode, drug-naïve Chinese patients with schizophrenia and controls in terms of their IAF as measured by MRI. They also found that 10 weeks of treatment with risperidone and chlorpromazine significantly increased this fat store.

Differences between the three studies may be explained by critical methodological deficits in the paper by Zhang et al. (66). Firstly, the SD for the controls was 50 years indicating that some subjects were elderly and the groups were not matched for gender. This is important as elderly males have higher amounts of IAF. Lifestyle parameters such as diet, exercise, smoking, and alcohol intake were not measured or indeed compared between the two groups. Secondly, we are not given any indication as to how an individual was selected for scanning, as all of the controls and patients recruited did not have an MRI scan. Thirdly, the authors did not use the same scanning techniques as Seidell et al. (67). Thus, there were large differences in terms of inversion and repetition times. Also, the most critical aspect of using a single scan to estimate IAF is to ensure that the scan is taken at the level of L4/5 which is located best by a (radiological) lateral scout and not palpation as the authors reported doing. Furthermore, in contrast to what the authors claim, MRI is not a "precise and reliable means of determining the two fat measures with better resolution than computed tomography" as it can erroneously estimate the amount of IAF by 22%. Finally, a one-way ANOVA should have been used to compare any differences among the three groups as the use of multiple *t* tests may have led to a type 2 error.

In short, conclusions are difficult to draw from the studies presented, though it is fair to say that first-episode, drug-naïve patients with schizophrenia appear to have higher rates of visceral fat distribution than appropriately matched controls and that neither olanzapine or risperidone significantly increase the levels of this fat deposit. These findings have not been supported by Zhang et al. (66), possibly due to differences in methodology.

POTENTIAL REASONS FOR EXCESS INTRA-ABDOMINAL FAT DISTRIBUTION IN FIRST-EPISODE SCHIZOPHRENIA

Lifestyle choices made by patients before they present to psychiatric services may have influenced IAF distribution in which they took less strenuous exercise and consumed less fiber and more saturated fat than matched controls. However, a positive energy balance correlates poorly with increased visceral fat stores and may not fully explain our findings (68). The role of stress axis disturbance in the pathogenesis of abdominal obesity has been increasingly recognized. In our studies we had measured cortisol, a crude biological correlate of stress and found that it was significantly higher in patients than in controls (62,65). Though not conclusive, there is considerable evidence that those with schizophrenia have hypothalamic–pituitary–adrenal (HPA) axis abnormalities. Feedforward disturbance is indicated by the following pieces of evidence, namely failure to lower plasma levels of cortisol between midnight and four hours, elevated CSF levels of corticotropin-releasing hormone (CRH), and pretreatment with dexamethasone (which normally suppresses the HPA axis) leading to an increase in corticotropin (ACTH) and cortisol in response to exogenously administered CRH (20–22,24,69–72). Feedback disturbance is indicated by the failure of a higher percentage of patients with schizophrenia to lower plasma levels of cortisol during the dexamethasone suppression test, which is an indicator of type 2 glucocorticoid receptor (GR) function (25,73). Further evidence of GR dysregulation is indicated by the fact that dexamethasone-induced growth hormone responses are blunted in those with schizophrenia (27,74). Dysregulation of this axis can result in hypercortisolaemia, as seen in our patients with schizophrenia, which can lead to metabolic disturbance including an increase in IAF deposition as previously documented in schizophrenia and major depression (28,29,62,65,75,76).

Though olanzapine and risperidone induced a clear rise in BMI, this was not accompanied by an increase in IAF deposition. This apparent discrepancy might be explained by the relatively short interval between the baseline and follow-up scans (six months), and by the fact that BMI does not correlate well with IAF distribution. This fact is borne out by the observation that nonpsychiatrically ill patients with obesity had a BMI of $32.1 \, kg/m^2$ and IAF deposits of $88.5 \, cm^2$ as detected by CT scanning, which was far less than our pretreatment group ($IAF = 116.8 \, cm^2$; $BMI = 24.6 \, kg/m^2$) (41). Furthermore, the decrease in plasma levels of cortisol and the increase in strenuous exercise taken may have mitigated against a significant increase in IAF (61).

In essence we have shown that first-episode patients with schizophrenia who are psychotropic naïve have on average normal BMIs though higher levels of visceral fat. In the general population it has been demonstrated that such individuals are hyperinsulinemic, insulin resistant, dyslipidemic, and predisposed to type 2 diabetes and are termed "metabolically obese" (77). It is clear from the articles of Heiskenan and Altmeras that patients with schizophrenia have a higher prevalence of the metabolic syndrome and a greater atherogenic risk profile, though both groups used a cross-sectional design and patients exposed to both typical and atypical antipsychotic medications (50,78). Therefore, a critical question that still requires an answer is whether the dyslipidemias, insulin resistance, hyperinsulinemia, and type 2 diabetes seen in schizophrenia predate the introduction of medication.

PREDIABETES AND TYPE 2 DIABETES AND SCHIZOPHRENIA

In recent years, there has been an increasing body of literature highlighting an association between atypical antipsychotic medication and type 2 diabetes in individuals with a diagnosis of schizophrenia (79,80). Though the evidence appears compelling, it must be placed in context with a medical literature reporting that schizophrenia and severe mental illness were associated with glucose dysregulation prior to the introduction of antipsychotic medication (81–84). Following the introduction of typical antipsychotics, further reports of glucose dysregulation and diabetes were reported in individuals with schizophrenia (85–91). In addition, animal studies demonstrated hyperglycemic properties of chlorpromazine, the first available antipsychotic (92). However, there were significant methodological problems with these studies, as the diagnoses of schizophrenia and diabetes mellitus were not standardized.

The latter has changed since the introduction of international standardized diagnostic schedules for psychiatric disorders, the current schedules being ICD-10 (WHO) and DSM-IV (APA) (93,94). Additional diagnostic criteria for diabetes were developed in 1979 and in 1980; the latter were updated in 1985 (95–97). In 1997, the American Diabetes Association approved new diagnostic criteria for diabetes mellitus (98). These internationally accepted criteria allow comparability between studies leading to greater clarity. The first study to use standardized oral glucose tolerance testing and WHO criteria to screen patients with schizophrenia for diabetes, following the introduction of typical antipsychotics, showed the prevalence of diabetes to be 8.8% among 420 patients and 5.0% among 312 sedentary office workers (99). These findings were statistically significant and further analysis of the data suggested that the effects of obesity, long-term antipsychotic treatment, and the illness of schizophrenia were all possible factors in the pathogenesis of diabetes. Another study by Mukherjee et al. (100) demonstrated an increased prevalence of diabetes (15.8%) among individuals with schizophrenia compared to the prevalence in the population (3.2%). The subjects were treated with typical antipsychotics and an interesting fact was that diabetes was more common in patients not receiving medication at the time of the study. An expected association was that diabetes was more common in the older age groups and did not occur in individuals under the age of 50 years (100).

In order to establish the true prevalence of diabetes among individuals with schizophrenia, it is important to examine some of the most recent literature on this topic. There has been a plethora of case reports and case series linking schizophrenia, atypical antipsychotic medication use, insulin resistance, diabetes, and diabetic ketoacidosis (52,79). The strongest association between medication and glucose dysregulation has been reported to be with clozapine and olanzapine, with some authors suggesting that there is a true drug-induced effect, implying that atypical antipsychotics are the main contributors to the increased risk (52,101). However, the authors qualify their conclusions by stating that diabetes is more common in those with schizophrenia regardless of any drug treatment (52). This fact was confirmed by a review finding diabetes mellitus to be more prevalent among individuals with schizophrenia than the general population prior to the widespread introduction of atypical antipsychotics (102). Dixon et al. (102) reported a lifetime prevalence for diabetes of 14.9% and a current prevalence of 10.9% in persons with schizophrenia compared to a national prevalence of 1.2% for persons aged 18 to 44 years and 6.3% for persons aged 45 to 64 years. In addition to diabetes, researchers have reported hyperinsulinemia and insulin resistance in association with schizophrenia and antipsychotic medication (103,104). In a study by Melkersson et al. (103) patients treated with clozapine had elevated insulin levels with normal blood glucose levels. Using a modified oral glucose tolerance test, Newcomer et al. (104) demonstrated hyperglycemia and hyperinsulinemia in schizophrenia patients treated with clozapine, olanzapine, and risperidone. The magnitude of glucose and insulin response was largest for patients treated with olanzapine and there was no difference between healthy controls and patients treated with typical antipsychotics. The groups were matched for BMI, thereby implying that body weight did not influence the results. A major criticism of this study is that glucose was only measured up to 75-minute postglucose load; thus there is a possibility that glucose levels may have normalized if the correct 120-minute follow-up was utilized. Moreover, others have been unable to replicate the findings of Newcomer et al. (104) and Melkersson et al. (103). For instance, Gupta et al. (105) have shown that the prevalence of diabetes, hypertension, and lipid disturbance is equal between, and among, typical and atypical medications. Furthermore, Koller et al. (106,107) and Koller and Doraiswamy (108) reviewed FDA Med "Watch surveillance data with regard to olanzapine, risperidone, and clozapine," and concluded that new cases of diabetes mellitus might be precipitated by such agents in already vulnerable individuals. Indeed, most of the data published thus far has come from case reports and cross-sectional epidemiological studies, with few prospective studies using subjects who had been chronically exposed to antipsychotic medications.

However, in terms of studies recruiting drug-naïve, first-episode subjects, there are three notable exceptions. The first is by Ryan et al. (109) who found that, in comparison to an age-, sex- and BMI-matched control group, over 15% of nonobese (BMI = 24.5 ±3.6) patients ($n = 26$) with first-episode, drug-naïve schizophrenia had impaired fasting glucose. Specifically, patients had higher fasting plasma levels of glucose (5.32 ± 0.94 mmol/L vs. 4.9 ± 0.29 mmol/L), insulin (70.3 ± 27.9 mmol/L vs. 55.25 ± 26.55 mmol/L), and cortisol (499.4 ± 161.4 nmol/L vs. 303.2 ± 10.5 nmol/L) than the healthy controls. Patients were also more insulin resistant compared to controls (2.3 ± 1.0 vs. 1.7 ± 0.7) as measured by the homeostasis model assessment. In addition, patients had significantly lower fasting plasma levels of cholesterol (4.02 mmol/L vs. 4.57 mmol/L) and LDL (2.39 mmoI/L vs. 2.91 mmoI/L), though there were no significant differences in plasma levels of triglycerides (0.99 nmol/L vs. 0.92 nmol/L) and HDL (1.20 mmol/L vs. 1.25 mmol/L) between the groups.

Lieberman et al. (110) studied the effects of chlorpromazine ($n = 80$) and clozapine ($n = 80$) in a Chinese cohort of treatment-naïve, first-episode patients with schizophrenia over 52 weeks. From a metabolic perspective, baseline levels of fasting plasma glucose were 4.8 (mmol/L) (chlorpromazine) and 4.7 (mmol/L) (clozapine) and were nonsignificantly increased to 5.5 and 5.3 mmol/L, respectively, at 52 weeks despite significant increases in weight from 60.3 to 68.8 kg for chlorpromazine and 61.6 to 71.5 kg for clozapine. This study is important in that it prospectively examined the effects of the prototypical neuroleptics chlorpromazine and clozapine (an agent which is believed to significantly increase weight and plasma glucose) over a one-year period and found no significant metabolic derangement. Shortcomings were the fact that there was no healthy control group and patients' diet and exercise habits were not recorded.

Zhang et al. (66) followed another Chinese cohort ($n = 46$) treated with risperidone ($n = 30$), chlorpromazine ($n = 15$), or quetiapine ($n = 1$) over a 10-week period. Although BMI increased with antipsychotic treatment from 20.5 to 22.2 kg/m^2, plasma levels of fasting glucose decreased from 5.01 to 4.91 mmol/L. Nonfasting glucose (samples taken two hours after breakfast) rose significantly from 6.34 to 7.18 mmol/L; this is a nonstandardized measure and at best approximates to a random glucose, thereby making it within normal limits. Though plasma levels of cholesterol (4.08–4.58 mmol/L), triglycerides (1.15–1.66 mmol/L), and LDL (2.19–2.63 mmol/L) were significantly increased at study endpoint, they were still within normal limits. Insulin levels increased from 18.65 to 25.65 mmol/L in the whole sample, but decreased in females from 30.53 to 25.92 mmol/L. Thus, the authors' conclusion of a drug-induced progression to the metabolic syndrome would seem to be incorrect as they demonstrated that fasting levels of glucose decreased in the subjects as a group and plasma insulin levels decreased in female subjects despite an increase in BMI.

In sum, the studies of prediabetes and type 2 diabetes conducted in first-episode schizophrenia patients have provided conflicting results, which may be due to methodological differences, and possibly flaws, as described above. These matters notwithstanding, it is clear that patients with schizophrenia are at a higher risk of developing type 2 diabetes.

POTENTIAL REASONS FOR INCREASED PREVALENCE OF TYPE 2 DIABETES IN FIRST-EPISODE SCHIZOPHRENIA

It has been found that 18% to 30% of patients with schizophrenia have a family history of type 2 diabetes, as opposed to 1.2% to 6.3% within the general population. Due to medication, these two illnesses may share a common pathophysiology beyond that (111). Although increasing age correlates with a higher risk of diabetes, a recent study showed that individuals with schizophrenia have a tendency to develop comorbid diabetes at a younger age (52,112). Sernyak et al. (112) found the prevalence of diabetes to be 8.75% in patients younger than 40 years and concluded that atypical antipsychotics may hasten the onset of diabetes in individuals with a diathesis for this disease rather than precipitating diabetes de novo. Yet another risk factor appears to be race; epidemiological studies have shown that the risks for diabetes in African Americans, Hispanics, and Native Americans are approximately 2, 2.5, and 5 times greater, respectively, than in Caucasians (113). Little research has examined the influence of race on the relationship between schizophrenia and diabetes. Physical activity plays a major role in glucose metabolism with exercise promoting leanness, lowering blood glucose levels, and improving insulin sensitivity (113). As discussed earlier, individuals with schizophrenia exercise less than the general population.

Various physiological mechanisms have been proposed to account for the increased risk of diabetes among individuals with schizophrenia. One such mechanism involves the satiety hormone leptin, which is produced by adipocytes and is elevated in patients receiving antipsychotics (114,115). As increased leptin levels are associated with insulin resistance, it is possible that increased leptin is another mechanism leading to type 2 diabetes (116). Serotoninergic systems are involved in glucose and insulin homeostasis; the impact of antipsychotic medication, particularly atypical antipsychotics, on this receptor system may contribute to glucose dysregulation as there is evidence from animal studies that antagonism of 5HT2 receptors elicits hyperglycemia and weight gain (117–119). However, conclusive evidence of a similar process occurring in humans is as yet lacking and the effects of blockade at multiple serotonin receptor sites on glucose metabolism are poorly understood (118).

Chronic activation of the HPA axis has been posited to increase the likelihood of hyperglycemia in schizophrenia as is seen within the general population (120). Importantly, this is not the same as stating that "acute stress of psychosis" is responsible for glucose dysregulation (121). The design of the study postulating this mechanism had major flaws, making it difficult to draw any firm conclusions from the findings presented. For instance, "acute psychotic stress" is not defined within DSM-4 and diagnostic criteria were not used to confirm the diagnoses of "chronic or paranoid schizophrenia" (94). Severity of illness was defined as a subjective impression of patients' "stress," as documented using a seven point Clinical Global Impression (CGI) scale, yet such a scale is without adequate validation. According to their CGI scores, patients were divided into "low and high" categories after which significant differences began to emerge. The "low and high" scores were either ≤6 or > 6 (the maximum being seven), respectively. Therefore, the authors compared the most extremely ill patients with all of the other patients and lastly, the cut-off figures were picked arbitrarily with no scientific reasons given for doing so.

Finally, much has been written about the positive association between low birth weight and the subsequent development of schizophrenia (122). This hypothesis of fetal origin is not exclusive to schizophrenia as those who develop the metabolic syndrome later in life also have a history of low birth weight, indicating that these phenotypes may share a common insulin-resistance genotype (123). Thus, both schizophrenia and glucose dysregulation may share a common pathophysiology which may become unmasked upon exposure to various iatrogenic factors or lifestyle choices.

SUMMARY

To date, evidence from the preantipsychotic era or first-episode psychosis patients does not allow us to categorically conclude exactly what mechanisms underlie the increasing incidence of obesity and diabetes observed in schizophrenia. What is clear is that visceral obesity and prediabetic states such as impaired fasting glucose and the metabolic syndrome may be present at the time of diagnosis, which implies that they may occur independently of the use of antipsychotic medication. This is important as it indicates the need for appropriate screening of patients with schizophrenia irrespective of the type of medication considered or used. Leaving aside the potential role of medication, the associations between schizophrenia and such metabolic dysregulation may be explicable in terms of lifestyle choices (diet, exercise), chronic stress as evidenced by the observed abnormalities of the HPA axis, low birth weight, and neurochemical disturbances.

REFERENCES

1. Fair W. Report upon the mortality of lunatics. J Stat Soc 1841; 4:17–33.
2. Malzberg B. Mortality among patients with mental disease. New York: New York State Hospital Press, 1934.
3. Ødegard Ø. Mortality in Norwegian psychiatric hospitals from 1916 to 1933. Acta Psychiatr Neurol 1936; 11:323–356.
4. Alstrom CH. Mortality in mental hospitals with especial regard to tuberculosis. Acta Psychiatr Neurol 1942; (suppl 42):1–432.
5. Craig TJ. Mortality among psychiatric in-patients. Age adjusted comparison of populations before and after psychotropic drug era. Arch Gen Psychiatry 1981; 38:935–938.
6. Harris EC, Barraclough B. Excess mortality of mental disorder. Br J Psychiatry 1998; 173:11–53.
7. Brown S. Excess mortality of schizophrenia. A meta-analysis. Br J Psychiatry 1997; 171:502–508.
8. Brown S, Inskip H, Barraclough B. Causes of the excess mortality of schizophrenia. Br J Psychiatry 2000; 177:212–217.
9. Hansen V, Jacobsen BK, Arnesen E. Cause-specific mortality in psychiatric patients after deinstitutionalisation. Br J Psychiatry 2001; 179:438–443.
10. Politi P, Piccinelli M, Klersy C, et al. Mortality in psychiatric patients 5 to 21 years after hospital admission in Italy. Psychol Med 2002; 32:227–237.
11. Mortensen PB, Juel K. Mortality and causes of death in first admitted schizophrenic patients. Br J Psychiatry 1993; 163:183–189.
12. Inskip HM, Harris C, Barraclough B. Lifetime risk of suicide for affective disorder, alcoholism and schizophrenia. Br J Psychiatry 1998; 172:35–37.
13. Miles CP. Conditions predisposing to suicide: a review. J Nerv Ment Dis 1977; 164:231–246.
14. Herrman HE, Baldwin JA, Christie D. A record-linkage study of mortality and general hospital discharge in patients diagnosed as schizophrenic. Psychol Med 1983; 13:581–593.

15. Allebeck P, Wistedt B. A ten-year follow-up based on the Stockholm County Inpatient Register. Arch Gen Psychiatry 1986; 43:650–653.
16. Baldwin JA. Schizophrenia and physical illness. Psychol Med 1979; 9:611–618.
17. Black DW, Warrack G, Winokur G. The Iowa record-linkage study. III. Excess mortality among patients with "functional" disorders. Arch Gen Psychiatry 1985; 42:82–88.
18. Martin RL, Cloninger R, Guze SB, Clayton PJ. Mortality in a follow-up of 500 psychiatric outpatients. II. Cause specific mortality. Arch Gen Psychiatry 1985; 42:58–66.
19. Ösby U, Correia N, Brandt L, Ekbom A, Sparen P. Time trends in schizophrenia mortality in Stockholm County Sweden: cohort study. Br Med J 2000; 321:483–484.
20. Ødegard Ø. Mortality in Norwegian mental hospitals 1926–1941. Acta Genet Stat Med 1951; 2:141–173.
21. Ødegard Ø. The excess mortality of the insane. Acta Psychiatri Neurol Scand 1952; 27:353–367.
22. Ødegard Ø. Mortality in Norwegian mental hospitals 1950–1962. Acta Genet Stat Med 1967; 17:137–153.
23. Chute D, Grove C, Rajasekhara B, Smialek JE. Schizophrenia and sudden death: a medical examiner case study. Am J Forensic Med Pathol 1999; 20: 131–135.
24. World Health Report 1999. Making a difference. Geneva: World Health Organisation, 1999.
25. Murray CJL, Lopez AD. Alternative projections of mortality and disability by cause 1990–2020: Global burden of disease study. Lancet 1997; 349:1498–1504.
26. Ruschena D, Mullen PE, Burgess P, et al. Sudden death in psychiatric patients. Br J Psychiatry 1998; 172:331–336.
27. Reilly JG, Ayis SA, Ferrier IN, Jones SJ, Thomas SH. QTc-interval abnormalities and psychotropic drug therapy in psychiatric patients. Lancet 2000; 355:1048–1052.
28. Reilly JG, Ayis SA, Ferrier IN, Jones SJ, Thomas SH. Thioridazine and sudden death in psychiatric in-patients. Br J Psychiatry 2002; 180:515–522.
29. Glassman AH, Bigger JT Jr. Antipsychotic drugs; prolonged QTc interval, torsade de pointes and sudden death. Am J Psychiatry 2001; 158:1774–1782.
30. Kitayama H, Kiuchi K, Nejima J, Katoh T, Takano T, Hayakawa H. Long-term treatment with antipsychotic drugs in conventional doses prolonged QTc dispersion, but did not increase ventricular tachyarrhythmias in patients with schizophrenia in the absence of cardiac disease. Eur J Clin Pharmacol 1999; 55:259–262.
31. Koranyi EK. Physical health and illness in a psychiatric outpatient department population. Can Psychiatr Assoc J 1972; 17(suppl 2):109–116.
32. Jeste DV, Gladsjo JA, Lindamer LA, Lacro JP. Medical comorbidity in schizophrenia. Schizophr Bull 1996; 22(3):413–430.
33. Goldman LS. Medical illness in patients with schizophrenia. J Clin Psychiatry 1999; 60(suppl 21):10–15.
34. Tsuang MT, Perkins K, Simpson JC. Physical diseases in schizophrenia and affective disorder. J Clin Psychiatry 1983; 44:42–46.

35. Harris AE. Physical disease and schizophrenia. Schizophr Bull 1988; 14:85–96.
36. Allebeck P. Schizophrenia: a life-shortening disease. Schizophr Bull 1989; 15:81–89.
37. Dixon L, Postrado L, Delahunty J, Fischer PJ, Lehman A. The association of medical comorbidity in schizophrenia with poor physical and mental health. J Nerv Ment Dis 1999; 187:496–502.
38. Adams PF, Marano MA. Current estimates from the National Health Interview Survey; 1994. National Center for Health Statistics. Vital Health Stat 1995; 10(193):1–260.
39. Lacro JP, Jeste DV. Physical comorbidity and polypharmacy in older psychiatric patients. Biol Psychiatry 1994; 36:146–152.
40. Haugland G, Craig TJ, Goodman AB, Siegel C. Mortality in the era of deinstitutionalisation. Am J Psychiatry 1983; 140:848–852.
41. Muck-Jorgensen P, Mors O, Mortensen PB, Ewald H. The schizophrenic patient in the somatic hospital. Acta Psychiatr Scand Suppl 2000; 102:96–99.
42. Koran LM, Sox HC, Marton KI, et al. Medical evaluation of psychiatric patients. Arch Gen Psychiatry 1989; 46:733–740.
43. D'Ercole A, Skodol AE, Struening E, Curtis J, Millman J. Diagnosis of physical illness in psychiatric patients using axis III and a standardized medical history. Hosp Commun Psychiatry 1991; 42:395–400.
44. Baxter DN. The mortality experience of individuals on the Salford case register. I. All cause mortality. Br J Psychiatry 1996; 168:772–779.
45. Joukamaa M, Heliovaara M, Knekt P, Aromaa A, Raitasalo R, Lehtinen V. Mental disorders and cause-specific mortality. Br J Psychiatry 2001; 179: 498–502.
46a. Lusis AJ. Atherosclerosis. Nature 2000; 407:233–241.
46b. Elisaf M. The treatment of coronary heart disease: an update. Part 1: An overview of the risk factors for cardiovascular disease. Curr Med Res Opin 2001; 17:18–26.
47. Wood D, Backer GD, Faergeman O, Graham I, Mancia G, Pyörälä K. Prevention of coronary heart disease in clinical practice: Recommendations of the Second Joint Task Force of European and other Societies on coronary prevention. Atherosclerosis 1998; 140:199–270.
48. Goldbourt U, Neufeld HN. Genetic aspects of arteriosclerosis. Arteriosclerosis 1988; 6:357–377.
49. Hansen BC. The metabolic syndrome X. Ann NY Acad Sci 1999; 892:1–24.
50. Heiskanen T, Niskanen L, Lyytikainen R, Saarinen PI, Hintikka J. Metabolic syndrome in patients with schizophrenia. J Clin Psychiatry 2003; 64:575–579.
51. American Diabetic Association. Consensus Development Conference on Antipsychotic Drugs and Obesity and Diabetes. Diabetes Care 2004; 27:596–601.
52. Mir S, Taylor D. Atypical antipsychotics and hyperglycemia. Int Clin Psychopharmacol 2001; 16:63–74.
53. Allison DB, Mentore JL, Moonseong H, et al. Antipsychotic-induced weight gain: a comprehensive research synthesis. Am J Psychiatry 1999; 156: 1686–1696.
54. Homel P, Casey D, Allison DB. Changes in body mass index for individuals with and without schizophrenia; 1987–1996. Schizophr Res 2002; 55:277–284.

55. Lawrence DM, Holman CDJ, Jablensky AV, Hobbs MST. Death rate from ischaemic heart disease in Western Australian psychiatric patients 1980–1998. Br J Psychiatry 2003; 182:31–36.
56. Feinleib M. Epidemiology of obesity in relation to health hazards. Ann Intern Med 1985; 103:1019–1024.
57. Larsson B. Obesity, fat distribution, and cardiovascular disease. Int J Obes 1991; 15:53–57.
58. Bjorntorp P. Obesity and the risk of cardiovasulart disease. Ann Clin Res 1985; 17:3–9.
59. Vague J. la differentiation sexuelle fateur determinant des formes de 1-obesite. Presse Med 1947; 55:339–340.
60. Enzi G, Busetto L, Inelmen EM, Coin A, Sergi G. Historical perspective: visceral obesity and related comorbidity in Joannes Baptista Morgagni's 'De sedibus et causis morborum per anatomen indagata'. Int J Obes Relat Metab Disord 2003; 4:534–535.
61. Wajchenberg LB. Subcutaneous and visceral adipose tissue: Their relation to the metabolic syndrome. Endocr Rev 2000; 21:697–738.
62. Thakore JH, Vlahoos J, Martin A, Reznek R. Increased visceral fat distribution in drug-naïve drug-free patients with schizophrenia. Int J Obes Relat Metab Disord 2002; 26:137–141.
63. Ackennan S, Nolan LJ. Body weight gain induced by psychotropic drugs. CNS Drugs 1998; 9:135–151.
64. Kraus T, Haack M, Schuld A, et al. Body weight gain and plasma leptin levels during treatment with antipsychotic drugs. Am J Psychiatry 1999; 156: 312–314.
65. Ryan MCM, Flanagan S, Kinsella U, Keeling F, Thakore JH. Atypical antipsychotics and visceral fat distribution in first episode, drug-naive patients with schizophrenia. Life Sci 2004; 74:1999–2008.
66. Zhang ZJ, Yao ZJ, Liu W, Fang Q, Reynolds GP. Effects of antipsychotics on fat deposition and changes in leptin and insulin levels: Magnetic resonance imaging study of previously untreated people with schizophrenia. Br J Psychiatry 2004; 184:58–62.
67. Seidell JC, Bjorntorp P, Sjostrom I, Sannerstedt R, KrotMewski M, Kvist H. Regional distribution of muscle and fat mass in men: new insight into the risk of abdominal obesity using computed tomography. Int J Obes 1989; 13:289–303.
68. Bouchard C, Despres J-P, Mauriege PO. Genetic and non-genetic determinants of regional fat distribution. Endocr Rev 1993; 14:72–93.
69. Van Cauter E, Linkowski P, Kerkhofs M, et al. Circadian and sleep-related endocrine rhythms in schizophrenia. Arch Gen Psychiatry 1991; 48:348–356.
70. Banki CM, Bissette G, Arato M, O'Connor L, Nemeroff CB. CSF corticotropin-releasing factor-like immunoreactiyity in depression and schizophrenia. Am J Psychiatry 1987; 144:873–877.
71. Banki CM, Karmasci L, Bissette G, Nemeroff CB. CSF corticotropin releasing hormone, somatostatin and thyrotropin releasing hormone in schizophrenia. Psychiatry Res 1992; 43:21–31.
72. Lammers CH, Garcia-Borrreguero D, Schmider J, Gotthardt U, Dettling M, Holsboer F. Combined dexamethasone/corticotropin-releasing hormone test

in patients with schizophrenia and in normal controls. Biol Psychiatry 1995;
38:803–807.

73. Dewan MJ, Pandurangi AK, Boucher ML, Levy BF, Major LF. Abnormal
dexamethasone suppression test results in chronic schizophrenic patients.
Am J Psychiatry 1982; 139:1501–1503.

74. Thakore JH, Dinan TG. Are blunted dexamethasone-induced growth hormone responses specific for depression? Psychol Med 1996; 26:1053–1059.

75. Thakore JH, Richards PJ, Reznek RH, Martin A, Dinan TG. Increased intra-
abdominal fat deposition in patients with major depressive illness as measured
by computed tomography. Biol Psychiatry 1997; 41:1140–1142.

76. Weber-Hamann B, Hentschel F, Kniest A, et al. Hypercortisolemic depression
is associated with increased intra-abdominal fat. Psychosom Med 2002;
64:274–277.

77. Ruderman N, Chrisholm D, Pi-Sunnyer FX, Schneider S. The metabolically
obese, normal-weight individuals re-visited. Diabetes 1988; 47:699–713.

78. Almeras N, Despres J-P, Villeneuve J, et al. Development of an atherogenic
metabolic risk profile associated with the use of atypical antipsychotics. J Clin
Psychiatry 2004; 65:557–564.

79. Henderson DC. Atypical antipsychotic-induced diabetes mellitus. How strong
is the evidence? CNS Drugs 2002; 16:77–89.

80. Koro CE, Fedder DO, L'Italien GJ, et al. An assessment of the independent
effects of olanzapine and risperidone exposure on the risk of hyperlipidemia
in schizophrenic patients. Arch Gen Psychiatry 2002; 59:1021–1026.

81. Kooy FH. Hyperglycaemia in mental disorders. Brain 1919; 42:214–288.

82. Lorenz WF. Sugar intolerance in dementia praecox and other mental disorders. Arch Neurol Psychiatry 1922; 8:184–196.

83. Freeman H, Looney JM, Hoskins RG, Dyer CF. Results of insulin and epi-
nephrine tolerance tests in schizophrenic patients and in normal subjects. Arch
Neurol Psychiatry 1943; 49:195.

84. Braceland FJ, Meduna LJ, Vaichulis JA. Delayed action of insulin in schizophrenia. Am J Psychiatry 1945; 102:108–110.

85. Charatan FBE, Bartlett NG. The effect of chlorpromazine ("Largactil") on
glucose tolerance. J Ment Sci 1955; 101:351–353.

86. Hiles BW. Hyperglycaemia and glycosuria following chlorpromazine therapy.
J Am Med Assoc 1956; 126:1651.

87. Arneson GA. Phenothiazine derivatives and glucose metabolism. J Neuropsychiatry 1964; 5:181–185.

88. Waitzkin L. A survey for unknown diabetics in a mental hospital. I. Men
under age fifty. Diabetes 1966; 15:97–104.

89. Schwarz L, Munro R. Blood sugar levels in patients treated with chlorpromazine. Am J Psychiatry 1968; 125:253–255.

90. Thonnard-Neumann E. Phenothiazines and diabetes in hospitalised women.
Am J Psychiatry 1968; 124:978–982.

91. Dynes JB. Diabetes in schizophrenia and diabetes in nonpsychotic medical
patients. Dis Nerv Sys 1969; 5:341–344.

92. Norman D, Hiestand WA. Glycemic effects of chlorpromazine in the mouse,
hamster, and rat. Proc Soc Exp Biol Med 1955; 90:89.

93. World Health Organization. Classification of mental and behavioral disorders. Geneva: WHO, 1992.
94. American Psychiatric Association. Diagnostic and statistical manual of mental disorders. 4th ed. Washington, DC: American Psychiatric Association 1994.
95. National Diabetes Data Group. Classification and diagnosis of diabetes mellitus and other categories of glucose intolerance. Diabetes 1979; 28:1039–1057.
96. World Health Organisation Expert Committee on Diabetes Mellitus. Second report. WHO Technical Report Series 646, 1980.
97. World Health Organisation Study Group. Diabetes mellitus. WHO Technical Report Series 1985; 727:1–104.
98. Expert Committee on the diagnosis and classification of diabetes mellitus. Report. Diabetes Care 1997; 20:1183–1197.
99. Tabata H, Kikuoka M, Kikuoka H, Bessho H. Characteristics of diabetes mellitus in schizophrenic patients. J Med Assoc Thailand 1987; 70(suppl 2): 90–93.
100. Mukherjee S, Decina P, Bocola V, Saraceni F, Scapicchio PL. Diabetes mellitus in schizophrenic patients. Compr Psychiatry 1996; 37:68–73.
101. Wirshing DA, Spellberg BJ, Erhart SM, Marder SR, Wirshing WC. Novel antipsychotics and new onset diabetes. Biol Psychiatry 1998; 44:778–783.
102. Dixon L, Weiden P, Delahunty J, et al. Prevalence and correlates of diabetes in national schizophrenia samples. Schizophr Bull 2000; 26:903–912.
103. Melkersson KI, Halting AL, Brismar KE. Different influences of classical antipsychotics and clozapine on glucose-insulin homeostasis in patients with schizophrenia or related psychoses. J Clin Psychiatry 1999; 60:783–791.
104. Newcomer JW, Haupt DW, Fucetola R, et al. Abnormalities in glucose regulation during antipsychotic treatment of schizophrenia. Arch Gen Psychiatry 2002; 59:337–345.
105. Gupta S, Steinmeyer C, Frank B, et al. Hyperglycaemia and hypertriglyceridemia in real world patients on antipsychotic therapy. Am J Ther 2003; 10: 348–355.
106. Koller E, Schneider B, Bennett K, et al. Clozapine-induced diabetes. Am J Med 2001; 111:716–723.
107. Koller E, Doraiswamy MP, Cross JT. Risperidone-induced diabetes. Diabetes, lipids an metabolism. San Francisco, CA: Endocrine Society Meeting, 2002.
108. Koller E, Doraiswamy MP. Olanzapine-induced diabetes. Pharmacotherapy 2002; 22:841–852.
109. Ryan MCM, Collins P, Thakore JH. Impaired fasting glucose and elevation of cortisol in drug-naïve first-episode schizophrenia. Am J Psychiatry 2003; 160:284–289.
110. Lieberman J, Phillips M, Gil H, et al. Atypical and conventional antipsychotic drugs in treatment-naïve first episode schizophrenia: A 52 week randomized trial of clozapine vs. chlorpromazine. Neuropsychopharmacology 2003; 28:99–1003.
111. Mukherjee S, Schnur DB, Reddy R. Family history of type-2 diabetes in schizophrenic patients. Lancet 1989; 8636:495.
112. Sernyak MJ, Leslie DL, Alarcon RD, Losonczy MF, Rosenheck R. Association of diabetes mellitus with use of atypical neuroleptics in the treatment of schizophrenia. Am J Psychiatry 2002; 159:561–566.

113. Hafiher SM. Epidemiology of type-2 diabetes: Risk factors. Diabetes Care 1998; 21(suppl 3):C3–C6.
114. Melkersson KI, Hutting AL, Brismar KE. Elevated levels of insulin, leptin, and blood lipids in olanzapine-treated patients with schizophrenia or related psychoses. J Clin Psychiatry 2000; 61:742–749.
115. Herran A, Garcia-Unzueta MT, Amado JA, de la Maza MT, Alvarez C, Vazquez-Barquero JL. Effects of long-term treatment with antipsychotics on serum leptin levels. Br J Psychiatry 2001; 179:59–62.
116. Hafmer SM, Miettinen H, Mykkanen L. Leptin concentrations and insulin sensitivity in normoglycaemic men. Int J Obes Relat Metab Disord 1997; 21:393–399.
117. Horacek J, Kuzmiakova M, Hoschl C, Andel M, Bahbonh R. The relationship between central serotoninergic activity and insulin sensitivity in healthy volunteers. Psychoneuroendocrinology 1999; 24:785–797.
118. Wozniak KM, Linnoila M. Hyperglycaemic properties of serotonin receptor antagonists. Life Sci 1991; 49:101–109.
119. Tecott LH, Sun LM, Alcana SF. Eating disorder and epilepsy in mice lacking 5-HT-sub (2C) serotonin receptors. Nature 1995; 374:542–546.
120. Rosmond R, Bjorntorp P. The hypothalamic–pituitary–adrenal axis activity as a predictor of cardiovascular disease, type-2 diabetes and stroke. J Intern Med 2000; 247:188–197.
121. Shiloah E, Witz S, Abramovitch Y, et al. Effect of acute psychotic stress in non-diabetic subjects on β-cell function and insulin sensitivity. Diabetes Care 2003; 26:1462–1467.
122. Wahlbeck K, Forsen T, Osmond C, et al. Association of schizophrenia with low maternal body mass index, small size at birth and thinness during childhood. Arch Gen Psychiatry 2001; 58:48–52.
123. Abel K. Foetal origins of schizophrenia: testable hypotheses of genetic and environmental influences. Br J Psychiatry 2004; 184:383–385.

3

Obesity and Mood Disorders

Susan L. McElroy, Renu Kotwal, and Erik B. Nelson
Psychopharmacology Research Program, Department of Psychiatry, University of Cincinnati College of Medicine, Cincinnati, Ohio, U.S.A.

Shishuka Malhotra
Private Practice and President of Neuro Behavioral Clinical Research, Inc., United Health Network, Canton, Ohio, U.S.A.

Paul E. Keck Jr.
Psychopharmacology Research Program, Department of Psychiatry, University of Cincinnati College of Medicine; General Clinical Research Center and Mental Health Care Line, Cincinnati Veterans Affairs Medical Center, Cincinnati, Ohio, U.S.A.

Charles B. Nemeroff
Emory University School of Medicine, Department of Psychiatry, Atlanta, Georgia, U.S.A.

Despite being a focus of scientific study for over 50 years, the nature of the relationship between obesity and mood disorders remains obscure (1–21). Thus, community studies of depressive symptoms and mood syndromes in persons with obesity have found normal, decreased, and increased rates, whereas studies of persons with mood disorders show that some have anorexia and weight loss while others have hyperphagia and weight gain (2,3,12,21–34).

The obscurity surrounding the relationship between obesity and mood disorders exists despite growing research showing that both conditions are increasingly severe public health problems that significantly overlap in treatment-seeking populations (21,35–49). Depressive symptoms and mood disorders are common in persons of all ages seeking treatment for obesity, and frequently co-occur with many of the general medical conditions associated with obesity, including type 2 diabetes, coronary artery disease, cerebrovascular disease, hypertension, chronic pain, and asthma (50–64). Conversely, weight gain, overweight, and obesity are common in children and adults seeking treatment for mood disorders (11,65,66).

The degree, nature, and causes of this overlap between obesity and mood disorders in clinical populations are not understood. Since obesity and mood disorders are each becoming increasingly severe public health problems, they may be co-occurring to a greater degree simply by chance alone. Since many of the drugs used to treat mood disorders are associated with weight gain, whereas some of the drugs used to treat the general medical conditions that co-occur with obesity may induce mood symptoms, iatrogenic factors may be contributing to the co-occurrence of obesity and mood symptoms (66–68). However, recent epidemiologic studies, which used modern definitions and assessments of obesity and major depressive episodes, have been more likely to find associations between obesity and depression in community samples than older studies, which did not use such methods (7,16,21). Since family history, twin, and genetic data indicate that obesity and mood disorders are each likely to be heterogeneous, complex genetic diseases, the findings of such obesity—major depressive episode associations in the community suggest that obesity and mood disorders could be related, including by shared inherited pathogenic factors (69–75).

Despite growing studies on the epidemiology of body weight on the one hand and mental disorders on the other, along with mounting clinical and epidemiologic evidence that these conditions frequently coexist, no major epidemiologic study has yet evaluated the co-occurrence of obesity, as assessed using the methods of the National Institutes of Health (NIH), with the full range of mood disorders, as defined by DSM-IV or other widely accepted operational diagnostic criteria (76,77). To elucidate present knowledge about the relationship between obesity and mood disorders, therefore, we first briefly compare studies of the epidemiology of these two conditions. We then review studies of mood (depressive and bipolar) disorders in obesity (and the obesity-related conditions overweight, abdominal obesity, and the metabolic syndrome) and, conversely, of obesity in mood disorders. We also compare studies of the phenomenology, psychiatric and general medical comorbidity, family history, neurobiology, and treatment response of obesity with similar studies of mood disorders. We conclude by discussing some of the implications of a relationship between obesity and mood disorders.

EPIDEMIOLOGY OF OBESITY AND MOOD DISORDERS:
A BRIEF OVERVIEW

Epidemiological studies consistently find that obesity and mood disorders are each highly prevalent in the general population (35–41,43,45,47–49). Importantly, estimates of the general population prevalence rates of both conditions are dependent on the diagnostic criteria applied and the ascertainment methods used. Thus, the behavioral risk factor and surveillance system, a national survey in which participants reported their weights, estimated that the combined incidence of obesity (BMI ≥ 30) and overweight (BMI 25–29.9) among adults in the United States increased from 12% and 45% in 1991 to 21% and 58% in 2001, respectively. The prevalence of severe (class 3) obesity (BMI ≥ 40) increased from 0.9% in 1991 to 2.3% in 2001. Using data from the National Health and Nutrition Examination Surveys (NHANES), in which respondents were weighed, obesity and overweight increased in prevalence from 22.9% and 55.9% in 1988–1994 to 30.5% and 64.5% in 1999–2000, respectively. Among adults aged at least 20 years in 2001–2002, 65.7% were overweight or obese, 30.6% were obese, and 5.1% were severely obese. Taken together, these data suggest obesity is common, increasing, and underreported in the general population.

Rates of obesity (defined as > 95th percentile of the sex specific BMI for age growth charts) have also increased in children and adolescents over the past decade (40,41). Although the percentages of obese children and adolescents were relatively stable over NHANES I (1971–1974) and II (1976–1980), they doubled to 11% during NHANES III (1988–1994) and increased to 15.5% during NHANES IV (1999–2000). Specifically, 15.5% of youths ages 6 to 19 were obese and 10.4% of children ages 2 to 5 were obese (41). As with adults, however, rates of overweight and obesity were stable between 1999–2000 and 2001–2002.

The first major epidemiologic study to assess the prevalence of mental disorders in the general population of the United States, the epidemiologic catchment area (ECA) study, conducted from 1980 to 1985, estimated the lifetime prevalence for any mood disorder in adults aged 18 and older to be 7.8% using the Diagnostic Interview Schedule (DIS) (43). The one-month and one-year prevalence rates were 2.4% and 3.7%, respectively. Mood disorders assessed were major depression, dysthymia, bipolar I disorder, and bipolar II disorder by DMS-III criteria; their lifetime prevalence rates were 5%, 3%, 0.8%, and 0.5%, respectively.

From 1990 through 1992, the first nationally representative survey of mental disorders, the National Comorbidity Survey (NCS), was conducted in the United States using a method similar to the ECA (45). The Composite International Diagnostic Interview (CEDI) was used to assess mental disorders by DSM-III-R criteria in 8098 respondents aged 15 to 54 years. The NCS estimated that more people had a mood disorder than the ECA did, with 17.1% of respondents meeting lifetime DSM-III-R criteria for a major depressive episode, 14.9% for a nonbipolar major depressive disorder, 1.6% for bipolar I disorder, and 19.3% for any mood disorder. The one-year prevalence rates of major depressive episodes and any mood disorder were 10.3% and 11.3%, respectively. The National Comorbidity Survey replication study (NCS-R) was conducted in 2001–2002 with a methodology similar to the first NCS, except DSM-IV criteria were used (49). The NCS-R found a lifetime prevalence of major depressive disorder of 16.2% in persons aged 18 years and older in the United States, with a one-year prevalence of 6.6%. (Rates for other mood disorders were not reported at the time this chapter went to press.) Similar to the ECA study, both the NCS and NCS-R found mood disorders to be chronic conditions associated with elevated rates of other Axis I disorders (especially anxiety and substance use disorders) and functional impairment. However, none of these major studies reported anthropometric measures.

Jonas et al. (48) used data from the NHANES-III to estimate the lifetime prevalences of major depressive episodes, dysthymia, and bipolar disorder in the United States general population from 1988 through 1994. During this period, 7667 (89.1%) of 8602 surveyed men and women 17 to 39 years of age completed DIS interviews. The following lifetime prevalence estimates were obtained: 8.6% for major depressive episodes; 7.7% for major depressive episodes "with severity"; 6.2% for dysthymia, 3.4% for severe major depressive episodes with dysthymia; 1.6% for bipolar I and II disorders combined; and 11.5% for any mood disorder. Although the same (DSM-III) diagnostic criteria were used, all estimates except those for major depressive episodes and severe major depressive episodes were higher than comparable ECA estimates. [As discussed later, this study also assessed anthropometric measures, but only reported the overlap of obesity and major depressive episodes (16)].

Epidemiologic studies suggest that major depression is rare among children, but common among adolescents, with up to a 25% lifetime prevalence by the end of adolescence (47,78). In the NCS, DSM-III-R major depression among adolescents aged 15 to 18 years was estimated to be 14%, with an additional 11% estimated to have minor depression (79). Moreover, pediatric bipolar disorder is probably more common than once realized, occurring with a 1% to 2% lifetime prevalence in older adolescents as currently defined by DSM criteria (47,80,81). Although the illness may present as bipolar I disorder in children and adolescents, one of the few epidemiologic studies conducted in this age group showed that it is much more likely to present as bipolar II disorder and cyclothymia, so-called soft spectrum forms of the illness (81). Moreover, in this study, Lewinsohn et al. (78–81) found an additional 5.0% of individuals had experienced subthreshold bipolar disorder—that is, a distinct period of elevated, expansive, or irritable mood plus one other core manic symptom without ever having met full criteria for a DSM-III-R bipolar disorder. Like adolescents with syndromal depressive and bipolar disorders, those with subthreshold bipolar disorder had high rates of other comorbid Axis I disorders, impaired functioning, and suicide attempts (80).

Of importance is that only one of the major American epidemiologic studies described above has reported information on hypomania, bipolar II disorder, and subthreshold manic/hypomanic symptoms in adults at this time. A reanalysis of the first 18,252 respondents in the ECA study showed that 5.1% of the subjects had lifetime subsyndromal manic/hypomanic symptoms—a number very similar to that found in Lewinsohn et al.'s (81) study in adolescents —thereby increasing the prevalence of the full spectrum of bipolar disorders in the ECA to 6.4% (82). These data, along with findings from other groups, have shown that hypomania, bipolar II disorder, and subthreshold forms of bipolarity (e.g., hypomania of two days duration) are substantially more common than mania and bipolar I disorder in adults as well as adolescents (83,84). In both age groups, these soft and subthreshold presentations of bipolar disorder are frequently misdiagnosed as major depressive disorder and other unipolar depressive disorders (80,85). Importantly, substantial epidemiologic, phenomenologic, course of illness, family history, genetic, and treatment response evidence has shown that recurrent major depression may be related to bipolar disorder, and that both conditions may belong to the larger diagnostic category of manic-depressive illness (72,84,86). Thus, it should be realized that the diagnostic and etiologic boundaries between recurrent major depression and bipolar disorder are not yet completely understood, and that the relationship between unipolarity and bipolarity may have important implications when interpreting research on the relationship between obesity and mood disorders. This is especially important when assessing community studies of depression in obesity, because the vast majority of these studies assessed depressive symptoms or episodes but not mood disorders.

Another important issue is that many major psychiatric epidemiology studies, including the ECA, NCS, and NCS-R, have found the cumulative lifetime prevalence of mood disorders to be significantly greater in persons born in earlier than later generations (42–45,48,49). Although age-related differential recall, differential willingness to disclose, differential mortality (persons with mood disorders are less likely to survive to older age), or other methodologic factors could account for this finding, a true increase in the prevalence of mood disorders in recent cohorts (a birth cohort effect) has not been disproven. Indeed, this trend has also been reported in epidemiologic studies from nine other countries and in the relatives of probands with depressive and bipolar disorders (44,87,88).

Taken together, these data suggest that, like obesity, mood disorders are common, probably under reported, and possibly increasing in prevalence. Yet another potential similarity between these conditions is their gender distribution. In the NHANES III, more women than men were in obesity classes two and three, whereas more men than women were overweight (BMI ≥ 25) (39). There was no difference in gender distribution in the prevalence of obesity in children and adolescents ages 6 to 19. Most psychiatric epidemiologic studies, including the ECA, NCS, and NCS-R, have shown that major depressive disorder is about two to three times more prevalent in females than in males, whereas bipolar disorder is equally common in the two genders (89). Of interest, this gender difference for depression emerges in early adolescence (ages 11 to 15 years) and persists through at least the mid-50s.

Despite the high prevalence of both obesity and mood disorders in the general population, the fact that the prevalence of obesity is increasing, the fact that a birth cohort effect has been consistently demonstrated for depressive and bipolar disorders, and the potentially similar gender distribution between the more severe forms of obesity and major depressive disorder, it is notable that no major epidemiologic study has yet assessed the co-occurrence of all classes of obesity and the full range of mood disorders using optimal techniques. The relationship between these two widely prevalent conditions at this time must therefore be gleaned from available studies of mood disorders in obesity and conversely, from studies of obesity in mood disorders. These studies, however, are limited by their methodologies—the former regarding the diagnosis of mood disorders, because the full range of mood disorders (especially the full spectrum of bipolar disorders and the milder forms of depressive disorders) was rarely determined, and the latter regarding the diagnosis of obesity and related conditions, because weight and other anthropometric variables were rarely measured. [Of note, although there have been many studies of depressive symptoms in obesity, we are focusing this chapter on studies of mood disorders and obesity because self-report screening scales significantly underdiagnose cases of major and minor depression (3,90,91). Moreover, they rarely assess manic or hypomanic symptoms.]

CLINICAL STUDIES OF MOOD DISORDERS IN PATIENTS WITH OBESITY

To date, at least 15 studies have evaluated syndromal mood disorders using operational diagnostic criteria in obese persons seeking weight loss treatment (Table 1) (50,54,92–104). The rates of mood disorders in these studies ranged from a low of 8% to a high of 60%, with a weighted average of 29%. Nine of these studies also used clinician-administered structured diagnostic interviews to assess mood disorders; 217 (33%) of 666 patients met criteria for a mood disorder in these studies, compared with 121 (25%) of 491 patients in the six studies that did not use such interviews (Table 1).

Only two of these studies used control groups as well as operationalized diagnostic criteria and clinician-administered structured interviews in

Table 1 Rates of Mood Disorders Defined by Diagnostic Criteria in Obese Patients

Study	Clinical population	Definition of obesity	Psychiatric diagnostic criteria	Findings
Wise & Fernandez, 1979 (92)	24 persons seeking ileal bypass	Massive: mean weight = 342 lb; averaged 232% of expected weight	Feighner et al.	2 (8%) had "secondary" affective disorder
Halmi et al., 1980 (93)	80 persons who had gastric bypass operations	Severe: mean weight ≥ 236% of ideal body weight at surgery	DSM-III	23 (29%) had a lifetime depressive disorder
Hopkinson & Bland, 1982 (94)	73 females seeking intestinal bypass surgery	Gross: ≥ 100 lb above or double ideal body weight	Feighner et al.	14 (28%) had a lifetime primary depressive disorder
Gertler & Ramsey-Stewart, 1986 (95)	153 persons seeking bariatric surgery	Morbid: ≥ 80% above ideal body weight	DSM-III	35 (23%) had a lifetime affective disorder
Hudson et al., 1988 (96)	70 obese females recruited for an obesity treatment study	Mild (20%) Moderate (67%) Severe (13%)	DSM-III[a]	42 (60%) had a lifetime major affective disorder
Marcus et al., 1990 (97)	50 subjects recruited for an obesity treatment study (fluoxetine)	BMI ≥ 30	DSM-III[a]	10 (20%) had a lifetime affective disorder; seven had major depression and three had dysthymia

(Continued)

Table 1 Rates of Mood Disorders Defined by Diagnostic Criteria in Obese Patients (*Continued*)

Study	Clinical population	Definition of obesity	Psychiatric diagnostic criteria	Findings
Black et al., 1992 (50)	88 persons seeking vertical banded gastroplasty	Morbid: 100% or 100lb over ideal body weight	DSM-III[a]	27 (31%) had a lifetime affective disorder; 17 (19%) had major depression, 7 (8%) had dysthymia, 3 (3%) had mania, and 1 (1%) had atypical bipolar disorder
Goldsmith et al., 1992 (98)	54 subjects presenting for an obesity treatment study (fluoxetine and CBT)	BMI ≥ 30; mean BMI = 40	DSM-III-R[a]	26 (48%) had a lifetime mood disorder; 3 (6%) had bipolar disorder
Specker et al., 1994 (99)	100 women presenting for weight loss treatment	Mean BMI = 36 (range 26–44)	DSM-IV[a]	38 (38%) had a lifetime mood disorder; 35 (35%) had lifetime major depression
Powers et al., 1997 (100)	131 persons presenting for gastric restriction surgery	MeanBMI=53	DSM-IV	37 (28%) had a lifetime mood disorder
Britz et al., 2000 (54)	47 adolescents and young adults receiving inpatient treatment	Extreme; mean BMI = 42	DSM-IV[a]	20 (43%) had a lifetime mood disorder; 14 (30%) had a depressive disorder and 5 (11%) had a bipolar disorder
Hsu et al., 2002[b] (101)	37 persons awaiting gastric bypass surgery	Extreme; mean BMI = 50	DSM-IV[a]	20 (56%) had lifetime major depression

Fontenelle et al., 2003[c] (102)	65 outpatients recruited for a weight loss program	BMI ≥ 30	DSM-IV[a]	15 (23%) had a lifetime mood disorder
Erermis S, et al., 2004 (103)	30 adolescents seeking weight loss treatment		DSM-IV	10 (33%) had major depressive disorder
Vila et al., 2004 (104)	155 consecutive pediatric patients presenting for weight loss treatment	BMI mean Z score = +6.1	DSM-IV[a]	19 (12%) had a current affective disorder; 9 (6%) had major depression and 10 (6%) had dysthymic disorder
Total[d]	1157			338 (29%) had a mood disorder

[a]Mood disorders evaluated with a clinician-administered structured diagnostic interview.

[b]Only 15% of eligible subjects were accepted into the study.

[c]Patients on psychotropics, those with current psychosis, substance abuse, or severe personality disorder, and those with a past history of anorexia or bulimia nervosa were excluded.

[d]In studies that used structured clinical interviews to assess syndromal mood disorders, 41% of patients (183 of 446) had lifetime mood disorders, compared with 24% of patients (111 of 461) in studies that did not use structured clinical interview.

Abbreviations: BMI, body mass index (mg/kg^2); CBT, cognitive behavior therapy.

Source: From Ref. 21.

assessing mood disorders in their subjects (50,54). Both studies found significantly elevated rates of mood disorders in severely obese patients compared with normal weight controls. In the first study, Black et al. (50) found significantly higher lifetime rates of major depression (19% vs. 5%) and any mood disorder (31% vs. 9%) by DSM-III criteria in 88 consecutive "morbidly" obese patients seeking bariatric surgery compared with 76 normal weight controls (50). Four (4.5%) of the obese patients had lifetime mania or atypical bipolar disorder compared with none of the control subjects. In the second study, Britz et al. (54) found that 20 (43%) of 47 adolescents and young adults receiving inpatient treatment for extreme obesity (mean BMI = 42.4) met DSM-IV criteria for a lifetime mood disorder, compared with eight (17%) of 47 obese population controls (mean BMI = 29.8) and 247 (15%) of 1608 general population controls (54). Among the obese patients, 14 (30%) had a depressive disorder (11 with major depression and three with dysthymia) and five (11%) had a bipolar disorder (one with bipolar I and four with bipolar II). The authors noted that bipolar II disorder was especially elevated in patients (8.5%) as compared to controls (0.5%). The rates of mood disorder between the obese patients and the obese population controls and, as discussed below, the obese controls and the general population controls did not differ. Of note, because the mean BMI of the obese patient group was significantly higher than that of the obese population controls, it is unknown if the higher rate of mood disorders in the patient group was related to their severe obesity or their treatment-seeking behavior.

COMMUNITY STUDIES OF MOOD DISORDERS IN OBESITY

To date, six studies have used operational diagnostic criteria to assess mood episodes or disorders in community samples with obese or overweight persons (7–10,13,16,54,105). Only one of these studies assessed the full range of lifetime DSM-IV mood disorders (54); the others assessed current, past-year, or lifetime major depressive episodes. An additional study evaluated major depressive episodes in persons with the metabolic syndrome (106). Each study is described in detail below.

In the largest study, Carpenter et al. (7) used the Alcohol Use Disorders And Associated Disabilities Interview Schedule (AUDADIS) to assess the relationships among weight, obesity, suicide ideation and attempts, and past-year DSM-IV major depressive episodes in 40,086 persons aged 18 years and older. The AUDADIS was administered by trained lay interviewers and weight and height were assessed by self-report. Bivariate analysis of weight data showed that BMI was significantly associated with past-year major depression via a U-shaped relationship, such that relatively high- and low-BMI values were associated with an increased probability of past-year depression.

Unadjusted analyses of weight status showed that, compared with average-weight respondents (BMI 20.78 to 29.99), obese respondents (BMI ≥ 30) had increased odds of suicide ideation (but not of major depression or suicide attempts), whereas underweight respondents (BMI < 20.77) had increased odds of past-year depression and suicide ideation. Adjusted analyses, however, showed that the relationship between weight and depression was affected by gender. Among women, increased BMI was associated with both depression and suicide ideation. Among men, decreased BMI was associated with depression, suicide attempts, and suicide ideation. Similarly, relative to average weight, obesity was associated with increased odds of past-year depression among women (OR = 1.37; 95% CI = 1.09, 1.73) but decreased odds of past-year depression among men (OR = 0.63; 95% CI = 0.60, 0.67). Furthermore, relative to average weight, underweight was associated with increased odds of suicide ideation and suicide attempts in men but not women. A limitation of the study was that 45% ($n = 12,737$) of the participants in the average-weight group would be categorized as overweight according to NIH Guidelines (76).

In the second largest study, conducted from 1988 to 1994, Onyike et al. (16) analyzed data from 8410 randomly chosen persons from the NHANES III survey aged 15 to 39 years who had been evaluated with the mood disorder section of the DIS, and who had their height and weight measured. Respondents were assigned diagnoses of past-month DSM-III major depression (the primary measure), past-year depression, and lifetime depression. They were also grouped into four or six BMI categories. The four-category division was underweight (BMI < 18.5), normal weight (BMI 18.5 to 24.9), overweight (BM 25.0 to 29.9), and obese (BM ≥ 30). In the six-category division, the obese category was subdivided into obesity class 1 (BMI 30.0 to 34.9), obesity class 2 (BMI 35.0 to 39.9), and obesity class 3 (BMI ≥ 40). The sample was 53.9% normal weight, 3.7% underweight, 26.1% overweight, and 16.3% obese.

The prevalence of past-month depression was higher in obese subjects (5.1%) than in normal-weight subjects (2.8%). Moreover, there was heterogeneity in the prevalence rates of depression in obese subjects, with the highest rates occurring in class 3 obesity (12.5%). Prevalence rates for depression in the underweight (3.2%) and overweight (2.4%) groups were similar to those in the normal-weight group (2.8%). Among women, depression rates increased with increasing levels of obesity. Among men, depression rates were lowest in class 2 obesity (0.8%) and highest in class 3 obesity (11.5%).

Unadjusted odds ratios showed that obesity (BMI ≥ 30) was associated with past-month major depression in women (OR = 1.82, 95% CI: 1.01, 3.3) but not in men (OR = 1.73, 95% CI = 0.56, 5.37), whereas class 3 obesity was associated with past-month major depression in women and men combined (OR = 4.98, 95% CI: 2.07, 11.99). The latter association remained strong after controlling for age, education, marital status, physician's health rating, dieting, psychiatric medication use, smoking, and drug use. Class 3 obesity was also associated with past-month major depression in women alone (OR = 3.78, 95% CI: 1.64, 8.68) and men alone (OR = 7.68, 95% CI: 1.03, 57.26), and with lifetime depression in women (OR = 2.15, 95% CI = 1.17, 3.92), though these odds ratios were not significant. In addition, there was a trend in women for higher odds ratios with increasing levels of obesity for past-month, past-year, and lifetime depression.

Adjusted odds ratios showed that class 3 obesity was significantly associated with depression (OR = 4.63, 95% CI: 2.06,10.42). Similar results were obtained for women but there were too few men with class 3 obesity and depression for multiple comparisons. Female gender, current smoking, and use of psychiatric medications were also associated with depression in these analyses. Post hoc analyses showed no evidence of interaction between gender or age and obesity in the association with depression.

In another study, Roberts et al. (8–10) used the Prime-MD, a self-report instrument, to evaluate 1886 survey respondents, aged 50 years and older, from Alameda County, Texas, in 1994 and 1999, to determine whether subjects met current (past two week) DSM-IV criteria for a major depressive episode. Height and weight were also determined by self-report. Obesity (BMI > 30) was associated with current major depressive episodes in both 1994 and 1999. Specifically, the prevalence ratio for depression among the obese was 1.83, with a 95% CI = 1.33,2.53. In addition, obesity in 1994 was associated with increased risk of depression in 1999, even after controlling for depression at baseline (OR = 2.01, 95% CI = 1.25,3.25). No gender differences were found in the relationship between obesity and depression.

To identify age-related developmental trajectories of obesity and their psychiatric correlates, Mustillo et al. (13) evaluated 991 rural white children-ages 9 to 16 years from the Great Smoky Mountains area annually over an eight-year period for weight, height, and psychiatric disorders. The Child and Adolescent Psychiatric Assessment was used to assess DSM-IV depressive disorders, as well as conduct disorder, oppositional defiant disorder, anxiety disorders, bulimia, substance abuse, and attention-deficit/hyperactivity disorder. Bipolar disorder was not assessed. Height and weight were measured. The authors identified four developmental trajectories of obesity: no obesity (72.8%), chronic obesity (14.6%), childhood obesity (5.1%), and adolescent obesity (7.5%). Bivariate analyses showed that those with childhood obesity and chronic obesity were significantly more likely than those without any history of obesity to have depression and oppositional defiant disorder. Depression was more common in chronically obese boys (OR: 37; 95% CI: 1.3 to 10.2), but not girls, and oppositional disorder was more common in chronically obese boys and girls (OR: 2.5; 95% CI: 1.36 to 4.61).

In a study of the correlates of binge eating behavior, Bulik et al. (105) reported that of 169 obese (self-reported BMI ≥ 30) women from a community sample of 2163 female twins, 34% met lifetime criteria for DSM-III-R major depression as assessed with a modified version of the Structured Clinical Interview for DSM-II1-R. Although this rate is higher than those reported in women in the ECA and NCS studies (7% and 21%, respectively), the rate of major depression for the entire sample was not provided.

In the only negative study, which we described earlier, Britz et al. (54) compared rates of DSM-IV mood (depressive and bipolar) disorders, assessed with the M-CIDI, across a clinical group of 47 extremely obese adolescent and young adult inpatients (mean BMI 42.4), a group of 47 gender-matched, population-based obese controls (mean BMI 29.8), and a population-based control group of the same age range ($n = 1608$; 788 males). Although the rate of mood disorders was significantly higher in the clinical group (42.6%) than in both control groups, there were no differences in the rates of mood disorders between the population-based obese control subjects (17.0%) and the population controls (15.4%). A limitation of this study was the fact that the mean BMI of the population-based obese controls was significantly lower than that of the clinically obese subjects.

In the study of mood disorder in metabolic syndrome, Kinder et al. (106) evaluated 3186 men and 3003 women from the NHANES III survey aged 17 to 39 years for the presence of a lifetime major depressive episode by DSM-III-R criteria with the DIS, and for the presence of the metabolic syndrome as defined by ATP III. Only subjects free of coronary heart disease and diabetes were analyzed. Women with a lifetime major depressive episode were twice as likely to have the metabolic syndrome compared with those with no history of depression. The relationship between depression and metabolic syndrome remained after controlling for age, race, education, smoking, physical inactivity, carbohydrate consumption, and alcohol use. By contrast, men with a lifetime major depressive episode were not significantly more likely to have the metabolic syndrome.

In sum, the most methodologically sound clinical studies of mood disorders in obesity have found a positive relationship between obesity and both major depressive and bipolar disorders in females and males (50,54). Three of the six community studies of mood episodes or disorders in obesity found a positive relationship between obesity and current or past-year major depressive episodes in women, but inconsistent results in men, with a negative relationship in men aged 18 years and older, no relationship in men aged 15 to 39 years, and a positive relationship in men aged 50 years and older (7–10,16). However, in the study with no relationship, further analysis showed an association between class 3 obesity and depressive episodes in men and women combined (16). The other three studies were possibly positive regarding a relationship between obesity and DSM-III-R major depression in women; positive regarding a relationship between chronic obesity and depression in boys; and negative regarding a relationship between the full spectrum of DSM-IV mood disorders and obesity in adolescents and young adults (13,54,105). The two prospective studies found positive relationships between obesity and depression—one in adults 50 years and older and the other in adolescent males (8–10,13). The one community study of mood disorder in persons with metabolic syndrome found a positive relationship with major depressive episodes in women but not in men (106).

The disparate results of these studies are likely due to methodological differences among the studies and to differential effects of various factors, and interactions among these factors, on the relationship between obesity and mood disorders (21). For example, both the definition of obesity and gender may affect the relationship between obesity and major depressive disorder. Thus, Onyike et al. (16) found that obesity defined as a BMI $\geq$ 30 was associated with past-month depression in women but not in men, whereas class 3 obesity (BMI > 40) was associated with past-month depression in women and men. Moreover, gender's effect on the relationship between obesity and mood disorders may be affected by age. Thus, a relationship between obesity and depression in males but not females was found by Mustillo et al. (13), who evaluated children 9 to 16 years of age, whereas the opposite was found by Carpenter et al. (7) and Onyike et al. (16), who assessed subjects aged 18 years and older and aged 15 to 39 years, respectively. By contrast, in the Roberts et al. (8–10) study, which included subjects aged 50 years and older, no gender effects were found.

STUDIES OF OBESITY IN MOOD DISORDERS

At least 20 studies have evaluated rates of obesity or obesity-related conditions (e.g., overweight, abdominal obesity, or visceral fat deposition) in persons with syndromal mood disorders. Twelve of these studies used clinical samples, eight used community samples, and five used prospective designs (4,8–11,17,27,33,107–116,119–122). These studies are described in detail below.

CLINICAL STUDIES OF OBESITY IN MOOD DISORDERS

One prospective and 11 cross-sectional studies evaluated obesity (or a related condition) in patients with mood disorders.

In the prospective study, Pine et al. (11) followed two age- and sex-matched groups of children 6 to 17 years old with major depression ($N = 90$) or no psychiatric disorder ($N = 87$) for 10 to 15 years with standardized psychiatric evaluations. Childhood major depression was significantly positively associated with adulthood BMI, and this association persisted after controlling for age, gender, substance use, social class, pregnancy, and medication exposure. Specifically, children with major depression had a higher mean BMI as adults (26.1) than control children (24.2). In addition, a bivariate logistic analysis showed that childhood depression predicted a two-fold increased risk for adult overweight status. Duration of depression between childhood and adulthood was associated with adult BMI, but this was not found for gender, change in eating patterns occurring with depressive episodes, diet, or medication use. Also, BMI did not differ between subjects who were or were not currently depressed at the time of the adult assessment.

The 11 cross-sectional studies are difficult to compare due to their different methodologies, including the use of different patient populations and different definitions of obesity and of mood disorders. Thus, nine studies reported rates of overweight or obesity in various mood disorder patients, whereas two explored visceral fat deposition in normal weight women with major depressive disorder (33,107–116). Rates of obesity in the first nine studies ranged from a low of 5.7% in a group of male and female patients with major depressive disorder participating in a phase IV antidepressant trial to a high of 67% in a group of mixed mood disorder patients, also of both genders, from Germany (Table 2) (33,107). Four of these studies, described below, used comparison groups.

In 1979, Muller-Oerlinghausen et al. (107) reported that 49 stable mood disorder patients receiving lithium maintenance therapy (29 with bipolar disorder) had a significantly higher rate of "severe obesity" (BMI > 30; 12%) than the expected general population rate (5.7%). In 2000, Elmslie et al. (110) compared the prevalence of overweight, obesity, and abdominal obesity in 89 euthymic outpatients with bipolar I disorder (87% of whom were receiving pharmacologic maintenance treatment) to that of 445 age- and sex-matched community control subjects in New Zealand. Female patients had significantly higher prevalence rates of overweight (44% vs. 25%), obesity (20% vs. 13%), and abdominal obesity (59% vs. 17%) than female control subjects. Male patients had significantly higher rates of obesity (19% vs. 10%) and abdominal obesity (58% vs. 35%), but the rates of overweight between male patients (29%) and control subjects (43%) were not significantly different. Similarly, in 2002, McElroy et al. (111) assessed the prevalence of overweight and obesity in 644 outpatients with bipolar disorder, types I and II, in both the United States and Europe; 57% of the total group was overweight or obese, with 31% overweight (BMI 25 to 29.9), 21% obese (BMI 30 to 39.9), and 5% extremely obese (BMI ≥ 40). Compared with rates from the NHANES III, female bipolar patients from the United States had higher rates of obesity and extreme obesity, but lower rates of overweight, than reference women. Male bipolar patients from the United States had higher rates of overweight and obesity, but not extreme obesity, than reference men.

Table 2 Clinical Studies of Obesity (and Related Weight Disorders) in Patients with Mood Disorders

Study	Patients	Definition of weight categories	Findings
Muller-Oerliaghausen et al., 1979 (107)	49 patients with bipolar disorder (N=26), major depression (N=14), SAD (N=8), and unclassified (N=1)	Obesity for females: BMI 24–30; Obesity for males = BMI 25–30; Severe obesity = BMI ≥ 30	33 (67%) were obese (43%) or severely obese (24%)
Berken et al., 1984 (108)	40 outpatients with major depression	Not provided	25% were obese prior to TCA therapy
Shiori et al, 1993 (109)	106 Japanese inpatients with DSM-III major depression	Not provided	Patients' body weight distribution on admission had significantly more individuals in the underweight groups compared with a standard distribution from the general population. Also, more patients with melancholia were in the underweight groups than expected. Rates of patients in body weight categories were not provided
Elmslie et al, 2000 (110)	89 euthymic outpatients with bipolar I disorder from New Zealand; 445 community controls	Overweight = BMI 25–29.9; Obesity = BMI ≥ 30; Abdominal obesity = WHR > 0.8 for females and > 0.9 for males	Female patients had significantly higher prevalence rates of overweight (44% vs. 25%), obesity (20% vs. 13%), and abdominal obesity (58% vs. 35%). Male patients had significantly higher rates of obesity (19% vs. 10%) and abdominal obesity (58% vs. 35%)

Study	Sample	BMI definitions	Results
McElroy et al., 2002 (111)	644 outpatients from United States and Europe with DSM-IV bipolar I and H disorders	Overweight = BMI 25–29.9; Obesity = BMI 30–39.9; Extreme obesity = BMI $\geq$ 40	57% were overweight or obese, with 31% overweight, 21% obese, and 5% extremely obese
Fagiolini et al., 2002 (112)	50 outpatients with DSM-IV bipolar I disorder	Overweight = BMI 25–29.9; Obesity = BMI $\geq$ 30	34 (68%) were overweight (36%) or obese (32%)
Fagiolini et al., 2003 (113)	175 outpatients with DSM-IV bipolar I disorder	Obesity = BMI $\geq$ 30	62 (35%) were obese
Berlin & Lavergne, 2003 (33)	1694 clinical trial subjects with DSM-IV major depressive disorder	Underweight = BMI $\leq$ 18.5%; Overweight = BMI 25 – 29.9; Obesity = BMI $\geq$ 30	144 (8.5%) were underweight. 456 (26.9%) were overweight (21.2%) or obese (5.7%)
Papkostas et al., 2004 (114)	369 outpatients with major depression enrolled in an eight-week trial of fluoxetine	Overweight = BMI 25 – 29.9; Obesity = BMI $\geq$ 30	190 (51.4%) were overweight (31.4%) or obese (20.0%); 47.2% of women and 56.5% of men were overweight whereas 25.1% of women and 14.1% of men were obese

Abbreviations: BMI, body mass index; SAD, schizoaffective disorder; TCA, tricyclic antidepressant.
Source: From Ref. 21.

By contrast, in 1993 in Japan, Shiori et al. (109) compared the frequency distribution of body weight of 106 patients hospitalized for DSM-III major depression with that of a standard group, and found that the patients' body weight distribution showed significantly more patients than expected in the underweight groups. This was particularly true for women and for patients with melancholia.

Taken together, these four studies suggest that bipolar patients are more likely to have overweight or obesity whereas those with melancholic unipolar depression are more likely to be underweight. Indeed, the only two cross-sectional studies reporting rates of underweight as well as obesity had similar findings. In one, Berlin and Lavergne found that among 1694 subjects with DSM-IV major depression participating in a phase IV antidepressant trial, more subjects were underweight (BMI < 18.5; 8.5%) than were obese (BMI > 30; 5.7%) (33). By contrast, Fagiolini et al. (112) reported that among 50 patients with bipolar I disorder entering a lithium-based maintenance trial, more patients were obese (BMI ≥ 30; 32%) than underweight (BMI < 18.5; 2%).

In the first study of visceral fat deposition, Thakore et al. (115) compared the body fat distribution [measured by abdominal computed tomography (CT)] of seven medication-free women (mean age 36.6 years; mean BMI 24.4) with DSM-III-R major depression, melancholic subtype, with that of seven healthy control women (mean age 32.7 years; mean BMI 23.6). None of the women had histories of obesity. Although patients and controls did not differ regarding weight, BMI, WHR, and total body fat, patients had significantly greater intra-abdominal fat stores than controls. Patients also had significantly higher baseline cortisol levels than controls, and their intra-abdominal fat stores correlated with both their WHRs and cortisol levels. In the second study, Weber-Hamann et al. (116) compared abdominal CT-determined intra-abdominal fat stores in 22 postmenopausal women with DSM-IV major depression (mean age 65.1; mean BMI 24.5) and 23 healthy control women (mean age 64.0; mean BMI 24.3) (116). Visceral fat stores did not differ between the depressed patients as a group and the healthy controls, or between the hypercortisolemic depressed patients and the controls. However, hypercortisolemic depressed patients had significantly more visceral fat than normocortisolemic depressed patients.

Several of the cross-sectional studies explored correlates of overweight and obesity in mood disorder patients. In a group of 369 patients with major depressive disorder receiving an eight-week trial of fluoxetine 20 mg/day, Papakostas et al. (114) found that obese patients did not differ from nonobese patients regarding severity of depression, anxiety, somatic complaints, hopelessness, or hostility. However, obese patients had worse somatic well-being scores. Also, greater relative body weight, but not obesity, predicted nonresponse to fluoxetine.

Factors associated with obesity in bipolar disorder have included treatment with antipsychotics, greater ingestion of carbohydrates, low levels of exercise, comorbid binge eating disorder, hypertension, type 2 diabetes, arthritis, and less coffee consumption, as well as variables suggestive of more severe bipolar illness (111,113,117). In a sample of 175 consecutive bipolar I patients receiving acute and long-term lithium-based treatment, Fagolini et al. (113) reported that, compared with nonobese patients, obese patients (35% of the group) had more previous depressive and manic episodes, higher baseline HAM-D scores, and required more time in acute treatment to achieve remission. During maintenance treatment, significantly more obese patients experienced a recurrence ($N = 25$, 54%) as compared to those who were not obese ($N = 28,35\%$). Also, the time to recurrence was significantly shorter for patients who were obese at baseline. When recurrence type was examined, the percentage of patients experiencing depressive recurrences was significantly greater for obese patients ($N = 15$, 33%) than for nonobese patients ($N = 11,14\%$). In a subsequent study on this group of patients, Fagiolini et al. (118) reported that higher BMI was significantly associated with more severe bipolar illness and a suicide attempt. Although preliminary and in need of replication, these observations suggest that increasing BMI, overweight, or obesity may be associated with poorer outcome and less favorable treatment response in patients with mood disorders.

COMMUNITY STUDIES OF OBESITY IN MOOD DISORDERS

To date, eight studies have evaluated body weight in community samples of persons with mood disorders. Detailed below, four studies used cross-sectional designs and four employed prospective designs (4,8–10,17,27,119–122).

In the first cross-sectional study, Kendler et al. (27) assessed depressive symptoms in a community-based registry of 1029 female twin pairs, and concluded that major depression consisted of at least three etiologically heterogeneous syndromes: mild typical depression, atypical depression, and severe typical depression. They found that twins with atypical depression were significantly more likely to be obese (BMI > 28.6; 28.9%) than those with mild typical depression (6.0%) or those with severe typical depression (3.1%). However, the rate of obesity in the twins as a group was not reported. Also, neither mania nor hypomania were evaluated.

In a study exploring the relationships between depression and the expression of inflammatory risk markers for coronary heart disease, Miller et al. (119) recruited 50 persons from the community with a major ($N = 32$) or minor ($N = 18$) depressive episode by DSM-IV criteria (established with the Depression Interview and Structured Hamilton Instrument) and 50 control subjects matched on demographic factors but free of lifetime psychiatric disorders. All subjects were in excellent general medical health, defined as having no acute infectious disease, chronic illness, or prescribed medical regimen. The depressed subjects showed a significantly greater mean BMI (30.5) than controls (25.9; $p < 0.003$), along with significantly higher levels of C-reactive protein and interleukin-6 (see Comorbidity section).

In the third cross-sectional study, Lamertz et al. (121) evaluated 3021 German adolescents and young adults ages 14 to 24 years for DSM-IV diagnoses with a modified version of the CIDI, and calculated BMI percentages for age and gender. Logistic regression analyses and MANCO-VAs showed no significant associations between mood disorders (or anxiety, substance use, or somataform disorders) and obesity or BMI. There were also no significant associations between any mental disorders and underweight. Of note, these findings may have been affected by the exclusion of subjects with eating disorders, who have elevated rates of mood and other mental disorders as well as weight disturbances.

In the fourth cross-sectional study, the purpose of which was to examine the relationship between psychiatric illness and physique, Wyatt et al. (120) compared the height, weight, and BMI of 7514 American active duty military personnel hospitalized for bipolar disorder, major depressive disorder, or schizophrenia with that of 85,954 healthy subjects matched for date of service entry. They found no consistent differences in height, weight, or BMI between patients and controls, or between patient groups. However, there was a diagnostic effect on BMI for white males: the mean BMI in patients with bipolar disorder was greater than the mean BMI in controls, which was equal to the mean BMI in patients with schizophrenia, which, in turn, was greater than the mean BMI in patients with major depressive disorder. An important limitation of this study was that service entry criteria (including mental health and weight status) were not described.

In the first prospective study, Pine et al. (4) evaluated 644 adolescents in 1983 (mean age 14 years) and again in 1992 (mean age 22 years) to assess the relationship between major depressive disorder and conduct disorder in youth and obesity in early adulthood. Diagnoses were assessed in 1992 with the DIS for Children (DISC); bipolar disorder was not determined. Univariate analyses showed that a higher BMI in adulthood was associated with increasing depressive and conduct symptoms in adolescence. Also, adulthood obesity was associated with adolescent depression in females, but not males, and with depression in adulthood in both genders. However, the latter association was positive in females and negative in males. Multivariate analyses showed that adulthood obesity was predicted by adolescent conduct disorder and the gender-by-adult depression interaction. Consistent with psychiatric epidemiologic studies showing significant comorbidity between mood disorders and conduct disorder, adolescent depression and conduct disorder scores were significantly positively correlated.

As discussed earlier, Roberts et al. (8–10) evaluated 1886 survey respondents who were aged 50 years or older and primarily examined depression in subjects with obesity. However, they also reported that the prevalence ratio for obesity among those with a current major depressive episode was increased at 1.65 (with a 95% CI = 1.28, 2.13), and concluded that there was a bidirectional association between obesity and depression (10). Moreover they reported that depression in 1994 predicted obesity in 1999 (OR = 1.92; 95% CI = 1.31,2.80), but not after controlling for obesity in 1994 (OR = 1.32; 95% CI = 0.65, 2.70). No other data regarding obesity in persons with depression were provided.

Richardson et al. (17) used data from a longitudinal study of a birth cohort of children ($N = 1037$) born between April 1, 1972 and March 31, 1973 in Dunedin, New Zealand to assess relationships between major depression in adolescence and the risk for obesity at age 26 years. Collected data included regular diagnostic mental health interviews and height and weight measurements obtained throughout childhood and adolescence. Major depression occurred in 7% of the cohort during early adolescence (11, 13, and 15 years of age) and 27% during late adolescence (18 and 21 years of age). Obesity occurred in 12% of the cohort at age 26 years. After adjusting for individuals' baseline BMI, depressed late adolescent girls were at a greater than two-fold increased risk for obesity in adulthood compared with their nondepressed female peers (relative risk 2.32, 95% CI: 1.29, 3.83). In addition, a dose–response relationship between the number of depressive episodes during adolescence and the risk for adult obesity was observed in late adolescent girls, but not in boys or early adolescent girls.

In the fourth prospective study (which to date has only been presented in abstract form) Hasler et al. (122) evaluated mood disorders in 591 young adults at ages 18 to 19 years from the general population of Zurich, Switzerland and followed them until age 40 years. Nineteen percent were classified as overweight, which was not defined. Atypical depression was positively associated with overweight in males and females; hypomanic symptoms were associated with overweight in males only. These associations remained significant after controlling for medication, social, and educational variables.

In sum, six of the eight community studies of obesity in mood disorders found positive relationships between the two conditions. Specifically, two of the four cross-sectional studies found relationships between depression, or a subtype of depression, and elevated body weight, and all four prospective studies found a relationship between a mood disorder or a major depressive episode and the development of overweight or obesity. Moreover, the latter relationship was found in two broad age groups: from adolescence to early or mid-adulthood; and from middle age to old age (4,10,17,27,119,122).

Taking the clinical and community studies of obesity in mood disorders together, they suggest that some forms of mood disorders may be

Table 3 Theoretical Relationships Between Mood Disorders and Weight Disorders

Mood disorder	Associated weight disorder
Major depressive disorder	Underweight, abdominal obesity, overweight, obesity
Atypical features	Overweight, obesity
Typical (melancholic) features	Underweight, abdominal obesity
Juvenile onset	Overweight, obesity
Bipolar disorder	Abdominal obesity, overweight, obesity

Source: From Ref. 21.

associated with overweight or obesity, whereas other forms may be associated with underweight (Table 3) (21). Subtypes associated with overweight or obesity might include major depressive disorder with atypical features, major depressive disorder with juvenile onset, and bipolar disorder, especially when depressive features predominate (4,11,17,27,107,110–113). Subtypes associated with underweight may include major depressive disorder with melancholic features (109). Moreover, major depressive disorder with hypercortisolemia, even when associated with normal body weight, may be associated with visceral fat deposition (115,116). Finally, prospective studies suggest onset of mood disorder may precede development of overweight or obesity in some persons, including patients with juvenile-onset major depression and young females in the community with major depression (4,11,11). However, these conclusions are preliminary and need to be verified in epidemiologic and longitudinal studies using validated assessments of both mood disorders and anthropometric measures.

PHENOMENOLOGY

Obesity and mood disorders share several important phenomenologic features, including abnormalities in appetite, eating behavior, and physical activity (21). Thus, numerous clinical and community studies have described increased appetite, overeating, and reduced physical activity in obese subjects (51,123–125). Indeed, modern studies have documented that obese persons of all ages eat more and are less physically active than their lean counterparts, including the subset of obese persons who report that their eating behavior and physical activity are normal or decreased (125,126). Moreover, although exceptions exist (123,127–129), many of the clinical and community studies that assessed depressive symptoms with standardized measures found increased levels of depressive symptoms in the obese groups compared with the normal weight or general medical clinical controls (51–53,55) or with the nonobese community controls [(7,130–133);

see Ref. (21) for review]. In addition, studies have found elevated levels of clinically meaningful behavioral problems in obese children; children with mood disorders, especially those with bipolar disorder, also have elevated rates of behavior problems (19,78–81,134).

For mood disorders, it is well established that depressive and manic syndromes are associated with anorexia, hypophagia, hyperactivity, and weight loss—factors associated with underweight (72,135,136). However, clinical and community studies have shown that a significant portion of persons with depressive syndromes have increased appetite, overeating, reduced physical activity, and weight gain—factors associated with obesity (21). Weissenburger et al. (22), for example, reported that of 109 medication-free outpatients with unipolar ($N = 93$) or bipolar depression ($N = 16$), 30% reported weight loss, 30% reported no weight change, and 40% described weight gain. In a prospective study of 53 outpatients with unipolar depression, Stunkard et al. (25) found that the direction of weight change was concordant for 45 (85%) patients across concurrent episodes: 23 patients lost weight during both episodes, 17 gained weight, and five showed no change. Changes in appetite paralleled those in body weight. More recently, Miller et al. found that both severe underweight and obesity predicted clinically relevant depressive symptoms, defined as a score ≥ 16 on the Center for Epidemiologic Studies Depression Scale (CES-D), among 998 community-dwelling African–Americans (137).

Regarding motor activity, Wolff III et al. (138)used wrist actigraphy to assess 27 affectively ill inpatients and 18 healthy control subjects. The patients showed less motor activity when depressed than when euthymic or manic. Even when euthymic, patients showed less daytime motor activity compared with controls. Volkers et al. (139) similarly compared the daily activity pattern of 67 unmedicated depressed inpatients with 64 control subjects, and found that the patients were significantly less active while awake (though they were more active during sleep). Consistent with these laboratory studies are cross-sectional community studies showing an inverse association between physical activity or exercise and depression scores (140–142).

As we noted in an earlier paper, several subtypes of depression have been delineated, in part, because of their association with increased appetite, overeating, weight gain, and reduced physical activity (21). These include atypical depression, somatic depression, seasonal affective disorder, perimenstrual depression, and possibly bipolar depression. Usually referred to as atypical or reversed neurovegetative features, increasing research has shown that these symptoms are common, distinct, and clinically relevant among patients with depressive syndromes. They have been associated with female preponderance, earlier onset, greater duration, familial aggregation, biological differences, and preferential response to monoamine oxidase inhibitors (MAOIs) over tricyclics (23,24,26–28,30–34,72,143).

We were unable to locate any studies that specifically examined atypical depressive features in obesity. Although very few studies have evaluated the relationship between atypical depressive features and actual body weight in mood disorders, we noted preliminary community data in an earlier paper suggesting that atypical depressive symptoms might be more likely to be associated with overweight than are typical depressive symptoms (21). In two latent-class analyses of depressive symptoms from two different population-based twin registries, Kendler et al. (27) and Sullivan et al. (31) each found that the "atypical" classes, characterized primarily by increased appetite and weight gain, and to a lesser extent psychomotor retardation, had significantly higher self-reported BMIs than the "typical" classes. By contrast, Berlin and Lavergne found no relationship between DSM-IV-defined atypical features and BMI in 1694 patients with major depression participating in a phase IV antidepressant trial (33). However, higher body weight was associated with less appetite reduction and fewer pessimistic thoughts. Limitations of this study were collection of data by 1185 psychiatrists and a number of exclusion criteria, including the presence of depressive disorder for more than one year, nonresponse to several antidepressants, and high suicidal risk.

COURSE OF MOOD SYMPTOMS AND WEIGHT CHANGE

Further supporting a relationship between obesity and mood disorders are at least six community studies that have prospectively shown a relationship between weight change and mood symptoms (21). Hallström and Noppa studied 800 women from the community, 38 to 54 years of age, and found no relationship between obesity and "depth of depression" upon cross-sectional analysis. Six years later, however, women who had gained $\geq 5\,kg$ had significantly higher baseline Ham-D scores than those who had gained $< 5\,kg$ (144). DiPietro et al. (145) assessed the effect of depressive symptoms on weight in 1794 adults, aged 25 to 74 years, from 1971 to 1975 and from 1982 to 1984. Overall, younger adults (< 55 years) gained weight, whereas older adults (≥ 55 years) lost weight. Depression at baseline was associated with additional weight gain in younger men, but a reduction in weight gain in younger women. Among older men and women, depression was associated with additional weight loss.

Barefoot et al. (146) assessed the relationship between depressive symptoms (assessed with the Minnesota Multiphasic Personality Inventory) and weight change in 3560 college students in the mid-1960s and again in the late 1980s, and found a statistically significant interaction between baseline BMI and weight change in depressed subjects. Specifically, depressed participants who were initially lean gained less weight than lean participants who were not depressed. Conversely, depressed participants who were initially heavy gained more weight than heavy participants who were not depressed.

Goodman and Whitaker evaluated 9374 adolescents in grades 7 to 12 in 1995 and one year later to determine whether depressed mood predicted the development and persistence of obesity in adolescence (147). Depressed mood was defined as a score of ≥ 24 for females and ≥ 22 for males on the CES-D, and obesity was defined as a BMI $\geq$ the 95th percentile. Baseline depressed mood independently predicted obesity at one-year follow-up, including among subjects who were not obese at baseline. Baseline depression, however, was not correlated with baseline obesity. Also, baseline obesity did not predict follow-up depression.

Sammel et al. (148) evaluated correlates of weight gain among 336 randomly selected women ages 35 to 47 years who were premenopausal and followed over a four-year period. Over 25% of the cohort gained ≥ 10lb during this time. Five of the 14 (36%) women who were considered menopausal gained weight. Women aged 45 to 47 were 61% less likely to gain ≥ 10lb compared with women aged 35 to 39 years (OR $= 0.39$, 95% CI: 0.18, 0.87). Depressed mood was a major correlate of weight gain (OR $= 1.9$, 95% CI: 1.09, 3,31). Anxiety and quality of life also correlated with weight gain, but sex hormone levels, recalled dietary factors, and self-reported measures of physical activity did not.

In sum, these studies suggest that depressive symptoms may be prospectively associated with long-term weight gain and obesity, as well as long-term weight loss (145–148). These studies also show that the relationship between depressive symptoms and weight gain or obesity may appear prospectively but not cross-sectionally in the same cohort of persons, and that the long-term relationship between depressive symptoms and weight may be affected by age (127,144,145,147,148).

COMORBIDITY

Two areas where obesity and mood disorders have each received relatively extensive study regarding comorbidity are their co-occurrence with eating disorders and with general medical disorders (21).

Comorbidity of Obesity and Mood Disorders with Eating Disorders

Considerable evidence indicates that obesity and mood disorders are each related to binge eating behavior in general, as well as DSM-IV-defined bulimia nervosa and binge eating disorder. Thus, obesity, major depressive disorder, and hypomania have each been shown to co-occur with binge eating behavior, bulimia nervosa, and/or binge eating disorder in community samples (149–163). Clinical and community studies have also found significantly higher rates of mood disorders in obese persons with binge eating behavior or binge eating disorder compared with obese persons without binge eating

(96,99,102,105,150). Thus, one possible relationship between obesity and mood disorders has been hypothesized to be due to their sharing a link with binge eating (21,150). Alternatively, others have hypothesized that binge eating is simply a nonspecific marker for psychopathology, including depressive symptoms, affective instability, and mood disorders (158).

General Medical Comorbidity of Obesity and Mood Disorders

Obesity and mood disorders also share similarities regarding general medical comorbidity (21). Like obesity and abdominal obesity, depressive symptoms and major depressive disorder have been associated with type 2 diabetes, hypertension, and cardiovascular disease in community studies (56,57,62,164–170). Both major depression and bipolar disorder have also been associated with elevated rates of type 2 diabetes in clinical studies (171–173). In addition, like obesity, abdominal obesity, and the metabolic syndrome, both major depressive disorder and bipolar disorder have been associated with increased mortality in community studies, including from coronary heart disease, stroke, and type 2 diabetes (174–176). Indeed, epidemiologic studies have suggested that obesity, abdominal obesity, the metabolic syndrome, depressive symptoms, and major depressive disorder are all independent risk factors for type 2 diabetes, hypertension, coronary heart disease, and stroke (56–62,166–170). Moreover, many of the metabolic and inflammatory abnormalities characteristic of obesity have been found in persons with mood disorders. These include insulin resistance and hyperglycemia, hypertriglyceridemia and decreased HDL cholesterol levels (with mixed evidence regarding LDL and total cholesterol levels), and elevated interleukin 6 and C-reactive protein levels (177–191).

Although the relationship between obesity and mood disorders as risk factors for general medical disorders has only begun to be explored, several studies have found associations between obesity and depression in patients with type 2 diabetes, cardiovascular disease, or cardiovascular risk factors (165,192–195). For example, in 1999, Nichols and Brown evaluated the prevalence of diagnosed depression in 16,180 health maintenance organization members with type 2 diabetes and in 16,180 nondiabetic comparison members matched for age and sex (166). They found depression was significantly more common in individuals with type 2 diabetes (17.9%) than among control subjects (11.2%; $P < 0.001$), and that this association remained strong after controlling for cardiovascular disease and obesity. Moreover, multivariate analysis showed gender differences in the relation among depression, diabetes, cardiovascular disease, and obesity. In men, younger age and cardiovascular disease were the strongest predictors of a depression diagnosis, followed by type 2 diabetes. Though statistically significant, body weight was the least important variable. By contrast, in women, body weight was by far the strongest predictor of depression.

Lesperance et al. (193) evaluated 481 patients two months after hospitalization for acute coronary syndromes for depression status and inflammatory markers. Compared with nondepressed patients, patients meeting DSM-IV criteria for major depression (7.3% of the group) had similarly increased BMIs (mean ± SD = 29.1 ± 4.9 vs. 28.2 ± 44), but significantly more abdominal obesity (60.9% vs. 43.9%), hypertriglyceridemia (74.3% vs. 47.8%), and significantly higher rates of metabolic syndrome (68.6% vs. 47.5%). Depressed patients not taking statins also had markedly higher C-reactive protein levels than did nondepressed patients.

Ladwig et al. (194) evaluated the effect of depressed mood on the association of C-reactive protein and obesity (BMI > 30) in a population-based sample of 3204 men aged 45 to 74 years. Stratification of the men into three levels of depressed mood showed a significant association between increased C-reactive protein in the obese group with the highest level of depression compared with the obese group with the lowest level of depression ($P = 0.013$). By contrast, in the nonobese group, there was no association between depressed mood and C-reactive protein concentrations. The authors concluded that obesity and depressed mood may have a synergistic effect on chronic low level inflammation that is important in the pathogenesis of atherosclerosis.

In a subsequent analysis of their findings that subjects with depressive episodes had higher mean BMIs and higher levels of inflammatory markers than healthy controls, Miller et al. (195) used structural equation modeling to examine the relationships among depression, adiposity, leptin, and inflammation. Their model showed that depressive symptoms were possibly associated with central adiposity, total adiposity, and inflammatory markers; that total adiposity was strongly associated with leptin while central adiposity was modestly associated with leptin; and that adiposity and leptin were positively associated with inflammatory markers. The authors concluded that their analysis was consistent with a "joint pathway model" in which depressive symptoms promoted adiposity which in turn activated the inflammatory response through at least two pathways—by increasing release of inflammatory molecules (from enhanced adipose stores) and by inducing leptin expression. They also concluded that their model did not support a sickness behavior model in which the inflammatory response arising from increased adiposity and leptin promoted the expression of depression.

In short, although obesity and mood disorders may be independent risk factors for many of the same general medical disorders, the effect of their co-occurrence on morbidity and mortality needs further study.

FAMILY HISTORY

Adoption and twin studies have established that heritable factors contribute substantially to the familiality of both obesity and mood disorders

(70,72–74). The familial co-aggregation of obesity and mood disorders, however, has received extremely little empirical attention. In the only controlled family history study of mood disorders in obese probands we were able to locate, Black et al. (196) evaluated 88 morbidly obese gastroplasty patients and a healthy comparison group using the family history method and family history-research diagnostic criteria (FH-RDC). Obese patients were significantly more likely than controls to have first-degree relatives with depression (18% vs. 4%) and bipolar disorder (3% vs. 0). More recently, Dong et al. (197) explored the relationship between depression and obesity in a sample of extremely obese individuals and their siblings and parents. Specifically, they evaluated BMI, history of treatment for depression, and several covariates in 1730 European Americans (mean BMI = 35.6) and 373 African Americans (mean BMI = 36.8) from 482 nuclear families segregating for extreme obesity and normal weight. Greater odds for depression were found for the obese, women, those with chronic medical illness, and the offspring of depressed parents. Multivariate analysis showed that BMI, along with race, marital status, and chronic medical conditions, predicted depression for both genders. Hierarchical analysis showed that BMI significantly increased the risk of depression above that predicted by the combined effects of all other variables. The authors concluded that extreme obesity was associated with an increased risk for depression across gender and racial groups, even after controlling for general medical disease, familial depression, and demographic risk factors.

We located no controlled studies of obesity in the family members of probands with mood disorders, but found two latent-class analyses of depressive symptoms of two separate community-based twin registries (one entirely female–female twin pairs and the other male–male and male–female twin pairs) that also assessed self-reported BMIs (21). Both analyses showed that, compared with co-twins in the nonclinical classes, atypical depressive symptoms (primarily increased appetite and weight gain) in one twin were significantly positively associated with self-reported BMI in the co-twin (27,31). In the all-female registry, mild typical depressive symptoms in one twin were also significantly associated with elevated BMI in the co-twin, but this increase was about half as large as seen in the co-twins with atypical depression (27).

Two other twin studies explored the relation between depressive symptoms and abdominal fat. In the first study, Marniemi et al. (198) evaluated 20 twin pairs discordant for obesity who were divided into two groups. In the first group, the visceral fat area of the obese co-twin was higher, and in the second group, the visceral fat area of the co-twin was lower than the gender-specific median value. Intra-pair differences showing distress in emotional reactions and lack of energy were seen only in the first group, in which a corresponding trend was also observed for depressive symptoms as measured by the BDI and HAM D. Furthermore, daily urinary cortisol and noradrenalin excretion were significantly higher in the obese than the lean co-twins in the pairs with high visceral fat, but not in the pairs with low visceral fat. The authors concluded that when genetic factors are identical, psychosocial stress induces hormonal changes that lead to intra-abdominal fat deposition. In the second twin study, McCaffery et al. (199) explored the extent that depressive symptoms, as evaluated with the CES-D, were associated with metabolic risk factors, including BMI, WHR, blood pressure, and serum triglycerides and glucose, among 87 monozygotic and 86 dizygotic male twin pairs. Depressive symptoms in a nonclinical range were associated with individual components of the metabolic syndrome (WHR, BMI, triglyceride level, glucose level, and mean arterial blood pressure) as well as the common variance among the components. Moreover, twin structural equation modeling indicated that these associations were due to unique environmental, rather than shared genetic, factors. The authors concluded that depressive symptoms, possibly from stress, increased the risk for "a pattern of physiological risk consistent with the metabolic syndrome."

Although extremely preliminary, taken together, some of these findings suggest that obesity and mood disorders, or perhaps certain subtypes of both conditions, might share common heritable pathogenic factors (27,31,196,199). Others suggest that, despite similar or common genetic factors, obesity may contribute to depression and that depressive symptoms may contribute to obesity, supporting the concept of a "bidirectional" relationship between obesity and mood disorders (197–199).

NEUROBIOLOGY

Although a number of central neurobiological systems impact the regulation of both feeding behavior and mood, no studies, to our knowledge, have directly compared the neurobiology of a group of persons with obesity (or an obesity-related disorder) with that of a group of persons with a mood disorder (21,200–203). Several neurobiological systems have received empirical attention in both conditions, but available studies are difficult to compare because of methodological differences. Importantly, many of these studies were limited by the fact that either mood (in the obesity studies) or weight (in the mood disorder studies) were not controlled for. Nonetheless, neurobiological abnormalities found in persons with obesity and those with mood disorders have involved the hypomalamic–pituitary–adrenocortical (HPAC) axis, the sympathetic nervous system, and some central monoamine and peptide neurotransmitter systems (143,201–215).

For example, we noted in an earlier paper that abdominal visceral fat deposition in both obesity and major depression has been hypothesized to be due in part to HPAC dysfunction, but that the profile of HPAC dysregulation found in abdominal obesity might be more similar to that seen in atypical depression (with normal or low morning cortisol levels and increased cortisol responsivity to social stressors) than in melancholic depression (with elevated corticotrophin releasing factor in cerebrospinal fluid and increased corticotrophin and cortisol levels in plasma) (143,202,203,208,209). The HPAC dysfunction of abdominal visceral fat deposition in obesity, in turn, has been attributed to the effects of psychosocial stress or to symptoms of depression and anxiety (204). Epel et al. (206), for example, reported that women with high WHRs secreted significantly more cortisol during a social stress test than did women with low WHRs. In a series of community studies, many, though not all, found significant positive correlations between depressive symptoms and WHR [reviewed in Ref. (21)]. Moreover, depressive symptom measures have been shown to correlate with measures of adiposity and metabolic disturbance. In a study of 90 middle-aged males with the "insulin resistance syndrome," high levels of "vital exhaustion and anger out" correlated with increased WHR as well as an augmented mean insulin response during an oral glucose tolerance test, increased triglyceride levels, and decreased HDL cholesterol levels (216). In a study of depressive symptoms and anthropometric and metabolic parameters in 59 middle-aged men from the community, those with WHRs > 1.0 ($N = 26$) had significantly higher scores on all depression scales used (HAM D, MADRS, and BDI) than those with WHRs < 1.0 ($N = 33$) (217). In addition, there were positive correlations between all depression scale scores and the WHR or the sagital abdominal diameter; BMI, insulin, and glucose levels were also significantly related to HAM D scores. By contrast, similar to some studies of atypical depression, morning cortisol levels were negatively related to BDI and MADRS scores (209).

Regarding other potential shared neurobiological abnormalities, melancholic major depression has been associated with sympathetic nervous system (SNS) activation, displayed by increased plasma norepinephrine metabolites, whereas obesity has been associated with regional heterogeneity in SNS activation involving the renal and skeletal muscle circulations, but not the heart (210,211). Serotonin, norepinephrine, dopamine, and neuropeptide Y are all involved in the regulation of feeding behavior and mood and have been implicated in the pathophysiology of obesity, major depression, and bipolar disorder. Although preliminary and sometimes inconsistent, studies have found abnormalities of these systems in persons with obesity and those with mood disorders (201–203,212–215).

RESPONSE TO TREATMENT: PHARMACOTHERAPY

No study has compared the pharmacotherapy of obesity with that of a mood disorder, and no controlled pharmacotherapy study has been conducted in patients with co-occurring obesity and a mood disorder. However, certain pharmacologic agents have received some study in both conditions

(218–220). Review of these studies suggest similarities and differences in the pharmacologic response of obesity and mood disorders.

Studies of Anti-Obesity Agents in Mood Disorders

Stimulants such as amphetamine and methylphenidate (which are no longer approved for obesity because of their abuse potential) have been the most extensively studied centrally active anti-obesity agents in major depression (221–223). Although many of the trials have limitations, taken together, they suggest stimulants are not generally effective as single agent antidepressants (222). However, limited controlled data suggest stimulants may be helpful in some depressed populations, including obese patients with anxious-depressive symptoms and those with medical illness (224,225). There also have been open-label reports of the successful use of stimulants to augment standard antidepressants in treatment-resistant patients (223,226).

There are no published controlled trials of other centrally acting anti-obesity agents in mood disorders, but preliminary data suggest that some of these agents may have antidepressant properties. The serotonergic agents fenfluramine and dexfenfluramine (which have been removed from the market for safety concerns) have been reported to improve depressed mood in patients with obesity, premenstrual depression, bipolar depression, seasonal affective disorder, and bulimia nervosa (224,227–230). Sibutramine, a serotonin–norepinephrine reuptake inhibitor (SNRI), has displayed antidepressant properties in animal models of depression, and has improved depressed mood (and binge eating and body weight) in patients with binge eating disorder (231,232). The novel anticonvulsants topiramate and zonisamide have each been shown superior to placebo in inducing weight loss in obesity (233–235). Although controlled trials of topiramate in acute bipolar I mania were negative, the drug has been reported to be superior to placebo in a prematurely discontinued trial of adolescent mania, as effective as bupropion in a single-blind controlled trial in bipolar depression, and beneficial for patients with soft spectrum bipolar disorders in numerous open-label trials (236,237). Zonisamide has also been reported to have therapeutic properties in some bipolar patients in several open trials (238,239).

Studies of Thymoleptics in Obesity

Established antidepressants studied in placebo-controlled trials in obesity include several serotonin selective reuptake inhibitors (SSRIs) and bupropion. In particular, the SSRI fluoxetine was shown to have dose-related, modest, short-term (e.g., six week to six month) weight-loss effects in obese patients that were also associated with improvement in obesity-related medical risk factors such as hyperglycemia and hypercholesterolemia. However, in several long-term studies most of the lost weight was regained by one year (218,240,241). Bupropion was shown superior to placebo in inducing weight loss in obesity in three double-blind, controlled trials (242–244). In one study, weight loss was maintained at 48 weeks (243). Although venlafaxine is an SNRI-like sibutramine, there are no published studies of venlafaxine in the treatment of obesity (245). In studies of depression, however, venlafaxine has been associated with anorexia and dose-related weight loss (246,247). Venlafaxine was also reported to induce weight loss in a clinical study of obese women with binge eating disorder, most of whom had a comorbid depressive disorder (248). Finally, although dopamine agonists are not formally considered antidepressants, three controlled trials have found pramipexole superior to placebo in major depression and bipolar depression (249–251). Similarly, bromocriptine was found superior to placebo for weight loss in one small study of obesity (252).

In short, major depression and obesity are similar in their pharmacotherapy response in that each responds acutely to SSRIs, bupropion, SNRIs, and possibly dopamine agonists. In addition, each condition shows maintenance of response to bupropion and SNRIs. However, they differ in their long-term response to SSRIs, with maintenance of response for one year and longer established for major depression but not for obesity. In addition, recent analyses of remission data from major depression comparator trials which show greater remission rates with venlafaxine than SSRIs suggest major depression may also share with obesity a better or more complete response to SNRIs than to SSRIs (21,253,254).

Behavioral Treatments

Extensive research has shown that both obesity and mood disorders may benefit from behavior therapy (especially cognitive-behavior therapy), physical activity (i.e., exercise), and various combinations of treatment approaches. For obesity, the NIH concluded that either behavior therapy or physical activity with a reduced-calorie diet were each modestly effective for weight loss, and that combining these approaches produced greater weight loss than either treatment alone (76). Similarly, cognitive-behavior therapy has been shown to be effective in the acute and maintenance treatment of mood disorders, particularly mild-to-moderate depression and chronic depression, and physical activity may have beneficial acute and long-term effects in outpatient depression, especially when used adjunctively (255–257). Interestingly, patients with depression, like those with obesity, can have poor exercise capacity, and major depression and obesity should each be considered in the differential diagnosis of the latter condition (258). Finally, controlled evidence suggests that combining behavioral and pharmacological treatments may be more effective than single modality treatment for both obesity (259,260) and mood disorders (261–264).

CONCLUSION

Although obesity and mood disorders are both increasingly serious public health problems, their relationship has been understudied and remains obscure. Nonetheless, based on the studies reviewed, several tentative conclusions can be made. First, the most methodologically sound clinical studies indicate that mood disorders, including both depressive and bipolar disorders, are common in persons of all ages seeking treatment for obesity, especially severe obesity. Conversely, obesity and the related conditions overweight and abdominal obesity are common in persons seeking treatment for certain mood disorders, especially childhood-onset major depressive disorder and bipolar disorder. By contrast, underweight may be more characteristic of major depressive disorder, especially when associated with melancholic features. Second, the more rigorous community studies suggest that obesity (BMI ≥ 30) is associated with major depressive episodes in females, severe obesity (BMI ≥ 40) is associated with major depressive episodes in females and males, and the metabolic syndrome (as defined by ATP criteria) is associated with major depressive episodes in women. Conversely, certain mood disorders, such as major depressive disorder in young females and major depressive disorder with atypical features in adults, may be associated with weight gain, overweight, or obesity.

Third, obesity and mood disorders share other similarities. Phenomenologically, each may be characterized by overeating, physical inactivity, weight gain, and in children, by behavioral problems. Obesity is often accompanied by depressive symptoms in persons of all ages. Obesity and mood disorders are each associated with binge eating behavior, as well as bulimia nervosa and binge eating disorder. General obesity, abdominal obesity, the metabolic syndrome, major depressive disorder, and bipolar disorder are each associated with elevated morbidity and mortality from cardiovascular disease and type 2 diabetes. Like mood disorders, extreme obesity has been characterized by elevated familial mood disorders. Similar biological systems appear to be deranged in both conditions. These include the HPAC axis, the sympathetic nervous system, central monoamine neurotransmitter systems, immune function, and glucose and lipid metabolism. Regarding treatment response, both obesity and depression respond to medications that selectively enhance central serotonin, norepinephrine and/or dopamine function, and to psychological treatments with cognitive behavioral components. Although both conditions may benefit from exercise, they are also each characterized by poor exercise capacity. Moreover, both conditions may respond better to combinations of psychological and pharmacological treatments than to either modality alone.

Taken together, these data suggest that there may be a relationship between mood disorders and obesity beyond that due to chance co-occurrence and iatrogenic factors. In an earlier paper, we proposed three hypothetical models to explain the relationship between obesity and mood disorders (Fig. 1) (21). In the first, obesity and mood disorders are separate entities with distinct, nonoverlapping pathophysiologies which co-occur by chance, but with significant frequency because they are both common conditions. This model seems unlikely, however, in light of the clinical, epidemiologic, longitudinal, comorbidity, family history, biological, and treatment response similarities between obesity and mood disorders reviewed in this chapter.

In the second model, obesity and mood disorders are the same disorder with the same fundamental pathophysiology (18). This model also seems unlikely in light of some of the phenomenologic and treatment response differences reviewed. In particular, melancholic depression is associated with weight loss and possibly underweight (at least in clinical samples), and obesity and depression may have a differential response to long-term SSRI treatment.

In the third model, obesity and mood disorders are separate but related disorders with distinct but overlapping pathophysiologies (Fig. 1). In this model, obesity and mood disorders, both heterogeneous, polygenetic illnesses, would share heritable, as well as acquired, factors. Thus, there would be forms of obesity and mood disorder that were pathogenically related, as well as forms that were not related. Moreover, the degree of pathophysiologic overlap in individuals with both conditions could theoretically vary, depending on the nature or amount of inherited or acquired pathogenic material. In addition, the "directionality" of the relationship could vary, with mood disorder preceding obesity, obesity preceding mood disorder, or the two conditions developing in tandem. This model could explain much of the clinical, epidemiologic, phenomenologic, comorbidity, family history, and treatment response similarities and differences between obesity and mood disorders.

A pathogenic relationship between obesity and mood disorders would have implications for understanding the etiology of both conditions. Thus, subtyping mood episodes according to the presence of pathological overeating, weight gain, or excess body weight, or to the degree of visceral fat deposition, might be a more valid classification method than by the broader DSM-IV concepts of atypical versus melancholic features. Similarly, subtyping obesity (or overweight or the metabolic syndrome) as being associated or not associated with a lifetime mood or related disorder, such as binge eating disorder or an affective spectrum disorder, might help explain some of the clinical and genetic heterogeneity seen among persons with obesity (150,265–267).

Indeed, we and others have hypothesized that individuals may engage in a variety of behaviors, including overeating, for the purpose of regulating their mood (268,269). Substantial evidence indicates that brain mechanisms mediating reward are involved in the regulation of eating and mood, as well as the response to drugs of abuse (270,271). Thus, some patients with mood

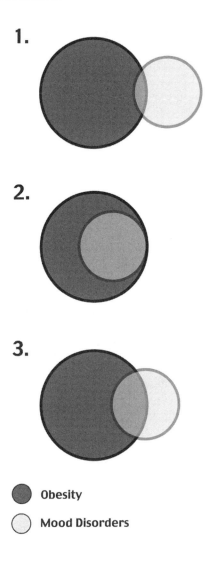

Key:
1. Obesity and mood disorders have separate pathophysiologies (they co-occur by chance)
2. Obesity and mood disorders have the same pathophysiologies (they are phenocopies)
3. Obesity and mood disorders have separate but overlapping pathophysiologies (they share pathogenic factors)

Figure 1 Three hypothetical models to explain the relationship between obesity and mood disorders. *Source*: From Ref. 21.

disorders may overeat to "self-medicate" their mood disorder symptoms. How effective overeating might be as a thymoleptic mechanism is unknown. Although food might be consumed for its mood-elevating or antidepressant properties, overeating might also have mood-destabilizing effects—as a consequence of repeated "withdrawals" from overeating-induced "highs," the physiologic effects of increased adiposity, or the psychosocial stigma of obesity. Nonetheless, until the pathophysiologies of obesity and mood disorders are understood, another possible means for subtyping at least some obesities could be by the pharmacologic responsiveness of the associated psychopathology (when it occurs). Thus, obesity associated with an antidepressant-responsive condition would be affective spectrum obesity; that associated with a mood-stabilizer-responsive bipolar spectrum disorder would be bipolar spectrum obesity; and that associated with a binge eating or addictive disorder responsive to an agent with anti-bingeing or anti-craving properties could be appetitive or addictive obesity (272–275,267).

A pathogenic relationship between obesity and mood disorders would also have implications for the treatment of both conditions (see chap. 10). In light of the different weight-loss profiles of available thymoleptics, persons seeking treatment for mood disorders who are obese might need to be managed differently from those who are normal weight or underweight. Similarly, in light of the potentially different thymoleptic profiles of anti-obesity agents, obese persons with mood disorders seeking weight loss treatment might need to be managed differently from those without mood disorders. A better understanding of the relationships among obesity, mood disorders, general medical illness, the beneficial and adverse effects of psychotropics on appetite, eating behavior, body weight, and metabolism, and the psychotropic effects of anti-obesity agents should improve the ability to treat both obesity and mood disorders. In addition, just as the weight and metabolic profiles of future psychotropics will need to be determined, so will the thymoleptic profiles of novel anti-obesity agents (21).

The above conclusions are preliminary because they are based on relatively few systematically acquired data. As noted, no large-scale psychiatric epidemiology study has also assessed anthropometric measures, and no epidemiologic study of body weight has also assessed the full range of mood disorders with structured interviews. There have been no published controlled studies directly comparing a group of patients with obesity with a group of patients with mood disorders, or a group of persons with obesity with and without mood disorders. Surprisingly few studies of mood disorders have included body weight as a factor, whereas relatively few studies of obesity have evaluated mood disorders as a factor. There are no controlled family history studies of psychopathology from nontreatment seeking populations of obese probands. Also, there are no controlled treatment studies in persons with both obesity and mood disorders. Moreover, there are important differences between obesity and mood disorders that may not be explained by a relationship between the two. In short, further research into the relationship between obesity and mood disorders is greatly needed.

REFERENCES

1. Richardson HB. Obesity as a manifestation of neurosis. Med Clin N Am 1946; 30:1187–1202.
2. Wadden TA, Stunkard AJ. Psychopathology and obesity. Ann NY Acad Sci 1987; 499:55–65.
3. Friedman MA, Brownell KD. Psychological correlates of obesity: moving to the next research generation. Psychol Bull 1995; 117:3–20.
4. Pine DS, Cohen P, Brook J, et al. Psychiatric symptoms in adolescence as predictors of obesity in early adulthood: a longitudinal study. Am J Public Health 1997; 97:1303–1310.
5. Rosmond R, Bjorntorp P. Psychiatric ill-health of women and its relationship to obesity and body fat distribution. Obes Res 1998; 6:338–345.
6. Mann JN, Thakore JH. Melancholic depression and abdominal fat distribution: a mini-review. Stress 1999; 3:1–15.
7. Carpenter KM, Hasin DS, Allison DB, et al. Relationships between obesity and DSM-IV major depressive disorder, suicide ideation, and suicide attempts: results from a general population study. Am J Public Health 2000; 90:251–257.
8. Roberts RE, Kaplan GA, Shema SJ, et al. Are the obese at greater risk for depression? Am J Epidemiol 2000; 152:163–170.
9. Roberts RE, Strawbridge WJ, Deleger S, et al. Are the fat more jolly? Ann Behav Med 2002; 24:169–180.
10. Roberts RE, Deleger S, Strawbridge WJ, et al. Prospective association between obesity and depression: evidence from the Alameda County Study. Int J Obes Relat Metab Disord 2003; 27:514–21.
11. Pine DS, Goldstein RB, Wolk S, et al. The association between childhood depression and adulthood body mass index. Pediatrics 2001; 107(5):1049–1056.
12. Faith MS, Matz, PE, Jorge MA. Obesity-depression associations in the population. J Psychosom Res 2002; 53:935–42.
13. Mustillo S, Worthman C, Erkanli A, et al. Obesity and psychiatric disorder: developmental trajectories. Pediatrics 2003; 111:851–859.
14. Dixon JB, Dixon ME, O'Brien PE. Depression in association with severe obesity. Changes with weight loss. Arch Intern Med 2003; 163:2058–2065.
15. Stunkard AJ, Faith MS, Allison KC. Depression and obesity. Biol Psychiatry 2003; 54:330–337.
16. Onyike CU, Crum RM, Lee HB, et al. Is obesity associated with major depression? Results from the Third National Health and Nutrition Examination Survey. Am J Epidemiol 2003; 158:1139–1147.
17. Richardson LP, Davis R, Poulton R, et al. A longitudinal evaluation of adolescent depression and adult obesity. Arch Pediatr Adolesc Med 2003; 157: 739–745.
18. Rosmond R. Obesity and depression: same disease, different names? Med Hypotheses 2004; 62:976–979.
19. Zametkin AJ, Zoon CK, Klein HW, et al. Psychiatric aspects of child and adolescent obesity: a review of the past 10 years. J Am Acad Child Adolesc Psychiatry 2004; 43:134–150.

20. Johnston E, Johnson S, McLeod P, et al. The relation of body mass index to depressive symptoms. Can J Public Health 2004; 95:179–183.
21. McElroy SL, Kotwal R, Malhotra S, et al. Are mood disorders and obesity related? A review for the mental health professional. J Clin Psychiatry 2004; 65:634–651.
22. Weissenburger J, Rush AJ, Giles DE, et al. Weight change in depression. Psychiatry Res 1986; 17:275–283.
23. Frank E, Carpenter LL, Kupfer DJ. Sex differences in recurrent depression: are there any that are significant? Am J Psychiatry 1988; 145:41–45.
24. Young MA, Scheftner WA, Fawcett J, et al. Gender differences in the clinical features of unipolar major depressive disorder. J Nerv Ment Dis 1990; 178:200–203.
25. Stunkard AJ, Fernstrom MH, Price A, et al. Direction of weight change in recurrent depression. Consistency across episodes. Arch Gen Psychiatry 1990; 47:857–860.
26. Horwath E, Johnson J, Weissman MM, et al. The validity of major depression with atypical features based on a community study. J Affect Disord 1992; 26:117–126.
27. Kendler KS, Eaves LJ, Walters EE, et al. The identification and validation of distinct depressive syndromes in a population-based sample of female twins. Arch Gen Psychiatry 1996; 53:391–399.
28. Levitan RD, LeSage A, Parikh SV, et al. Reversed neurovegetative symptoms of depression: a community study of Ontario. Am JPsychiatry 1997; 154:934–940.
29. Michelson D, Amsterdam JD, Quitkim FM, et al. Changes in weight during a 1-year trial of fluoxetine. Am J Psychiatry 1999; 156:1170–1176.
30. Angst J, Gamma A, Sellaro R, et al. Toward validation of atypical depression in the community: results of the Zurich cohort study. J Affect Disord 2002; 72:125–138.
31. Sullivan PF, Prescott CA, Kendler KS. The subtypes of major depression in a twin registry. J Affect Disord 2002; 68:273–284.
32. Posternak MA, Zimmerman M. Partial validation of the atypical features subtype of major depressive disorder. Arch Gen Psychiatry 2002; 59:70–76.
33. Berlin I, Lavergne F. Relationship between body-mass index and depressive symptoms in patients with major depression. Eur Psychiatry 2003; 18:85–88.
34. Korszun A, Moskvina V, Brewster S, et al. Familiality of symptom dimensions in depression. Arch Gen Psychiatry 2004; 61:468–474.
35. Mokdad AH, Serdula MK, Dietz WH, et al. The spread of the obesity epidemic in the United States, 1991–1998. JAMA 1999; 282:1519–1522.
36. Mokdad AH, Serdula MK, Dietz WH, et al. The continuing epidemic of obesity in the United States [letter]. JAMA 2000; 284:1650–1651.
37. Mokdad AH, Bowman BA, Ford ES, et al. The continuing epidemics of obesity and diabetes in the United States. JAMA 2001; 286:1195–1200.
38. Mokdad AH, Ford ES, Bowman BA, et al. Prevalence of obesity, diabetes, and obesity-related health-risk factors, 2001. JAMA 2003; 289:76–79.
39. Flegal KM, Carroll MD, Ogden CL, et al. Prevalence and trends in obesity among US adults, 1999–2000. JAMA 2002; 288:1723–1727.
40. Ogden CL, Flegal KM, Carroll MD, et al. Prevalence and trends in overweight among US children and adolescents, 1999–2000. JAMA 2002; 288:1728–1732.

41. Hedley AA, Ogden CL, Johnson CL, et al. Prevalence of overweight and obesity among US children, adolescents, and adults, 1999–2002. JAMA 2004; 291:2847–2850.
42. Klerman GL, Weissman MM. Increasing rates of depression. JAMA 1989; 261:2229–2235.
43. Robins LN, Regier DA. Psychiatric disorders in America. In: The epidemiologic catchment area study. New York, NY: The Free Press, 1991.
44. Cross-National Collaborative Group. The changing rate of major depression: cross-national comparisons. JAMA 1992; 268:3098–3105.
45. Kessler RC, McGonagle KA, Zhao S, et al. Lifetime and 12-month prevalence of DSM-III-R psychiatric disorders in the United States. Arch Gen Psychiatry 1994; 51:8–19.
46. Murray CJL, Lopez, eds. The global burden of disease: a comprehensive assessment of mortality and disability from diseases, injuries and risk factors in 1990 and projected to 2020. Harvard School of Public Health on behalf of the World Health Organization and the World Bank. Cambridge, Vol. 1, MA: 1996.
47. Kessler RC, Avenevoli S, Merikangas KR. Mood disorders in children and adolescents: an epidemiologic perspective. Biol Psychiatry 2001; 49:1002–1014.
48. Jonas BS, Brody D, Roper M, et al. Prevalence of mood disorders in a national sample of young American adults. Soc Psychiatry Psychiatr Epidemiol 2003; 38:618–624.
49. Kessler RC, Berglund P, Dermier O, et al. The epidemiology of major depressive disorder. Results from the National Comorbidity Survey Replication (NCS-R). JAMA 2003; 289:3095–3105.
50. Black DW, Goldstein RB, Mason EE. Prevalence of mental disorders in 88 morbidly obese bariatric clinic patients. Am J Psychiatry 1992; 149:227–234.
51. Sullivan M, Karlsson J, Sjörstöm L, et al. Swedish obese subjects (SOS)—an intervention study of obesity. Baseline evaluation of health and psychosocial functioning in the first 1743 subjects examined. Int J Obes Relat Metab Disord 1993; 17:503–512.
52. Goldstein LT, Goldsmith SJ, Anger K, et al. Psychiatric symptoms in clients presenting for commercial weight reduction treatment. Int J Eat Disord 1996; 20:191–197.
53. Cugini P, Cilli M, Salandri A, et al. Anxiety, depression, hunger and body composition: III. Their relationships in obese patients. Eat Weight Disord 1999; 4:115–120.
54. Britz B, Siegfried W, Ziegler A, et al. Rates of psychiatric disorders in a clinical study group of adolescents with extreme obesity and in obese adolescents ascertained via a population based study. Int J Obes Relat Metab Disord 2000; 24:1707–1714.
55. Csabi G, Tenyi T, Molnar D. Depressive symptoms among obese children. Eat Weight Disord 2000; 5:43–45.
56. Thakore J. Physical consequences of depression. Petersfield: Wrightson Biomedical Publishing, 2001.
57. Musselman DL, Betan E, Larsen H, et al. Relationship of depression to diabetes types 1 and 2: epidemiology, biology, and treatment. Biol Psychiatry 2003; 54:317–329.

58. Musselman DL, Evans DL, Nemeroff CB. The relationship of depression to cardiovascular disease: Epidemiology, biology, and treatment. Arch Gen Psychiatry 1998; 55:580–592.
59. Lett HS, Blumenthal JA, Babyak MA, et al. Depression as a risk factor for coronary artery disease: evidence, mechanisms, and treatment Psychosom Med 2004; 66:305–315.
60. Larson SL, Owens PL, Ford D, et al. Depressive disorder, dysthymia, and risk of stroke: thirteen-year follow-up from the Baltimore epidemiologic catchment area study. Stroke 2001; 32:1979–1983.
61. Jones DJ, Bromberger JT, Sutton-Tyrrell K, et al. Lifetime history of depression and carotid atherosclerosis in middle-aged women. Arch Gen Psychiatry 2003; 60:153–160.
62. Bosworth HB, Bartash RM, Olsen MK, et al. The association of psychosocial factors and depression with hypertension among older adults. Int J Geriatr Psychiatry 2003; 18:1142–2248.
63. Ohayon MM, Schatzberg AF. Using chronic pain to predict depressive morbidity in the general population. Arch Gen Psychiatry 2003; 60:39–47.
64. Calabrese JR, Hirschfeld RMA, Reed M, et al. Impact of bipolar disorder on a US community sample. J Clin Psychiatry 2003; 641:425–432.
65. Keck PE, Jr, McElroy SL. Bipolar disorder, obesity, and pharmacotherapy-associated weight gain. J Clin Psychiatry 2003; 64:1426–1435.
66. Arrone LJ, Segal KR. Weight gain in the treatment of mood disorders. J Clin Psychiatry 2003; 64(suppl 18):22–29.
67. Brown TM, Stoudemire A. Psychiatric side effects of prescription and over the counter drugs. Washington, DC: American Psychiatric Press, 1998.
68. Patten SB, Barbui C. Drug-induced depression: a systematic review to inform clinical practice. Psychother Psychosom 2004; 73:207–215.
69. Barsh GS, Farooqui S, O'Rabilly S. Genetics of body-weight regulation. Nature 2000; 404:644–651.
70. Bouchard C, Perusse L, Rice T, et al. Genetics of human obesity. In: Bray GA, Bouchard C, eds. Handbook of obesity. New York, NY: Marcel Dekker, 2004:157–200.
71. Snyder EE, Walts B, Perusse L, et al. The human obesity gene map: the 2003 update. Obes Res 2004; 369–439.
72. Goodwin FK, Jamison KR. Manic-depressive illness. New York: Oxford University Press, 1990.
73. Sullivan PF, Neale MC, Kendler KS. Genetic epidemiology of major depression: review and meta-analysis. Am J Psychiatry 2000; 157:1552–1562.
74. Kelsoe JR. Arguments for the genetic basis of the bipolar spectrum. J Affect Disord 2003; 73:183–197.
75. Becker KG. The common variants/multiple disease hypothesis of common complex genetic disorders. Med Hypotheses 2004; 62:309–317.
76. National Institutes of Health National Heart, Lung, and Blood Institute. Clinical guidelines on the identification, evaluation, and treatment of overweight and obesity in adults. The Evidence Report. NIH Publication No. 98–4083,1998.
77. American Psychiatric Association. Diagnostic and statistical manual of mental disorders. 4th ed. Text Revision. Washington, DC: American Psychiatric Association, 2000.

78. Lewinsohn PM, Róhde P, Seeley JR. Major depressive disorder in older adolescents: prevalence, risk factors, and clinical implications. Clin Psychol Rev 1998; 18:765–794.
79. Kessler RC, Walters EE. Epidemiology of DSM-III-R major depression and minor depression among adolescents and young adults in the National Comorbidity Survey. Depress Anxiety 1998; 7:3–14.
80. Faedda GL, Baldessarini RJ, Glovinsky IP, et al. Pediatric bipolar disorder: phenomenology and course of illness. Bipolar Disord 2004; 6:305–313.
81. Lewinsohn PM, Klein DN, Seeley JR. Bipolar disorders hi a community sample of older adolescents: prevalence, phenomenology, comorbidity, and course. J Am Acad Child Adolesc Psychiatry 1995; 34:454–463.
82. Judd LL, Akiskal HS. The prevalence and disability of bipolar spectrum disorders in the US population: re-analysis of the ECA database taking into account subthreshold cases. J Affect Disord 2003; 73:123–131.
83. Angst J. The emerging epidemiology of hypomania and bipolar II disorder. J Affect Disord 1998; 50:143–151.
84. Angst J, Gamma A, Benazzi F, et al. Toward a redefinition of subthreshold bipolarity: epidemiology and proposed criteria for bipolar II, minor bipolar disorders and hypomania. J Affect Disorder 2003; 73:133–146.
85. Hantouche EG, Akiskal HS, Lancrenon S, et al. Systematic clinical methodology for validating bipolar-II disorder: data in mid-stream from a French national multi-site study (EPIDEP). J Affect Disord 1998; 50:163–173.
86. Cassano GB, Rucci P, Frank E, et al. The mood spectrum in unipolar and bipolar disorder: arguments for a unitary approach. Am J Psychiatry 2004; 161:1264–1269.
87. Klerman GL, Lavori PW, Rice J, et al. Birth-cohort trends in rates of major depressive disorder among relatives of patients with affective disorder. Arch Gen Psychiatry 1985; 42:689–693.
88. Gershon ES, Hamovit JH, Guroff JJ, et al. Birth-cohort changes in manic and depressive disorders in relatives of bipolar and schizoaffective patients. Arch Gen Psychiatry 1987; 44:314–319.
89. Kessler RC. Epidemiology of women and depression. J Affect Disord 2003; 74:5–13.
90. Myers JK, Weissman MM. Use of a self-report symptom scale to detect depression in a community sample. Am J Psychiatry 1980; 137:1081–1084.
91. Eaton WW, Neufield K, Chen LS, et al. A comparison of self-report and clinical diagnostic interviews for depression: diagnostic interview schedule and schedules for clinical assessment in neuropsychiatry in the Baltimore epidemiologic catchment area follow-up. Arch Gen Psychiatry 2000; 57:217–222.
92. Wise TN, Fernandez F. Psychological profiles of candidates seeking surgical correction for obesity. Obes Bariatr Med 1979; 8:83–86.
93. Halmi KA, Long M, Stunkard AJ, et al. Psychiatric diagnosis of morbidly obese gastric bypass patients. Am J Psychiatry 1980; 137:1470–1472.
94. Hopkinson LC, Bland RC. Depressive syndromes in grossly obese women. Can J Psychiatry 1982; 27:213–215.

95. Gertler R, Ramsey-Stewart G. Pre-operative psychiatric assessment of patients presenting for gastric bariatric surgery (surgical control of morbid obesity). Aust NZ J Surg l986; 56:157–161.
96. Hudson JI, Pope HG Jr, Wurtman J, et al. Bulimia in obese individuals. Relationship to normal weight bulimia. J Nerv Ment Dis 1988; 152:144–152.
97. Marcus MD, Wing RR, Ewing L, et al. Psychiatric disorders among obese binge eaters. Int J Eat Disord 1990; 9:69–77.
98. Goldsmith SJ, Anger-Friedfeld K, Beren S, et al. Psychiatric illness in patients presenting for obesity treatment. Int J Eat Disord 1992; 12:63–71.
99. Specker S, deZwaan M, Raymond N, et al. Psychopathology in subgroups of obese women with and without binge eating disorder. Comp Psychiatry 1994; 35:185–90.
100. Powers PS, Rosemurgy A, Boyd F, et al. Outcome of gastric restriction procedures: Weight, psychiatric diagnoses, and satisfaction. Obes Surg 1997; 7:471–477.
101. Hsu LK, Mulliken B, McDonagh B, et al. Binge eating disorder in extreme obesity. Int J Obes 2002; 26:1398–1403.
102. Fontenelle LF, Vltor Mendlowicz M, de Menezes GB, et al. Psychiatric comorbidity in a Brazilian sample of patients with binge-eating disorder. Psychiatry Res 2003; 119:189–194.
103. Erermis S, Cetin N, Tamar M, et al. Is obesity a risk factor for psychopathology among adolescents? Pediatr Int 2004; 46:296–301.
104. Vila G, Zipper E, Dabbas M, et al. Mental disorders in obese children and adolescents. Psychosom Med 2004; 66:3287–3394.
105. Bulik CM, Sullivan PF, Kendler KS. Medical and psychiatric morbidity in obese women with and without binge eating. Int J Eat Disord 2002; 32:72–78.
106. Kinder LS, Carnethon MR, Palaniappan LP, et al. Depression and the metabolic syndrome in young adults: findings from the Third National Health and Nutrition Examination Survey. Psychosom Med 2004; 66:316–322.
107. Müller-Oerlinghausen B, Passoth P-M, Poser W, et al. Impaired glucose tolerance in long-term lithium-treated patients. Int Pharmacopsychiatry 1979; 14:350–362.
108. Berken GH, Weinstein DO, Stern WC. Weight gain. A side effect of tricyclic antidepressants. J Affect Disord 1984; 7:133–135.
109. Shiori T, Kato T, Murashita J, et al. Changes in the frequency distribution pattern of body weight in patients with major depression. Acta Psychiatr Scand 1993; 88:356–360.
110. Elmslie JL, Silverstone JT, Mann JI, et al. Prevalence of overweight and obesity in bipolar patients. J Clin Psychiatry 2000; 61:179–184.
111. McELroy SL, Frye MA, Suppes T, et al. Correlates of overweight and obesity in 644 patients with bipolar disorder. J Clin Psychiatry 2002; 63:207–213.
112. Fagiolini A, Frank E, Houck PR, et al. Prevalence of obesity and weight change during treatment in patients with bipolar I disorder. J Clin Psychiatry 2002; 63:528–533.
113. Fagiolini A, Kupfer DJ, Houck PR, et al. Obesity as a correlate of outcome in patients with bipolar I disorder. Am J Psychiatry 2003; 60:112–17.

114. Papakostas GI, Peterson T, Iosifescu DV, et al. Obesity among outpatients with major depressive disorder. Int J Neuropsychopharmacol 2004; 7:1–5.
115. Thakore JH, Richards PJ, Rezuek RH, et al. Increased abdominal fat deposition in patients with major depressive illness as measured by computed tomography. Biol Psychiatry 1997; 41:1140–1142.
116. Weber-Hamann B, Hentschel F, Kniest A, et al. Hypercortisolemic depression is associated with increased intra-abdominal fat. Psychosom Med 2002; 64:274–277.
117. Elmslie JL, Mann JI, Silverstone JT, et al. Determinants of overweight and obesity in patients with bipolar disorder. J Clin Psychiatry 2001; 62:486–491.
118. Fagiolini A, Kupfer DJ, Rucci P, et al. Suicide attempts and ideation in patients with bipolar I disorder. J Clin Psychiatry 2004; 65:509–514.
119. Miller GE, Stetler CA, Carney RM, et al. Clinical depression and inflammatory risk markers for coronary heart disease. Am J Cardiol 2002; 90:1279–1283.
120. Wyatt RJ, Henter ID, Mojtabai R, et al. Height, weight, and body mass index (BMI) in psychiatrically ill US Armed Forces personnel. Psychol Med 2003; 33:363–368.
121. Lamertz CM, Jacobi C, Yassouridis A, et al. Areobese adolescents and young adults at higher risk for mental disorders? A community survey. Obes Res 2002; 10:1152–1160.
122. Hasler G, Merikangas K, Eich D, et al. Psychopathology as a risk factor for being overweight. American Psychiatric Association 156th Annual Meeting New Research Abstracts, San Francisco, CA, May 17–22, 2003, NR 106:39–40.
123. Holland J, Masling J, Copely D. Mental illness in lower class normal, obese and hyperobese women. Psychosom Med 1970; 32:351–357.
124. Jacobs SB, Wagner MK. Obese and nonobese individuals: behavioral and personality characteristics. Addict Behav 1984; 9:223–226.
125. Faith MS, Johnson SL, Allison DB. Putting the behavior into the behavior genetics of obesity. Behav Genet 1997; 27:423–439.
126. Lichtman SW, Pisaraka K, Berman ER, et al. Discrepancy between self-reported and actual caloric intake and exercise in obese subjects. N Engl J Med 1992; 327:1893–1898.
127. Hällström T, Noppa H. Obesity in women in relation to mental illness, social factors and personality traits. J Psychosom Res 1981; 25:75–82.
128. Wadden TA, Foster GD, Stunkard AJ, et al. Dissatisfaction with, weight and figure in obese girls: discontent but not depression. Int J Obes 1989; 13:89–97.
129. Palinkas LA, Wingard DL, Barret-Connort E. Depressive symptoms in overweight and obese older adults: a test of the "jolly fat" hypothesis. J Psychosom Res 1996; 40:59–66.
130. Istvan J, Zavela K, Weidner O. Body weight and psychological distress in the NHANES I. Int J Obes 1992; 16:999–1003.
131. Erickson SJ, Robinson TN, Haydel KF, et al. Are overweight children unhappy? Body mass index, depressive symptoms, and overweight concerns in elementary school children. Arch Pediatr Adolesc Med 2000; 154:931–935.
132. Pesa JA, Syre TR, Jones E. Psychological differences associated with body weight among female adolescents: the importance of body image. J Adolesc Health 2000; 26:330–337.

133. Siegel JM, Yancery AK, McCarthy WJ. Overweight and depressive symptoms among African American women. Prev Med 2000; 31:232–340.
134. Lumeng JC, Gannon K, Cabral HJ, et al. Association between clinically meaningful behavior problems and overweight in children. Pediatrics 2003; 112: 1138–1145.
135. Cassidy WL, Flanagan NB, Spellman M, et al. Clinical observations in manic-depressive disease; a quantitative study of one hundred manic depressive patients and fifty medically sick controls. J Am Med Assoc 1957; 164: 1534–1546.
136. Sobin C, Sackeim HA. Psychomotor symptoms of depression. Am J Psychiatry 1997; 154:4–17.
137. Miller DK, Mahmstrom TK, Joshi S, et al. Clinically relevant levels of depressive symptoms in community-dwelling middle aged African Americans. J Am Geriatr Soc 2004; 51:741–748.
138. Wolff III EA, Putnam FW, Post RM. Motor activity and affective illness. The relationship of amplitude and temporal distribution to changes in affective state. Arch Gen Psychiatry 1985; 42:288–294.
139. Volkers AC, Tulen JHM, vd Broek WW, et al. Motor activity and autonomic cardiac function in major depressive disorder. J Affect Disord 2003; 76:23–30.
140. Camacho TC, Roberts RE, Lazarus NB, et al. Physical activity and depression: evidence from the Almeda County Study. Am J Epidemiol 1991; 134:220–231.
141. Kritz-Silverstein D, Barret-Connor E, Corbeau C. Cross-sectional and prospective study of exercise and depressed mood in the elderly. The Rancho Bernardo study. Am J Epidemiol 2001; 153:596–603.
142. Yancy AK, Wold CM, McCarthy WJ, et al. Physical inactivity and overweight among Los Angeles County adults. Am J Prev Med 2004; 27:146–152.
143. Gold PW, Chrousos GP. Organization of the stress system and its dysregulation in melancholic and atypical depression: high vs low CRH/NE states. Mol Psychiatry 2002; 7:254–275.
144. Noppa H, Hällström T. Weight gain in adulthood in relation to socioeconomic factors, mental illness and personality traits: a prospective study of middle-aged women. J Psychosom Res 1981; 25:83–89.
145. DiPietro L, Anda RF, Williamson DF, et al. Depressive symptoms and weight change in a national cohort of adults. Int J Obes 1992; 16:745–753.
146. Barefoot JC, Heitmann BL, Helms MJ, et al. Symptoms of depression and changes in body weight from adolescence to mid-life. Int J Obes 1998; 22:688–694.
147. Goodman E, Whitaker RC. A prospective study of the role of depression in the development and persistence of adolescent obesity. Pediatrics 2002; 109: 497–504.
148. Sammel MD, Grisso JA, Freeman EW, et al. Weight gain among women in the late reproductive years. Fam Pract 2003; 20:401–409.
149. Spitzer RL, Devlin M, Walsh BT, et al. Binge eating disorder: a multisite field trial of the diagnostic criteria. Int J Eat Disord 1992; 11:191–203.
150. Yanovski SZ, Nelson JE, Dubbert BK, et al. Association of binge eating disorders and psychiatric comorbidity in obese subjects. Am J Psychiatry 1993; 150:1472–1479.

151. Fairbum CG, Welch SL, Doll HA, et al. Risk factors for bulimia nervosa: a community based case-control study. Arch Gen Psychiatry 1997; 54:509–517.
152. Fairbum CG, Doll HA, Welch SL, et al. Risk factors for binge eating disorder. A community-based, case-control study. Arch Gen Psychiatry 1998; 55:425–432.
153. Smith DE, Marcus MD, Lewis CE, et al. Prevalence of binge eating disorder, obesity, and depression in a biracial cohort of young adults. Ann Behav Med 1998; 20:227–232.
154. French SA, Jeffery RW, Sherwood NE, et al. Prevalence and correlates of binge eating in a nonclinical sample of women enrolled in a weight gain prevention program. Int J Obes 1999; 23:576–585.
155. Bulik CM, Sullivan PF, Kendler KS. An empirical study of the classification of eating disorders. Am J Psychiatry 2000; 157:886–895.
156. Fairburn CG, Cooper Z, Doll HA, et al. The natural course of bulimia nervosa and binge eating disorders in young women. Arch Gen Psychiatry 2000; 57:659–665.
157. Ackard DM, Neumark-Sztainer D, Story M, et al. Overeating among adolescents: prevalence and associations with weight-related characteristics and psychological health. Pediatrics 2003; 111:67–74.
158. Stunkard AJ, Allison KC. Two forms of disordered eating in obesity: binge eating and night eating. Int J Obes Relat Metab Disord 2003; 27:1–12.
159. Kendler KS, MacLean C, Neale M, et al. The genetic epidemiology of bulimia nervosa. Am J Psychiatry 1991; 148:1627–1637.
160. Vollrath M, Koch R, Angst J. Binge eating and weight concerns among young adults. Results from The Zurich Cohort Study. Br J Psychiatry 1992; 160: 498–503.
161. Garfinkel PE, Lin E, Goering P. Bulimia nervosa in a Canadian community sample: prevalence and comparison of subgroups. Am J Psychiatry 1995; 152:1052–1058.
162. Wittchen H-U, Mühlig S, Pezawas L. Natural course and burden of bipolar disorders. Int J Neuropsychopharmacol 2003; 6:145–154.
163. McElroy SL, Kotwal R, Keck PE Jr, et al. Comorbidity of bipolar and eating disorders: distinct or related disorders with shared dysregulations? J Affect Disord, 2005; 86:107–127.
164. Anderson RJ, Freedland KE, Clouse RE, et al. The prevalence of comorbid depression in adults with diabetes: a meta-analysis. Diabetes Care 2001; 24:1069–1078.
165. Nichols GA, Brown JB. Unadjusted and adjusted prevalence of diagnosed depression in type 2 diabetes. Diabetes Care 2003; 26:744–749.
166. Golden SH, Williams JE, Ford DE, et al. Depressive symptoms and the risk of type 2 diabetes: The Atherosclerosis Risk in Communities study. Diabetes Care 2004; 27:429–435.
167. Markowitz JH, Jonas BS, Davidson K. Psychological factors as precursors to hypertension. Curr Hypertens Rep 2001; 3:25–32.
168. Ferketich AK, Schwartzbaum JA, Frid DJ, et al. Depression as an antecedent to heart disease among women and men in the NHANES I study. Arch Intern Med 2000; 160:1261–1268.

169. Jonas BS, Mussolino ME. Symptoms of depression as a prospective risk factor for stroke. Psychosom Med 2000; 62:463–471.
170. Ohira T, Iso H, Satoh S, et al. Prospective study of depressive symptoms and risk of stroke among Japanese. Stroke 2001; 32:903–908.
171. Lilliker SL. Prevalence of diabetes in a manic-depressive population. Compr Psychiatry 1980; 21:270–275.
172. Cassidy F, Ahearn E, Carroll BJ. Elevated frequency of diabetes mellitus in hospitalized manic-depressive patients. Am J Psychiatry 1999; 156:1417–1420.
173. Regenold WT, Thapar RK, Marano C, et al. Increased prevalence of type 2 diabetes mellitus among psychiatric inpatients with bipolar I affective and schizoaffective disorders independent of psychotropic drug use. J Affect Disord 2002; 70:19–26.
174. Hoyer EH, Mortensen PB, Olesen AV. Mortality and causes of death in a total national sample of patients with affective disorders admitted for the first time between 1973 and 1993. Br J Psychiatry 2000; 176:76–82.
175. Osby U, Brandt L, Correia N, et al. Excess mortality in bipolar and unipolar disorder in Sweden. Arch Gen Psychiatry 2001; 58:844–850.
176. Penninx BW, Beekman ATF, Honig A, et al. Depression and cardiac mortality. Results from a community-based longitudinal study. Arch Gen Psychiatry 2001; 58:221–227.
177. Bray GA, Bouchard C, eds. Handbook of Obesity. Etiology and Pathophysiology. 2nd ed. Marcel Dekker New York 2004.
178. National Cholesterol Education Program (NCEP) Expert Panel: Executive summary of the third report of the NCEP Expert Panel on detection, evaluation, and treatment of high blood cholesterol in adults (adult treatment panel). JAMA 2001; 285:2486–2497.
179. Das UN. Is obesity an inflammatory condition? Nutrition 2001; 17:953–966.
180. Ghanim H, Aljada A, Hofmeyer D, et al. Circulating mononuclear cells in the obese are in a proinflammatory state. Circulation 2004; 110:1564–1571.
181. Okamura F, Tashiro A, Utsumi A, et al. Insulin resistance in patients with depression and its changes during the clinical course of depression: minimal model analysis. Metabolism 2000; 49:1255–1260.
182. Lustman PJ, Anderson PJ, Freedland KB, et al. Depression and poor glycemic control: a meta-analytic review of the literature. Diabetes Care 2000; 23:934–942.
183. Ramasubbu R. Insulin resistance: a metabolic link between depressive disorder and atherosclerotic vascular diseases. Med Hypotheses 2002; 59:537–551.
184. Kopf D, Westphal S, Luley CW, et al. Lipid metabolism and insulin resistance in depressed patients: significance of weight, hypercortisolism, and antidepressant treatment. J Clin Psychopharmacol 2004; 24:527–531.
185. Horsten M, Wamala SP, Vingerhoets A, et al. Depressive symptoms, social support, and lipid profile in healthy middle-aged women. Psychosom Med 1997; 59:521–528.
186. Ledochowski M, Murr C, Sperner-Unterweger B, et al. Association between increased serum cholesterol and signs of depressive mood. Clin Chem Lab Med 2003; 41:821–824.

187. Huang TL, Chen JF. Lipid and lipoprotein levels in depressive disorders with melancholic feature or atypical feature and dysthymia. Psychiatry Clin Neurosci 2004; 58:295–299.
188. Kop WJ, Gottdiener JS, Tangen CM, et al. Inflammation and coagulation factors in persons > 65 years of age with symptoms of depression but without evidence of myocardial ischemia. Am J Cardiol 2002; 89:419–424.
189. Penninx BW, Kritchevsky SB, Yaffe K, et al. Inflammatory markers and depressed mood in older persons: results from the health, aging and body composition study. Biol Psychiatry 2003; 54:566–572.
190. Ford DE, Erlmger TP. Depression and C-reactive protein in U.S. adults: data from the Third National Health and Nutrition Examination Survey. Arch Intern Med 2004; 164:1010–1014.
191. Panagiotakos DB, Pitsaros C, Chrysohoou C, et al. Inflammation, coagulation, and depressive symptomatology in cardiovascular disease-free people; ATTICA study. Eur Heart J 2004; 25:492–499.
192. Katon W, von Korff M, Ciechanowski P, et al. Behavioral factors associated with depression among individuals with diabetes. Diabetes Care 2004; 27: 914–920.
193. Lespérance F, Frasure-Smith N, Theroux P, et al. The association between major depression and levels of soluble intercellular adhesion molecule 1, interleukin-6, and c-reactive protein in patients with acute coronary syndromes. Am J Psychiatry 2004; 161:271–277.
194. Ladwig K-H, Marten-Mittaq B, Löwel H, et al. Influence of depressive mood on the association of CRP obesity in 3205 middle aged healthy men. Brain Behav Immun 2003; 17:268–275.
195. Miller GE, Freedland KE, Carney RM, et al. Pathways linking depression, adiposity, and inflammatory markers in healthy young adults. Brain Behav Immun 2003; 17:276–285.
196. Black DW, Goldstein RB, Mason EE, et al. Depression and other mental disorders in the relatives of morbidly obese patients. J Affect Disord 1992; 25:91–95.
197. Dong C, Sanchez LE, Price RA. Relationship of obesity to depression: a family based study. Int J Obes Relat Metab Disord 2004; 28:790–795.
198. Marniemi J, Kronhahn E, Aunola S, et al. Visceral fat and psychosocial stress in identical twins discordant for obesity. J Int Med 2002; 251:35–43.
199. McCaffery JM, Niaura R, Todaro JF, et al. Depressive symptoms and metabolic risk in adult male twins enrolled in the National Heart, Lung, and Blood Institute twin study. Psychosom Med 2003; 65:490–497.
200. Leibowitz SF, Hoebel BG. Behavioral neuroscience and obesity. In: Bray GA, Bouchard C, eds. Handbook of obesity. Etiology pathophysiology. 2nd ed. New York: Marcel Dekker, 2004:301–371.
201. Redrobe JP, Dumont Y, Quirion R. Neuropeptide Y(NPY) and depression: from animal studies to the human condition. Life Sci 2002; 71:2921–2937.
202. Garlow SJ, Nemeroff CB. The neurochemistry of depressive disorders: clinical studies. In: Charney DS, Nestler EJ, eds. Neurobiology of mental illness. 2nd ed. New York: Oxford, 2004:440–460.

203. Flores BH, Musselman DL, De Battista C, et al. Biology of mood disorders. In: Schatzberg AF, Nemeroff CB, eds. The american psychiatric publishing textbook of psychopharmacology. 3rd ed. Washington, DC: American Psychiatric Publishing, 2004:717–763.
204. Björntorp P, Rosmond R. Hypothalamic origin of the metabolic syndrome X. Ann NY Acad Sci 1999; 892:297–307.
205. Vincennati V, Pasquali R. Abnormalities of the hypomalamic–pituitary–adrenal axis in nondepressed women with abdominal obesity and relations with insulin resistance: evidence for a central and a peripheral alteration. J Clin Endocrinol Metab 2000; 85:4093–4098.
206. Epel ES, Me Ewen B, Seeman T, et al. Stress and. body shape: stress induced cortisol secretion is consistently greater among women with central fat. Psychosom Med 2000; 62:623–632.
207. Duclos M, Gatta B, Corcuff J-B, et al. Fat distribution in obese women is associated with subtle alterations of the hypothalamic–pituitary–adrenal axis activity and sensitivity to glucocorticoids. Clin Endocrinol 2002; 55:447–454.
208. Casper RC, Kocsis J, Dysken M, et al. Cortisol measures in primary major depressive disorder with hypersomnia or appetite increase. J Affect Disord 1988:131–140.
209. Anisman H, Ravindran AV, Griffiths J, et al. Endocrine and cytocrine correlates of major depression and dysthymia with typical or atypical features. Mol Psychiatry 1999; 4:182–188.
210. Davy KP. The global epidemic of obesity: are we becoming more sympathetic? Curr Hypertens Rep 2004; 6:241–246.
211. Veith RC, Lewis N, Linares OA, et al. Sympathetic nervous system activity in major depression. Basal and desipramine-induced alterations in plasma norepinephrine kinetics. Arch Gen Psychiatry 1994; 51:411–422.
212. Strombom U, Krotkiewski M, Blennow K, et al. The concentrations of monoamine metabolites and neuropeptides in the cerebrospinal fluid of obese women with different body fat distribution. Int J Obes 1996; 20:361–368.
213. Lambert GW, Vaz M, Cox HS, et al. Human obesity is associated with chronic elevation in brain 5-hydroxytryptamine turnover. Clin Sci 1999; 96:191–197.
214. Wang GJ, Volkow ND, Logan J, et al. Brain dopamine and obesity. Lancet 2001; 357:354–357.
215. Zahorska-Marklewicz B, Obuchowicz E, Waluga M, et al. Neuropeptide Y in obese women during treatment with adrenergic modulation drugs. Med Sci Monit 2001; 7:403–408.
216. Räikkönen K, Keltikangas-Järvinen L, Adlercreutz H, et al. Psychosocial stress and the insulin resistance syndrome. Metabolism 1996; 45:1533–1538.
217. Ahlberg AC, Ljung T, Rosmond R, et al. Depression and anxiety symptoms in relation to anthropometry and metabolism in men. Psychiatry Res 2002; 112: 101–110.
218. Bray GA, Greenway FL. Current and potential drugs for treatment of obesity. Endoc Rev 1999; 20:805–875.
219. Bays HE. Current and investigational antiobestiy agents and obesity therapeutic treatment targets. Obes Res 2004; 12:1197–1111.

220. Appolinario JC, Bueno JR, Coutinho W. Psychotropic drugs in the treatment of obesity: what promise? CNS Drugs 2004; 18:629–651.
221. Chiarello RJ, Cole JO. The use of psychostimulants in general psychiatry. A reconsideration. Arch Gen Psychiatry 1987; 44:286–295.
222. Satel SL, Nelson JC. Stimulants in the treatment of depression: a critical overview. J Clin Psychiatry 1989; 50:241–249.
223. Fawcett J, Busch KA. Stimulants in psychiatry. In: Schatzberg AF, Nemeroff CB, eds. Textbook of Psychopharmcology. 2nd. Washington, DC: American Psychiatric Press, 1998:503–522.
224. Rickels K, Hesbacher P, Fisher E, et al. Emotional symptomatology in obese patients treated with fenfluramine and dextroamphetamine. Psychol Med 1976; 6:623–630.
225. Wallace AE, Kofoed LL, West AN. Double-blind, placebo-controlled trial of methyphenidate in older, depressed, medically ill patients. Am J Psychiatry 1995; 152:929–931.
226. Carlson PJ, Merlock MC, Suppes T. Adjunctive stimulant use in patients with bipolar disorder: treatment of residual depression and sedation. Bipolar Disord 2004; 6:416–420.
227. O'Rourke D, Wurtman JJ, Wurtman RJ, et al. Treatment of seasonal depression with D-fenfluramine. J Clin Psychiatry 1989; 50:343–347.
228. Brzezinski AA, Wurtman JJ, Wurtman RJ, et al. D-Fenfluramine suppresses the increased calorie carbohydrate intakes and improves the mood of women with premenstrual depression. Obstet Gynecol 1990; 76:296–301.
229. Murphy DL, Slater S, de la Vega CE, et al. The serotonergic neurotransmitter system in the affective disorders—a preliminary evaluation of the antidepressant and antimanic effects of fenfluramine. In: Deniker P, Radonco-Thomas C, Villeneuve A, eds. Neuropsychopharmacology. New York: Pergamon Press, 1978:675–682.
230. Blouin AG, Blouin JH, Perez EL, et al. Treatment of bulimia with fenfluramine and desipramine. J Clin Psychopharmacol 1988; 8:261–269.
231. Buckett WR, Thomas PL, Luscombe GP. The pharmacology of sibutramine hydrochloride (BTS 54 524), a new antidepressant which induces rapid noradrenergic down-regulation. Prog Neuropsychopharmacol Biol Psychiatry 1988; 12:575–584.
232. Appolinario JC, Bacaltchuk J, Sichieri R, et al. A randomized, double-blind, placebo-controlled study of the treatment of binge-eating disorder. Arch Gen Psychiatry 2003; 60:1109–1116.
233. Bray GA, Hollander P, Klein S, et al. A 6-month randomized, placebo-controlled, dose-ranging trial of topiramate for weight loss in obesity. Obes Res 2003; 11:722–733.
234. Wilding J, Gaal LV, Rissanen A, et al. A randomized double-blind placebo-controlled study of the long-term efficacy and safety of topiramate in the treatment of obese subjects. Int J Obes Relat Metab Disord 2004; 28:1399–1410.
235. Gadde KM, Franciscy DM, Wagner II HR, et al. Zonisamide for weight loss in obese adults. A randomized, controlled trial. JAMA 2003; 289:1820–1825.

236. McElroy SL, Keck PE Jr. Topiramate. In: Schatzberg AF, Nemeroff CB, eds. American Psychiatric Publishing Textbook of Psychopharmacology. 3rd ed. Arlington, VA: American Psychiatric Publishing, 2004:627–636.
237. McIntyre RS, Mancini DA, McCann S, et al. Topiramate vs bupropion SR when added to mood stabilizer therapy for the depressive phase of bipolar disorder: a preliminary single-blind study. Bipolar Disord 2002; 4:207–213.
238. Kanba S, Yagi G, Kamijima K, et al. The first open study of zonisamide, a novel anticonvulsant, shows efficacy in mania. Prog Neuropsychopharmacol Biol Psychiatry 1994; 18:707–715.
239. McElroy SL, Suppes T, Keck PE, et al. Open-label adjunctive zonisamide in the treatment of bipolar disorders: a prospective trial. J Clin Psychiatry, 2005; 66:617–624.
240. Wise SD. Clinical studies with fluoxetine in obesity. Am J Clin Nutr 1992; 55(suppl 1):181S–184S.
241. Sayler ME, Goldstein DJ, Roback PJ, et al. Evaluating success of weight- loss programs, with an application to fluoxetine weight-reduction clinical trial data. Int J Obes Relat Metab Disord 1994; 18:742–751.
242. Gadde KM, Parker CB, Maner LG, et al. Bupropion for weight loss: an investigation of efficacy and tolerability in overweight and obese women. Obes Res 2001; 9:544–551.
243. Anderson JW, Greenway FL, Fujioka K, et al. Bupropion SR enhances weight loss: a 48-week double-blind, placebo-controlled trial. Obes Res 2002; 10:633–641.
244. Jain AK, Kaplan RA, Gadde KM, et al. Bupropion SR vs placebo for weight loss in obese patients with depressive symptoms. Obes Res 2002; 1049–1056.
245. Harvey AT, Rudolph RL, Preskom SH. Evidence of the dual mechanisms of action of venlafaxine. Arch Gen Psychiatry 2000; 57:503–509.
246. Rudolph RL, Fabre LF, Feighner JP, et al. A randomized, placebo-controlled, dose–response trial of venlafaxine hydrochloride in the treatment of major depression. J Clin Psychiatry 1998; 59:116–122.
247. Kraus T, Haack M, Schuld A, et al. Body weight, the tumor necrosis factor system, and leptin production during treatment with mirtazepine or venlafaxine. Pharmacopsychiatry 2002; 35:220–225.
248. Malhotra S, King KH, Welge JA, et al. Venlafaxine treatment of binge eating disorder associated with obesity: a series of 35 patients. J Clin Psychiatry 2002; 63:802–806.
249. Corrigan MH, Denahan AQ, Wright CE, et al. Comparison of pramipexole, fluoxetine, and placebo in patients with major depression. Depress Anxiety 2000; 11:58–65.
250. Goldberg JF, Burdick KE, Endick CJ. Preliminary randomized, double-blind, placebo-controlled trial of pramipexole added to mood stabilizers for treatment- resistant bipolar depression. Am J Psychiatry 2004; 161:564–66.
251. Zarate CA Jr, Payne JL, Singh J, et al. Pramipexole for bipolar II depression: a placebo-controlled proof of concept study. Biol Psychiatry 2004; 56:54–60.
252. Cincotta AH, Meieer AH. Bromocriptine (Ergoset) reduces body weight and improves glucose tolerance in obese subjects. Diabetes Care 1996; 19:667–670.

253. Thase ME, Entsuah AR, Rudulph RL. Remission rates during treatment with venlafaxine or selective serotonin reuptake inhibitors. Br J Psychiatry 2001; 178:234–241.

254. Stahl S, Entsuah R, Rudolph RL. Comparative efficacy between venlafaxine and SSRIs: a pooled analysis of patients with depression. Biol Psychiatry 2002; 52:1166–1174.

255. Wright JH, Beck AT, Thase ME. Cognitive therapy. In: Hales RE, Yudofsky SC, Talbott JA, eds. The American Psychiatric Publishing Textbook of Clinical Psychiatry. 4th ed.. Washington, DC: American Psychiatric Publishing, 2003:1245–1284.

256. Hensley PL, Nadiga D, Uhlenhuth EH. Long-term effectiveness of cognitive therapy in major depressive disorder. Depress Anxiety 2004; 20:1–7.

257. Craft LL, Perna FM. The benefits of exercise for the clinically depressed. Prim Care Comparison. J Clin Psychiatry 2004; 6:104–111.

258. Ruo B, Rumsfeld JS, Pipkin S, et al. Relation between depressive symptoms and treadmill exercise capacity in the Heart and Soul Study. Am J Cardiol 2004; 94:96–99.

259. Wadden TA, Berkowitz RI, Sarwer DB, et al. Benefits of lifestyle modification in the pharmacologic treatment of obesity: a randomized trial. Arch Intern Med 2001; 161:218–227.

260. Phelan S, Wadden TA. Combining behavioral and pharmacological treatments for obesity. Obes Res 2002; l0:560–574.

261. Keller MB, McCullough JP, Klein DN, et al. A comparison of nefazodone, the cognitive-behavioral analysis system of psychotherapy, and their combination for the treatment of chronic depression. N Engl J Med 2000; 342:1462–1470.

262. Lam DH, Watkins ER, Hayward P, et al. A randomized controlled study of cognitive therapy for relapse prevention for bipolar affective disorder: outcome of the first year. Arch Gen Psychiatry 2003; 60:145–152.

263. March J, Silva S, Petrycki S, et al. Treatment for Adolescents with Depression Study (TADS) Team. Fluoxetine, cognitive-behavioral therapy, and their combination for adolescents with depression: treatment for adolescents with depression study (TADS) randomized controlled trial. JAMA 2004; 292:807–820.

264. Pampallona S, Bollini P, Tibaldi G, et al. Combined pharmacotherapy and psychological treatment for depression. A systematic review. Arch Gen Psychiatry 2004; 61:714–719.

265. Branson R, Potoczna N, Kral J, et al. Binge eating as a major phenotype of melanocortin 4 receptor gene mutations. N Engl J Med 2003; 348:1096–1103.

266. Shinohara M, Mizushima H, Hirano M, et al. Eating disorders with binge eating behavior are associated with the s allele of the 3'-UTR VNTR polymorphism of the dopamine transporter gene. Rev Psychiatr Neurosci 2004; 29:134–137.

267. Hudson JL, Mangweth B, Pope HG Jr, et al. Family study of affective spectrum disorder. Arch Gen Psychiatry 2003; 60:170–177.

268. Christensen L. Effects of eating behavior on mood: a review of the literature. Int J Eat Disord 1993; 14:171–183.

269. McElroy SL, Pope HG Jr, Keck PE Jr, et al. Are impulse control disorders related to bipolar disorder? Compr Psychiatry 1996; 37:229–240.

270. Tremblay LK, Naranjo CA, Cardenas L, et al. Probing brain reward system function in major depressive disorder: altered response to dextroamphetamine. Arch Gen Psychiatry 2002; 59:409–416.
271. Wang G-J, Volkow ND, Telang F, et al. Exposure to appetitive food stimuli markedly activates the human brain. Neuro Image 2004; 21:1790–1797.
272. McElroy SL. Diagnosing and treating comorbid (complicated) bipolar disorder. J Clin Psychiatry 2004; 65(suppl 15):35–44.
273. McElroy SL, Arnold LM, Shapira NA, et al. Topiramate in the treatment of binge eating disorder associated with obesity: a randomized, placebo-controlled trial. Am J Psychiatry 2003; 160:255–261.
274. Johnson BA, Ait-Daoud N, Bowden CL, et al. Oral topiramate for treatment of alcohol dependence: a randomized controlled trial. Lancet 2003; 361: 1677–1685.
275. LeFoll B, Goldberg SR. Cannabinoid CB_1 receptor antagonists as promising new medication for drug dependence. J Pharmacol Exp Ther 2005; 312:875–883.

4

Eating Disorders in Obesity

L. K. George Hsu

Department of Psychiatry, Tufts-New England Medical Center,
Boston, Massachusetts, U.S.A.

Clinical experience suggests that eating disturbances are very common among obese individuals, although there is no epidemiological survey to confirm this. In 1959, Stunkard described three abnormal eating patterns among the obese population: binge eating, night eating, and eating without satiation (1). In the intervening years only the first two disturbances have received much attention, and this chapter is therefore devoted to binge eating disorder and night eating syndrome.

BINGE EATING DISORDER

Clinical Features

Currently, a binge is defined in behavioral terms. According to the DSM-IV-TR, there are two characteristics to a binge (2). First, eating a definitely larger amount of food in a discrete period of time than most people would in a similar period of time under similar circumstances. Second, presence of a feeling of lack of control over eating during the episode. Neither of these terms is subject to precise definition or measurement.

The concept of a binge eating episode is derived from the Greek term bulimia, or ox-appetite, a form of hunger first recognized by Hippocrates as definitely pathological (3). The shift of definition from abnormal appetite to abnormal behavior is interesting and presumably made to facilitate more precise definition and measurement, although as pointed out, this aim is far from having been achieved. Binge eating disorder (BED) is currently included as a diagnostic category for further study in Appendix B of the DSM-IV-TR, and can be technically diagnosed as an eating disorder not otherwise specified (EDNOS) (2). Diagnostically, according to the DSM-IV-TR, the duration and binge frequency of BED are currently somewhat arbitrarily set at six months and two days a week, respectively. The duration of an individual binge episode has not been precisely defined. Although the duration of two hours is given as an example in the DSM criteria, some 25% of subjects reported much longer periods of bingeing (4). Also, the amount of food consumed during an episode has not been precisely defined, and as reviewed later, is highly variable. In addition, the loss of control over eating during the episode is rated as present or absent according to the subject's subjective response, and may be problematic for a clinician or researcher to decide if it is really present. With all these problems of definition, perhaps it is not surprising that a recent study found that 66% of 38 carefully diagnosed non-BED women to report one or more binge episodes in a six-day period [Ref. (5); discussed in the section "Eating Disturbances in BED".]

Nevertheless, the validity of the construct of BED has been confirmed by several studies. Fairburn et al. (6,7) and Wilfley et al. (8) identified relatively distinct risk factors, clustering of symptoms, and course and outcome for the disorder. Bulik et al. (9) applied latent class analysis to nine eating disorder symptoms of some 2000 female twins and found a category of eating disorder broadly resembling BED. Furthermore, BED individuals have higher medical and psychiatric comorbidity than non-BED individuals, including suicidal ideation, although the level of psychopathology is less than those with bulimia nervosa (10–12). Medical morbidity includes increased reports of headaches, joint pains, gastrointestinal symptoms, menstrual problems, shortness of breath, chest pain, and type II diabetes (13). Comorbid psychopathology includes depression, anxiety, somatoform symptoms, and personality disturbances (14,15). The subjective distress of binge eaters is independent of their overweight status (16). BED is also associated with impaired quality of life, but whether this impairment is related to weight status, depression, or binge eating is still debatable (17,18). Unexpectedly, one study found no increase in eating or other psychiatric disorders among the first-degree relatives of BED subjects in comparison with their non BED obese counterparts, but more studies are needed (19). Despite some contrary opinions, the category of BED is probably here to stay, although it is likely that the diagnostic criteria will be refined (20,21). Changes will likely focus on how to delineate the disorder from generalized overeating on the one hand, and from bulimia nervosa, particularly the nonpurging subtype, on the other (22).

BED occurs mainly in obese subjects and its prevalence in this population is around 8% (12). Among those seeking weight loss treatment, the prevalence is around 30% (2). In the U.S. general population, where some 60% are overweight or obese, the prevalence is 0.7% to 4% (2). Onset is in the early 20s, and the female-to-male ratio is about three to two. In contrast to anorexia nervosa and bulimia nervosa, BED affects blacks as well as whites (23). Risk factors include childhood and family history of obesity, negative comments by others regarding weight, shape and eating, low self-esteem, and family history of parental depression (6). The onset of binge eating may precede that of dieting in at least one-third of BED individuals, particularly among those with an early onset of binge eating (24–27). This suggests that characterological impulsivity may be another risk factor, at least for a subgroup of BED subjects who also have personality disturbances (27). Dietary restraint has been implicated as a risk factor for binge eating for some time, but recent data on this issue are conflicting [Refs. (27–30); also discussed in the next section]. One study found emotional eating to be more common in BED (31). Mood disturbance as a risk factor is reviewed in the following section on eating disturbances.

Eating Disturbances in BED

By self-report, BED individuals have higher food intake than non-BED individuals, are more prone to emotional eating, i.e., eating when distressed or anxious, and are more prone to eating after a period of dietary restraint (28,31,32). However, self-reports of food intake are notoriously inaccurate, as subjects of all age groups and weight status have been found to be unreliable in reporting food intake (33). Attempts to improve accuracy and reliability in assessment of food intake have included the use of hand-held computers (ecological momentary recall), feeding laboratories, and doubly labeled water.

For example, Greeno et al. (5) used hand-held computers to measure mood, appetite, and setting of eating episodes in 41 BED and 38 non-BED women. This momentary assessment is probably less prone to recall bias associated with weekly or daily self-reports. As mentioned earlier, 25 of 38 (66%) non-BED women reported of having at least one binge episode during the six days of the study. This was unexpected since BED status was carefully diagnosed by a two-stage strategy including the use of the Eating Disorder Examination, a well-validated, state-of-the-art interview instrument (34). The calories consumed during the BED and non BED binges were similar. However, the antecedents of binge episodes differed between the two groups. As expected, antecedents to BED binges consisted of low mood, low alertness, feelings of poor eating control, and craving for sweets. Among non-BED binges, the antecedents consisted of only feelings of poor eating control and sweet cravings. Le Grange et al. (35), in a separate study using similar methodology, confirmed these findings. These studies highlight the difficulties in the diagnosis of BED and the study of eating behaviors in obese subjects, but they confirm the occurrence of emotional eating in BED.

Earlier feeding laboratory studies of BED have been reviewed by Walsh and Boudreau (36). This direct observation approach to study feeding under controlled circumstances circumvents some of the shortcomings of self-report studies. The findings may be summarized as follows. Obese BED individuals consistently ate more calories than their non-BED counterparts, regardless of whether they were instructed to binge eat or just eat normally. Among BED subjects, amount of calories consumed was positively correlated with body mass index (BMI). Studies on precipitants of binge eating have produced less consistent findings. Induction of negative mood and longer period of food deprivation did not precipitate larger binges, but a greater amount and variety of foods offered did. However, these results may be related to methodological differences among the studies. Three recent feeding laboratory studies have extended these findings. Geliebter et al. (37) found that amount of intake in overweight women was correlated with stomach volume, which was larger in BED than non-BED subjects. Nasser et al. (38) found impulsivity scores to be higher in BED subjects, and mood disturbance and impulsivity to be related to amount of test meal intake. Our group used a liquid meal to study obese patients for 24 hours, before and after gastric bypass surgery, and found BED subjects to consume more of the liquid meal before surgery (39). After surgery, consumption decreased significantly in both groups.

Doubly labeled water is a technique used to study total energy expenditure in weight stable subjects, in whom energy intake is equal to energy expenditure. Thus, it can be used to study energy intake in these subjects. Our group used the doubly labeled water technique to study severely obese subjects before and after gastric bypass and found energy expenditure to be correlated with BMI in both BED and non-BED subjects (39). The significance of these findings is discussed below.

Pathogenesis of BED

Very little is known about the pathogenesis of BED. Quantitative genetic studies of BED are rare. In the Virginia population-based sample of 2163 female twins, Bulik et al. (40) conducted bivariate twin modeling to study the relationship between genetic and environmental risk factors for obesity and binge eating. They found substantial heritability for obesity (86%), moderate heritability for binge eating (49%), and modest overlap in the genetic risk factors that increase liability for each condition. In a study of 8045 twins of same and opposite sex from a Norwegian twin registry, Reichborn-Kjennerud et al. (41), using the best fitting biometrical model, found heritability of binge eating to be 41%. Clearly, more studies are needed.

Molecular genetic studies of BED are also rare. Mutations in the melanocortin 4 receptor gene (MC4R) may be associated with binge eating and obesity (42,43). Because the anorexigenic neuropeptide alpha-MSH is a potent agonist of MC4R, this finding is particularly exciting but needs replication (44). Various peptides have been recently identify, which may play a role in the central control of eating (45,46). Although the field is advancing rapidly, the neuropeptide control of eating behavior and energy metabolism is likely to be complex.

Brief reference was already made to our group's study of energy expenditure in severe obesity (39). Our findings suggest that obesity and binge eating appear not to be related to a disturbance in energy expenditure. If confirmed, it would appear that more disturbances may occur on the side of energy intake.

Treatment and Outcome

The psychological and nutritional treatment of BED has been the subject of a recent review (47). Briefly, psychological treatments that are effective for bulimia nervosa are also effective for BED. Thus, cognitive behavioral therapy (CBT) is effective in BED, in which about 40% of patients became abstinent, 20% drop out, and 40% show a decrease in bingeing frequency. This improvement is maintained at one-year follow-up. However, there is no significant weight loss even in those who have achieved abstinence, although a small amount of weight loss may occur with time. Interpersonal therapy produces improvement rates similar to CBT. Dietary treatments such as very low calorie diets (VLCDs) and behavioral self-management strategies are also effective in the short term; 50% of subjects achieve and maintain abstinence at one year. Moreover, VLCDs result in significant weight loss in BED subjects of 15 to 20 kg. Long-term outcome of dietary treatments for weight loss, however, appears less favorable, as much of the weight is regained.

Pharmacological treatment has also been the subject of a recent review (48). Briefly, serotonergic antidepressants are somewhat effective in decreasing binge eating, but are not as effective in producing weight loss. The appetite suppressant sibutramine is effective in decreasing binge frequency and producing weight loss, but the data are more limited relative to those for serotonergic antidepressants. Topiramate, an anticonvulsant, has been found in several open trials and one double-blind trial to be significantly more effective than placebo in decreasing binge frequency and in inducing weight loss. Its side effects may limit more widespread use.

Antidepressants, including the serotonergic agents, do not add effectiveness to CBT in the treatment of BED, but whether topiramate or sibutramine will is not known.

Bariatric surgery is effective in producing weight loss and abstinence in severely obese BED patients (49). Available long-term follow-up data suggest that a recurrence of binge eating sometimes occurs at two years after surgery and is more likely with gastric banding than bypass.

These treatment data need to be reviewed in the context of diagnostic difficulties and the naturalistic outcome of BED. First, BED may be an unstable diagnosis. Self-reports of binge eating are unreliable (see section on eating disturbances) and its assessment may contaminate treatment findings. Second, binge-eating decreases significantly even among those assigned to weight list control groups (50). The naturalistic five-year outcome of BED is quite encouraging, with only 10% of subjects diagnosed with BED at the beginning of one community survey still receiving the diagnosis five years later (6). Finally, the response rate of BED to placebo treatment is very high (51). Perhaps the issue is that we need more effective treatments for obesity, and not for BED per se.

NIGHT EATING SYNDROME

Night eating syndrome (NES) is not included in the DSM-IV-TR. The prevalence of NES is probably very low in the general population, but it apparently increases with increasing BMI. One study found that 27% of obese subjects seeking bariatric surgery suffer from NES (52). Our own study found that only 5% had NES by self-report, but many subjects consumed significant amounts of a liquid meal during the midnight to 8 A.M. time period during their stay in a clinical study unit (53). Furthermore, clinical experience suggests that many severely obese BED subjects may develop NES after they have stopped binge eating and successfully lost weight, and that NES in these individuals may be difficult to treat since eating often occurs in total or partial unconsciousness (54).

In recent provisional criteria, morning anorexia and evening hyperphagia have been added as defining features (51,55). NES subjects awaken on average 3.6 times per night, and consume large amounts of food during half of such awakenings (55). One intriguing feature is the marked blunting of plasma melatonin levels at night of NES subjects.

There are no published data on the treatment of NES. Stunkard (51) has suggested that serotonergic agents may be helpful.

REFERENCES

1. Stunkard AJ. Eating patterns and obesity. Psychiatr Quart 1959; 33:284–294.
2. American Psychiatric Association. Diagnostic and Statistical Manual of Mental Disorders. 4th ed. Text Revision. Washington D.C., American Psychiatric Association, 2000.
3. Stunkard AJ. A history of binge eating. In: Fairburn CG, Wilson GT, eds. Binge Eating: Nature Assessment, and Treatment. New York: Guilford, 1993:15–34.
4. Marcus MD, Smith D, Santelli R, et al. Characterization of eating disordered behavior in obese binge eaters. Int J Eat Disord 1992; 12:249–255.

5. Greeno CG, Wing RR, Shiffman S. Binge antecedents in obese women with and without binge eating disorder. J Consult Clin Psychol 2000; 68:95–102.
6. Fairburn CG, Doll HA, Welch SL, Hay PJ, Davis BA, O'Connor ME. Risk factors for binge eating disorder: A community based, case-control study. Arch Gen Psychiatry 1998; 55:425–432.
7. Fairburn CG, Cooper Z, Doll HA, Norman PA, O'Connor ME. The natural course of bulimia nervosa and binge eating disorder in young women. Arch Gen Psychiatry 2000; 57:659–665.
8. Wilfley DE, Friedman MA, Dounchis JZ, et al. Comorbid psychopathology in binge eating disorder: Relation to eating disorder severity at baseline and following treatment. J Consult Clin Psychol 2000; 69:383–388.
9. Bulik CM, Sullivan PF, Kendler KS. An empirical study of the classification of eating disorders. Am J Psychiatry 2000; 157:886–895.
10. Bulik CM, Sullivan PF, Kendler KS. Medical and psychiatric morbidity in obese women with and without binge eating. Int J Eat Disord 2002; 32:72–78.
11. Johnsen LA, Gorin A, Stone AA, et al. Characteristics of binge eating among women in the community seeking treatment for binge eating or weight loss. Eat Behav 2003; 3:295–305.
12. Dingemans AF, Bruna MJ, van Furth EF. Binge eating disorder: A review. Int J Obes Relat Metab Disord 2002; 26:299–307.
13. Bulik CM, Reichborn-Kjennerud T. Medical morbidity in binge eating disorder. Int J Eat Disord 2003; 34:S39–S46.
14. Picot AK, Lilenfeld LR. The relationship between binge severity, personality pathology, and body mass index. Int J Eat Disord 2003; 34:98–107.
15. van Hanswijck de Jonge P, van Furth EF, Lacey JH, waller G. The prevalence of personality pathology among individuals with bulimia nervosa, binge eating disorder, and obesity. Psychol Med 2003; 33:1311–1317.
16. Didie ER, Fitzgibbon M. Binge eating and psychological distress: Is the degree of obesity a factor? Eat Behav 2005; 6:35–41.
17. Masheb RM, Grilo CM. Quality of life in patients with binge eating disorder. Eat Weight Disord 2004; 9:194–199.
18. Kolotkin RL, Westman EC, Ostbye T, et al. Does binge eating disorder impact weight-related quality of life? Obes Res 2004; 12:999–1005.
19. Lee YH, Abbott DW, Seim H, et al. Eating disorders and psychiatric disorders in the first-degree relatives of obese probands with binge eating disorder and obese non-binge eating disorder controls. Int J Eat Disord 1999; 26:322–332.
20. Stunkard AJ, Allison KC. Binge eating disorder: Disorder or marker? Int J Eat Disord 2003; 34:S107–S116.
21. Devlin MJ, Goldfein JA, Dobrow I. What is this thing called BED? Current status of binge eating disorder nosology. Int J Eat Disord 2003; 34:S2–S18.
22. Cooper Z, Fairburn CG. Refining the definition of binge eating disorder and nonpurging bulimia nervosa. Int J Eat Disord 2003; 34:S89–S95.
23. Striegel-Moore RH, Franko DL. Epidemiology of binge eating disorder. Int J Eat Disord 2003; 34:S19–S29.
24. Grilo CM, Marsheb RM. Onset of dieting vs. binge eating in outpatients with binge eating disorder. Int J Obes 2000; 24:404–409.

25. Mussell MP, Mitchell JE, Weller CL, Raymond NC, Crow SJ, Crosby RD. Onset of binge eating, dieting, obesity and mood disorders among subjects seeking treatment for binge eating disorder. Int J Eat Disord 1995; 17:395–401.
26. Marcus MD, Moulton MM, Greeno CG. Binge eating onset in obese patients with binge eating disorder. Addict Behav 1995; 20:747–755.
27. Spurrell EB, Wilfley DE, Tanofsky MB, Brownell KD. Age of onset for binge eating: Are there different pathways to binge eating? Int J Eat Disord 1997; 21:55–65.
28. Herman CP, Polivy J. From dietary restraint to binge eating: Attaching causes to effects. Appetite 1990; 14:123–125.
29. Marcus MD, Wing RR, Hopkins J. Obese binge eaters: Affect, cognitions, and response to behavioral weight control. J Consult Clin Psychol 1988; 56:433–439.
30. Masheb RM, Grilo CM. On the relation of attempting to lose weight, restraint, and binge eating in outpatients with binge eating disorder. Obes Res 2000; 8:638–645.
31. Pinaquy S, Chabrol H, Simon C, Louvet JP, Barbe P. Emotional eating, alexithymia, and binge eating disorder in obese women. Obes Res 2003; 11:195–201.
32. Raymond NC, Neumeyer B, Warren CS, Lee SS, Peterson CB. Energy intake patterns in obese women with binge eating disorder. Obes Res 2003; 11:869–879.
33. Schoeller DA, Fjeld CF. What have we learned from the doubly labeled water method? Ann Rev Nutr 1991; 11:355–375.
34. Fairburn CG, Cooper Z. The eating disorder examination. In: Fairburn CG, Wilson GT, eds. Binge Eating: Nature, Assessment, and Treatment. New York: Guilford, 1993:317–360.
35. Le Grange D, Gorin A, Catley D, Stone AA. Does momentary assessment detect binge eating in overweight women that is denied at interview? Eur Eating Disord Rev 2001; 9:309–324.
36. Walsh BT, Boudreau G. Laboratory studies of binge eating disorder. Int J Eat Disord 2003; 34:S30–S38.
37. Geliebter A, Yahav EK, Gluck ME, Hashim SA. Gastric capacity, test meal intake, and appetitive hormones in binge eating disorder. Physiol Behav 2004; 81:735–740.
38. Nasser JA, Gluck ME, Geliebter A. Impulsivity and test meal intake in obese binge eating women. Appetite 2004; 43:303–307.
39. Das SK, Roberts SB, Me Crory MA, et al. Long-term changes in energy expenditure and body composition following massive weight loss induced by gastric bypass surgery. Am J Clin Nutr 2003; 78:22–30.
40. Bulik CM, Sullivan PF, Kendler KS. Genetic and environmental contributions to obesity and binge eating. Int J Eat Disord 2003; 33:293–298.
41. Reichborn-Kjennerud T, Bulik CM, Tambs K, Harris JR. Genetic and environmental influences on binge eating in the absence of compensatory behaviors: a population based study. Int J Eat Disord 2004; 36:307–314.
42. Farooqi IS, Keogh JM, Yeo GSH, Lank EJ, Cheetham T, O'Rahilly S. Clinical spectrum of obesity and mutations in the melanocortin 4 receptor gene. NEJM 2003; 348:1085–1095.

43. Branson R, Potoczna N, Kral JG, Lentes KU, Hoehe MR, Horber FF. Binge eating as a major phenotype of melanocortin 4 receptor gene mutation. NEJM 2003; 348:1096–1103.
44. List JF, Habener JF. Defective melanocortin 4 receptors in hyperphagia and morbid obesity. NEJM 2003; 348:1160–1163.
45. Hokfelt T, Bartfei T, Bloom F. Neuropeptides: Opportunity for drug discovery. Lancet Neurol 2003; 2:463–472.
46. Neary NM, Small CJ, Bloom SR. Gut and mind. Gut 2003; 52:918–921.
47. Wonderlich SA, de Zwaan M, Mitchell JE, Peterson C, Crow S. Psychological and dietary treatments of binge eating disorder: Conceptual implications. Int J Eat Disord 2003; 34:S58–S73.
48. Carter WP, Hudson JI, Lalonde JK, Pindyk L, McElroy SL, Pope HG. Pharmacologic treatment of binge eating disorder. Int J Eat Disord 2003; 34: S74–S88.
49. Hsu LKG, Benotti PN, Dwyer J, et al. Non-surgical factors that influence that outcome of bariatric surgery. Psychosom Med 1998; 60:338–346.
50. Carter JC, Fairburn CG. Cognitive behavioral self help for binge eating disorder. A controlled effectiveness study. J Consult Clin Psychol 1998; 66:616–623.
51. Stunkard AJ. Binge eating disorder and night eating syndrome. In: Wadden TA, Stunkard AJ, eds. Handbook of Obesity Treatment. New York: Guilford, 2002:107–124.
52. Rand CSW, Macgregor MD, Stunkard A. The night eating syndrome in the general population and among post-operative obesity surgery patients. Int J Eat Disord 1997; 22:65–69.
53. Hsu LKG, Mulliken B, McDonagh B, et al. Binge eating disorder in extreme obesity. Int J Obes 2002; 22:65–69..
54. Schenk CH, Mahowald MW. Review of sleep-related eating disorders. Int J Eat Disord 1994; 16:343–356.
55. Birketvedt G, Florholmen J, Sundsfjord J, et al. Behavioral and neuroendocrine characteristics of the night eating syndrome. JAMA 1999; 282:657–663.

5

Obesity and Substance Use Disorders

Mark S. Gold, Helen C. Oppenheim, and Kimberly Frost-Pineda
Department of Psychiatry, Neuroscience, Anesthesiology, and Community Health and Family Medicine, University of Florida, Gainesville, Florida, U.S.A.

> *"Never get too hungry, angry, lonely or tired"*
> —*Alcoholics Anonymous advice for avoiding a drug relapse.*

Hunger stimulates drug taking, so do not become too hungry warns the HALT acronym at the 12 step meetings around the globe. Hunger, anger, loneliness, and insomnia can all trigger bouts of eating or drug taking. Also heard at the 12 step meetings around the United States: "No one uses drugs of abuse after Thanksgiving dinner." Thus, the relationship among food, overeating, drugs, and moods has been established for the recovering community. Since neurobiological research often confirms the axioms and wisdom in the Big Book, we have been investigating these relationships for the past decade.

INTRODUCTION

Obesity and substance use disorders (SUDs) are both major public health issues in the United States and other industrialized nations of the world. Both obesity and SUDs cause preventable premature death, disability, and contribute to an ever-expanding health care budget (1). Tobacco use is still the number one cause of death at 435,000 per year; however, poor diet and sedentary lifestyle may soon displace tobacco as the leading cause of premature death in the United States (2). Indeed, other studies suggest that obesity is overtaking smoking as the number one cause of early death with the largest increase in the last 10 years (3). While obesity is now considered a disease, comorbidity with depression, certain medical disorders, personality disorders, and addiction are still in question (4). Addiction is also considered a disease, and was accepted recently as a disease of the brain (5). Obesity may also become recognized as a brain disease. Use of a drug, like cocaine or heroin may initially be under voluntary control, but insidiously over time becomes more automatic. Loss of control and continued use despite social, economic, and health consequences has become the hallmark of addictive diseases. Similarly, replace the drug of choice with food and the DSM-TV substance use disorders appear similar if not identical to the DSM-IV eating disorders characterized by binge eating (Table 1). Though research focusing on the relationships among substance abuse, obesity, and eating disorders is limited, recent studies suggest a strong correlation among certain aspects of these disorders (1,6,7).

EATING DISORDERS/SUBSTANCE ABUSE COMORBIDITY

The Road from Naïve to Obsessed

A critical question is how a person progresses from drug naive or normal weight to drug or food obsessed with cravings, continued and compulsive use regardless of consequence, and loss of control. For opiates, even a single use has been shown to cause important changes in the brain that might be seen as early evidence of motivational toxicity or changes (8). Opiates stimulate opioid receptors and produce neuroadaptive changes in multiple areas of the brain. However, the mesolimibic dopamine system has been increasingly seen as the critical site for the motivational changes produced by drugs of abuse. Naive animals respond differently compared to those who have had prior drug experiences. The dopamine rich ventral tegmental area may be the site for a switch process from dopamine independent to dopamine dependent reward (9). Distinct brain mechanisms underlie illicit drug use in the preabuse state and in those who have lost control and are dependent. Just as the brain is unprepared by evolution for powerful drugs of abuse like heroin or cocaine, it may also be unprepared for gourmet, preprocessed, and energy dense foods. However, many drugs were tried by our ancestors to produce euphoria and the current drugs of abuse are all known by their ability to stimulate self-administration, so too, foods have been "improved" on the basis of their ability to induce self-administration or increase sales receipts. The more rewarding and compelling the foods are, the more we go to certain restaurants or choose certain foods.

Link Between Eating Disorders and Substance Use Disorders

Research focused on eating disordered patients has reported high rates of co-occurring SUDs. Thus, persons suffering from binge eating disorder

Table 1 Comparison of DSM-IV Binge Eating and Substance Dependence Criteria

DSM-IV criteria for SUD	DSM-IV criteria for binge eating

A maladaptive pattern of substance use leading to clinically significant impairment or distress, manifested by three or more of the following, occurring within a 12-month period:
 Tolerance
    Need for increased amount to achieve the desired effect
    Diminished effect with continued use of the same amount
 Withdrawal
    Characteristic withdrawal symptom for the substance
    The same or similar substance is taken to avoid withdrawal symptoms
 Substance is taken in larger amounts or over a longer period than intended
 Persistent desire or unsuccessful attempts to cut down or control use
 Great deal of time is spent obtaining, using, or recovering from the substance
 Important activities are reduced or given up because of the substance
 Continued use despite adverse consequences
	Recurrent episodes of binge eating characterized by both
	 Eating in a discrete period of time (e.g., two hours) an amount of food that is much larger than most people would eat in a similar time period under similar circumstances
	 A sense of lack of control over eating during the episode
	 Episodes include three or more of the following:
	 Eating much more rapidly than normal
	 Eating until feeling uncomfortably full
	 Eating large amounts of food when not feeling physically hungry
	 Eating alone because of being embarrassed by how much one is eating
	 Feeling disgusted with oneself, depressed or very guilty after overeating
	 Marked distress regarding binge eating is present
	 The binge eating occurs on an average of at least two days a week for six months
	 The binge eating is not associated with the regular use of inappropriate compensatory

Abbreviation: SUD, substance use disorders.

are significantly more likely to have first degree relatives with a substance abuse disorder (10–12). Studies have also found that substance abuse rates in families of bulimic patients and in the morbidly obese are significantly higher than in families of controls (4,7,10). Hudson et al. (13) evaluated

386 consecutive patients hospitalized for SUDs for co-occurring eating disorders, and found that 15% of the women had a lifetime diagnosis of anorexia or bulimia nervosa. Women with eating disorders had significantly higher rates of stimulant abuse and lower rates of opioid abuse when compared to women without eating disorders. Furthermore, bulimia was found to be elevated in alcohol-dependent persons with rates of 6.17% and 1.35% in women and men, respectively (13). Initiation of disordered eating normally begins before substance abuse problems, according to retrospective reports of patients with concurrent disorders. A 10-year follow-up study on 18 binge-eating patients without a pre-existing substance abuse disorder found that 50% developed a dual diagnosis by the end of the study (14). Another study found that binge eaters were more likely to use all types of substances, with a high rate of cannabis use (11).

Obesity and Substance Use

Obesity, substance abuse, and substance dependence have increased alarmingly in adolescents (15). We suspect and have hypothesized that these increases are related (1). Currently, it has been estimated that one in five adolescents in the United States can be classified as overweight, while another one in four adolescents is at risk of becoming overweight (16–18). The centers for disease control and prevention describes adolescent obesity as an epidemic responsible for the dramatic increase in childhood type II diabetes (17). What was once "adult onset diabetes" is now called Type II diabetes in recognition of the ever increasing numbers of children and adolescents with this body mass-related disease (18).

Weight and substance abuse in adolescence have been shown to be good predictors of adult weight and substance abuse, respectively (1,19). This has suggested that early experience with either drugs or highly rewarding, energy-rich foods can change the brain and modify behavior, making continued use and abuse more likely. Drugs of abuse and food appear to compete for brain sites, and abstinence from drug use causes craving for drugs and also for food. As noted earlier, in drug treatment meetings it is said that no one uses cocaine after Thanksgiving dinner. Thus, there appears to be a neurochemical reason for why overeating and satiety reduce drug use. In animals, drug self-administration rates are increased by starvation and decreased by overfeeding (20). Competition between food and drugs of abuse at brain sites, critical for reward and pleasure, may explain the common comorbidities of starvation or bingeing and purging and drug use on the one hand and morbid obesity and lack of drug use on the other hand (21). While tobacco use causes weight loss and has effects on leptin, cessation of tobacco use has the opposite effects and has been associated with increased eating, weight gain, and the risk of obesity (22). Recent studies suggest that tobacco-cessation related weight gain is related to increased food reward (23). Supervised abstinence from any type of substance dependence causes a rebound in drug and food cravings. Adolescents often experience significant weight gain while abstinent from alcohol and illicit drugs (1,17). While it is successful in treating the primary drug addiction, drug rehabilitation programs must include preventative diet and exercise programs to avoid replacing addiction with another. These data along with others suggest that early drug use and drug addiction may sensitize and change the brain in such a way that it makes drug relapse, overeating, and other co-occurring disorders more likely.

Correlations with Depression

Studies of patients with obesity and those with substance abuse patients commonly find positive correlations with depressive symptoms and mood disorders. Drugs of abuse produce depression so reliably that they are used as model systems to test new antidepressants (24). Each Amphetamine withdrawal, cocaine withdrawal, and nicotine withdrawal produce chemical states identical to naturally occurring major depression. Moreover, drug-induced depression stimulates more drug self-administration, and drug-induced depression during abstinence drives relapse. Thus, the co-occurrence of drug abuse and depression is the rule rather than the exception.

Alcohol use also dramatically increases the risk of suicidal behavior among alcohol-dependent and alcohol-independent individuals (25–28). Glassman et al. (29). documented a strong positive correlation between nicotine dependence and depression. Furthermore, individuals with personal or family histories of depression are at increased risk for depressive episodes during smoking abstinence and are more likely to relapse (29). This correlation has been posited to be due to nicotine's antidepressant capability. Cigarette smoking is seen in eating disorders, including those with depression or dysphoria. In addition, depressed patients frequently smoke cigarettes and drink alcohol, while those who smoke and drink commonly have depression. One out of every three suicide victims has a history of substance abuse and higher rates of substance abuse are observed in teenage suicides (30).

Obese individuals also show higher rates of major depression and depressive symptoms than nonobese individuals in many clinical and some epidemiological studies (discussed in chap. 10). Studies have found lower self efficacy ratings in overweight binge eaters when compared to overweight nonbinge eaters. Furthermore, women consistently report greater binge eating, greater depression, and lower self-efficacy (31). However, the relationship between obesity and depressive disorders is difficult to ascertain because of confounding diagnosis criteria. Symptoms for obesity including irregular sleep patterns, increased appetite, and decreased sex drive may be interpreted as false positives for the DSM IV criteria for depression. Indeed, in contrast to the many studies reporting high rates of depression in bariatric surgery patients, we have found a remarkable sense of well-being reported by patients at our bariatric clinic with morbid obesity. Suicide is often seen in individuals suffering from substance abuse but is generally not observed in obese patients. Another possibility, therefore, is that overeating is a better "antidepressant" than drug abuse.

The Role of Culture in Comorbid Disorders

Finally, culture appears to play a role in the relationship between obesity and substance abuse, because patients with eating disorders in Western countries have higher rates of comorbid substance abuse (32,33). Substance-related disorders were found in 9% to 55% of patients with bulimia, 0% to 19% of patients with anorexia, and 10% to 44% of obese binge eaters (34–39). Thus, eating disorders are far more common in cultures with plentiful food supplies and few individuals eat in response to hunger alone. Culture and food availability likely play a role in the variable concepts of hunger, satiation, and satiety. Hunger is defined as both the physiological drive to eat and the perceived desire to eat, while satiation is the process that ends eating. Satiety is the state after the completion of eating behavior in which further eating is inhibited. Eating disorders and obesity may be divided into related groups that affect either aspect of the eating process. Feeding is regulated by a complex coordinated system designed to meet an organism's metabolic needs by integrating peripheral afferent signals, reward, endocrine response, energy states, drive and mood states, micronutrient intake and supply, neurotransmitter responses, and efferent motor commands within the central nervous system (40). Disruptions of this primitive reward system can cause self-perpetuating maladaptive behaviors which are seen in both eating disorders and substance abuse disorders (40).

NEUROTRANSMITTERS AND PEPTIDES

Neurotransmitters and the Reward System

The role of neurotransmitters may provide valuable insight to the common, primitive reward pathway, which is disrupted in both eating disorders and substance abuse disorders (Table 2). The primary function of the neurotransmitters, which are "hijacked" by drugs of abuse is the regulation and control of eating. If drug addiction undermines survival instincts and changes the brain, as it appears, the question is, where in the brain? Naturally, the initial candidates for the effect of drugs of abuse are endogenous ligands which are related to the drug itself. So, it follows that opiates stimulate endogenous opioid systems, cannabis stimulates the endogenous cannabinoid systems, and so on. All of these systems appear to be involved in a coordinated effort to maintain the species through the reinforcement of eating (and other behaviors such as sexual procreation). The more we learn

Table 2 Orexigenic and Anorexigenic Neuropeptides and Neurotransmitters

Orexigenic	Anorexigenic
NPY	Serotonin
AgrP	α-MSH, TSH
GABA	CART
Ghrelin	Insulin
Galanin	Leptin
β-Endorphin	Cholescystokinin
Dynorpbin	Dopamine
GHRH	Neurotensin
Norepinephrine	CRF
Anandamide	Glucagon, enterostatin, calcitonin, amylin, bombesin, somatostatin, cytokines

Abbreviations: AgrP, agouti related peptide; CART, cocaine and amphetamine regulating transcript; CRF, corticotrophin-releasing-factor; GABA, γ-aminobutyric acid; GHRH, growth hormone releasing hormone; α-MSH, alpha-melanocyte-stimulating hormone; NPY, neuropeptide Y; TSH, thyroid stimulating hormone.

about the sites where drugs of abuse act, the more they appear to overlap with those used to regulate and reinforce eating. This may be the link between overeating and drug abuse.

The Hypothalamus

Control of feeding behavior has been localized to the hypothalamus using various techniques including brain lesions, microinjections of drugs and neuropeptides, and microdialysis studies of neurotransmitter levels (40–42). Appetite regulation primarily involves the appetite regulating network (ARN) which consists of distinct orexigenic and anorexigenic circuitries operating in the arcuate nucleus-paraventricular nucleus (PVN) axis of the hypothalamus (Table 2). Appetitive drive is modulated by excitatory messages from the lateral hypothalamus and inhibitory messages from the ventromedial nucleus (41–43). Disrupted communication between these two sites results in unabated hyperphagia and abnormal weight gain (40,44,45). Short-term energy homeostasis is regulated by opposing humoral signals including anorexigenic leptin from adipocytes and orexigenic ghrelin from the stomach (46–49). Understanding of the ARN provides insight related to appetitive drive in patients with eating disorders and obesity and parallel drug cravings in substance abuse patients (44).

Dysfunctional Regulation

Eating disorders and obesity are both suspected to represent dysfunctional regulation of neurotransmitters such as dopamine (DA) and serotonin

(5HT), and endogenous opioids and other neuropeptides (40). As food has changed from a human version of Purina Lab Chow to 5 Star cuisine and fast food, its rewarding quality has become more evident. Eating for pleasure has become commonplace. Food has evolved to smell, look, taste, and feel great. Food is presented on the plate in a way that resembles art. Hedonic food is appreciated by all of the senses and acts in the brain as if it is a drug of abuse. The gourmet experience in a 5 Star restaurant looks, smells, and feels like a Beverly Hills drug party with a set of sights, smells, sounds, and expectations aimed at stimulating the brain's reward pathways. The hedonic reward pathway for food ingestion begins processing in the brainstem, and animal models of food intake show opioid mediation of the reward value of food. The lateral hypothalamus, ventral striatum, shell of the nucleus accumbens, and the central amygdala are all structures related to the endogenous opioid system (50,51). Opioid agonists specific for the mu receptor have been shown to induce a strong increase in food intake, while opioid antagonists, such as naltrexone, have been shown to block the pleasure derived from food intake (51). Opioid and DA systems are related and much of the work in humans relating obesity to substance abuse has involved the study of the human DA system by PET imaging. The dopaminergic system appears to provide a common crucial link in the brain reward pathway of addiction. Anticipation of food, sex, or drug reward induces a dopaminergic priming to enhance the experience. Drugs of abuse may be in competition with food at brain sites responsible for species survival reinforcement, but as the experiences at Woodstock demonstrated, they do not compete with sex. Consider the casual associations among food, sex, and drugs; individuals commonly desire a cigarette or coffee after a good meal, or alcohol use before sex, and a cigarette afterwards. Furthermore, patients frequently substitute binge eating for alcohol during early recovery from alcoholism. While DA has been the focus of initial study, neuropeptides may be key in the relationship between food and substance abuse (40).

Other Neuropeptides

Neurotensin: Neurotensin (NT) is an inhibitory neuropeptide which has an important relationship with DA and the regulation of appetite and drug use. NT-containing neurons are found within title mesencephalon and diencephatlon. Within the former structure, NT-containing neurons originate in the ventral tegmental area (VTA) and end in the substantia nigra pars compacta (SNC), the nucleus accumbens (nAC), the caudate, the putamen, the prefrontal cortex, and the central median amygdale; in the latter structure NT-containing neurons are found within the zona incerta and median eminence (40,52).

Studies show that chronic cocaine administration and withdrawal disrupts normal NT–DA interactions from the nerve cell bodies to the nerve cell terminals. Cocaine use up-regulation of postsynaptic NT receptors followed by increased NT binding in the prefrontal cortex and the SNC. This phenomenon is believed to be caused by the depletion of NT from NT–DA nerve terminals from VTA projections to the prefrontal cortex and SNC. Thus, enhanced DA levels cause a selective depletion of NT and an imbalance in the NT–DA system (40,53).

Neuropeptide Y: Neuropeptide Y (NPY), one of the most abundant and widely distributed neuropeptides, is a potent orexigenic compound that has been shown to induce uncontrolled hyperphagia leading to obesity. NPY is a member of the pancreatic polypeptide family and is involved in the regulation of other hormones and neurotransmitters and appears involved in circadian rhythms. Administration of NPY into the PVN induces massive carbohydrate intake, while administration of anti-NPY agents decreases spontaneous carbohydrate intake in animals. NPY has been demonstrated as a viable model for hyperphagia and obesity in which chronic NPY administration produces an obesity syndrome (40,54). Methamphetamine alters the expression of neuropeptide Y and changes leptin, ghrelin, and insulin (Satya Kalra, personal communication). Inhibition of NPY expression may underlie the weight loss effects of psychostimulants. Amphetamine and other stimulants release DA and other neurotransmitters, which in turn have effects that inhibit appetite and eating. Stimulation of D2 dopamine receptors, for example, decreases NPY expression and microinjection of amphetamine or fenfluramine into the paraventricular region inhibits NPY-induced feeding.

The opioid antagonist naloxone blocks the orexigenic effects of NPY when injected intracerebroventricularly, peripherally, and when placed in the fourth ventricle. These data suggest that the NPY has numerous receptors within the brain, though the particular NPY receptor responsible for increased carbohydrate intake remains unknown (55). One theory suggests that NPY and galanin reinforce existing macronutrient preference by increasing the attraction for carbohydrates and fats by enhancing specific tastes, smells, or textures (40).

VTA and nAC are considered the neural centers modulating positive reinforcement. Processes within the VTA and nAC reinforce survival behaviors such as feeding and sex (56). Numerous authors have reported an increase in the extracellular level of DA in the nAC during food ingestion (57–62) and use of cocaine and other self-administered drugs (63–65). This evidence implies a relationship between food intake and the mesolimbic dopamine system similar to that of illicit drug reinforcement (40).

THE PROCESS OF ADDICTION

The process of addiction for substances including drags, tobacco, and alcohol is modulated by reinforcement and neuroadaptation. The general reward pathway includes the VTA and the basal forebrain, and the use of drugs has been shown to change the neural processes around these connections. The mesolimbic dopamine system connects the VTA to the basal forebrain and is critical for the self-administration of psychomotor stimulants (1,66).

Dopamine deficiency has been suggested to be a common characteristic of individuals who are prone to drug or food addiction (1). Thus, studies have shown that obese individuals have abnormalities in brain dopamine activity, where striatal dopamine receptor (DRD2) availability is significantly lower than in control groups. Also, body mass index (BMI) was shown to correlate inversely with measures of D2 receptors (67). Thanos et al. (68) examined ethanol preferring rats over-expressing DRD2, and found that an increase in striatal dopamine receptors resulted in reductions in alcohol preference and alcohol intake.

Studies examining BMI and alcohol usage provide strong support for the theory that overeating and drugs compete for common brain reward sites. Kleiner et al. (21) found an inverse relationship between BMI and rates of alcohol use in women. This study also showed that BMI increased during alcohol abstinence.

Primary reinforcers, including feeding, drinking, copulation, and drugs of abuse, have a direct effect upon the medial forebrain bundle (40). Normal feeding behavior is typically induced by hunger. Studies show that food deprivation-induced hunger enhances the reward effects of both feeding and illicit drugs. Food ingestion or drug use, in turn, produces satiation. Thus, illicit drugs such as cocaine compete with food for the same hunger–reward–satiation pattern and become an acquired primary drive equated with survival (40).

Common Reward Pathways

Obesity, eating disorders, and SUDs may share a common neuroanatomical and neurochemical basis. SUDs may access brain reward through exogenous, illicit drugs, while obesity and eating disorders may access the same pathways through dietary and environmental manipulations. A thorough understanding of the relationship among obesity, eating disorders, and SUDs may be essential for developing more effective and focused treatment strategies (40).

Thus, recent imaging studies have shown that medial prefrontal circuits appear to be activated by inappropriate stimuli (such as a disgust response to food stimuli) in those with eating disorders and those who are addicted (69). As noted earlier, neurotransmitter release, including DA, in the nucleus accumbens has been associated with self-administration, anticipatory changes, and learning similar to that seen with drugs of abuse. Significant hyperphagia and weight gain is observed during supervised and confirmed drug abstinence, lending support to the aforementioned common pathway theory. Thus, subjects use food as a replacement for drugs of choice (1). Amphetamines, cocaine, and substituted amphetamines like MDMA cause weight loss for appetite suppression in certain doses, and are important reinforcing drugs of abuse. Cannabis and alcohol stimulate eating at low doses and have an opposite effect among addicts who prefer and prioritize drug self-administration to eating, hygiene, and other behaviors. Drugs of abuse have important and consistent effects on eating, and eating disturbances are frequent problems in the treatment of patients with addictions.

Eating Disorders and Obesity as Addictions

Recent advances have led to an expansion of the definition of addiction to encompass overeating and obesity as addictions to food. As discussed earlier, imaging studies support the notion that food and drugs of abuse share common neurological reward pathways. Addictions involving both food and drugs also share similar etiologies and behavioral symptoms. Furthermore, various pharmacological agents used to treat drug abuse have also been effective in treating obesity: these include topiramate, bupropion, and to a lesser extent, naltrexone and naloxone (70). Finally, treatment strategies need to focus on treating food and drug addictions concurrently or else one disorder may worsen as the other improves.

Hyperphagia Induced by Abstinence

Numerous studies confirm the strong, positive correlation of smoking cessation with hyperphagia resulting in weight gain and an increase in BMI in both adults and adolescents (71). Hyperphagia induced by abstinence may be a mechanism to replenish the release of neurotransmitters in the reward system (1). Recent studies suggest that drug self-administration is correlated with taste and diet preference, since human adults and animals substitute carbohydrates, fats, and sweets for alcohol and cocaine (72–74). This evidence further supports the notion of a common drug/food reward system (1,74).

Models of Addiction

Neuroscience studies, clinical experience, and functional magnetic resonance imaging studies support the hypothesis that overeating and obesity can be viewed as SUDs (4). Formerly, addiction was believed to result from an individual avoiding distress from substance withdrawal. This model considered addiction treatment equivalent to treating drug withdrawal. However, this theory was called into question when significant improvements in antiwithdrawal agents did little to improve outcome for addiction. Withdrawal and its associated distress have increasingly become recognized as not central to the understanding and treatment of addictive diseases. Drug use and ultimately addiction is now viewed as a progressive disease with underlying neuroadaptations in which the experience of drug use overtakes the endogenous sites used to reinforce species survival. In this model, smoking a cigarette might be interpreted as saving the species. Similarly, overeating might cause similar changes in the brain and behavior. Pathological attachment to food is certainly a problem for the 21st century where food is highly palatable, abundant, and energy dense. Expansions of the former withdrawal theory of addiction have therefore led to inclusion of cocaine and other drugs with minor withdrawal syndromes and new substances, including food into the model of abuse (40). Essentially, in eating disorders and obesity, food is the substance of abuse. A vast scientific literature and clinical experience supports the model of food as an addictive substance that may become subject to abuse.

Loss of control: Patients who feel unable to control food consumption report food as being addicting or extremely rewarding (40). Animal studies show that activation of the hedonic food reward system depends in part on palatability (64,65). Given a more palatable diet, animals display hyperphagia and become obese (75–77). While passive drug administration is not addicting, active drug seeking behavior for their euphoric effects is addicting. Similarly, merely eating cake does not suggest an eating disorder, while eating cake secretly raises concerning questions. The development of a pathological attachment to food makes binge eating or obesity fall into the category of addiction (40). Thus, behavioral patterns in eating disorders and obesity closely parallel those of addictive disorders (40).

Impulsive and compulsive behavior: Eating disorders, including those associated with obesity, are characterized by impulsive and compulsive features strikingly similar to those found in SUDs. Thus, patients with binge eating behavior display symptoms similar to substance abusers in which they describe craving for specific foods or urges to binge, and report of being unable to control their consumption. Indeed, part of the diagnostic criteria for bulimia nervosa and binge eating disorder is the inability to control food intake (Table 1). Similar to substance abuse patients, eating disorders cause cognitive dysfunction and food is used to alleviate negative affect (78). Eating disordered behaviors are frequently viewed as habit forming and serve the purpose of relieving tension or stress in certain individuals. For example, subjects suffering from bulimia nervosa and binge-eating disorder commonly report that unpleasant affect is decreased while they are bingeing or purging (79). Both disorders commonly include social isolation to prevent others from learning their abnormal eating patterns (80,81). Patients with binge eating are often secretive about their disorder, when they are alone, and may hide or hoard food for bingeing (82).

Denial: Patients with obesity or eating or SUDs show similar stubbornness in maintaining and denying "abusive" behavior despite the presence and severity of the disorder. Just as an alcoholic will continue to drink with endstage liver disease, an anorexic patient will continue to starve herself despite emaciation. Similarly, a person with obesity will continue to overeat or binge eat despite full awareness of the adverse health effects of their obesity and overeating. Moreover, the chronic effects of both overeating and drug abuse are commonly different from those originally achieved. Binge eating is often initially associated with reduced dysphoria, but when done chronically it induces dysphoric states. Similarly, chronic use of alcohol may produce anxiety, despite the user's original intended use for sedation and relaxation.

Modes of Treatment

If obesity and eating disorders were similar to addictions, we might expect treatments used for one to be efficacious in the other. Abstinence approaches, though effective for substance use disorders, are not an option for obesity and eating disorders. We must eat to survive. Even strict restriction tends to create the potential for loss of control over eating in eating disorders (78). While diet-related abstinence tends to undermine effective treatment, patients can learn to maintain a healthy balanced diet without strict abstinence from certain foods.

In the past, patients diagnosed with both eating disorder and substance abuse were usually treated separately for each disorder. However, this treatment strategy has proven ineffective, as when both problems are not treated concurrently, the patient will substitute one substance for the other. Given two primary, similarly severe disorders, concurrent and aggressive treatment is essential (79,80). However if the two disorders differ in severity, the primary condition should be prioritized in treatment (79).

Pharmacotherapy: Several psychopharmacologic treatment strategies are used in obesity, eating disorders, and SUDs. Treatments that may be effective in dual diagnosed disorders include topiramate, naltrexone, and benzodiazepines. Topiramate is an antiepileptic drug which has been shown to be effective in placebo-controlled trials for treatment of obesity, binge-eating disorder, bulimia nervosa, and alcohol dependence. Naltrexone is used in the treatment of opioid addiction and alcoholism, causes weight loss, and may have beneficial effects in bulimia nervosa. Benzodiazepines are used for alcohol withdrawal and to lessen preprandial anxiety in anorexia nervosa.

Naloxone, melanocortin MC-4 receptor agonists, and leptin specifically suppress carbohydrate and fat intake (83). Δ^9-THC encourages fat and carbohydrate intake while a study by Rinaldi-Carmona et al. (84) showed that the cannabinoid antagonist SR 141716 blocks carbohydrate-rich food intake (85). Other studies suggest that cannabinoid receptor antagonism reduces food intake by reducing the reward value of the food (86–88). Verty et al. (88) presented evidence that the CB_1 antagonist SR 141716

[*N*-piperidino-5-(4-chlorophenyl)-l-(2,4-dichlorophenyl)-4-methylpyrazole-3-carboxamide, Sanofi-Synthelabo] suppresses food intake irrespective of food palatability in nondeprived rats. This agent appears to have efficacy in weight loss as well as smoking cessation through the cannabinoid system (89).

Phentermine and fenfluramine are amphetamine analogs used in combination in the past (as PHEN/FEN) for the treatment of obesity (90). Though both drugs are proven appetite suppressants their mechanisms of action differ. Phentermine produces amphetamine-like stimulant effects, increases extracellular DA in the brain (91–95), and is self-administered by animals. Unlike phentermine, fenfluramine does not produce stimulant effects, is not self-administered by animals, and is rarely abused by humans (96). Fenfluramine administration leads to release of 5-HT from neurons (94,97). Of note, the combination of phentermine and fenfluramine has been shown to decrease cravings, alleviate withdrawal symptoms, and prolong drug abstinence in cocaine addicts (97). Also, individuals often self-administer drugs of abuse, such as amphetamines, for their weight loss effects.

12-step groups: 12-step treatments are widely used, with success, for all SUDs. They are especially helpful in overcoming shame, depression, and guilt that comes with addictive and eating disorders. Though abstinence is commonly used in the 12-step treatment for drug abuse, abstinence from eating is impossible. Rather, a more effective treatment for obesity and eating disorders involves building recognition as to how behaviors are used for self-soothing, substituting alternative, less-destructive coping mechanisms, and re-establishing healthful patterns of eating (79).

CONCLUSIONS

It has become increasingly apparent that there is a strong relationship among obesity, eating disorders, and SUDs. Addictions involving both food and drugs share similar etiologies and behavioral symptoms. Current treatment programs for alcohol, tobacco, and illicit drug abuse tend to focus on the SUDs while ignoring the effects of abstinence on weight gain. Specifically, little, if any attention, is given to nutritional counseling, exercise, and education concerning the substitution of food for substances of abuse. Effective treatment protocols are needed for comorbid obesity, SUDs, and eating disorders. Research is also necessary to delineate the neuroanatomical and neuropharmacological relationships between overeating and addictions.

REFERENCES

1. Hodgkins CC, Cahill KS, Seraphine AE, Frost-Pineda K, Gold MS. Adolescent drug addiction treatment and weight gain. J Addict Dis 2004; 23(3):55–65.

2. Marshall E. Public enemy number one: tobacco or obesity. Science 2004; 7:804.
3. Mokdad AH, Marks JS, Stroup DF, Gergerding JL. Actual causes of death in the United States, 2000. JAMA 2004; 291:1238–1245.
4. Liu Y, Gold MS. Human functional magnetic resonance imaging of eating and satiety in eating disorders and obesity. Psychiatr Ann 2003; 33(2):127–132.
5. World Health Organization. Neuroscience of Psychoactive Substance Use and Dependence, Switzerland, 2004.
6. Kaye WH. Understanding eating disorders. Psychiatry Today. MS Gold, ed. Available online at: http://www.psychiatry.ufl.edu/Newsletters/Content/ kaye.pdf. Last Accessed July 6, 2004.
7. Krahn DD, Kurth C, Demitrack M, Drewnowski A. The relationship of dieting severity and bulimic behaviors to alcohol and other drug use in young women. J Subst Abuse 1992; 4:341–353.
8. Schulteis G, Heyser CJ, Koob GF. Opiate withdrawal signs precipitated by naloxone following a single exposure to morphine: potentiation with a second morphine exposure. Psychopharmacology 1997; 129:56–65.
9. Laviolette SR, Gallegos RA, Henriksen SJ, van der Kooy D. Opiate state controls bidirectional reward signaling via GABA-A receptors in the ventral tegmental area. Nat Neurosci 2004; 7:160–169.
10. Yanovski SZ, Nelson JE, Dubbert BK, Spitzer RL. Association of binge eating disorder and psychiatric comorbidity in obese subjects. Am J Psychiatry 1993; 150(10):1472–1479.
11. Ross HE, Ivis F. Binge eating and substance use among male and female adolescents. Int J Eat Disord 1999; 26:245–260.
12. Bulik CM, Sullivan PF, ICendler KS. Medical and psychiatric morbidity in obese women with and without binge eating. Int J Eat Disord 2002; 32(l):72–78.
13. Hudson JL, Pope HG, Jonas JM et al. Family history study of anorexia nervosa and bulimia. Br J Psychiatry 1983; 17:883–890.
14. Halmi K, Eckert E, Marchi P, Sampugnaro V, Apple R, Cohen J. Comorbidity of psychiatric diagnoses in anorexia nervosa. Arch Gen Psychiatry 1991; 48:712–718.
15. Hedley AA, Ogden CL, Johnson CL, Carroll MD, Curtin LR, Flegal KM. Prevalence of overweight and obesity among US children, adolescents, and adults, 1999–2002. JAMA 2004; 291:2847–2850.
16. Dietz W. Childhood obesity. In: Shils M, Olsen J, Sbike M et al., eds. Modem Nutrition in Health and Disease. 9th ed. Baltimore: Williams and Wilkins, 1999:1071–1080.
17. Hodgkins CC, Jacobs WS, Gold MS. Weight gain after adolescent drug addiction treatment and supervised abstinence. Psychiatr Ann 2003; 33(2):112–115.
18. CDC. Youth risk behavioral surveillance. Atlanta: Centers for Disease Control, 2000.
19. Whitaker RC, Wright JA, Pepe MS. Predicting obesity in young adulthood from childhood and parental weight. NEJW 1997; 337:869–873.
20. Miller CC, Murray TF, Freeman KG, Edwards GL. Cannabinoid agonist, CP 55,940, facilitates intake of palatable foods when injected into the hindbrain. Physiol Behav 2004; 80(5):611–616.

21. Kleiner KD, Gold MS, Frost-Pineda K, Lenz-Brunsman B, Perri MG, Jacobs WS. Body mass index and alcohol use. J Addict Dis 2004; 23(3):108–115.

22. Filozof C, Fernandez Pinilla MC, Fernandez-Cruz A. Smoking cessation and weight gain. Obes Rev 2004; 5(2):95–103.

23. Lerman C, Berrettni W, Pinto A, et al. Changes in food reward following smoking cessation: a pharmacogenetic investigation. Psychopharmacology 2004; 174(4):571–577.

24. Cryan JF, Markou A, Lucki I. Assessing antidepressant activity in rodents: recent developments and future needs. Trends Pharmacol Sci 2002; 23(5):238–245.

25. Murphy GE, Wetzel RD. The lifetime risk of suicide in alcoholism. Arch Gen Psychiatry 1990; 47(4):383–392.

26. Roy A, Linnoila M. Alcoholism and suicide. Suicide Life Threat Behav 1986; 16(2):244–273.

27. Borges G, Rosovsky H. Suicide attempts and alcohol consumption in an emergency room sample. J Stud Alcohol 1996; 57(5):543–548.

28. Young MA, Fogg LF, Scheflner WA, Fawcett JA. Interactions of risk factors in predicting suicide. Am J Psychiatry 1994; 151(3):434–435.

29. Glassman AH, Covey LS, Stetner F, Rivelli S. Smoking cessation and the course of major depression: a follow-up study. Lancet 2001; 357(9272): 1929–1932.

30. Gold MS. Adolescent suicide and drugs. Addict Recov 1991:15.

31. Linde JA, Jeffery RW, Levy RL, Sherwood NE, Utter J, Prank NP, Boyle RG. Binge eating disorder, weight control self-efficacy, and depression in overweight men and women. Int J Obes Relat Metab Disord 2004; 28(3):418–425.

32. Holderness CC, Brooks-Gunn J, Warren MP. Co-morbidity of eating disorders and substance abuse: review of the literature. Int J Eat Disord 1994; 16:1–34.

33. Lilenfeld LR, Kaye WH, Greeno CG, et al. Psychiatric disorders in women with bulimia nervosa and their first-degree relatives: effects of comorbid substance dependence. Int J Eat Disord 1997; 22:253–264.

34. Krahn DD. The relationship of eating disorders and substance abuse. J Subst Abuse 1991; 3:239–253.

35. Mitchell JE, Specker SM, deZwaan M. Comorbidity and medical complications of bulimia nervosa. J Clin Psychiatry 1991; 52:13–20.

36. Bulik CM, Sullivan PF. Comorbidity of bulimia and substance abuse: perceptions of family or origin. Int J Eat Disord 1993; 13:49–56.

37. Mitchell JE, Pyle RL, Specker S, Hanson K. Eating disorders and chemical dependency. In: Yager J, Gwirtsman HE, Edelstein CK, eds. Special Problems in Managing Eating Disorders. Washington, DC: American Psychiatric Press, 1992.

38. Wilson GT. The addiction model of eating disorders: a critical analysis. Adv Behav Res Ther 1991; 13:27–72.

39. Kanter RA, Williams BE, Cummings C. Personal and parental alcohol abuse, and victimization in obese binge eaters and non-bingeing obese. Addict Behav 1992; 17:439–445.

40. Gold MS, Star J. Eating disorders in substance abuse a comprehensive textbook. 2nd ed. In: Lowinson JH, Ruiz P, Mailman RB eds. York, PA Williams and Wilkins, chapter 27, 2004:469–488.

41. Bray, GA. Historical framework for the development of ideas about obesity. In: George A. Bray, Claude Bouchard, James WPT, eds. Handbook of Obesity, Vol. 1. New York: Marcel Dekker, 1998:1–29.
42. Kalra SP, Dube MG, Pu S, Xu B, Horvath TL, Kalra PS. Interacting appetite-regulating pathways in the hypothalamic regulation of body weight. Endocr Rev 1999; 20:68–100.
43. Anand BK, Brobeck JR. Hypothalmic control of food intake in rats and cats. Yale J Biol Med 1951; 24:123–146.
44. Kalra SP, Kalra PS. Overlapping and interactive pathways regulating appetite and craving. J Addict Dis 2004; 23(3):5–21.
45. Weingarten HP, Parkinson W. Ventromedial hypothalamic lesions eliminate acid secretion elicited by anticipated eating. Appetite 1988; 10:205–219.
46. Friedman JM, Halaas JL. Leptin and the regulation of body weight in mammals. Nature 1998; 395:763–770.
47. Kojima M, Hosoda H, Date Y, Nakazato M, Matsuo H, Kangawa K. Ghrelin is a growth-hormone-releasing acylated peptide from stomach. Nature 1999; 402:656–660.
48. Tschop M, Smiley DL, Heiman ML. Ghrelin induces adiposity in rodents. Nature 2000; 407:908–913.
49. Nakazato M, Murakami N, Date Y, Kojima M, Matsuo H, Kangawa K, Matsukura S. A role for ghrelin in the central regulation of feeding. Nature 2001; 409:194–198.
50. Holland PC, Petrovich GD, Gallagher M. The effects of amygdala lesions on conditioned stimuls-potentiated eating in rats. Physiol Behav 2002; 76:117–129.
51. Kelley AE, Bakshi VP, Haber SN, Steininger TL, Will MJ, Zhang M. Opioid modulation of taste hedonics within the ventral striatum. Physiol Behav 2002; 76:365–377.
52. Kaschow J, Nemeroff CB. The neurobiology of neurotensin: focus on neurotensin-dopamine interactions. Regul Pept 1991; 26:153–164.
53. Gold MS. Are eating disorders addictions? Adv Biosci 1993; 90:455–463.
54. Sahu A, Kaka SP. Neuropeptide regulation of feeding behavior: neuropeptide Y. TEM 1993; 4(7):217–224.
55. Kotz, CM, Grace MK, Briggs J, Levine AS, Billington CJ. Effects of opioid antagonists naloxone and naltrexone on neuropeptide Y-induced feeding and brown fat thermogenesis in the rat. J Clin Invest 1995; 96:163–170.
56. Gold MS. Clinical implications of the neurobiology of addiction. In: ASAM Official Manual, Basic Science. Bethesda: American Society of Addiction Medicine 1994, Section 1, Chapter 4.
57. Hernandez L, Hoebel B. Feeding and hypothalamic stimulation increase dopamine turnover in the accumbens. Physiology 1988; 44:599–606.
58. Hernandez L, Hoebel BG. Feeding can enhance dopamine turnover in the prefrontal cortex. Brain Res Bull 1990; 24:975–979.
59. Mogenson GJ. Studies of the nucleus accumbens and its mesolimbic dopaminergic affects in relation to ingestive behaviors and reward. In: Hoebel GB, Noving D, eds. Neural Basis of Feeding and Reward. Brunswick: Haer Institute, 1982: 275–506.

60. Radhakishun FS, van Ree JM, Westerink BH. Scheduled eating increases dopamine release in the nucleus accumbens of food-deprived rata as assessed with on-line brain dialysis. Neurosci Lett 1988; 82:351–356.
61. Yoshida M, Yokoo H, Mizoguchi K, Kawahara H, Tsuda A, Nishikawa T, Tanaka M. Eating and drinking cause increased dopamine release in the nucleus accumbens and ventral tegmental area in the rat: Measurement by in vivo microdialysis. Neurosci Lett 1992; 139:73–76.
62. Young AM, Joseph MN, Gray JA. Increased dopamine release in vivo in nucleus accumbens and caudate nucleus of the rat during drinking: A microdialysis study. Neuroscience 1992; 48:871–876.
63. Miller NS, Gold MS. A hypothesis for a common neurochemical basis for alcohol and drug disorders. Psychiatr Clin North Am 1993; 16:105–117.
64. Fantino M. Properties sensorielles des aliments et controle de la prise alimentaire. Sci Alim 1987; 7:5–16.
65. Grill HJ, Berridge KC. Taste reactivity as a measure of the neural control of palatability. Prog Psychobiol Physiol Psychol 1985; 11:1–61.
66. Roberts AJ, Koob GF. The neurobiology of addiction: An overview. Alcohol Health Res World 1997; 21:101–106.
67. Wang GJ, Volkow ND, Logan J, et al. Brain dopamine and obesity. Lancet 2001; 357:354–357.
68. Thanos PK, Volkow ND, Freimuth P, et al. Overexpression of dopamine D2 receptors reduces alcohol self-adrninistration. J Neurochem 2001; 78:1094–1103.
69. Uher R, Murphy T, Brammer MJ, et al. Medial prefrontal cortex activity associated with symptom provocation in eating disorders. Am J Psychiatry 2004; 161(7):1238–1246.
70. Bay HE. Current and investigational antiobesity agents and obesity therapeutic treatment targets. Obes Res 2004; 12:1197–1211.
71. Klesges RC, Robinson LA, Zbikowski SM. Is smoking associated with lower body mass in adolescents? A large-scale biracial investigation. Addict Behav 1998; 23:109–113.
72. Krahn DD, Kurth C, Demitrack M, Demitrack M, Drewnowski A. The relationship of dieting severity and bulimic behaviors to alcohol and other drug use in young women. J Subst Abuse 1992; 4:341–353.
73. Gosnell BA, Krabn DD, Yracheta JM, Harasha BJ. The relationship between intravenous cocaine self-administration and avidity for saccharin. Pharmacol Biochem Behav 1998; 60:229–236.
74. Gosnell BA, Krahn DD. Taste and Diet Preferences as Predictors of Drug Self-administration. Washington DC, National Institute on Drug Abuse, 2001: 154–175.
75. Louis-Sylvestre J, Giachetti I, Le Magnen J. Sensory vs. dietary factors in cafeteria-induced overweight. Physiol Behav 1984; 32:901–905.
76. Rolls BJ. Palatability and food preference. In: Diaffi AL et al., eds. The Body Weight Regulatory System: Normal and Disturbed Mechanisms. New York: Raven Press, 1981:271–278.
77. Sclafani A, Berner CN. Influence of diet palatability on the meal taking behavior of hypothalamic hyperphagic and normal rats. Physiol Behav 1976; 16: 355–363.

78. Krahn DD. The relationship of eating disorders and substance abuse. J Subst Abuse 1991; 3:239–253.
79. Becker A. Update on eating disorders. Psychiatry Today. MS Gold, ed. Available online at: http://www.psychiatry.ufl.edu/Newsletters/Content/becker.pdf. Last Accessed July 6, 2004.
80. Butterfield PS, LeClair S. Cognitive characteristics of bulimic and drug-abusing women. Addict Behav 1988; 13:131–138.
81. Marcus MD, Wing RR, Ewing L, Kern E, Gooding W, McDermott M. Psychiatric disorders among obese binge eaters. Int J Eating Disord 1990; 9:69–77.
82. Zweben JA. Eating disorders and substance abuse. J Psychoactive Drugs 1987; 19:181–191.
83. Marks-Kaufman R, Kanarek RB. Modifications of nutrient selection induced by naloxone in rats. Psychopharmacology (Berl) 1981; 74(4):321–324.
84. Rinaldi-Carmona M, Barth F, Heaulme M, et al. SR141716A, a potent and selective antagonist of the brain cannabinoid receptor. FEBS Lett 1994; 350(2–3):240–244.
85. Koch JE, Matthews SM. Delta9-tetrahydrocannabinol stimulates palatable food intake in Lewis rats: effects of peripheral and central administration. Nutr Neurosci 2001; 4(3):179–187.
86. Higgs S, Williams CM, Kirkham TC. Cannabinoid influences on palatability: microstructural analysis of sucrose drinking after delta(9)-tetrahydrocannabinol, anandamide, 2-arachidonoyl glycerol and SR141716. Psychopharmacology (Berl). 2003; 165(4):370–377. Epub 2002 November 22.
87. Freedland CS, Poston JS, Porrino LJ. Effects of SR141716A, a central cannabinoid receptor antagonist, on food-maintained responding. Pharmacol Biochem Behav 2000; 67(2):265–270.
88. Verty AN, McGregor IS, Mallet PE. Consumption of high carbohydrate, high fat, and normal chow is equally suppressed by a cannabinoid receptor antagonist in non-deprived rats. Neurosci Lett 2004; 354(3):217–220.
89. Anthenelli RM. On behalf of the study investigators, using a cannabinoid receptor antagonist as an aid to smoking cessation: STRATUS-US. Poster presented at The Metabolic Syndrome, Type II Diabetes and Atherosclerosis Congress Meeting, Marrakech, Morocco, May 2004.
90. Baumann MH, Ayestas MA, Dersch CM, Brockington, Rice KC, Rothman RB. Effects of phentermine and fenfluramine on extracellular dopamine and serotonin in rat nucleus accumbens: therapeutic implications. Synapse 2000; 36(2):102–113.
91. Cox RH Jr, Maickel RP. Comparison of anorexigenic and behavioral potency of phenylethylamines. J Pharmacol Exp Ther 1972; 181(l):1–9.
92. Griffiths RR, Brady JV, Snell JD. Relationship between anorectic and reinforcing properties of appetite suppressant drugs: implications for assessment of abuse liability. Biol Psychiatry 1978; 13(2):283–290.
93. Shoaib M, Baumann MH, Rothman RB, Goldberg SR, Schindler CW. Behavioural and neurochemical characteristics of phentermine and fenfluramine administered separately and as a mixture in rats. Psychopharmacology (Berl) 1997; 131(3):296–306.

94. Balcioglu A, Wurtman RJ. Effects of phentennine on striatal dopamine and serotonin release in conscious rats: in vivo microdialysis study. Int J Obes Relat Metab Disord 1998; 22(4):325–328. .

95. Rowland NE, Carlton J. Neurobiology of an anorectic drug: fenfluramine. Prog Neurobiol 1986; 27(1):13–62.

96. Berger UV, Gu XF, Azmitia EC. The substituted amphetamines 3,4-meihylene-dioxymeibamphetarnine, methamphetamme, *p*-chloroamphetamine and fenfluramine induce 5-hydroxytryptamine release via a common mechanism blocked by fiuoxetine and cocaine. Eur J Pharmacol 1992; 215(2–3):153–160.

97. Rothman RB, Gendron T, Hitzig P. Hypothesis that mesolimbic dopamine (DA) plays a key role in mediating the reinforcing effects of drugs of abuse as well as the rewarding effects of ingestive behaviors. J Subst Abuse Treat 1994; 11(3):273–275.

6

Obesity and Smoking

Jaimee L. Heffner
Mental Health Care Line, Cincinnati Veterans Affairs Medical Center, Cincinnati, Ohio, U.S.A., and Department of Psychology, Ohio University, Athens, Ohio, U.S.A.

Suzan Winders-Barrett
Mental Health Care Line, Cincinnati Veterans Affairs Medical Center, and Department of Psychology and Psychiatry, University of Cincinnati College of Medicine, Cincinnati, Ohio, U.S.A.

Robert M. Anthenelli
Department of Psychiatry and Neuroscience, Tri-State Tobacco and Alcohol Research Center and Addiction Sciences Division, University of Cincinnati College of Medicine and Cincinnati Veterans Affairs Medical Center, Cincinnati, Ohio, U.S.A.

Based on the definition of obesity established by the World Health Organization (i.e., body mass index of $30 \, kg/m^2$ or greater), approximately one-quarter of the United States population aged 20 or older are classified as obese (1). The prevalence of obesity in the United States has nearly doubled since the early 1970s (2). If this figure is not sufficiently disquieting, consider the projected prevalence of obesity among United States adults if we extrapolate from the current trends reported by Schiller et al. (1): Given that obesity rates rose an average of 0.81% per year from 1997 to 2004, a continued increase at this same rate over the next 30 years would result in one-half of the United States adult population being classified as obese.

The increasing prevalence of obesity is quite alarming from a public health perspective, as obesity increases the risk of morbidity and mortality. More specifically, obese individuals are at higher risk than normal weight individuals for developing and dying from diabetes, cardiovascular disease, and several forms of cancer (3–8). An estimated 365,000 people in the United States die from overweight- and obesity-related causes each year (9). From an economic standpoint, the health care costs attributable to obesity represent a substantial proportion (5.5–7.0%) of annual health care expenditures in the United States, totaling around $70 billion per year (10,11). Considering that these figures do not even include indirect costs, such as the loss of productivity, that can be associated with obesity-related functional impairments, the economic cost of obesity is clearly significant.

Cigarette smoking, much like obesity, is a burden upon the health care system and accounts for a substantial number of preventable deaths in the United States and worldwide each year. Examining figures from the United States alone, over 430,000 deaths per year are attributable to the direct effects of smoking (9). Like obesity, smoking has been linked to cardiovascular disease, several forms of cancer, and type 2 diabetes (12). Additionally, smoking has been causally linked to respiratory diseases (e.g., chronic obstructive pulmonary disease and pneumonia), reproductive problems (e.g., reduced fertility), and a variety of other health problems such as cataracts and low bone density (12). Smoking is associated with increased risk of all-cause mortality as well as risk of death from cancer, cardiovascular disease, and chronic obstructive pulmonary disease (13). In terms of economic costs, health care expenditures that can be directly attributed to smoking account for 6% to 8% of national health care costs, or over $70 billion (12). Again, this estimate does not include indirect costs such as loss of productivity, which may even surpass the direct costs according to some estimates (12). Fortunately, unlike obesity, the rates of smoking in the United States have been decreasing steadily in recent years from 24.7% in 1997 to 20.1% in 2004 (1).

Given the aforementioned negative health consequences of both obesity and smoking, one would intuitively predict increased risk of mortality associated with combined obesity and smoking as opposed to either obesity or smoking alone. Consistent with this prediction, Peeters et al. (14) calculated life expectancies for middle-aged smokers and found that those who were obese lost an additional seven years of life as compared to smokers of a normal weight. It appears, then, that the combined effects of obesity and smoking are more hazardous than either alone, placing the estimated 17.8% of smokers who are classified as obese at high risk for early death and disease (6).

In this chapter, we discuss the relationship between smoking and obesity by supplementing the findings of a previous review by Klesges et al. (15) that covered a vast body of literature on smoking and body weight with more current research on this topic. More specifically, we examine the effects of smoking cessation on weight gain and discuss the effectiveness of interventions to reduce or prevent weight gain following smoking cessation. We conclude, then, by summarizing the status of current research related to smoking and obesity and identifying areas that have not received adequate empirical attention.

SMOKING AND WEIGHT GAIN

Klesges et al. (15) concluded in their comprehensive review of the literature on smoking and weight that the majority of both cross-sectional and prospective studies conducted between 1970 and 1988 indicated that (i) current smokers weigh less than nonsmokers, and (ii) individuals tend to gain weight when they quit smoking. Because more recent evidence also supports these conclusions, the findings can be characterized as robust (16–19). Although it seems clear that weight gain following smoking cessation is the norm rather than the exception, research indicates that there is a great deal of variability in the amount of weight gained following smoking cessation. In this section, we explore the current status of research investigating the amount of weight gained as a result of smoking cessation and factors associated with greater postcessation weight gain. We also address the relationship between smoking cessation and obesity and examine how the health risks of postcessation weight gain compare with the benefits of quitting smoking.

What Factors Influence Postcessation Weight Gain?

In their classic review, Klesges et al. (15) reported an average weight gain of 6.4 lb following smoking cessation, with a range of 0.5 to 18.1 lb. The substantial variability in the average postcessation weight gain reported in the studies reviewed by Klesges et al. (15) is likely to be a result of both methodological variability across the studies and individual difference factors (e.g., gender, heaviness of smoking) that influence the magnitude of weight gain. Understanding these sources of variability is critical in evaluating the findings of studies reporting on postcessation weight gain and, as such, they will be explored in more detail in this section.

Methodological Differences

Several methodological differences may account for some of the variability in the amount of weight gained following smoking cessation. One methodological source of variability is the amount of time elapsed from the point of smoking cessation to the point at which weight is measured. Estimates of the amount of weight gained following smoking cessation can be expected to vary as a result of the length of smoking abstinence. In fact, some research has indicated that most of the weight gain observed after smoking cessation occurs within approximately one year of abstinence, with the sharpest increases noted in the first one to six months after cessation (20–23). Weight may still increase over a longer period of time, albeit at a slower pace, before finally leveling off (19,21). Given that the follow-up periods in the Klesges et al. (15) review ranged from 4 days to 40 years, then, one would expect to find a great deal of variability in the amount of postcessation weight gain reported.

Another important methodological source of variability is whether the estimate is based on continuous abstinence (i.e., absolutely no smoking since the identified quit date) or point prevalence abstinence (i.e., no smoking within a few days of the assessment). Klesges et al. (24) reported that smokers who were continuously abstinent for one year gained an average of 13 lb, whereas smokers who were considered abstinent using point prevalence criteria gained only half that amount (i.e., 6.7 lb). Thus, the operational definition of abstinence can have a significant impact on estimates of postcessation weight gain. As the Klesges et al. (24) study suggests, investigations utilizing more lenient definitions of abstinence (i.e., point prevalence) may underestimate the amount of weight gained as a result of discontinuing smoking.

Finally, a third methodological factor to consider is whether quitters achieved smoking abstinence with the aid of pharmacotherapies found to attenuate postcessation weight gain, such as sustained-release buproprion or nicotine gum (25,26). Clearly, studies in which participants have utilized treatments that are efficacious for both smoking cessation and postcessation weight control can be expected to produce results that are biased in the direction of underestimating weight gain, particularly during the period in which the treatment is used. As such, information regarding the type and duration of any pharmacological treatments used by study participants becomes critical to the interpretation of the results.

Individual Differences

Several longitudinal analyses have reported on individual difference variables that appear to moderate the relationship between smoking cessation and weight gain. Moderating variables that have received the most support are age, heaviness of smoking, race, and exercise behavior. The results of several studies indicate that people who are younger, heavier smokers, African American, and less physically active gain more weight following smoking cessation (15,19,21,27). Evidence regarding the relationship between precessation body weight and postcessation weight gain is mixed. Two studies demonstrated that smokers with higher pre-quit BMIs gained more weight than smokers with lower pre-quit BMIs, whereas another study suggested that only underweight female smokers are more likely to gain weight (19,21,26). Gender may also be a determining factor, although studies showing that women gain more weight than men appear to be outnumbered by those showing no gender differences in weight gain (16,19,21,28–30). Women may gain weight over a longer period of time, however. Nides et al. (31), for example, demonstrated that men's weight gain peaked within one year following smoking cessation while women's weight continued to increase throughout the two-year follow-up period, resulting in a greater overall gain for women at the two-year mark. Another factor to be taken into consideration when examining gender as a moderator of postcessation weight gain is that even where weight gain for men and women is demonstrated to be approximately equal, women are typically gaining a greater percent of their body weight than men due to the fact that men are, on average, heavier than women (21).

How Is Smoking Cessation Related to Obesity Trends?

There is some evidence that smokers are beginning to experience more post-cessation weight gain than they have in the past. For example, data from NHANES I (1971–1974) showed that 9.8% of male smokers and 13.4% of female smokers gained more than 13 kg (28.7 lb) within 10 years of quitting (19). In the NHANES III (1988–1994) sample, 16% of males and 21% of females reported more than a 15 kg (33.1 lb) weight increase within 10 years of their quit date (32). This observed increase in the frequency of large weight gains following smoking cessation seems even more significant when one takes into consideration the fact that NHANES III participants had access to pharmacological aids to smoking cessation that may attenuate or delay postcessation weight gain, such as nicotine gum, whereas NHANES I participants did not. Taken together with the finding that the prevalence of obesity in the United States is increasing while the prevalence of smoking is decreasing, these data might be interpreted as an indication that smoking cessation is contributing to increasing rates of overweight and obesity (1). It is unclear from the NHANES data alone, however, to what extent the increase in the frequency of significant weight gain following smoking cessation is attributable to the discontinuation of smoking as opposed to the general trend of increasing overweight and obesity in the United States.

Flegal et al. (32) addressed this issue empirically by using logistic regression models to calculate the expected prevalence of overweight in the NHANES III sample assuming that men and women who quit smoking in the past 10 years had continued to smoke. The expected prevalence for each sex was then compared to the actual prevalence to obtain a percentage difference, which was interpreted as the percentage increase in the prevalence of overweight and obesity attributable to smoking cessation. In this study, the authors determined that one-quarter of the increased prevalence of overweight and obesity in men and one-sixth of the prevalence in women between the NHANES II and NHANES III samples can be accounted for by smoking cessation (32). On the basis of these findings, then, it appears that smoking cessation has probably contributed to, but does not fully account for, the increasing prevalence of overweight and obesity in the United States. Even more compelling is the fact that the authors utilized a BMI cut-off for overweight (i.e., $27.8 \, kg/m^2$ for men and $27.3 \, kg/m^2$ for women) that is higher than the current standards of the World Health Organization ($25.0 \, kg/m^2$). As a result, the figures reported by Flegal et al. (32) may underestimate the influence of smoking cessation on the prevalence of overweight and obesity in the United States.

Does the Risk of Postcessation Weight Gain Outweigh the Benefits of Smoking Cessation?

Several authors have directly or indirectly posed the question as to whether a cost–benefit analysis of smoking cessation would result in the conclusion that the potential health risks of postcessation weight gain outweighed the potential benefits of continued smoking (i.e., benefits related to weight maintenance) (22,33,34). In a study examining risk of developing cardiovascular disease during menopause, Burnette et al. (33) concluded that women who gained weight following smoking cessation were not at greater risk than nonsmokers for cardiovascular problems despite the fact that they tended to gain more weight. In fact, the ex-smokers showed an increase in high-density lipoprotein cholesterol (HDL), a protective factor for cardiovascular disease, in spite of the weight gain.

Noting that smoking cessation can lead to obesity and that obesity can have a significant detrimental effect on pulmonary health, Wise et al. (22) investigated the impact of postcessation weight gain on lung condition. These authors found that the effects of weight gain on pulmonary functioning observed in smokers who quit were minimal compared with the negative effects of continued smoking. Wise et al. (22) estimated that a weight gain of 38 to 60 kg (i.e., 84–132 lb) would be required to rival the impact of continued smoking on lung functioning.

Finally, Wannamethee et al. (34) looked at the relationship between postcessation weight gain and risk for the development of type 2 diabetes. The results of this prospective study indicated that smokers who quit between the baseline measurement period and the five-year follow-up period (recent ex-smokers) were more likely than never smokers, continuing smokers, or long-term ex-smokers to gain weight and had the highest risk of developing type 2 diabetes. The authors reported, however, that the risk of type 2 diabetes among recent ex-smokers was similar for individuals who gained weight and those who did not gain weight. Despite the greater average weight gain observed in recent ex-smokers, then, the authors conclude that the increased risk of diabetes in this group is better explained by lingering effects of smoking.

In conclusion, the available evidence does not suggest that potential risks associated with postcessation weight gain are sufficient to warrant continued smoking. Even though the majority of smokers gain some weight when they quit, the amount of weight gain required to offset the benefits of smoking appears to be considerably greater than the amount gained by the average smoker following cessation. Nevertheless, there are some smokers who experience a significant amount of postcessation weight gain and, as a consequence, are at increased risk for developing weight-related health problems such as type 2 diabetes. As such, the availability of efficacious interventions to prevent or reduce large weight gains following smoking cessation is critical. In the next section, we review the current status of the interventions literature.

INTERVENTIONS TO PREVENT OR REDUCE WEIGHT GAIN FOLLOWING SMOKING CESSATION

In their earlier review of studies examining smoking and weight gain, Klesges et al. (15) were able to locate only nine studies that examined the effectiveness of treatments to reduce weight gain following smoking cessation. Since that time, the number of investigations of interventions that either focus on weight gain prevention or incorporate discussion of weight gain into treatment outcome analyses has grown substantially to include approximately 50 studies. The reason for this increased attention to weight gain prevention is not entirely clear, but it is likely that the increasing prevalence of overweight and obesity in the United States as well as the recognition that weight gain may interfere with attempts to quit smoking have elevated the importance of isolating effective treatments for smoking that decrease the probability of gaining weight (1,35).

Because Klesges et al. (15) included a discussion of the efficacy of interventions to prevent or reduce weight gain following smoking cessation, we will provide brief summaries of the conclusions derived from this paper and focus primarily on studies that have not appeared in that review. We also focused our literature search on studies in which the prevention of weight gain following smoking cessation was the primary focus of the research, although we supplemented the review with studies that did not specifically target the topic of weight gain if such information was useful in terms of clarifying trends or if it represented the only information regarding the relationship between that form of treatment and change in body weight. For studies examining the efficacy of medications, we did not include studies involving treatments that have not been approved by the FDA for smoking cessation or recommended by the Clinical Practice Guideline for Treating Tobacco Use and Dependence (36).

Studies that have sought to prevent or reduce weight gain following smoking cessation can be conceptualized as falling into two categories: pharmacological treatments and behavioral treatments. Pharmacological treatments include nicotine replacement therapies and buproprion SR.

Behavioral treatments include programs that provide information and/or assistance in modifying dietary intake and exercise behaviors and in restructuring beliefs about weight. In this section, we review the current status of the literature pertaining to the efficacy of both pharmacological and behavioral interventions to prevent or reduce postcessation weight gain.

Nicotine Replacement Therapies

Nicotine Gum

Nicotine gum has shown some promise in reducing weight gain in the short term in previous reviews, and the results of more recent studies tend to support this finding. On the basis of the scant early studies of nicotine gum as an agent for minimizing weight gain while treating tobacco use or dependence, Klesges et al. (15) were unable to generate solid conclusions about the efficacy of this form of nicotine replacement in their review of the literature (26,37,38). Using the data available at the time, they concluded that nicotine gum had some potential to reduce weight gain, but these effects were limited to heavy smokers and those who used heavier doses of the gum. It should be noted, however, that the two studies from which this conclusion was drawn suffered from serious methodological limitations (e.g., lack of randomization, no control groups, reliance on self-report to determine abstinence and treatment adherence, and failure to report gum dose) that made it difficult to draw firm conclusions (37,38). Data from the third study, which was more methodologically sound, showed significantly less weight gain at the end of the 10-week treatment period for abstinent smokers who used nicotine gum as compared to those using placebo gum (26). This difference had disappeared by the three-month follow-up period, however, when the participants were no longer using the gum.

Three of the five studies of nicotine gum located for this review [and not covered in Klesges et al. (15) review] were randomized controlled trials (RCTs) that incorporated procedures to monitor treatment adherence (i.e., returning used and/or unused gum) and to verify abstinence (i.e., expired carbon monoxide). Two of these three RCTs reported less weight gain among users receiving nicotine gum as opposed to placebo gum (28,39). Specifically, Doherty et al. (28) found that, after 13 weeks of treatment with either 0-, 2-, or 4-mg gum, men and women in the group using the 4-mg gum had gained significantly less weight than subjects in the placebo group (1.7 kg vs. 3.7 kg). Leischow et al. (39) reported that four weeks of treatment with either 0-, 2-, or 4-mg gum resulted in significant weight change differences among women, but not among men. Women chewing the 4-mg gum actually lost an average of 0.26 kg, while the 2- and 0-mg groups gained 0.33 and 1.69 kg, respectively. Thus, the effectiveness of the gum appeared to be dependent on higher dose and female gender (28,39). The third RCT reported no significant differences in weight gain among male and female users of 0-, 2-, or 4-mg gum but did suggest that the percentage of baseline cotinine levels replaced by the nicotine gum predicted weight change at the three follow-up periods (6, 9, and 12 months) (40). More specifically, replacement of cotinine (the major metabolite of nicotine) at levels that were closer to their cotinine levels while smoking was associated with less weight gain. This finding was also reported by Doherty et al. (28).

Hajek et al. (41) demonstrated that smokers who remained abstinent for one year gained an average of 5.2 kg if they were not using gum at that time and 3.1 kg if they were, but the study's lack of methodological rigor (e.g., no randomization, no control group, poor monitoring of abstinence) makes conclusions drawn from these findings tentative at best. Killen et al. (42) also demonstrated that individuals who used at least five pieces of nicotine gum per day after quitting smoking gained significantly less weight than individuals who did not use the gum over a period of two months, although the practical significance of the difference between users and nonusers was small (1.8 kg vs. 1.1 kg).

In summary, nicotine gum has demonstrated a capacity to reduce weight gain during its period of use, but its efficacy in attenuating weight gain seems to be limited to that period (26). In addition, the degree to which weight gain is limited appears to be proportional to the percentage of cotinine replaced by the gum. At least one study has demonstrated that adherence to this form of nicotine replacement decreases as dosage increases, however, making it difficult to achieve high levels of cotinine replacement, especially in heavier smokers who are at higher risk of weight gain (19,43).

Nicotine Patch

No studies that focused on weight change associated with the use of the nicotine patch were available at the time of the Klesges et al. (15) review. Of the five studies examining the efficacy of the nicotine patch in preventing postcessation weight gain that are currently available, three of the studies are RCTs. The results of these studies were mixed, with one demonstrating no difference between treatment and control groups after eight weeks of treatment, one suggesting that the patch significantly reduced weight gain after five weeks of treatment, and one indicating that the patch reduced weight gain over the first six weeks of treatment but that differences between the active and placebo groups had disappeared by the 10th week of treatment (44–46). The other two studies, although not controlled, showed nicotine patch users gaining an average of 2.5 and 4.7 kg following six and seven weeks of treatment (47,48). Without a control group for comparison, however, solid conclusions about the potential for the nicotine patch to attenuate or prevent postcessation weight gain cannot be made on the basis of these findings.

Because the results of the three RCTs described previously were mixed with respect to the weight-attenuating effects of the nicotine patch, we examined the findings of other investigations of the efficacy of the patch that did not focus on weight gain as a primary outcome measure in an attempt to obtain further clarification. This search produced an additional six studies (49–54). None of these studies showed a significant difference in weight gain between users of the active versus placebo patch following treatment periods ranging from 6 to 18 weeks, indicating that the active patch was not effective in limiting postcessation weight gain. Given the robustness of this null finding, it is possible that the results of the two previously described studies that reported a weight-attenuating effect of the nicotine patch may be an artifact of the methods of sampling or analyzing data (45,46). For example, the sample utilized by Hill et al. (46) was a group of primarily Mexican–American Hispanic adults, making the generalizability of the findings questionable.

Taken together, the findings of these investigations suggest that the nicotine patch is largely ineffective in preventing or limiting postcessation weight gain. The reason for the difference in efficacy between the nicotine patch and nicotine gum is unclear at this time, although it seems reasonable to suggest that the variability in the pharmacokinetic properties of the two treatments may be partially responsible. More specifically, the profile of plasma cotinine levels following nicotine gum use more closely resembles the profile associated with cigarette smoking (i.e., a sharp increase followed by a gradual decrease) as opposed to the nicotine patch, in which plasma cotinine increases gradually to a steady state that is maintained throughout the day (55). Another possibility is that the nicotine patch may delay postcessation weight gain for a brief period of time (e.g., two to three weeks) and that this effect has not been detected or reported up to this point due to a tendency to report weight change only after completion of treatment, which is usually five or six weeks at a minimum.

Nicotine Nasal Spray

No studies of the effectiveness of nicotine nasal spray in limiting postcessation weight gain were available at the time of the Klesges et al. (15) review. Although prevention of weight gain was not a stated purpose of a study conducted by Sutherland et al. (29), these authors demonstrated that the nicotine nasal spray significantly reduced weight gain following 52 weeks of treatment in smokers who were continuously abstinent, with users of the active form of the spray gaining an average of 3.0 kg as compared to the 5.8 kg average gain observed in the placebo spray users. Participants who discontinued use of the active form of the spray, however, gained an average of 5.5 kg, placing them right on course with the placebo group. It appears, then, that the weight gain was slowed through the use of the nicotine nasal spray but not reduced significantly in the long term. Despite the general methodological soundness of this study, more research is needed in order to determine the extent to which nicotine nasal spray reliably attenuates postcessation weight gain, particularly following discontinuation of its use.

Nicotine Inhaler

Klesges et al. (15) found no studies examining the weight-control properties of the nicotine inhaler. Only one investigation of the nicotine inhaler that discussed weight change following smoking cessation was located for this review, although the primary focus of this study was not on weight gain. Tonnesen et al. (56) offered participants nicotine inhalers for six months (i.e., three months of using 2 to 10 inhalers per day as desired, followed by a three-month tapering period) and measured weight change after six weeks and again after one year. Results indicated that the mean weight gain for the placebo and active inhaler groups did not differ significantly at either point in time. At six weeks, both groups had gained 1.8 kg. At one year, participants using the nicotine inhaler gained 4.5 kg and the participants using the placebo inhaler gained 4.0 kg. Consequently, the lone investigation addressing the potential to reduce weight gain through the use of the nicotine inhaler suggests that this treatment is not effective for that purpose.

Buproprion SR

Buproprion SR, which, in addition to the variety of nicotine replacement therapies available, is listed as a first-line pharmacological treatment for tobacco use and dependence in the report of the Clinical Guideline panel, has not been studied extensively in terms of its capacity to curtail postcessation weight gain (36). In the one study that focused primarily on examining this capacity, the authors reported that buproprion was not significantly more effective than the nicotine patch in preventing weight gain, with buproprion users gaining an average of 4.4 kg and patch users gaining an average of 4.7 kg (48). Unfortunately, the study did not include a control group against which changes in weight associated with treatment could be compared.

Hays et al. (23) found that a one-year trial of buproprion SR (300 mg) as a method of preventing relapse following smoking cessation resulted in less weight gain in the group receiving the active treatment than in the placebo group at both the end of the one-year treatment period and the two-year follow-up. Similarly, Hurt et al. (25) found that daily use of buproprion SR (300 mg) attenuated weight gain over the seven-week treatment period. However, by the six-month follow-up, there was no significant difference in weight gain between the active and placebo groups.

The results of the limited studies available to determine the efficacy of buproprion SR in limiting weight gain following smoking cessation indicate that the drug seems to be effective during its period of use. It is unclear, however, whether this attenuating effect is maintained beyond the treatment period, as the results of studies incorporating long-term follow-ups are equivocal (23,25). Additional research is needed to make definitive conclusions about both the short-term and long-term efficacy of buproprion SR in minimizing postcessation weight gain.

Behavioral/Cognitive-Behavioral Treatments
Targeting Both Weight and Smoking

At the time of the Klesges et al. (15) review, studies that involved behavioral or cognitive-behavioral interventions to simultaneously facilitate smoking cessation and prevent weight gain were more prevalent in the literature than were pharmacological intervention studies. Six of the nine studies discussed by these authors incorporated behavioral or cognitive-behavioral components to address both smoking and weight-control. The results of these studies were mixed, with some indicating that the provision of weight-control information resulted in less weight gain and some indicating that it did not [see Klesges et al. (15) for a complete review].

In the past 15 years, four additional studies have reported on the efficacy of behavioral or cognitive-behavioral weight control interventions incorporated into treatment for smoking. Hall et al. (57) provided participants with two weeks of a cognitive-behavioral smoking cessation program followed by four weeks of one of the following: (i) a weight control intervention consisting of weight and dietary intake monitoring, an individualized exercise plan, and cognitive-behavioral strategies to control eating ("innovative intervention"); (ii) an intervention promoting insight into eating behavior and offering information about nutrition and exercise ("nonspecific control"); or (iii) provision of written information about exercise and diet not specific to prevention of postcessation weight gain ("standard treatment control"). Results of this study indicated that there was no significant difference in weight change among the three groups following the six-week treatment. Further analyses demonstrated that participants in the innovative intervention group showed reduced dietary intake compared to the other two groups at the end of the six-week treatment period but that no significant difference between groups was detected at the 12-, 26-, or 52-week marks. Likewise, there were no differences among the three groups in physical activity level at any measurement point. Thus, it appears that the efficacy of the intervention may have been undermined by poor compliance with the key behavioral components of the program.

Marcus et al. (58) offered female smokers a smoking cessation intervention that included information about diet and weight control followed by 12 weeks of either a supervised exercise program (30–40 min of aerobic exercise three times per week) or a nonspecific wellness program that provided information about a variety of general health issues. At the end of the treatment period, participants in the exercise program had gained significantly less weight than participants in the control group (3.1 kg vs. 5.4 kg). At the 20- and 60-week follow-up periods, however, the differences in weight gain between the two groups were no longer significant, leading the authors to conclude that exercise can delay but not prevent postcessation weight gain. They did note, however, that only 10% of the participants in the exercise condition reported continuing with a regular exercise regimen in the 12 months following the conclusion of the supervised exercise program, suggesting that the failure to find differences between the exercise and control groups at the follow-up periods may have been a result of reduction or discontinuation of regular exercise. Much like the Hall et al. (57) study, then, the results of this study demonstrate the need to monitor and address problems with treatment adherence.

Perkins et al. (59) compared a seven-week program accompanying a cognitive-behavioral smoking cessation intervention that represented either (i) a behavioral weight control treatment that consisted of monitoring and reducing caloric intake as well as identifying strategies to avoid overeating, (ii) a cognitive-behavioral treatment (CBT) to reduce concerns about postcessation weight gain that involved discouragement of dietary restriction and restructuring of beliefs about the ideal body size and shape, or (iii) a control condition involving a support group that focused on general discussion of smoking cessation without reference to weight gain. Both the behavioral weight control program and the CBT weight concerns intervention minimized weight gain at the end of treatment when compared to the control condition. Paradoxically, only the participants in the CBT group differed from control participants at the 6- and 12-month follow-ups in terms of weight gain. At the 12-month follow-up, the CBT group had gained only 2.5 kg, whereas the weight management group and the control group gained 5.4 and 7.7 kg, respectively. Interestingly, despite the superiority of the CBT condition in terms of reducing postcessation weight gain, the data did not support the efficacy of the intervention for its intended purpose (i.e., reducing weight concerns). The method by which the intervention attenuated weight gain, then, is unclear.

Finally, Spring et al. (60) investigated an eight-week behavioral treatment for weight control incorporated into a 16-week behavioral smoking cessation program. These authors were interested in determining how the timing of the weight control intervention would affect the treatment efficacy for both of the targeted areas (i.e., smoking cessation and weight management). Thus, participants in the treatment groups were assigned to complete the weight control portion of the program either in the first eight weeks of the program (early diet) or the second eight weeks (late diet). Participants assigned to the control group did not receive any assistance with weight control. Results indicated that neither of the two treatment groups differed from the control group at the end of treatment or at the nine-month follow-up in terms of average weight gain. In a supplemental analysis, the authors found that participants in the late diet condition who attended a higher number of treatment sessions demonstrated less weight gain than controls, whereas participants who attended a lower number of sessions did not significantly differ from control participants. This finding may reflect the possibility that weight can be minimized among a select group of smokers who demonstrate greater motivation and adherence to weight control interventions.

In summary, the findings of the behavioral/CBT studies have not been promising, especially with respect to long-term efficacy. Only one study demonstrated any sustained reduction of weight gain due to treatment, and it is unclear how this intervention helped to prevent weight gain given that it did not achieve its primary goal (i.e., to reduce weight concerns). If the Perkins et al. (59) findings can be successfully replicated, it would appear to be important to determine the components of the cognitive-behavioral intervention utilized in that study that were associated with reduced weight gain. The findings of Marcus et al. (58) provide some hope that exercise may limit postcessation weight gain but suggest that, in order to maintain the benefits, one must make exercise a life-long endeavor.

Combined Treatments for Weight Control and Smoking Cessation

Several studies have examined the efficacy of combining behavioral weight control interventions with nicotine replacement therapy. Three of these investigations involved nicotine gum and one involved the nicotine patch. Danielsson et al. (61) conducted a study in which female smokers who had previously quit but resumed smoking due to weight gain were provided with nicotine gum for 16 weeks (2 mg initially, increased to 4 mg if chewing more than 20 pieces per day) and given behavioral recommendations to facilitate smoking cessation. Half of the participants were also provided with low-calorie meals to be eaten in three two-week intervals (i.e., weeks 1–2, 7–8, and 13–14 of the study). Despite the fact that adherence to the low calorie diet decreased steadily from weeks 1 to 2 (75% of participants compliant) through weeks 13 to 14 (18% of participants compliant), the diet group had lost 2.1 kg of body weight by the end of the 16-week treatment, whereas the control group gained an average of 1.6 kg. At the 12-month follow-up, however, the difference in weight change between the diet and control groups was no longer statistically significant. Unfortunately, the authors did not report on the participants' dietary intake over the course of the follow-up period, but it seems probable to assume that the participants in the diet group did not continue to follow to the same low-calorie diet that was provided by the researchers during the 16 weeks of treatment. If it is, in fact, safe to make such an assumption, then participants in the diet group most likely gained weight due to the discontinuation of this method of weight control.

Nides et al. (31) offered a 12-week behavioral smoking cessation program that included information about preventing postcessation weight gain (i.e., cognitive-behavioral strategies to avoid increased energy intake). Study participants were also encouraged to use nicotine gum and were provided with 2-mg gum for a period of six months. After 12 months of abstinence, male subjects had gained an average of 5.5 kg, and females gained an average of 5.3 kg. Gum dose was inversely related to weight gain through 12 months, but not at the 24-month follow-up. Because this study was not a RCT, strong conclusions about the efficacy of this combined form of treatment cannot be made. Nevertheless, the results suggest that the use of nicotine gum along with behavioral recommendations for weight control does not prevent postcessation weight gain in the long run, as the weight gain following one year of abstinence is similar to or greater than the amount gained by individuals using placebo gum or no gum in the studies of the efficacy of nicotine gum reviewed in a previous section.

Pirie et al. (62) conducted a RCT in which the treatment groups received either a behavioral weight-control intervention, nicotine gum (2 mg), or both in combination with a cognitive-behavioral smoking cessation program (62). The behavioral weight-control program consisted of ongoing counseling to assist participants in reducing caloric intake and increasing exercise to at least one hour of walking three times per week. Participants were also provided with materials to monitor energy intake. In this study, there were no significant differences among the treatment groups and the control group in terms of weight gain at the end of the eight-week treatment period or at the 12-month follow-up. It is important to note, however, that compliance with the nicotine gum ranged from 93% to 99%, whereas compliance with the food record component of the behavioral weight control program ranged from 23% to 69%. It seems, then, that problems with adherence limited the potential efficacy of the weight control intervention.

Ussher et al. (63) also reported the results of a RCT in which smokers participated in a seven-week smoking cessation program that included a nicotine replacement component (i.e., daily use of a 15-mg nicotine patch). Participants were randomized into either an exercise condition or a general health education (control) condition. Participants in the exercise condition were provided with five minutes of individualized exercise planning during the first session and approximately two minutes of goal monitoring and encouragement for further exercise at each subsequent session, whereas the control group received equivalent contact time during which the researchers provided general health advice that included information about diet. After six weeks of abstinence from smoking, there were no significant differences in weight gain between the control group and the exercise group (2.0 kg vs. 1.8 kg) even though measures of treatment adherence suggested that participants in the exercise condition engaged in more physical activity than the control group. This finding was based solely on self-reported exercise behavior, however, and should be interpreted with some caution.

In general, data from the studies of combined treatments indicate that the addition of a behavioral or cognitive-behavioral weight control treatment in conjunction with nicotine replacement therapy does not result in less weight gain than nicotine replacement alone. The Danielsson et al. (61) study is one notable exception, however, as participants who reduced dietary intake significantly for two-week periods during the treatment phase of the study in addition to chewing nicotine gum actually lost more weight over the course of the 16-week study period than participants who used the gum only. These weight-control benefits were not maintained in the long term, however, probably due to discontinuation of the treatment. The conclusions derived from combined intervention studies should also be interpreted with some caution in light of evidence that adherence to behavioral components of the treatment may be problematic.

CONCLUSIONS AND RECOMMENDATIONS
FOR FURTHER RESEARCH

Despite the known health consequences of both smoking and obesity, the prevalence of these two risk factors for disease and early death remains alarmingly high in the United States. Obese smokers appear to be particularly vulnerable to developing health problems due to the combined effects of the two risk factors, yet little headway has been made in establishing effective interventions to address both smoking and obesity. Complicating the combined treatment of these two conditions is the fact that most people who quit smoking actually gain weight.

Although most smokers do tend to gain weight when they quit, estimates of the amount of postcessation weight gain vary as a result of both methodological and individual differences across studies that report these data. Methodological factors contributing to variability in estimates of weight gain following smoking cessation include the time period over which the gain is measured, the operational definition of abstinence, and the type and duration of adjunctive pharmacotherapies. Individual-level differences that appear to moderate postcessation weight gain are age, heaviness of smoking, race/ethnicity, physical activity level, precessation body weight, and gender.

A number of investigations have focused on both societal-level and individual-level consequences of weight gain following smoking cessation. On a societal level, there has been some suggestion that smoking cessation may be contributing to the increased prevalence of overweight and obesity in the United States. By one estimate, approximately one-quarter of the increased prevalence in men and one-sixth of the increased prevalence in women can be attributed to smoking cessation (32).

On an individual level, weight gain following smoking cessation may increase the risk of morbidity and mortality. There is no evidence to suggest, however, that the benefits of smoking cessation are, on average, outweighed by the risks associated with increased body weight. In fact, metabolic profiles appear to improve in ex-smokers in spite of postcessation weight gain. Such findings may be due to the fact that weight gain following smoking cessation is, in most cases, not large enough to produce negative health consequences that are comparable to the consequences of continued smoking. Major weight gains do occur, however, and can result in increased health risks for former smokers. In such cases, the availability of treatments that are effective in reducing postcessation weight gain becomes particularly important.

The major finding that emerged from the review of literature focusing on pharmacological, behavioral, and combined therapies for smoking cessation and weight control is that weight gain can be attenuated over the course of treatment but that, following discontinuation of treatment, weight is gained to the point where it would be expected to climb if the individual had not received treatment. Of the pharmacological interventions reviewed, nicotine gum, nicotine nasal spray, and buproprion SR have demonstrated the most promise in terms of reducing weight gain during the period of use, although these benefits do not seem to last following treatment discontinuation. The nicotine patch and the nicotine inhaler, by contrast, have not shown much potential for limiting postcessation weight gain.

Behavioral or cognitive-behavioral interventions involving dietary modifications and exercise appear to have some capacity to reduce weight gain in recent ex-smokers when they are compliant with the treatments. Treatments that combine nicotine replacement therapy with behavioral or cognitive-behavioral interventions do not appear to be superior to nicotine replacement alone, however, in terms of limiting postcessation weight gain, particularly in the long term. Importantly, the efficacy of the behavioral/cognitive-behavioral weight control component of these programs appears to be a function of adherence to the treatment regimen, which is typically moderate to poor during the active treatment period and markedly poor by the point at which long-term follow-ups are conducted. These studies seem to suggest, then, that the modified diet and exercise regimen must be continued indefinitely in order to maintain the associated weight-control benefits. Further research is needed to empirically validate the long-term efficacy of such an approach, however.

Because of the high probability that some increase in body mass will occur as a result of smoking cessation and the finding that pharmacological, behavioral, and combined interventions designed to prevent postcessation weight gain have had limited success, perhaps more attention should be paid to developing and evaluating effective interventions to prevent large, longer-term weight gains following smoking cessation that have more severe negative health consequences. Such interventions would be particularly important for individuals who are already overweight or obese and are consequently at higher risk for weight-related health problems. Unfortunately, this population of smokers has been largely overlooked in the treatment literature. As such, future research on interventions for smoking cessation and weight management that target overweight and obese smokers in particular is encouraged.

Perkins (64) has also suggested that interventions which minimize unwarranted concerns about the weight gain that occurs frequently after smoking cessation and assist recent exsmokers in coping with increases in body mass may be beneficial which to help prevent smoking relapse, particularly for individuals who are at risk to resume smoking as a consequence of postcessation weight gain. Such interventions may also reduce postcessation weight gain (59). The mechanism(s) by which this effect was achieved in the Perkins et al. (59) study are unclear, however, and should be investigated further.

ACKNOWLEDGMENTS

Support for this work was provided by the Department of Veterans Affairs and grants #AA013307 and AA013957 from the National Institute on Alcohol Abuse and Alcoholism.

REFERENCES

1. Schiller JS, Nelson C, Hao C, et al. Early release of selected estimates based on data from the January–June 2004 National Health Interview Survey. National Center for Health Statistics 2004. www.cdc.gov/nchs/nhis.htm.
2. Flegal KM, Carroll MD, Kuczmarski RJ, et al. Overweight and obesity in the United States: prevalence and trends, 1960–1994. Int J Obes Relat Metab Disord 1998; 22:39–47.
3. Dyer AR, Stamler J, Garside DB, et al. Long-term consequences of body mass index for cardiovascular mortality: the Chicago Heart Association Detection Project in Industry study. Ann Epidemiol 2004; 14:101–108.
4. Calle EE, Thun MJ, Petrelli JM, et al. Body-mass index and mortality in a prospective cohort of U.S. adults. N Engl J Med 1999; 341:1097–1105.
5. Calle EE, Rodriguez C, Walker-Thurmond K, et al. Overweight, obesity, and mortality from cancer in a prospectively studied cohort of U.S. adults. N Engl J Med 2003; 348:1625–1638.
6. Mokdad AH, Ford ES, Bowman BA, et al. Prevalence of obesity, diabetes, and obesity-related health risk factors, 2001. JAMA 2003; 289:76–79.
7. Rogers RG, Hummer RA, Krueger PM. The effect of obesity on overall, circulatory disease- and diabetes-specific mortality. J Biosoc Sci 2003; 35:107–129.
8. Shaper AG, Wannamethee SG, Walker M. Body weight: implications for the prevention of coronary heart disease, stroke, and diabetes mellitus in a cohort study of middle aged men. BMJ 1997; 314:1311–1317.
9. Mokdad AH, Marks JS, Stroup DF, et al. Actual causes of death in the United States, 2000. JAMA 2004; 291:1238–1245.
10. Thompson D, Wolf AM. The medical-care cost burden of obesity. Obes Rev 2001; 2:189–197.

11. Field AE, Barnoya J, Colditz GA. Epidemiology and health and economic consequences of obesity. In: Wadden TA, Stunkard AJ, eds. Handbook of obesity treatment. New York: The Guildford Press, 2002:3–18.
12. Surgeon General. United States Department of Health and Human Services. The health consequences of smoking. Washington, DC: Department of Health and Human Services, Centers for Disease Control and Prevention, National Center for Chronic Disease Prevention and Health Promotion, Office on Smoking and Health, 2004.
13. Jacobs DR Jr, Adachi H, Mulder I, et al. Cigarette smoking and mortality risk: twenty-five-year follow-up of the Seven Countries Study. Arch Intern Med 1999; 159:733–740.
14. Peeters A, Barendregt JJ, Willekens F, et al. Obesity in adulthood and its consequences for life expectancy: a life-table analysis. Ann Intern Med 2003; 138:24–32.
15. Klesges RC, Meyers AW, Klesges LM, et al. Smoking, body weight, and their effects on smoking behavior: a comprehensive review of the literature. Psychol Bull 1989; 106:204–230.
16. Klesges RC, Ward KD, Ray JW, et al. The prospective relationships between smoking and weight in a young, biracial cohort: the Coronary Artery Risk Development in Young Adults Study. J Consult Clin Psychol 1998; 66:987–993.
17. Sempos CT, Durazo-Arvizu R, McGee DL, et al. The influence of cigarette smoking on the association between body weight and mortality. The Framingham Heart Study revisited. Ann Epidemiol 1998; 8:289–300.
18. Wannamethee SG, Shaper AG, Walker M. Weight change, body weight and mortality: the impact of smoking and ill health. Int J Epidemiol 2001; 30:777–786.
19. Williamson DF, Madans J, Anda RF, et al. Smoking cessation and severity of weight gain in a national cohort. N Engl J Med 1991; 324:739–745.
20. Froom P, Melamed S, Benbassat J. Smoking cessation and weight gain. J Fam Pract 1998; 46:460–464.
21. O'Hara P, Connett JE, Lee WW, et al. Early and late weight gain following smoking cessation in the Lung Health Study. Am J Epidemiol 1998; 148: 821–830.
22. Wise RA, Enright PL, Connett JE, et al. Effect of weight gain on pulmonary function after smoking cessation in the Lung Health Study. Am J Respir Crit Care Med 1998; 157:866–872.
23. Hays JT, Hurt RD, Rigotti NA, et al. Sustained-release bupropion for pharmacologic relapse prevention after smoking cessation, a randomized, controlled trial. Ann Intern Med 2001; 135:423–433.
24. Klesges RC, Winders SE, Meyers AW, et al. How much weight gain occurs following smoking cessation? A comparison of weight gain using both continuous and point prevalence abstinence. J Consult Clin Psychol 1997; 65:286–291.
25. Hurt RD, Sachs DP, Glover ED, et al. A comparison of sustained-release bupropion and placebo for smoking cessation. N Engl J Med 1997; 337:1195–1202.
26. Gross J, Stitzer ML, Maldonado J. Nicotine replacement: effects of postcessation weight gain. J Consult Clin Psychol 1989; 57:87–92.

27. Swan GE, Carmelli D. Characteristics associated with excessive weight gain after smoking cessation in men. Am J Public Health 1995; 85:73–77.
28. Doherty K, Militello FS, Kinnunen T, et al. Nicotine gum dose and weight gain after smoking cessation. J Consult Clin Psychol 1996; 64:799–807.
29. Sutherland G, Stapleton JA, Russell MA, et al. Randomised controlled trial of nasal nicotine spray in smoking cessation. Lancet 1992; 340:324–329.
30. Vander Weg MW, Klesges RC, Clemens LH, et al. The relationships between ethnicity, gender, and short-term changes in energy balance following smoking cessation. Int J Behav Med 2001; 8:163–177.
31. Nides M, Rand C, Dolce J, et al. Weight gain as a function of smoking cessation and 2-mg nicotine gum use among middle-aged smokers with mild lung impairment in the first 2 years of the Lung Health Study. Health Psychol 1994; 13:354–361.
32. Flegal KM, Troiano RP, Pamuk ER, et al. The influence of smoking cessation on the prevalence of overweight in the United States. N Engl J Med 1995; 333:1165–1170.
33. Burnette MM, Meilahn E, Wing RR, et al. Smoking cessation, weight gain, and changes in cardiovascular risk factors during menopause: the Healthy Women Study. Am J Public Health 1998; 88:93–96.
34. Wannamethee SG, Shaper AG, Perry IJ. Smoking as a modifiable risk factor for type 2 diabetes in middle-aged men. Diabetes Care 2001; 24:1590–1595.
35. Borrelli B, Mermelstein R. The role of weight concern and self-efficacy in smoking cessation and weight gain among smokers in a clinic-based cessation program. Addict Behav 1998; 23:609–622.
36. Fiore MC. Treating tobacco use and dependence: an introduction to the US Public Health Service Clinical Practice Guideline. Respir Care 2000; 45:1196–1199.
37. Emont SL, Cummings KM. Weight gain following smoking cessation: a possible role for nicotine replacement in weight management. Addict Behav 1987; 12:151–155.
38. Fagerstrom KO. Reducing the weight gain after stopping smoking. Addict Behav 1987; 12:91–93.
39. Leischow SJ, Sachs DP, Bostrom AG, et al. Effects of differing nicotine-replacement doses on weight gain after smoking cessation. Arch Fam Med 1992; 1:233–237.
40. Nordstrom BL, Kinnunen T, Utman CH, et al. Long-term effects of nicotine gum on weight gain after smoking cessation. Nicotine Tob Res 1999; 1:259–268.
41. Hajek P, Jackson P, Belcher M. Long-term use of nicotine chewing gum. Occurrence, determinants, and effect on weight gain. JAMA 1988; 260:1593–1596.
42. Killen JD, Fortmann SP, Newman B. Weight change among participants in a large sample minimal contact smoking relapse prevention trial. Addict Behav 1990; 15:323–332.
43. Gross J, Johnson J, Sigler L, et al. Dose effects of nicotine gum. Addict Behav 1995; 20:371–381.
44. Dale LC, Schroeder DR, Wolter TD, et al. Weight change after smoking cessation using variable doses of transdermal nicotine replacement. J Gen Intern Med 1998; 13:9–15.

45. Jorenby DE, Hatsukami DK, Smith SS, et al. Characterization of tobacco withdrawal symptoms: transdermal nicotine reduces hunger and weight gain. Psychopharmacology (Bed) 1996; 128:130–138.
46. Hill AL, Roe DJ, Taren DL, et al. Efficacy of transdermal nicotine in reducing post-cessation weight gain in a Hispanic sample. Nicotine Tob Res 2000; 2: 247–253.
47. Assali AR, Beigel Y, Schreibman R, et al. Weight gain and insulin resistance during nicotine replacement therapy. Clin Cardiol 1999; 22:357–360.
48. Botella-Carretero JI, Escobar-Morreale HF, Martin I, et al. Weight gain and cardiovascular risk factors during smoking cessation with bupropion or nicotine. Horm Metab Res 2004; 36:178–182.
49. Fiore MC, Kenford SL, Jorenby DE, et al. Two studies of the clinical effectiveness of the nicotine patch with different counseling treatments. Chest 1994; 105:524–533.
50. Hughes JR, Hatsukarni DK. Effects of three doses of transdermal nicotine on post-cessation eating, hunger and weight. J Subst Abuse 1997; 9:151–159.
51. Muller P, Abelin T, Ehrsam R, et al. The use of transdermal nicotine in smoking cessation. Lung 1990; 168(suppl):445–453.
52. Sachs DP, Sawe U, Leischow SJ. Effectiveness of a 16-hour transdermal nicotine patch in a medical practice setting, without intensive group counseling. Arch Intern Med 1993; 153:1881–1890.
53. Tonnesen P, Norregaard J, Simonsen K, et al. A double-blind trial of a 16-hour transdermal nicotine patch in smoking cessation. N Engl J Med 1991; 325:311–315.
54. Transdermal nicotine for smoking cessation. Six-month results from two multicenter controlled clinical trials. Transdermal Nicotine Study Group. JAMA 1991; 266:3133–3138.
55. Rigotti NA. Clinical practice. Treatment of tobacco use and dependence. N Engl J Med 2002; 346:506–512.
56. Tonnesen P, Norregaard J, Mikkelsen K, et al. A double-blind trial of a nicotine inhaler for smoking cessation. JAMA 1993; 269:1268–1271.
57. Hall SM, Tunstall CD, Vila KL, et al. Weight gain prevention and smoking cessation: cautionary findings. Am J Public Health 1992; 82:799–803.
58. Marcus BH, Albrecht AE, King TK, et al. The efficacy of exercise as an aid for smoking cessation in women: a randomized controlled trial. Arch Intern Med 1999; 159:1229–1234.
59. Perkins KA, Marcus MD, Levine MD, et al. Cognitive-behavioral therapy to reduce weight concerns improves smoking cessation outcome in weight-concerned women. J Consult Clin Psychol 2001; 69:604–613.
60. Spring B, Pagoto S, Pingitore R, et al. Randomized controlled trial for behavioral smoking and weight control treatment: effect of concurrent versus sequential intervention. J Consult Clin Psychol 2004; 72:785–796.
61. Danielsson T, Rossner S, Westin A. Open randomised trial of intermittent very low energy diet together with nicotine gum for stopping smoking in women who gained weight in previous attempts to quit. BMJ 1999; 319:490–493.
62. Pirie PL, McBride CM, Hellerstedt W, et al. Smoking cessation in women concerned about weight. Am J Public Health 1992; 82:1238–1243.

63. Ussher M, West R, McEwen A, et al. Efficacy of exercise counselling as an aid for smoking cessation: a randomized controlled trial. Addiction 2003; 98: 523–532.
64. Perkins KA. Issues in the prevention of weight gain after smoking cessation. Ann Behav Med 1994; 16:46–52.

7

Obesity and Impulsive and Compulsive Disorders

Latha V. Soorya

*Department of Psychiatry, Seaver and New York Autism Center of Excellence,
Mount Sinai School of Medicine, New York, New York, U.S.A.*

Bryann R. Baker and Lisa Sharma

*Compulsive, Impulsive and Anxiety Disorders Program, Mount Sinai School of
Medicine, New York, New York, U.S.A.*

Eric Hollander

*Department of Psychiatry, Clinical Psychopharmacology, and Compulsive,
Impulsive and Anxiety Disorders Program, Seaver and New York Autism Center of
Excellence, Mount Sinai School of Medicine, New York, New York, U.S.A.*

INTRODUCTION

This chapter examines the relationship between impulsive and compulsive disorders as well as select obsessive-compulsive spectrum disorders (OCSDs). Although there is no direct link between impulsive and compulsive disorders and obesity, individual disorders are associated with both weight loss and weight gain. OCSD disorders with the strongest association with clinical obesity include binge-eating disorder (BED) and Prader–Willi Syndrome (PWS). The compulsive eating associated with these disorders and the links between binge eating, PWS, and obsessive-compulsive disorder (OCD) will be explored closely in this chapter. Obesity and weight gain may be directly related to other impulse control disorders as a result of generalized problems with impulse control or may be indirectly related due to sedentary lifestyles (e.g., pathological gambling) and/or medication side effects. The associated features and medication side effects can result in clinically significant weight gain. This chapter will review the weight gain issues associated with select compulsive, impulsive, and developmental disorders comprising OCSD. In addition to reviews of extant literature, data on baseline weight will be presented across our own clinical populations.

In recent years, OCD and related conditions have emerged as a distinct spectrum of disorders (1). This has led to OCSDs being proposed as a distinct diagnostic category in the research planning agenda for the DSM-V and ICD-10. While the breadth of the inclusion criteria may be of some debate, the OCSD and OCD overlap in many respects including clinical symptoms (demographics, repetitive thoughts, and behaviors), comorbidity, etiology, and preferential response to antiobsessional treatments such as selective serotonin reuptake inhibitors (2,3). A seemingly diverse group of psychiatric disorders may share the defining features of OC spectrum disorders including disorders characterized by obsessive thoughts about appearance, health, and eating (anorexia nervosa, body dysmorphic disorder, and hypochondriasis); disorders characterized by stereotyped, ritualistic behaviors (Tourette's syndrome, trichotillomania, autism, and Prader–Willi); and impulse control problems (e.g., pathological gambling, compulsive shopping, and binge eating disorder) (4).

Conceptualization of OCSD from a dimensional, rather than categorical perspective, has advanced diagnostic treatment and etiological investigations of many conditions. As we have written elsewhere, dimensional views include conceptualization on a spectrum of risk averse versus risk seeking, with risk aversion associated with compulsive disorders and risk seeking observed with impulse-control disorders (1). Compulsions are thought to reduce anxiety related to overestimation of risks. Alternatively, individuals with impulse-control disorders, may grossly underestimate the risk involved with their behaviors and over-value fulfilling their pleasure-seeking drive.

OCSDs may also share common neurobiological foundations. For example, OCSDs may be characterized on a dimension of serotonin sensitivity and frontal lobe activity, with impulsive disorders characterized by hypofrontality and decreased presynaptic serotonergic levels, and compulsive disorders associated with hyperfrontality and increased serotonergic sensitivity (4). Serotonergic dysfunction in OCSDs is indirectly supported by the wide use and efficacy of SRI treatments across spectrum disorders including OCD, autism, pathological gambling, and eating disorders. Baxter et al. (5), also suggest that OC spectrum may share an underlying dysfunction in the corticostriatal system, with the specific area of dysfunction within the system differing across disorders.

OBSESSIVE COMPULSIVE DISORDER

OCD is estimated to affect approximately 2.3% of the United States population and its symptomalogy provides the basis for classification of OCSDs (6). OCD is characterized by complaints of persistent or repetitive thoughts (obsessions) or behaviors (compulsions). Those who suffer from this disorder feel compelled to continue these actions despite an awareness that the thoughts or behaviors may be excessive or inappropriate, and feel distress if they stop them (7). Treatment regimens for OCD vary according to the severity and course of the disorder. The most common forms of treatment are serotonin reuptake inhibitors, which typically produce at least some clinical benefit in most patients with OCD (8). Other forms of treatment include cognitive behavioral approaches such as exposure + response (ERP), SRIs with adjunctive treatment (i.e., atypicals), and more recently, deep brain stimulation (9–11).

No studies to date have documented a link between obesity and OCD. As previously indicated, compulsive eating can be a characteristic of OCD and the prevalence of OCD in disorders characterized by compulsive eating (BED, PWS) is high (12,13). In addition, some antipsychotic medications which may be used as adjuncts to SRIs, are associated with significant weight gain (14–17). Newer atypical antipsychotics such as ziprasidone and quetiapine, however, show less weight gain (18). Clinical considerations in treating obesity in patients with OCD include the risk of exacerbating patients' obsessions by emphasizing potential health risks associated with obesity and weight gain.

BODY DYSMORPHIC DISORDER

Body dysmorphic disorder (BDD) is defined as an intense preoccupation with a defect in appearance, in which the defect is either imagined, or, if a slight physical anomaly is present, the individuals concern is markedly excessive. These excessive concerns characteristically cause clinically significant distress or impairment in social, occupational or other important areas of functioning and are devastating to individuals with BDD. The true prevalence of BDD is unknown, however, estimates range from 0.7% to 1.9% in the United States population (19–21).

BDD is considered to be an OC spectrum disorder due to its similarities in phenomology and possible treatment response with OCD. According to McElroy et al. (22), "BDD preoccupations are 'structurally' similar to OCD obsessions in which they are often experienced as repetitive intrusive thoughts that are associated with anxiety or distress and are usually difficult to control." Most individuals with BDD exhibit compulsive-like behaviors, such as mirror checking, excessive grooming, skin picking, and frequent requests for reassurance related to their fixations. The most common treatment approach to BDD is medication, with SRI medications being the most promising. SRI medications can significantly relieve BDD symptoms by diminishing bodily preoccupation, distress, depression, and anxiety, significantly increasing control over one's thoughts and behaviors and improving overall functioning (23). Cognitive behavioral approaches are also used to treat BDD through the use of response prevention of checking behaviors and cognitive restructuring to help a person with BDD to develop a more realistic view of their appearance. This type of therapy has so far proved quite effective in the treatment of BDD (24).

With regards to the possible relationship between obesity and BDD, no studies to date have sought to determine a link between the two. However, since individuals with BDD are extremely fixated on their appearance, a causative link between the two is unlikely. Obesity can be comorbid with BDD, however, if an individual with BDD is obese, the individual will focus not only on his/her weight, but also on specific body parts (e.g., calves). When a clinician treats an obese patient, special consideration should be made not to over-emphasize the physical aspect of the obesity, lest it become an obsession.

EATING DISORDERS

Since a more comprehensive review of eating disorders is found in the previous chapter, this chapter focusses on the obsessive and compulsive features of eating disorders. The three major eating disorders, anorexia nervosa, bulimia nervosa, and BEDs, have features consistent with the OC spectrum profile. A study by Speranza et al. (25) found current and lifetime prevalence of OCD in eating disordered individuals to be significantly higher than in the general population (15.7% and 19% vs. 0% and 1.1%, $p = 0.05$). Individuals with bulimia nervosa, a condition characterized by episodes of binge eating followed by recurrent inappropriate compensatory behavior in order to prevent weight gain, exhibit obsessive–compulsive symptoms insofar as their inability to control their compulsive overeating, compensatory behavior, and the repetitiveness of their eating behavior. Anorexia nervosa is defined as a refusal to maintain body weight at or above a minimally normal weight for age and height coupled with intense fear of getting fat or gaining weight. Individuals with anorexia often exhibit OC spectrum symptoms including obsessions and rituals with food, meticulous detail of caloric intake, and extreme concern with body shape, size, and weight.

BED is the only eating disorder associated with obesity. BED is a newly recognized eating disorder characterized by recurrent episodes of binge eating without extreme behaviors to lose weight characteristic of bulimia nervosa or anorexia nervosa (such as vomiting, misuse of laxatives, fasting, or excessive exercise) (26,27). BED is not a formal diagnosis within the DSM-IV, although it is a generally accepted condition in clinical practice. Prevalence rates of BED range from 2% to 5% in community samples (28,29).

Individuals with BED are often overweight or obese (30,31). In weight control clinics, individuals with binge eating patterns are on average more obese and have a history of more marked weight fluctuations than individuals without this pattern. Moreover, the prevalence of BED seems to increase with the degree of obesity (32). Of note, a study by Becker et al. (33) showed obese women in their representative sample to have the highest rates of anxiety disorder, affective disorders, somatoform disorders, and disorders of childhood. In some cases (i.e., anxiety and somatoform disorders) prevalence rates for obese women were almost double the rates of the normal weight group.

As outlined by McElroy et al. (34) in their article "Obsessive Compulsive Spectrum Disorders" several lines of evidence suggest that BED is related to OCD insofar as phenomology, secrecy, course of illness, and comorbidity. Beginning with phenomology, individuals with BED exhibit an extreme preoccupation with food, body weight, and the urge to binge eat similar to OCD obsessions. Similarities to OCD compulsions involve the actual binge eating behavior: eating very rapidly, eating large amounts of food until uncomfortably full, and feeling disgust, guilt or depression after overeating. Likewise, "the lack of satiety individuals with BED described during bingeing is similar to the lack of completeness some persons with OCD experience while ritualizing" (34). Course of illness for BED and OCD is also similar, with onset of both disorders typically beginning in adolescence or early adulthood; among those presenting for treatment, the course appears to be chronic. Binge eating is often a secretive disorder, as many individuals eat alone due to embarrassment about how much they are eating.

Numerous studies have outlined the occurrence of psychopathology (including OCD symptomology) in individuals with BED. In a study of Brazilian BED patients, Fontenelle et al. (35) found that Brazilian obese binge eaters (OBE) are significantly more likely to be affected than obese non-binge eaters (OBNE) during their lifetime by Axis I disorders (59.3% vs. 24.2%), mood disorders (34.3% vs. 12.1%) (including current or past MDD), and anxiety disorders (43.7% vs. 21.2%). Similar rates of Axis I disorders were also found in North American OBE populations (36,37).

In a study by Bulik et al. (38) binge eating was associated with elevated scores on depression, anxiety/phobia, and neurovegetative symptoms (i.e., insomnia, agitation, retardation, and obsessive–compulsive traits). Similarly, in a study by Fassino et al. (39), researchers found that obese patients with BED show greater levels of hostility, criticism, and externalized anger, independent of depression levels; additionally, in obese patients with BED, anger was strongly correlated to impulsivity. In a review of impulsivity in eating disorders, Dawe and Loxton (40) found heightened impulsivity in binge eating women from clinical and nonclinical settings. A positive relationship between measures of bulimic behavior and a component of impulsivity was also found, which lends support to a specific relationship between binge eating and rash-spontaneous impulsivity, especially in response to negative affect.

CBT is the most widely investigated treatment for BED and is often the treatment of choice for the disorder (41). Psychopharmacological treatments have also been investigated in controlled clinical trials for BED including SRIs, anti-obesity medications such as sibutramine, and anti-convulsants such as topiramate. SRIs have been the most widely studied, but all three classes of drugs have been shown to be effective in reducing binging and body weight in short-term trials (42).

IMPULSE-CONTROL DISORDERS AND BORDERLINE PERSONALITY DISORDER

Within the DSM-IV TR, pathological gambling, kleptomania (compulsive stealing), intermittent explosive disorder, pyromania (compulsive firesetting), and trichotillomania (compulsive hair pulling) are classified as impulse-control disorders (ICDs) not otherwise specified. Within the obsessive-compulsive spectrum, people afflicted with an impulse control disorder act on their impulses, despite the long-term consequences of their actions. As a group, these disorders are relatively understudied in terms of epidemiology and targeted treatments. Currently, there are other disorders such as sexual compulsivity, internet addiction, and compulsive shopping, which are not in the DSM-IV-TR, yet may fit under the heading of impulse control disorders not otherwise specified. These disorders may be considered as impulsive–compulsive disorders for the DSM-V. This section covers both DSM-IV impulse disorders and those not yet classified in the diagnostic system.

There are no statistics on obesity in relation to any of the ICDs; therefore, we assessed rates of obesity in our clinical sample (Table 1). Within this sample, all patients responded to a newspaper ad, flyer, website, or were referred to us by another physician for participation in one of our programs for pathological gambling, internet addiction, sexual compulsivity, or borderline personality disorder (BPD). The pathological gambling and BPD patients met criteria for a DSM-IV diagnosis. The internet addiction and sexual compulsivity patients met our criteria for their respective disorders. We recorded the height and weight of all the participants and calculated their body mass index (BMI). Analyses of interest will be discussed in relation to each disorder.

Within the impulse control disorders, the most studied disorder is pathological gambling (PG). According to the DSM-IV-TR, pathological

Table 1 BMI in Our Clinical Sample

Diagnosis	Percent of sample				
	Under-weight (BMI < 20)	Normal weight (BMI: 20–24.99)	Overweight (BMI: 25–29.99)	Obese (BMI > 30)	Overweight and obese combined (BMI > 25)
Pathological gambling (n = 105)	10.5 %	26.7 %	26.7 %	36.2 %	62.9%
Sexual compulsivity (n = 31)	0.0 %	32.3 %	41.9 %	25.8 %	67.7%
Internet addiction (n = 21)	4.8 %	61.9 %	14.3 %	19.0 %	33.3%
BPD (n = 33)	12.1%	24.2 %	27.3 %	36.4 %	63.7%
ICDs population (n = 190)					

Abbreviations: BMI, body mass index; BPD, boderline personality disorder; ICDS, impulse-control disorders.

gambling is characterized by "persistent and recurrent maladaptive gambling behavior that disrupts personal, family, or vocational pursuits" (DSM-IV). The distinction between a pathological gambler and a recreational or professional gambler, is that a pathological gambler's habit causes severe negative consequences such as deterioration of relationships with family and friends, and illegal actions to obtain money that may lead to imprisonment. PG has a prevalence of 1.6% in United States adults, a chronic and progressive course, and is associated with up to 20% suicide attempt rate (43,44). Comorbidity is common, particularly with substance abuse, OCD, anxiety, attention-deficit/hyperactivity, mood disorders, and binge eating. Additionally, men are twice as likely to be afflicted with pathological gambling than women (45).

Pharmacological and cognitive behavioral treatments have been efficacious in treating a PG population (46). Clomipramine, fluvoxamine, citalopram, paroxetine, and fluoxetine have all alleviated gambling symptoms. In gamblers with bipolar spectrum features, lithobid has reduced gambling symptoms and mood swings (47–53).

There is a shortage of literature pertaining to obesity and gambling. In a sample of college students, one study found significantly higher rates of binge eating in problem and pathological gamblers when compared to nongamblers and social gamblers (54). However, there was no distinction as to the role obesity played in this population. Within our clinical sample of 105 patients that met criteria for pathological gambling, 11 (10.5%)

had a BMI under 20, 28 (26.7%) had a BMI between 20 and 24.99, 28 (26.7%) had a BMI between 25 and 29.99, and 38 (36.2%) had a BMI over 30 (Table 1). In comparison to the other ICDs, sexual compulsivity and internet addiction, the pathological gambling population had much higher BMIs that were classified as overweight or obese (Table 1). Similar rates were found in our BPD population. However, these analyses are limited by sample size and program seeking nature of the population. One possible reason for the higher BMIs in this population could be due to the sedentary nature of the disorder. PG is also comorbid with BED, which can lead to obesity (54).

Kleptomania, or compulsive stealing, is rare in the general population, although exact prevalence rates are unknown (DSM-IV TR). There is no recommended treatment for kleptomania. In a sample of 22 patients diagnosed with kleptomania, 3 (13.6%) had comorbid binge eating (55). In a Swedish sample, 43% of kleptomaniacs had "food issues," although the types of food issues were not specified (56).

Persons diagnosed with intermittent explosive disorder (IED) experience specific periods in which they cannot control their aggressive impulses. According to the DSM-IV TR, IED is a rare disorder, although there are no prevalence studies to provide an estimate. SRIs, mood stabilizers, and atypical antipsychotics are clinically useful for the treatment of IED. Clozapine has been efficacious in treating adolescents with IED, although this treatment does cause weight gain in some patients (57). There are no obesity statistics in an IED population.

Pyromania, or compulsively setting fires, is relatively rare within the population and there is no targeted treatment for this disorder. The prevalence rates of trichotillomania, or compulsive hair pulling, are also unknown, however it appears to be a rare disorder. Behavioral therapies have been reported to be effective and there have been mixed results with different pharmacological treatments (58–69). Rates of obesity within these populations are unavailable.

Patients afflicted with sexual compulsivity, or problematic sexual behavior, frequently engage in episodes of anonymous sexual behavior with multiple partners without regard to the consequences (70). There are no prevalence rates for this population and there is a shortage of literature on targeted treatments, although fluoxetine has been shown to be efficacious in men with comorbid sexual compulsivity and depression (71). In our clinical sample of patients with sexual compulsivity (Table 1), rates of obesity were lower than the general population (25.8% in our sample and 30% in the general population), while rates of overweight individuals was higher in our clinical sample than in the general population (41.9% in our clinical sample and 34% in the general population). Further research in a larger sample is needed to clarify the relationship between sexual compulsivity and obesity.

Internet addiction or problematic internet use is not in the DSM-IV TR and its prevalence is unknown. Internet addiction is thought to be characterized by both impulsive and compulsive features. While some patients report the difficulties in resisting the urge to be online, others report that they "zone out" during internet use. Patients with Internet addiction often neglect household or work responsibilities. There are currently no treatments for Internet addiction. In a sample of 20 patients diagnosed with Internet addiction, two (10%) had a current diagnosis of comorbid binge eating and four (20%) had a lifetime diagnosis of binge eating (72). In our clinical sample, the vast majority of patients diagnosed with Internet addiction were of normal weight (Table 1).

Compulsive shopping is characterized by an overwhelming urge to buy items that are not needed, which results in financial issues, and psychological distress (73). Selective serotonin reuptake inhibitors have shown mixed results in treating compulsive shopping (74–77). Although there are no rates of obesity in a compulsive shopping population, Ninan et al. (78) assessed a sample of 42 compulsive shoppers and found that four (9.5%) had comorbid binge eating. Further research is needed to illuminate the relationship between impulse control, lifestyle, and weight.

The three key symptom domains of BPD are emptiness, anger, and impulsivity. Patients afflicted with BPD engage in problematic relationships, perform impulsive behavior that can lead to harmful consequences, cannot control their anger, frequently experience affective instability, and feel chronic feelings of emptiness. Within the obsessive–compulsive spectrum, BPD patients act on their impulsive urges without regard to the cost of their actions. Approximately 2% of the population is afflicted with BPD (DSM-IV TR). Dialectical Behavioral Therapy (DBT), developed by Marsha Linehan, is an effective therapy (79,80). Pharmacotherapies such as clozapine, risperidone, divalproex sodium have shown efficacy (81–86). Olanzapine has been effective in treating BPD, however, it does cause some weight gain (87).

Several studies have found a link between BPD and obesity (88–91). Sansone et al. (92) assessed a sample of obese women with the diagnostic interview for borderline patients. Seven percent of the sample met the criteria for BPD, which is a much higher rate than in the general population. The authors hypothesize that the relationship between obesity and BPD may be due in part to "self-regulatory deficits" which may result in overeating (93). These self-regulatory deficits can also be conceptualized as an impulse control problem within the obsessive compulsive spectrum. In our clinical sample (Table 1), 36.4% of the patients were obese, which is a higher rate than the general population.

DEVELOPMENTAL DISORDERS

Obesity is a part of the clinical presentation of a number of developmental disorders including PWS, Cohen syndrome, and Bardet-Biedl syndrome (94). Of these conditions, PWS also has impulsive and compulsive behaviors that are considered core features of the syndrome. PWS is a complex, multi-system genetic disorder caused by genetic abnormalities on chromosome 15q on a region known as the Prader–Willi/Angelman critical region (PWACR). PWS has an estimated prevalence of 1/10,000 to 1/15,000 with an approximately equal male:female ratio.

The clinical features of PWS vary by age. The cardinal symptom of PWS in infancy is severe hypotonia. A number of failure to thrive symptoms are associated with the hypotonia including feeding difficulties as a result of poor suckling response, slow weight gain, and impaired growth. Between two and four years, the other defining feature of the disorder, hyperphagia, emerges and results in rapid weight gain and extreme obesity. Dysmophic and other physical features of PWS include short stature, almond shaped eyes, smaller hands and feet, and hypogonadism. PWS is also associated with mild to moderate mental retardation, characteristic behavior problems that persist into adulthood (e.g., temper tantrums and aggression), and a number of psychiatric conditions including OCD, bipolar disorder, and severe affective disorder with psychosis (94).

Compulsive behaviors in PWS include compulsive eating, insistence on sameness, perseverations, hoarding, and skin-picking (95). Clarke et al. (96) conducted a population-based study of compulsions in individuals with PWS. The authors found that the majority of individuals exhibited a greater number and severity of compulsive symptoms than a comparison group of individuals with similar intellectual disabilities and BMIs. The need to ask or confess (49.1%) and adherence to routines (29.8%) were the most commonly reported compulsions by caregivers. The more classic OCD behaviors such as hand washing and checking, and obsessions are less prevalent than the other compulsions. Other studies have found skin-picking to be prevalent in individuals with PWS, occurring in 78% of the sample in one study (95). Factor analytic studies evaluating the relationships between compulsive behaviors in PWS suggest that skin-picking is not strongly associated with other compulsive behaviors (97). These investigations suggest that skin-picking in PWS, may represent the pleasure-seeking or impulsive behaviors, rather than the anxiety-reduction dimension of the OC spectrum.

Although the motor problems, compulsions, and disruptive behaviors cause significant impairment in PWS, obesity is the most prominent feature and the leading cause of death, with approximately 90% of individuals with PWS meeting criteria for clinical obesity (98). The average BMI for individuals with PWS was found to be 31.6 kg in the previously cited population-based investigation (96). Individuals with PWS frequently experience common obesity-related problem such as Type II diabetes, heart disease, and skin problems on the legs such as chronic edema and thrombophlebitis (94). In addition, the food-seeking behaviors in PWS cause distress for families and the individuals. Individuals with PWS have an extreme obsession with food and have impairments in their sense of satiety. Clinical observations commonly include significant efforts and time spent in food-seeking activities such as hoarding and sneaking food, gorging food, and eating unappetizing foods such as pet food, garbage, and sticks of butter. The eating behaviors in PWS are thought to be related with compulsivity, with more ritualized eating behaviors observed in PWS compared to obese individuals matched for intellectual functioning (99).

Although the etiology and mechanisms for the hyperphagia in PWS is not known, studies indicate that the chromosomal abnormalities in 15q11 result in hypothalamic dysfunction (100). A number of hypothalamic deficits are observed in PWS including the lack of sense satiety, severe growth hormone deficiency resulting in short stature and medical complications, hypoganadism, and sleep and temperature regulation difficulties. Zipf et al. (101) reported that impaired polypeptide release after a meal might be related to the hypothalamic dysfunction in PWS. Delparigi et al. (102) suggests that ghrelin, a novel orexigenic hormone, is elevated in PWS. Ghrelin is an endogenous hormone released by the stomach and is involved in maintaining energy, initiating meals, and decreasing fat utilization in rodents. Ghrelin levels are found to be high before a meal and decrease afterwards. Delparigi et al. (102) found that individuals with PWS did not have variations in ghrelin levels before and after meals which may be an explanation for the hyperphagia and lack of satiety.

Given the complexity of the disorder, a multi-disciplinary medical and behavioral treatment approach in PWS is necessary. A targeted symptom approach is used in PWS for treating the obesity, compulsive behaviors, behavior disorders, and hormone regulation deficiencies individually. Obesity in PWS has been treated with both behavioral and medical interventions. Behavioral treatments include environmental controls such as close supervision, locking cabinets, refrigerator doors, and diet controls including low-calorie, low-fat diets. Many individuals with PWS are placed in residential settings because of the environmental modifications required to control their diets (103). Growth hormone treatment has also been used to successfully modify body composition in PWS, resulting in reduced body fat and increased lean body mass (100). Finally, several studies have attempted the use of Topiramate in individuals with PWS. Topiramate is a novel antiepileptic, which has shown preliminary efficacy in the treatment of BED, in individuals with PWS. One study found Topiramate was effective in reducing skin-picking, improving mood, and stabilizing weight (104). However, Shapira et al. (105) confirmed the beneficial effects of tompiramate on skin-picking, but found no improvements in weight gain. In summary, the current treatments for obesity in PWS appear to be moderately effective in controlling hyperphagia. Research on treatments for PWS is in its nascent stages and will hopefully explore combined behavioral and medical treatments for the condition as the field advances.

Another developmental disorder with OC spectrum features is autism spectrum disorders (ASDs). Autism is one of the most severe neuropsychiatric developmental disorders defined by impairments in three cores symptom domains: communication, socialization, and repetitive behaviors/restricted interests. ASDs include autistic disorder, Asperger's disorder, and pervasive developmental disorder, not otherwise specified (PDD-NOS) and are distinguished by differences in severity and number of the core symptoms. While prevalence rates are currently debated, conservative estimates suggest prevalence rates of 27.5/10,000 for the combined spectrum disorders (10/10,000 for the full condition of autistic disorder, 1.7/10,000 for Asperger's, and 15/10,000 for PDD-NOS), although some studies provide prevalence estimates almost twice as high (106). Currently, there is no FDA approved treatment for the syndrome of autism. Currently, a multi-modal treatment approach is recommended for ASD with educational (e.g., applied behavior analysis), medical interventions (e.g., SSRI treatments for repetitive behaviors, atypical and anticonvulsants for disruptive behaviors), and social skills interventions used to treat the core and associated symptoms of autism.

ASD shares commonalities in terms of symptom presentation, treatment, and possibly genetic etiology with PWS. Both disorders have also been associated with abnormalities on chromosome 15q (107). Furthermore, both disorders also share compulsive (e.g., need for sameness), impulsive (self-injury), and impaired social behaviors. The compulsive core of ASD, a diagnostic symptom domain, includes stereotyped movements such as hand flapping and rocking; maintenance of rigid routines; repetitive, nonfunctional toy play; restricted eating patterns; repetitive questions or verbal rituals; and immediate and delayed echolalia. Although impulsivity is not a core feature, it is commonly associated with ASD and includes behaviors such as self-injury (e.g., head banging and skin-picking), aggressivity, and hyperactivity. It has been hypothesized that the stereotyped and repetitive behaviors in autism may actually span across the dimension of risk-averse versus risk-seeking in OC spectrum conditions. Lower-order behaviors, such as self-stimulatory hand flapping, may serve more of a pleasure-seeking, self-reinforcement function and thus may be more akin to impulse control disorders. Alternatively, higher-order behaviors, such as the need for sameness and verbal rituals, may serve an anxiolytic function, and be more akin to compulsive behaviors in anxiety disorders such as OCD Anagnostou E (personal communication).

Although obesity is not a commonly associated feature in ASD, excessive weight gain during administration of atypical neuroleptics in children with ASD is a growing concern. Risperidone is the most widely used and studied neuroleptic in ASD and has been effective in reducing aggression, irritability, and other impulsive behaviors associated with autism in an eight-week, randomized, double-blind placebo controlled trial conducted by the Research Units on Pediatric Psychopharmacology Autism Network

(108). Weight gain is a commonly reported side effect in both open-label and controlled evaluations of risperidone (109). The RUPP network found clinically and statistically significant weight gain in the eight-week trial, with an average increase of approximately 5.9 lbs for the treatment group and 1.76 lbs for placebo [$p < 0.001$ for each comparison, (108)]. In a long-term (6 mo) follow-up trial, the RUPP studies reported absolute weight and BMI increases of 16.7%, which was more than expected based on developmentally normative growth during that period. Martin et al. (110) found a curvilinear effect, with rate of weight gain slowing over time.

Our own studies with the atypical antipsychotic, olanzapine, suggests olanzapine is also associated with significant weight gain. Hollander et al. (111) evaluated the effects of olanzapine on the impulsive behaviors in nine children with ASD in a randomized, short-term (eight-week), double-blind, placebo controlled trial. The average weight gain for children taking olanzapine was 9 lbs (sd = 3.5) compared to 1.5 lbs (sd = 1.47) in the placebo group ($t = 3.935$, $p = 0.006$). The weight gain associated with olanzapine in our trial is supported by open-label studies (112).

The mechanism by which atypical antipsychotics produce weight gain is currently unknown. Some studies suggest that the weight gain results from increased appetite, possibly from desensitization of leptin receptors such that the satiety centers do not receive adequate feedback (113). Evidence for temporary or permanent changes in metabolism are not available and are considered unlikely.

The rapid and sudden weight gain associated with atypical antipsychotic use in ASD is of serious clinical concern, given the wide use of this class of drugs in children with ASD. Anecdotal reports and the long-term RUPP trial suggest that weight gain within the first few weeks of administration could be predictive of overall weight gain. As such, clinicians using atypical antipsychotics may consider alternatives when rapid weight gain is observed during the initial phase of treatment. In addition to the long-term health risks (e.g., diabetes), clinical reports of increased frustration and aggression related to food may also create immediate problems in family functioning. As such, future investigations of atypical antipsychotics in this population should specifically evaluate the hypothesized mechanisms for weight gain, albeit, leptin receptor desensitization, or increased insulin levels. Identifying such mechanisms may provide avenues to use this powerful treatment in a safer and clinically meaningful manner.

SUMMARY

Our review of the literature exposes the paucity of information available on the relationship between OC spectrum conditions and obesity. Compulsive eating is clearly related to some cases of obesity, particularly in the cases of BED and PWS. The nature of compulsive eating in these disorders is akin to other compulsions such as those reported in OCD, in which compulsions are associated with a drop in anxiety and sense of temporary relief. The high co-morbidity of OCD and other compulsive behaviors also suggests an important commonality in the phenomology of these disorders. Further investigations of the comorbidity of compulsive eating in other OC spectrum disorders are needed to evaluate the true prevalence and nature of this problem.

Obesity also appears to be related to OC spectrum conditions as a secondary effect of medication and lifestyle. That is, obesity is found in higher rates than expected in our compulsive gambling and borderline personality disorder populations. Exploring the relationships between compulsive eating and lifestyle issues such as activity level and diet are warranted to better understand the rates of obesity found in our sample. Finally, the rates of obesity observed in studies of atypical antipsychotics used with children with autism spectrum disorders merit attention. Although various atypicals have been found to reduce incidence of weight gain in other mental disorders, the rapid weight gain associated with atypical antipsychotic use in some patients with autism should be investigated in longitudinal studies.

REFERENCES

1. Hollander E. Obsessive-Compulsive-Related Disorder. Washington, DC: American Psychiatric Press, 1993.
2. Rasmussen. Obsessive compulsive spectrum disorders. J Clin Psychiatry 1994; 55:89–91.
3. Hollander E. Treatment of obsessive-compulsive spectrum disorders with SSSRIs. Br J Psychiatry 1998; 173(suppl 35):7–12.
4. Allen A, King A, Hollander E. Obsessive compulsive spectrum disorders. Dialog Clin Neurosci, Anxiety II 2003; 5(3):259–271.
5. Baxter LR, Schwartz JM, Guze BH, Bergman K, Szuba MP. Neuroimaging in obsessive-compulsive disorders: seeking the mediating neuroanatomy. In: Jenike MA, Baer L, Minichiello W, eds. Obessive Compulsive Disorders: Practical Management. 2nd ed. Chicago, Ill: Year Book Medical Publishers, 1990:167–188.
6. Narrow WE, Rae DS, Regier DA. NIMH epidemiology note: prevalence of anxiety disorders. One-year prevalence best estimates calculated from ECA and NCS data. Population estimates based on U.S. Census estimated residential population age 18 to 54 on July 1, 1998. Unpublished.
7. American Psychiatric Association. Diagnostic and Statistical Manual of Mental Disorders. 4th ed. Washington, DC: American Psychiatric Association; 1994.
8. Greenberg BD, Altemus M. The role of neurotransmitters and neuropeptides in obsessive-compulsive disorder. Greenberg and Altemus. Int Rev Psychiatry 1997; 9:31–34.
9. Rabheru K, Persad E. A review of continuation and maintenance electroconvulsive therapy. Can J Psychiatry 1997; 43:305–306.

10. Anderson D, Ahmed A. Treatment of patients with intractable obsessive-compulsive disorder with anterior capsular stimulation. J Neurosurg 2003; 98:1104–1108.

11. Nuttin BJ, Gabriels LA, Cosyns PR, et al. Long-term electrical capsular stimulation in patients with obsessive-compulsive disorder. Neurosurgery 2003; 52:1263–1274.

12. Speranza M, Corcos M, Godart N, et al. Obsessive compulsive disorders in eating disorders. Autumn 2001; 2:193–207.

13. Wigren M, Hansen S. Rituals and compulsivity in Prader-Willi syndrome: profile and stability. J Intell Dis Res 2003; 47(6):428–438.

14. Metin O, Yazici K, Tot S, Yazici AE. Amisulpiride augmentation in treatment resistant obsessive-compulsive disorder: an open trial. Hum Psychopharmacol 2003; 18:463–467.

15. Bystritsky A, Ackerman DL, Rosen RM, et al. Augmentation of serotonin reuptake inhibitors in refractory obsessive–compulsive disorder using adjunctive olanzapine: a placebo-controlled trial. J Clin Psychiatry 2004; 65:565–568.

16. Bogetto F, Bellino S, Vaschetto P, Ziero S. Olanzapine augmentation of fluvoxamine-refractory obsessive-compulsive disorder (OCD): a 12-week open trial. Psychiatry Res 2000; 96:91–98.

17. Fava M, Judge R, Hoog SL, Nilsson ME, Koke SC. Fluoxetine versus sertraline and paroxetine in major depressive disorder: changes in weight with long term treatment. J Clin Psychiatry 2000; 61:863–867.

18. Allison DB, Mentore JL, Heo M, et al. Antipsychotic induced weight gain: a comprehensive research synthesis. Am J Psychiatry 1999; 156:1686–1696.

19. Otto MW, Wilhelm S, Cohen LS, Harlow BL. Prevalence of body dysmorphic disorder in a community sample of women. Am J Psychiatry 2001; 158:2061–2063.

20. Phillips KA, Atala KD, Pope HG. Diagnostic instruments for body dysmorphic disorder. In: New Research Program and Abstracts, American Psychiatric Association 148th Annual Meeting. Miami: American Psychiatric Association, 1995:157.

21. Rich N, Rosen JC, Orosan PG, Reiter JT. Prevalence of body dysmorphic disorder in non-clinical populations. Presented at: Association for the Advancement of Behavior Therapy; Boston, Massachusetts: November 2, 1992.

22. McElroy SL, Phillips KA, Keck PE Jr. Obsessive compulsive spectrum disorder. J Clin Psychiatry 1994; 55(suppl: 33–51); discussion 52–53.

23. Phillips KA, Albertini RS, Siniscalchi JM, Khan A, Robinson M. Effectiveness of pharmacotherapy for body dysmorphic disorder: a chart review study. J Clin Psychiatry 2001; 62:721–727.

24. Neziroglu F, Khemlani-Patel S. A review of cognitive and behavioral treatment for body dysmorphic disorder. CNS Spectr 2002; 7:464–471.

25. Speranza M, Corcos M, Godart N, et al. Obsessive compulsive disorders in eating disorders. Autumn 2001; 2:193–207.

26. de Zwaan M, Mitchell JE, Raymond NC, Spitzer RL. Binge eating disorder: clinical features and treatment of a new diagnosis. Harv Rev Psychiatry 1999; 1:310–325.

27. Agras WS. Treatment of binge-eating disorder. In: Gabbard GO, ed. Treatment of Psychiatric Disorders. Washington, DC: American Psychiatric Press, 2001:2209–2219.
28. Spitzer RL, Yanovski S, Wadden T, et al. Binge eating disorder: its further validation in a multisite study. Int J Eat Disord 2003; 13:137–153.
29. American Psychiatric Association Work Group on Eating Disorders. Practice guideline for the treatment of patients with eating disorders (revision). Am J Psychiat 2000; 157(suppl 1):1–39.
30. de Zwaan M. Binge eating disorder and obesity. Int J Obes Relat Metab Disord 2001; 25(suppl 1):S51–S55.
31. Telch CF, Agras WS, Rossiter EM. Binge eating increases with increasing adiposity. Int J Eat Disord 1988; 7:115–119.
32. Dingemans AE, Bruna MJ, van Furth EF. Binge eating disorder: a review. Int J Obes 2002; 26:299–307.
33. Becker ES, Margraf J, Turke V, Soeder U, Neumer S. Obesity and mental illness in a representative sample of young women. Int J Obes 2001; 1(suppl 25):S5–S9.
34. McElroy SL, Phillips KA, Keck PE Jr. Obsessive compulsive spectrum disorder. J Clin Psychiatry 1994; 55(suppl: 33–51); discussion 52–53.
35. Fontenelle LF, Mendlowicz MV, Bezerra de Menezes G, et al. Psychiatric comorbidity in a Brazilian sample of patients with binge-eating disorder. Psychiatry Res 2003; 119:189–194.
36. Yanovski SZ, Nelson JE, Dubbert BK, Spitzer RL. Association of binge eating disorder and psychiatric comorbidity in obese subjects. Am J Psychiatry 1993; 150:1472–1479.
37. Marcus MD, Wing RR, Ewing L, Kern E, Gooding W, McDermott M. Psychiatric disorders among obese binge eaters. Int J Eat Disord 1990; 9:69–77.
38. Bulik CM, Sullivan PF, Kendler KS. Medical and psychiatric morbidity in obese women with and without binge eating. Int J Eat Disord 2002; 32:72–78.
39. Fassino S, Leombruni P, Piero A, Abbate-Daga G, Rovera GG. Mood, eating attitudes and anger in obese women with and without binge eating disorder. J Psychosom Res 2003; 54:559–566.
40. Dawe S, Loxton NJ. The role of impulsivity in the development of substance use and eating disorders. Neurosci Biobehav Rev 2004; 28:343–351.
41. Wifley DE, Cohen LR. Psychological Treatment of bulimia nervosa and binge eating disorder. Psychopharmac Bull 1997; 33:437–454.
42. Appolinario JC, McElroy SL. Pharmacological approaches in the treatment of binge eating disorder. Curr Drug Targets 2004; 5:301–307.
43. Shaffer HJ, Hall MN, Vander Bilt J. Estimating the prevalence of disorder gambling behavior in the United States and Canada: a research synthesis. Am J Public Health 1999; 89:1369–1376.
44. Hollander E, Buchalter AJ, DeCaria CM. Pathological gambling. Psychiatr Clin North Am 2000; 23:629–642.
45. Volberg RA. The prevalence and demographics of pathological gamblers: implications for public health. Am J Pub Health 1994; 84:237–241.
46. Volberg RA, Abbott MW. Gambling and problem gambling among indigenous peoples. Subst Use Misuse 1997; 32:1525–1538.

47. Grant JE, Kim SW, Potenza MN. Advances in the pharmacological treatment of pathological gambling. J Gambl Stud 2003; 19:85–109.
48. Hollander E, Frenkel M, DeCaria C, Trungold S, Stein DJ. Treatment of pathological gambling with clomipramine [letter]. Am J Psychiatry 1992; 149:710–711.
49. Hollander E, DeCaria CM, Mari E, et al. Short-term single-blind fluvoxamine treatment of pathological gambling. Am J Psychiatry 1998; 155:1781–1783.
50. Hollander E, DeCaria CM, Finkell JN, Begaz T, Wong CM, Cartwright C. A randomized double-blind fluvoxamine/placebo crossover trial in pathological gambling. Biol Psychiatry 2000; 47:813–817.
51. Zimmerman M, Breen R. An open-label study of citalopram in the treatment of pathological gambling. J Clin Psychiatry 2002; 63:44–48.
52. Kim SW, Grant JE, Adson DE, Shin YC, Zaninelli RM. A double-blind, placebo-controlled study of the efficacy and safety of paroxetine in the treatment of pathological gambling. J Clin Psychiatry 2002; 63:501–507.
53. De la Gandara JJ. Fluoxetine: open-trial in pathological gambling. 152nd Annual Meeting of the American Psychiatric Association, Washington, DC: May 16–21, 1999.
54. Hollander E, Pallanti S, Allen A, Sood E, Baldini Rossi N. Sustained–release lithium reduces impulsive gambling and affective instability vs. placebo in bipolar spectrum pathological gamblers. Am J Psychiatry 2005; 162:137–145.
55. Engwall D, Hunter R, Steinberg M. Gambling and other risk behaviors on university campuses. J Am Coll Health 2004; 52:245–255.
56. Grant JE, Kim SW. Clinical characteristics and associated psychopathology of 22 patients with kleptomania. Comp Psychiatry 2002; 43:378–384.
57. Sarasalo E, Bergman B, Toth J. Personality traits and psychiatric and somatic morbidity among kleptomaniacs. Acta Psychiatr Scand 1996; 94:358–364.
58. Kant R, Chalansani R, Chengappa R, Dieringer MF. The off-label use of clozapine in adolescents with bipolar disorder, intermittent explosive disorder, or posttraumatic stress disorder. J Child Adolesc Psychopharmacol 2004; 14:57–63.
59. van Minnen A, Hoogduin KAL, Keijsers GPJ, Hellenbrand I, Hendriks GJ. Treatment of trichotillomania with behavioral therapy or fluoxetine. Arch Gen Psychiatry 2003; 60:517–522.
60. Rosenbaum MS, Allyon T. The habit reversal technique in treating trichotillomania. Behav Ther 1981; 12:473–481.
61. Vitulano LA, King RA, Scahill L, Cohen DJ. Behavioral treatment of children and adolescents with trichotillomania. J Am Acad Child Adolesc Psychiatry 1992; 31:139–146.
62. Rothbaum BO. The behavioral treatment of trichotillomania. Behav Psychother 1992; 20:85–89.
63. Mouton SG, Stanley MA. Habit reversal training for trichotillomania: a group approach. Cogn Behav Pract 1996; 3:159–182.
64. Lerner J, Franklin ME, Meadows EA, Hembree E, Foa EB. Effectiveness of a cognitive behavioral treatment program for trichotillomania. Behav Ther 1998; 29:157–171.

65. Salama SA, Salama AA. New behavioral approach to trichotillomania [letter]. Am J Psychiatry 1999; 156:1469–1470.
66. Pollard CA, Ibe IO, Krojanker DN, Kitchen AD, Bronson SS, Flynn TM. Clomipramine treatment of trichotillomania: a follow-up report on four cases. J Clin Psychiatry 1991; 52:128–130.
67. Stein DJ, Hollander E. Low-dose pimozide augmentation of serotonin reuptake blockers in the treatment of trichotillomania. J Clin Psychiatry 1992; 53:123–126.
68. Koran LM, Ringold A, Hewlett W. Fluoxetine for trichotillomania: an open clinical trial. Psychopharmacol Bull 1992; 28:145–149.
69. Stanley MA, Bowers TC, Swann AC, Taylor DJ. Treatment of trichotillomania with fluoxetine [letter]. J Clin Psychiatry 1991; 52:282.
70. Winchel RM, Jones JS, Stanley B, Molcho A, Stanley M. Clinical characteristics of trichotillomania and its response to fluoxetine. J Clin Psychiatry 1992; 53:304–308.
71. Raymond NC, Coleman E, Miner MH. Psychiatric comorbidity and compulsive/impulsive traits in compulsive sexual behavior. Compr Psychiatry 2003; 44:370–380.
72. Kafka MP, Prentky R. Fluoxetine treatment of nonparaphilic sexual addictions and paraphilias in men. J Clin Psychiatry 1992; 53:351–358.
73. Shapira NA, Goldsmith TD, Keck PE Jr, Khosla UM, McElroy SL. Psychiatric features of individuals with problematic internet use. J Affect Disord 2000; 57:267–272.
74. Christenson GA, Faber RJ, De Zwaan M, et al. Compulsive buying: descriptive characteristics and psychiatric comorbidity. J Clin Psychiatry 1994; 55:5–11.
75. Koran LM, Chuong HW, Bullock KD, Smith SC. Citalopram for compulsive shopping disorder: an open-label study followed by double-blind discontinuation. J Clin Psychiatry 2003; 64:793–798.
76. Black DW, Gabel J, Hansen J, Schlosser S. A double-blind comparison of fluvoxamine versus placebo in the treatment of compulsive buying disorder. Ann Clin Psychiatry 2000; 12:205–211.
77. Black DW, Monahan P, Gabel J. Fluvoxamine in the treatment of compulsive buying. J Clin Psychiatry 1997; 58:159–163.
78. Ninan PT, McElroy SL, Kane CP, et al. Placebo-controlled study of fluvoxamine in the treatment of subjects with compulsive buying. J Clin Psychopharmacol 2000; 20:363–366.
79. Linehan MM. Dialectical behavior therapy: a cognitive-behavioral approach to parasuicide. J Personal Disord 1987; 1:328–333.
80. Linehan MM. Cognitive-behavioral Treatment of Borderline Personality Disorder. Guilford: New York, 1993.
81. Chengappa KNR, Ebeling T, Kang JS, Levine J, Parepally H. Clozapine reduces severe self-mutilation and aggression in psychotic patients with borderline personality disorder. J Clin Psychiatry 1999; 60:477–484.
82. Parker GF. Clozapine and borderline personality disorder. Psychiatr Serv 2002; 53:348–349.

83. Rocca P, Marchiaro L, Cocuzza E, Bogetto E. Treatment of borderline personality disorder with risperidone. J Clin Psychiatry 2002; 63:241–244.
84. Townsend MH, Cambre KM, Barbee JG. Treatment of borderline personality disorder with mood instability with divalproex sodium: series of ten cases. J Clin Psychopharmacol 2001; 21:249–251.
85. Frankenburg FR, Zanarini MC. Divalproex sodium treatment of women with borderline personality disorder and bipolar II disorder: a double-blind, placebo-controlled pilot study. J Clin Psychiatry 2002; 63:442–446.
86. Hollander E, Allen A, Lopez RP, et al. A preliminary double-blind, placebo-controlled trial of divalproex sodium in borderline personality disorder. J Clin Psychiatry 2001; 62:199–203.
87. Bogenschutz MP, George Nurnberg H. Olanzapine versus placebo in the treatment of borderline personality disorder. J Clin Psychiatry 2004; 65:104–109.
88. Grana AS, Coolidge FL, Merwin MM. Personality profiles of the morbidly obese. J Clin Psychol 1989; 45:762–765.
89. Black DW, Yates WR, Reich JH, Bell S, Goldstein RB, Mason EE. DSM-III personality disorder in bariatric clinic patients. Ann Clin Psychiatry 1989; 1:33–37.
90. Berman WH, Berman ER, Heymsfield S, Fauci M, Ackerman S. The incidence and comorbidity of psychiatric disorders in obesity. J Pers Disord 1992; 6:168–175.
91. Yanovski SZ, Nelson JE, Dubbert BK, Spitzer RL. Association of binge eating disorder and psychiatric comorbidity in obese subjects. Am J Psychiatry 1993; 150:1472–1479.
92. Sansone RA, Sansone LA, Fine MA. The relationship of obesity to borderline personality, self-harm behaviors, and sexual abuse in female subjects in a primary-care setting. J Pers Disord 1995; 1:254–265.
93. Sansone RA, Sansone LA, Wiederman MW. The comorbidity, relationship and treatment implications of borderline personality and obesity. J Psychosom Res 1997; 43:541–543.
94. Gunay-Aygun M, Cassidy SB, Nicholls RD. Prader-Willi and other syndromes associated with obesity and mental retardation. Beh Genet 1997; 27(4):307–324.
95. Wigren M, Hansen S. Rituals and compulsivity in Prader-Willi syndrome: profile and stability. J Intellec Disab Res 2003; 47(6):428–438.
96. Clarke DJ, Boer H, Whittington J, Holland A, Butler J, Webb T. Prader-Willi syndrome, compulsive and ritualistic behaviors: the first population based survey. Brit J Psychiatry 2002; 180:358–362.
97. Feurer ID, Dimitropoulos A, Stone WL, Roof E, Butler MG, Thompson T. The latent variable structure of the Compulsive Behavior Checklist in people with Prader-Willi syndrome. J Intel Disab Res 1998; 42(6):472–480.
98. Delparigi A., Tschöp M, Heiman ML, et al. High circulating ghrelin: A potential cause for the hyperphagia and obesity in Prader-Willi Syndrome. J Clin Endocrinol Metab 2002; 87(12):5461–5464.
99. Dimitropoulous A, Feurer ID, Roof E, et al. Appetitive behavior, compulsivity, and neurochemistry in Prader-Willi Syndrome. Mental Ret Dev Dis Res Rev 2000; 6:125–130.

100. Hoybye C, Hilding A, Jacobsson H, Thorén M. Metabolic profile and body composition in adults with Prader-Willi Syndrome and severe obesity. J Clin Endocrinol Metab 2002; 87(8):3590–3597.
101. Zipf WB, O'Dorisio TM, Cataland S, Dixon K. Pancreatic polypeptide responses to protein meal challenges in obese but otherwise normal children and obese children with Prader-Willi syndrome. J Clin Endocrinol Metab 1983; 57(5):1074–1080.
102. Delparigi A., Tschöp M, Heiman ML, et al. High circulating ghrelin: A potential cause for the hyperphagia and obesity in Prader-Willi Syndrome. J Clin Endocrinol Metab 2002; 87(12):5461–5464.
103. Greenswag LR. Adults with Prader-Willi syndrome: a survey of 232 cases. Dev Med Child Neurol 1987; 29:145–152.
104. Smathers SA, Wilson JG, Nigro MA. Topiramate effectiveness in Prader-Willi syndrome. Ped Neurology 2003; 28(2):130–133.
105. Shapira NA, Lessig MC, Lewis MH, Goodman WK, Driscoll DJ. Effects of topiramate in adults with Prader-Willi Syndrome. Am J Mental Retard 2004; 109(4):301–309.
106. Fombonne E. Epidemiological surveys of autism and other pervasive developmental disorders: an update. J Autism Develop Disord 2003; 33(4):365–382.
107. Schanen C. Dosage analysis of choromosome 15q duplications in autism by array CGH. Symposia presented at the CPEA-STAART Annual Meeting, Bethesda, MD: May 17–20, 2004.
108. McCracken JT, McGough J, Shah B, et al. Risperidone in children with autism and serious behavioral problems. N Engl J Med 2002; 347(5):314–321.
109. Masi G, Cosenza A, Mucci M, Brovedani P. A 3-year naturalistic study of 53 preschool children with pervasive developmental disorders treated with risperidone. J Clin Psychiatry 2003; 64(9):1039–1047.
110. Martin A, Scahill L, Anderson GM, et al. Weight and leptin changes among risperidone-treated youths with autism: 6-month prospective data. Am J Psychiatry 2004; 161:1125–1127.
111. Hollander E, Wasserman S, Swanson E, Zagursky K, Chaplin W. Olanzapine vs. placebo in childhood and adolescent autism: a double blind placebo controlled study. Submitted to The International Journal of Neuropsychopharmacology.
112. Kemner C, Willemsen-Swinkels SH, de Jonge M, Tuynman-Qua H, van Engeland H. Open label study of olanzapine in children with pervasive developmental disorder. J Clin Psychopharmacol 2002; 22(5):455–460.
113. Gothelf D, Falk B, Singer P, et al. Weight gain associated with increased food intake and low habitual activity levels in male adolescent schizophrenic inpatients treated with olanzapine. Am J Psychiatry 2002; 159:1055–1057.

8

Metabolic Syndrome: Overview and Relationship with Psychiatric Disorders

Richard A. Bermudes

Department of Psychiatry and Behavioral Sciences, University of California Davis Medical Center, Sacramento, California, U.S.A.

Anna Guerdjikova

Department of Psychiatry, University of Cincinnati College of Medicine, Cincinnati, Ohio, U.S.A.

INTRODUCTION

Obesity and diabetes are worldwide epidemics (1,2). The medical community is keenly aware of the heightened risk for these two disorders in the general population. However, many psychiatrists and mental health providers are unaware of the particular risk psychiatric patients face for obesity and its complications. One such complication of obesity is the metabolic syndrome. It is also known as "syndrome X." The metabolic syndrome is a grouping of risk factors predisposing individuals to type 2 diabetes and cardiovascular disease (CVD).

The association of central obesity with changes in metabolism has been described in the medical literature for the last 50 years. In 1988, Dr. Gerald Reaven noted that persons with CVD often had three other conditions: dylipidemia, hypertension, and hyperglycemia, and linked this constellation of features with the android pattern of fat distribution (3). He named this phenotype "syndrome X." Subsequently, other names for syndrome X appeared in the medical literature, including "Reaven's syndrome," "dysmetabolic syndrome," and "insulin resistance syndrome." In 1998, a working group on the definition of diabetes organized by the World Health Organization (WHO) first proposed a definition for syndrome X, naming it the "metabolic syndrome" (4). In 2001, a report from the National Cholesterol Education Program-Adult Treatment Panel III (NCEP-ATP III), identified the metabolic syndrome as an independent risk factor for CVD and proposed clinical criteria for the diagnosis, recommending "intensive lifestyle modification" as first line treatment (5).

DEFINING FEATURES OF THE METABOLIC SYNDROME

The fundamental components of the metabolic syndrome include abdominal obesity, insulin resistance, elevated blood pressure, dyslipidemia (elevated triglycerides and/or low high-density lipoprotein (HDL) cholesterol), and abnormalities in prothrombotic and proinflamatory factors. Table 1 lists the two major criteria sets used today to make the clinical diagnosis of the metabolic syndrome. There are subtle differences between the NCEP-ATP III and WHO criteria although they are similar in structure. The WHO criteria require patients to have direct evidence of insulin resistance which can be verified by oral glucose tolerance testing, measurement of insulin itself, or a diagnosis of type 2 diabetes. In contrast, the NCEP-ATP III criteria rely upon simple measurement of fasting glucose to define impaired glucose metabolism. The NCEP-ATP III criteria do not include weight or body mass index (BMI) as a defining feature, whereas the WHO criteria use either a measure of waist size or BMI as one criterion. The WHO includes microalbuminuria (indicative of a proinflamatory state), while NCEP-ATP III does not. Despite these differences, there are a number of similarities and many are identified with the syndrome regardless of the criteria used. Neither definition, for example, excludes patients with type 2 diabetes.

Research suggests that the metabolic syndrome is associated with a proinflamatory/prothrombotic state, although it is not part of the clinical criteria. Elevated C-reactive protein, endothelial dysfunction, hyperfibrinogenemia, increased plasminogen activator inhibitor 1, elevated uric acid, microalbuminuria, and a shift toward small, dense particles of low-density lipoprotein (LDL) cholesterol have been all associated with the metabolic syndrome. Similar to the other components highlighted in the WHO and NCEP-ATP III criteria, these factors increase one's risk for CVD and type 2 diabetes (6–14).

SIGNIFICANCE OF METABOLIC SYNDROME

People with the metabolic syndrome are at increased risk for type 2 diabetes, CVD, as well as increased mortality from CVD and all causes (15–17). In a prospective study, Lakka et al. (18) followed healthy Finnish men with and

Table 1 ATP and WHO Criteria for Metabolic Syndrome

	ATP III	WHO
Criteria	Presence of 3 of 5 criteria	Presence of disturbance in glucose metabolism plus two other criteria.
Glucose metabolism	High fasting glucose ($\geq$110 g/dL or $\geq$6.1 mmol/L)	Presence of diabetes, impaired glucose tolerance, impaired fasting glucose, or insulin resistance
Obesity	Abdominal obesity (waist circumference: >102 cm in men, >88 cm in women)	Central obesity: waist to hip ratio of >0.90 in men or >0.85 in women and/or BMI >30 kg/m^2
Lipids	Hypertriglyceridemia: $\geq$150 mg/dL (1.695 mmol/L) Low HDL cholesterol: <40 mg/dL (1.036 mmol/L) in men <50 mg/dL (1.295 mmol/L) in women	Hyperlipidemia: triglycerides $\geq$150 mg/dL (1.695 mmol/L) and/or HDL cholesterol <35 mg/dL (0.9 mmol/L) in men and <39 mg/dL (1.0 mmol/L) in women
Blood pressure	High blood pressure: $\geq$130/85 mmHg	High blood pressure: $\geq$160/90 mmHg
Albumin		Microalbuminuria: urinary albumin excretion rate $\geq$20 μg/min or an albumin to creatinine ratio $\geq$20 mg/g

Abbreviations: ATP, adult treatment panel; BMI, body mass index; HDL, high-density lipoprotein; WHO, World Health Organization

without the metabolic syndrome over an average of 11.4 years and measured death due to coronary heart disease, CVD, and any cause. Subjects with the metabolic syndrome were more likely to die from coronary heart disease, CVD, and all causes, even after adjustment for conventional cardiovascular risk factors. In the absence of baseline CVD, diabetes, or other illnesses, persons with the metabolic syndrome were at an elevated risk for CVD and all cause mortality.

Individuals with diabetes and/or coronary heart disease as well as the metabolic syndrome are at increased risk for complications from their medical disorders. Costa et al. (19) conducted a cross-sectional study of patients with type 2 diabetes mellitus (DM) and compared comorbidity and complications with the metabolic syndrome to those without the metabolic syndrome. Those with type 2 diabetes and metabolic syndrome had a higher prevalence of peripheral vascular disease (35% vs. 18%), retinopathy (44% vs. 20%), distal sensory neuropathy (44% vs. 24%), and coronary artery disease (53% vs. 36%). Furthermore, the more metabolic components an individual accumulated, the higher the proportion of diabetic complications the person suffered. In patients with vascular disease of any kind, the presence of the metabolic syndrome resulted in more extensive vascular damage. Olijhoek et al. (20) conducted a cross-sectional survey of patients with various manifestations of vascular disease, including coronary heart disease, stroke, peripheral arterial disease, and abdominal aorta aneurysm, and compared carotid intima media thickness (IMT), ankle brachial pressure index (ABPI), and albuminuria (non-invasive markers of vascular damage) in patients with and without the metabolic syndrome. Patients with the metabolic syndrome had increased mean IMTs, decreased ABPIs, and increased alminuria as compared to those without the metabolic syndrome. Thus, in patients with vascular disease of any manifestation or diabetes, the metabolic syndrome is associated with more extensive disease, co-morbidity, and increased mortality.

PATHOPHYSIOLOGY OF METABOLIC SYNDROME—THE ROLE OF VISCERAL OBESITY

Each component of the metabolic syndrome independently increases the risk for adverse cardiovascular events. However, there is evidence to suggest abdominal (visceral) obesity as a major underlying risk factor for the metabolic syndrome. Indeed, even normal weight individuals who are abdominally obese can have a compromised metabolic profile with insulin resistance and dyslipidemia (21).

The widely accepted measurement of abdominal obesity—waist circumference—reflects both abdominal visceral adipose tissue and abdominal subcutaneous adipose tissue (22). Visceral adipose tissue stores are highly correlated with metabolic and cardiovascular complications of obesity as compared to BMI and/or subcutaneous adipose tissue (23). Expert panels on obesity estimate that waist circumferences of at least 102 cm in men and 89 cm in women increase the risk for cardiovascular complications. However, Han et al. (24) suggested that even smaller waist circumferences (between 94 and 102 cm in men and 80 and 88 cm in women) are associated with having one or more cardiovascular risk factors. Individuals with normal weights but high visceral fat levels have significant risk for the metabolic syndrome, diabetes, and CVD (21). Moreover, favorable metabolic changes have been observed in obese patients whose weight loss was mainly attributable to a reduction in visceral fat (25).

Why does the accumulation of visceral fat predispose individuals to the metabolic syndrome? One theory suggests that abdominal fat is more insulin resistant than lower body adipose tissue (26). Another concept is that the accumulation of abdominal fat leads to increased visceral adipose tissue products, such as free fatty acids (FFA) and their metabolites in the systemic circulation (27). This in turn elicits various changes throughout the body which contributes to the development of the metabolic syndrome components, such as insulin resistance, decreased glucose tolerance, elevated blood pressure, and dyslipidemia (Fig. 1). Although FFA levels correlate with the amount of total body fat, increased visceral fat in particular, along with intramuscular fat deposits, stimulate lipolysis and cause greater increases in FFA. For example, the release of FFA from adipose tissues is greater in women with visceral fat that in non-obese or subcutaneously obese women (28). Considering the central role of FFAs in the development of the metabolic syndrome, we briefly discuss the pathophysiological mechanisms underlying the other components of this syndrome with regards to visceral obesity and increased FFA levels.

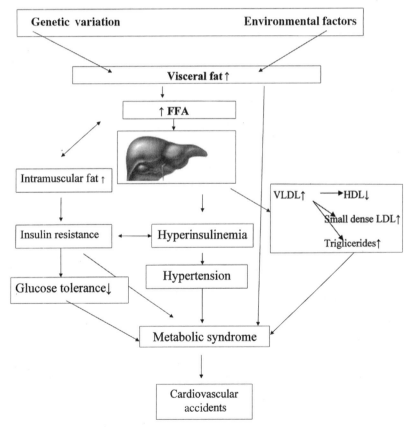

Figure 1 The role of visceral obesity in the pathophysiology of the metabolic syndrome.

VISCERAL FAT AND GLUCOSE INTOLERANCE

Obesity in general and abdominal obesity in particular alter glucose metabolism in skeletal muscle, liver, and pancreas by increasing FFA production
from adipose tissue. In skeletal muscle, circulating FFAs impair glucose
uptake and insulin signaling, resulting in insulin resistance and glucose intolerance. In the liver, increased hepatic FFA accumulation, along with other
factors, stimulates gluconeogenesis and provokes insulin resistance and
glucose intolerance. Finally, chronic over production of adipose products
(i.e., FFAs, inflammatory cytokines, and leptin) and decreased adiponec-
tines interferes with pancreatic beta cell functioning, further impairing insulin metabolism and resulting in glucose intolerance (29).

VISCERAL FAT AND DYSLIPIDEMIA

Visceral fat accumulation is associated with atherogenic dyslipidemia which
consists of increased triglycerides, apolipoprotein B (apo B), small LDL
particles, and decreased HDL particles. Similar to elevated LDL cholesterol,
atherogenic dyslipidemia promotes the development of atherosclerosis and
ultimately CVD. The key abnormality of this dylipidemia is an increase of
apo B containing lipoproteins [i.e., very low density lipoproteins (VLDL)
large LDL, and small LDL] in the circulation. Visceral fat is the body's
central storage site for triglycerides. During fasting states triglycerides are
broken down at a rapid rate releasing nonesterified fatty acids (NEFA) into
circulation. As NEFAs inundate the liver, they are re-esterified into triglycerides for incorporation into VLDL. Consequently, obese persons have
high levels of VLDL triglycerides and triglycerides (29).

Small, dense LDL and HDL particles result from excess VLDL triglycerides in the circulation. With the presence of VLDL triglycerides in the
circulation, special proteins facilitate the exchange of triglycerides from
VLDL particles for cholesterol ester in LDL and HDL. Ultimately, this
triglyceride-rich LDL and HDL undergo lipolysis resulting in small, dense
LDL and HDL. HDL concentrations are further decreased by hepatic lipase
which is found at higher than normal concentrations in obese individuals
(30). Smaller and denser LDL is associated with increased risk for myocardial
infarction and increased severity of coronary artery disease (31,32). Low
HDL predisposes individuals to coronary artery disease independent of triglyceride levels (33). Thus, excess FFAs, resulting from abdominal obesity,
undergo extensive hepatic remodeling resulting in increased LDL and triglycerides and decreased HDL characteristic of artherogenic dyslipidemia.

VISCERAL FAT AND ELEVATED BLOOD PRESSURE

Consensus guidelines consider increased blood pressure to be part of the metabolic syndrome, although many investigators do not consider hypertension to

be a metabolic risk factor per se. High blood pressure is a risk factor for CVD but the relationship between metabolic abnormalities and hypertension is less certain. Blood pressure regulation is a complex process, so it is not surprising that there are multiple ways in which the metabolic changes induced by obesity may lead to hypertension. Several changes related to hyperinsulinemia may cause increased blood pressure in individuals with the metabolic syndrome. Hyperinsulinemia is associated with increased sympathetic tone and has been linked to increased sodium reabsorption by the kidney (29). Moreover, smooth muscle and myocardial cells have been shown to be stimulated by insulin and insulin-like growth factors, further contributing to hypertension development (25). Insulin resistance reduces endothelial nitric oxide which under normal circumstances causes vasodilatation; this also leads to hypertension (25).

Other factors that strengthen the relationship among visceral fat, metabolic changes, and hypertension include changes in cytokines, increases in FFAs, and renal fat accumulation. Cytokines, such as adiponectin and plasminogen-activator inhibitor, released in large quantities with visceral fat accumulation may inhibit nitric oxide release by endothelial cells, thereby impairing vasodilatation (34,35). FFAs may lead to hypertension by two pathways. The observation that FFA infusion increases blood pressure and heart rate while decreasing heart rate variability suggests that excess FFA might contribute to increased sympathetic activity. FFAs are also thought to impair normal endothelial function (36,37). Lastly, mechanical compression of the kidneys from fat accumulation may decrease renal function leading to subsequent hypertension (29).

Several prospective studies demonstrate that obesity increases risk for CVD (38–40). This association appears to be mediated in part via visceral fat accumulation and subsequent metabolic changes (38,41–43). Visceral adipose tissue negatively affects glucose and lipid metabolism, factors that regulate blood pressure, and inflammatory and thrombotic factors. Despite the strength of these associations, visceral fat or obesity alone is unlikely to be sufficient to cause metabolic syndrome. Rather, other factors such as genetics or aging may need to be present (29). Nonetheless, visceral adiposity is highly predictive of metabolic abnormalities, diabetes, and CVD (29).

MAGNITUDE OF THE PROBLEM

Prior to the publication of the NCEP-ATP III, prevalence estimates of the metabolic syndrome in the United States varied widely due to the use of different diagnostic criteria to define the syndrome. Estimates therefore ranged from 4.6% among Caucasian women in the Atherosclerosis Risk in Communities Study to 29.4% in Caucasian men in the Framingham Offspring Study (44,45).

Since publication of the NCEP-ATP III criteria, studies have confirmed the prevalence of the metabolic syndrome has reached epidemic proportions although variations were found across age, race, and gender. The largest study, the Third National Health and Nutrition Examination Survey (NHANES III), was a cross-sectional health survey of a nationally representative sample of the U.S. adult population conducted from 1988 to 1994. This study found the age-unadjusted prevalence of the metabolic syndrome was 21.8%, while the age-adjusted prevalence was 23.7% (46). The prevalence varied from 6.7% among participants 20 to 29 years of age to 43.5% among persons 60 to 69 years of age. Prevalence rates were highest among Mexican Americans (31.9%) and lowest among whites (23.8%) and African Americans (21.6%). Across ethnic groups, the age adjusted prevalence was similar for men and women (24.0% vs. 23.4%). However, African American women had a 57% higher prevalence compared with African American men and Mexican American women had a 26% higher prevalence compared with Mexican American men. This study confirmed that the metabolic syndrome is common in the U.S. adult population. Approximately 20% of all individuals age 20 or older met criteria for the metabolic syndrome, and 40% of all individuals older than 40 years of age met criteria. Application of the age-specific prevalence rates to U.S. census data from 2000 suggests that up to 47 million U.S. adults may meet criteria for the metabolic syndrome.

The prevalence rate of the metabolic syndrome is also high in U.S. adolescents. Utilizing cross-sectional data from the Third National Health and Nutrition Examination Survey (47), male and female respondents age 12 to 19 showed an overall prevalence of 4.2%. Male gender and obesity predicted the greatest risk in this cohort. Males had a rate of 6.1% as compared to 2.1% in females ($p = 0.01$). In addition, 28.7% of overweight adolescents (BMI > 95th percentile) met criteria for the syndrome compared with 6.8% of at risk adolescents (BMI, 85th to < 95th percentile) and 0.1% of those with a BMI below the 85th percentile ($p < 0.001$). Adolescents in the West and Midwest were at highest risk compared to other U.S. regions and Mexican Americans were at higher risk than Caucasians and African Americans. With a similar distribution across all American adolescents, estimates are that approximately 910,000 meet the criteria for the metabolic syndrome.

The metabolic syndrome is also a significant world wide health problem. Similar to the situation in the U.S., the prevalence of the metabolic syndrome world wide varies by definition and population studied. For example, one study conducted in Finnish men found a rate of 11.4% using the NCEP-ATP III criteria and 22% using the WHO criteria (48). Rates less than 10% have been found in France and as high as 46% in India utilizing the same criteria (49,50). Despite this variation, studies have documented rates greater than 20% in a number of countries including India, Iran, Mexico, Ireland, Turkey, England, Denmark and others (50–56).

THE METABOLIC SYNDROME IN PSYCHIATRIC POPULATIONS

Studies indicate that psychiatric patients are at increased risk for the metabolic syndrome. For example, in Finland the rate of the syndrome is approximately 14% in the general population but has been measured at 37% in a cohort of patients with schizophrenia (18,57). Studies conducted in the U.S. among patients with schizophrenia or schizoaffective disorder found rates from 42.4% to 63% compared with a prevalence rate of approximately 22% in the general population (46,58,59). One multi-center naturalistic study assessed inpatients and outpatients with schizophrenia or schizoaffective disorder and found that 51% of outpatients and 22.2% of inpatients met criteria for the metabolic syndrome (60). These preliminary studies therefore suggest that there is a high prevalence of the metabolic syndrome in patients with schizophrenia and schizoaffective disorder.

Patients with depression also appear to share a liability for the metabolic syndrome. Using a nationally representative sample from the U.S. (the NHANES III), Kinder et al. (61) found an association between the metabolic syndrome and depression in women. In a study among monozygotic and dizygotic male twin pairs, depressive symptoms were associated with individual components of the metabolic syndrome (62). Moreover, Raikkonen et al. (63) followed an American population-based cohort of women for an average of 7.4 years and found women with elevated levels of depression, anxiety, current perceived stress, tension, and anger at baseline, and increased anger during the follow-up period were at increased risk for the metabolic syndrome.

Prospective data suggest that children and adolescents with psychological traits such as anger and hostility are at increased risk for the metabolic syndrome. One study prospectively followed African American and Caucasian children and adolescents and found that those with high hostility ratings at baseline were more likely to have the metabolic syndrome at three years follow-up (64). In two other prospective studies, children and adolescents with high levels of aggression, anger, hyperactivity, and responsivity to others had an increased risk for the metabolic syndrome (65,66).

METABOLIC ABNORMALITIES IN PSYCHIATRIC PATIENTS

Although investigation of the metabolic syndrome is recent, evidence has accumulated since the early 20th century indicating that psychiatric patients have high rates of abnormal glucose metabolism and other metabolic disturbances. Thus, there have been a number of reports of impaired glucose tolerance, insulin resistance, overt diabetes, central obesity, and dyslipidemia among psychiatric patients. These associations persist in drug-free and drug-naïve subjects, as well as in studies that control for medication and other traditional risk factors for diabetes. Furthermore, incident diabetes or metabolic disturbances are increasingly associated with psychiatric symptoms, such as depressive symptoms in otherwise healthy adults in general community samples.

Abnormalities in metabolism and weight were first described in schizophrenia prior to the introduction and wide spread use of antipsychotic medications, with the majority of reports indicating an increased rate of insulin resistance in drug-naïve patients (67–69). Four recent studies confirmed this association. In one study, first-episode drug-naïve patients with schizophrenia had a higher prevalence of impaired fasting glucose, were more insulin resistant, and had higher levels of glucose, insulin, and cortisol compared with matched controls (70). Another study found that drug-free and drug-naïve subjects with schizophrenia had over three times as much intra-abdominal fat as measured by abdominal computerized tomography (CT), and higher waist to hip ratios compared with matched controls (71). In a retrospective chart review, Regenold et al. (72) found that compared with national norms, diabetes rates were significantly elevated in hospitalized older (age 50–74) adults with bipolar I affective and schizoaffective patients. The association persisted after controlling the effects of age, race, gender, BMI, and psychotropic medications. Severe psychotic stress in non-diabetic subjects with chronic schizophrenia may also adversely affect glucose control. In a group of patients with no previous exposure to atypical antipsychotics, Shiloah et al. (73) found that those with the higher scores for psychotic stress had greater fasting glucoses and insulin levels compared with those with lower psychotic stress scores.

Several reports describe metabolic changes and weight gain associated with major depression and symptoms of depression or mental distress. Three large prospective epidemiological studies have shown depressive symptoms or major depression predict incident type 2 diabetes in otherwise healthy adults (74–76). This relation persisted after adjustment for stress-associated lifestyle factors (smoking, physical activity, and caloric intake) and metabolic covariates (fasting insulin and glucose, lipids, blood pressure, and adiposity) (74). In a small cross sectional study of drug-naïve and drug-free female subjects with major depression, Thakore et al. (77) found those diagnosed with depression had an increased intra-abdominal fat as measured by CT scanning compared with matched controls.

Of note, associations between major depression and changes in inflammatory and coagulation factors have also been reported, further supporting the association between depression and metabolic disturbances that elevate cardiovascular risk. Thus, depression has been associated with increases in the following inflammatory markers: C-reactive protein, interleukin-6, tumor necrosis factor-α, serum amyloid A, and increased white blood cells (78–81). Depression has also been associated with alteration in coagulation factors such as homocysteine and fibrinogen (80).

PSYCHIATRIC TREATMENTS AND METABOLIC ABNORMALITIES

Weight Gain

Weight gain, particularly central obesity, may be the most noticeable sign a patient is at increased risk for the metabolic syndrome. Many psychiatric medications cause weight gain. However, little is known about the different liabilities of medications for centralized weight gain or visceral fat accumulation, a key element of the metabolic syndrome. Two studies examined the effect of second generation antipsychotics (SGAs) on visceral fat distribution in drug-naïve patients with schizophrenia. Zhang et al. (82) studied drug-naïve, first-episode patients with schizophrenia and compared weight, waist and hip circumferences, abdominal subcutaneous fat, and intra-abdominal fat measurements before and after 10 weeks of antipsychotic drug treatment. Thirty patients received risperidone at a mean does of 4.77 mg, 15 patients were treated with cholorpromazine at a mean dose of 480 mg, and one patient was treated with quetiapine at a dose of 600 mg a day. After 10 weeks of antipsychotic treatment, patients as a group showed statistically significant increases in waist-to-hip ratio, subcutaneous fat, and intra-abdominal fat as measured by magnetic resonance imaging.

Ryan et al. (83) studied the effects of SGAs on visceral fat distribution, in drug-naïve subjects with schizophrenia. Sixteen drug-naïve patients treated with risperidone or olanzapine for six months were compared with controls matched in terms of age, gender, exercise and smoking habits, alcohol intake, and BMI, At baseline, the drug-naïve patients with schizophrenia had significantly more intra-abdominal fat and subcutaneous fat as measured by CT scanning compared with controls. However, after six months of treatment, intra-abdominal and subcutaneous fat stores did not significantly increase in the treated group, although they remained elevated compared with the control group. Thus, although it is clear that SGAs cause or contribute to significant weight gain in patients treated with these agents, it is still undetermined how much and at what rate intra-abdominal and subcutaneous fat stores are affected by these agents.

Hyperglycemia and Insulin Resistance

A simple explanation for the changes in glucose metabolism associated with SGAs is to ascribe them to drug-induced increased weight gain. For example, clozapine and olanzapine have the highest liability for weight gain and are highly associated with hyperglycemia and insulin resistance (84,85). However, patients receiving SGAs can develop changes in glucose metabolism without significant weight gain (86). One study compared nondiabetic patients with schizophrenia taking SGAs with matched controls and found that they had increased glucose levels after oral glucose tests independent of adiposity (87). Another study examined the acute effects of clozapine, olanzapine, and risperidone on insulin resistance in a group of nonobese patients with schizophrenia (88). Clozapine produced significantly higher glucose levels as compared to risperidone, while risperidone was associated with higher insulin sensitivity measures versus olanzapine or clozapine. These observations suggest that the hyperglycemia associated with some SGAs may be independent of weight gain and thus possibly due to a direct effect on glucose metabolism.

Dyslipidemia

Dyslipidemia is common in certain SGAs, most noteably olanzapine and clozapine. The pattern of dyslipidemia associated with SGAs—elevated triglycerides, increased LDL cholesterol, and decreased HDL cholesterol—is the same pattern found in the metabolic syndrome. There is a debate as to whether these changes are secondary to the weight gain these agents promote, or if they are direct effects of the agents themselves. Most available studies suggest that the changes in serum lipids are concordant with weight gain.

In a prospective study, Lindenmayer et al. (89) assessed the effects of clozapine, olanzapine, risperidone, and haloperidol on cholesterol levels in hospitalized patients with schizophrenia or schizoaffective disorder. Lipid profiles were assessed at baseline and after 8 and 14 weeks of treatment. Cholesterol levels were significantly higher at 8 weeks for both clozapine and olanzapine subjects and at 14 weeks for olanzapine subjects. In another prospective study, weight, triglycerides and cholesterol were measured at baseline and then after eight weeks of treatment with olanzapine or risperidone in patients with schizophrenia or schizoaffective disorder (90). Compared with baseline measurements, both risperidone and olanzapine subjects had significant increases in weight. However, olanzapine subjects had higher triglycerides compared to baseline measures and had significantly greater weight gain and triglycerides compared with the risperidone group. In Pfizer's 054 study summarized by Casey et al. (91) the effects of five different antipsychotics on serum lipids were compared in patients with schizophrenia. After three weeks, olanzapine (+31%) and quetiapine (+18.3%) subjects had significant increases in fasting triglycerides, while thioridazine (+7.9%) and risperidone (−6.7%) had nonsignificant changes, and ziprasidone (−28%) and haloperidol (−18%) had significant decreases in fasting triglycerides.

Other studies have confirmed the differential effects of certain SGAs on lipid profile. In contrast to clozapine, olanzapine, and quetiapine; risperidone, ziprasidone, and ariiprazole are not associated with changes in lipid profile. In a large case-control study involving 18,000 individuals diagnosed with schizophrenia, Koro et al. (92) evaluated the effect of olanzapine, risperidone, conventional antipsychotics, and no antipsychotic exposure on the risk for hyperlipidemia. Olanzapine subjects had a five-fold increase in the odds of developing hyperlidemia, in contrast to risperidone subjects, who had no increase in risk. Results of pooled safety data from aripiprazole trials showed subjects treated with aripiprazole had no significant differences in total cholesterol when compared with placebo (93). In a review of ziprasidone's effects on serum lipids, ziprasidone was shown to have neutral or favorable effects on patients' serum lipid profiles in placebo-controlled, active-comparator, and in open label switch studies (91,94–99).

MONITORING FOR THE METABOLIC SYNDROME IN PSYCHIATRIC SETTINGS

Given that psychiatric patients are at increased risk for the metabolic syndrome whether due to an underlying predisposition, unhealthy lifestyle choices, or the effects of psychiatric medications, what should psychiatrists do about this syndrome in their patients? There is substantial evidence the metabolic syndrome is associated with premature development of diabetes and cardiovascular disease. Psychiatrists and other mental health providers should consider identifying individuals with goals to prevent and reverse disease progression. There is evidence that treating the metabolic syndrome can prevent or delay development of diabetes or cardiovascular disease.

The first step in evaluating patients for the metabolic syndrome is to identify patients who are at increased risk for cardiovascular disease and diabetes. Comorbid medical conditions, lifestyle factors, and genetic predisposition should be categorized for each patient and included in each patient's initial risk assessment. Patients with diabetes, cardiovascular disease, cerebral vascular disease, dyslipidemia, obesity, and hyperglycemia should be clearly identified. Patients smoking, exercise, and dietary habits should be assessed. Family history of metabolic-associated conditions and ethnicity should be noted for each patient as well. Based on history and ethnicity alone, most psychiatric patients can be categorized into high, medium, or low risk for future metabolic complications and disease.

Second, psychiatrists should obtain regular measurements of weight, BMI, waist circumference, and blood pressure. These parameters are the "routine vitals" that should be completed at each patient encounter. These values should be clearly documented and accessible for mental health providers in the medical record. This would ensure a minimum measurement of two of the five parameters of the metabolic syndrome with each patient visit. Although BMI is not part of the criteria for the metabolic syndrome per NCEP-ATP III, a BMI greater than 30 dramatically increases one's risk for the metabolic syndrome. Making these measures part of standard clinical practice in psychiatric settings is the first step in addressing the metabolic syndrome.

Several reviews make recommendations regarding the frequency of metabolic monitoring in patients receiving SGAs. However to date, no outcome, effectiveness, or costeffectiveness studies exist comparing the different recommendations. Most guidelines recommend obtaining baseline values of blood pressure, weight, height, BMI, waist circumference, fasting serum lipids (total, LDL, HDL, and triglycerides), and a fasting glucose level prior to initiating an antipsychotic medication or when changing to a new antipsychotic medication. After the initial phase of treatment (i.e., 12 weeks) follow-up monitoring of the above parameters should be obtained. Subsequent frequency of monitoring should be determined by the patient's established risk for metabolic disturbances (i.e., high risk patients monitored quarterly) or on dramatic changes in the patient's metabolic profile (i.e., weight gain ≥ 5%, waist circumference increase, increase in fasting glucose).

Why then are these measures not routinely obtained in psychiatric settings? Equipment which measures height, weight, and blood pressure is not a traditional fixture in psychiatric settings. Calculating BMI requires scales in the office that weigh heavier patients (up to 200 kg) and a standiometer that can accurately measure height. Measuring blood pressure requires a calibrated sphygmomanometer and trained staff to obtain readings. Measuring waist circumference requires a flexible tape measure and trained staff to perform the measurement accurately and reliably. Lack of trained personal and adequate equipment is potentially one barrier to metabolic monitoring in psychiatric patients. Furthermore, getting weighed and measured may be an anxiety provoking event for some patients. Some providers may feel assessing waist size and weight in certain patients constitutes an invasion of privacy or a boundary crossing that would not be therapeutic. However, designating specific staff trained to perform these measurements with privacy and respect may address this barrier to metabolic assessment.

Patients' health values, level of concern, and motivation may be a third barrier to metabolic assessment. Although the mentally ill are often aware of their weight problems, their level of concern may not directly correlate and they may be reluctant to choose dieting as a remedy. Myer (100) studied awareness and concern of obesity and weight issues in chronically mentally ill inpatients. In this study, state hospital patients completed an anonymous questionnaire concerning obesity, weight gain variables, concern about weight, and methods to control weight. In addition to the surveys, data regarding each individual's sex, age, weight, and height were collected. Although there was a significant correlation between BMI and awareness of current weight status, there was not an association between BMI and level of concern about weight among the respondents. Only 10% of obese patients requested to be placed on a mandatory monitored diet. Lack of insight, cognitive deficits, and loss of initiative are common symptoms in patients with severe and chronic mental illness and may be a further barrier to metabolic monitoring. Even in highly supervised psychiatric settings, it can be difficult to coordinate care between physical and mental health problems and for patients to follow up on potential physical health interventions.

TREATMENT RECOMMENDATIONS

If treatment-related weight gain, dyslipidemia, hyperglycemia, or hypertension emerges, switching to another psychotropic agent with less propensity for metabolic side effects should be considered. Generally, discussion with the patient to discontinue the offending agent should be initiated prior to adding a treatment for the metabolic disturbance. However, practically this may not be possible in all clinical situations, given a patient's symptomatic response or personal preference for a particular medication that may have metabolic side effects. Periodic assessment of benefits as well as risks, including metabolic risks for each medication, should be routinely reviewed with patients.

Although there is a growing consensus that psychiatrists should monitor for the metabolic syndrome, particularly with SGA pharmacotherapy, there is no current consensus regarding treatment of the metabolic syndrome. Data are available suggesting that lifestyle modification and/or some medications may be efficacious treatment strategies.

First line therapy for the metabolic syndrome is intensive lifestyle modification aimed at reducing weight, increasing levels of physical activity, and changing diet composition to reduce risk of CVD and diabetes. Small changes in diet and exercise can produce modest weight loss and significantly lower patients' risk for diabetes. One prospective study randomly assigned obese adult subjects with impaired glucose tolerance to individualized diet and exercise program aimed at reducing weight or a control group which consisted of oral and written information about diet (a two-page leaflet) and exercise (101). Participants in the intervention group had seven sessions with a nutritionist during the first year and then one session every three months after for the remaining two years of the study. The mean amount of weight lost between baseline and at the end of years 1 and 2 was significantly greater for the intervention group. Furthermore, the cumulative incidence of diabetes after four years was 11% in the intervention group and 23% in the control group. During the trial the risk for diabetes was reduced by 58% ($p < 0.001$) in the intervention group.

Regular exercise, even at modest levels, improves metabolic risk factors including HDL, triglyceride levels, blood pressure, and insulin resistance (102–104). Even exercise without dietary change is beneficial for the metabolic syndrome. In one prospective study, the prevalence of the metabolic syndrome was determined before and after 20 weeks of supervised aerobic training consisting of supervised sessions on a cycle ergometer (105). Participants received counseling at baseline and at midway through the study not to alter their usual health and lifestyle habits outside the study. The prevalence of the metabolic syndrome prior to the exercise program was 16.9% (105/621) and decreased to 11.8% after the training. Almost one third (30.5%) of the original 105 participants with the metabolic syndrome no longer met the criteria after the exercise program. Modest changes in aerobic exercise and diet with the goal of weight loss improves individual components and reverses the metabolic syndrome.

Adjusting diet composition may specifically target metabolic parameters compared with simple weight reduction via reduction in caloric intake (106,107). Stern et al. (107) compared the effects of a low-carbohydrate diet to a conventional weight loss diet in severely obese adults with diabetes or the metabolic syndrome. Study participants received counseling to either restrict carbohydrate intake <30 g per day (low-carbohydrate) or to restrict caloric intake by 500 calories per day with <30% of calories from fat (conventional). At one year, there was no significant difference in mean weight change between the groups. However, persons on the low-carbohydrate diet had significant decreases in triglycerides levels, higher HDL levels, and more improvement in hemoglobin A1C levels as compared to persons on the conventional diet. Thus, certain diets, such as low carbohydrate diets, may be more specific for targeting metabolic risk factors, but this area needs further study.

When metabolic risk factors are not reduced by lifestyle changes, drug therapies will be needed to treat their blood pressure and lipid levels. Although unresolved for healthy patients with the metabolic syndrome, aggressive pharmacologic management of cardiovascular risk factors has been shown to be more effective than routine care in preventing CVD in patients with type 2 diabetes (108). The metabolic syndrome alone does not require drug treatment per se, but many with the metabolic syndrome will require drug treatment per existing treatment guidelines for hypertension, dyslipidemia, and/or diabetes.

An important unresolved question is whether insulin sensitizing agents should be employed in persons with the metabolic syndrome to prevent the development of type 2 diabetes. The diabetes prevention program research group studied this issue by randomly assigning otherwise healthy individuals with elevated fasting and post-load plasma glucose concentrations to placebo, metformin, or a lifestyle-modification program (109). Lifestyle changes and treatment with metformin both reduced the incidence of diabetes in this high risk sample (58% and 31%, respectively). However, the lifestyle intervention was more effective than metformin.

Thiazolidinediones (glitazones) are the only compounds that specifically target tissue insulin resistance. The glitazones regulate genetic transcription and translation of numerous proteins, including many that are involved in glucose and lipid metabolism (110). These drugs (rosiglitazone and pioglitazone) are currently approved for treatment of type 2 diabetes, although the therapeutic potential of this class in treating insulin resistance and preventing type 2 diabetes has stirred considerable interest. For example, in a prospective study of individuals with fasting glucose levels of 100 to 125 mg/dL and two hours postprandial glucose levels of 140 to 200 mg/dL, Durbin found that patients treated with a thiazolidinedione had decreased mean hemoglobin A1C levels and a 88.9% lower incidence of diabetes after three years compared to the control group (111). Although preliminary data for metformin and the thiazolidinediones are encouraging, all available data involve the impact of these agents on surrogate markers rather than the metabolic syndrome itself. Moreover, while these agents may also impact blood pressure, triglycerides, and HDL, there are therapies available with more data proving their efficacy and safety in these parameters (112).

SUMMARY

The metabolic syndrome is a grouping of risk factors predisposing individuals to type 2 diabetes and cardiovascular disease. There is accumulating evidence that psychiatric patients, including those with psychotic and mood disorders, are particularly at high risk for this syndrome. A number of factors may predispose psychiatric patients to the metabolic syndrome including high rates of obesity, unhealthy life style choices, psychiatric treatments, and the psychiatric disorders themselves. Monitoring for the metabolic syndrome begins by identifying high risk patients based on age, ethnicity, and history. Blood pressure, waist circumference, and weight should be assessed at regular intervals and increases in these measures should trigger further evaluation for dyslipidemia and glucose intolerance. The NCEP-ATP III identified metabolic syndrome as an indication for vigorous lifestyle interventions including changes in diet and exercise. Weight loss improves all components of the metabolic syndrome, and exercise, even without weight loss, can also improve components of the syndrome. In the absence of improvement with lifestyle changes, pharmacologic treatments for elevated blood pressure and dyslipidemia are indicated and have decreased the risk of cardiovascular events.

REFERENCES

1. World Health Organization. Diabetes: the cost of diabetes. Fact sheet No 236: (at www.who.int/medicacentre/factsheets/fs236).
2. World Health Organization. Global strategy diet & physical activity. Obesity and overweight document. (at www.who.int/dietphysicalactivity/publications/facts/obesity/en/).

3. Reaven GM. Banting lecture 1988. Role of insulin resistance in human disease. Diabetes 1988; 37:1595–1607.
4. Alberti KG, Zimmet PZ. Definition, diagnosis and classification of diabetes mellitus and its complications. Part 1: diagnosis and classification of diabetes mellitus, provisional report of a WHO consultation. Diab Med 1998; 15: 539–553.
5. National Institutes of Health: Third Report of the National Cholesterol Education Program Expert Panel on Detection, Evaluation, and Treatment of High Cholesterol in Adults (Adult Treatment Panel III). Executive Summary of the Third Report of the National Cholesterol Education Program (NCEP). Expert Panel on Detection, Evaluation, and Treatment of High Blood Cholesterol in Adults (Adult Treatment Panel III). JAMA 2001; 285: 2486–2497.
6. Ridker PM, Buring JE, Cook NR, Rifai N. C-reactive protein, the metabolic syndrome, and risk of incident cardiovascular events: an 8-year follow-up of 14719 initially healthy American women. Circulation 2003; 107(3):391–397.
7. Hsueh WA, Lyon CJ, Ouinones MJ. Insulin resistance and the endothelium. Am J Med 2004; 15(2):109–117.
8. Imperatore G, Riccardi G, Iovine C, Rivellese AA, Vaccaro O. Plasma fibrinogen: a new factor of the metabolic syndrome. A population-based study. Diab Care 1998; 21(4):649–654.
9. Bastard JP, Pieroni L, Hainque B. Relationship between plasma plasminogen activator inhibitor 1 and insulin resistance. Diab Metab Res Rev 2000; 16(3):192–201.
10. Bonara E, Targher G, Zenere MB et al. Relationship of uric acid concentration to cardiovascular risk factors in young men. Role of obesity and central fat distribution. The Verona Young Men Atherosclerosis Risk Factors Study. Int J Obes Relat Metab Disord 1996;20(11):975–980.
11. Rosenbaum P, Gimeno SG, Sanudo A, Franco LJ, Ferreira SR. Japanese-Brazilian Diabetes Study Group. Independent impact of glycemia and blood pressure in albuminuria on high-risk subjects for metabolic syndrome. Clin Nephrol 2004; 61(6):369–376.
12. Krauss RM, Siri PW. Metabolic abnormalities: triglycerides and low-density lipoprotein. Endocrinology and Metabolism Clin North Am 2004; 33(2): 405–415.
13. Willerson JT, Ridker PM. Inflammation as a cardiovascular risk factor. Circulation 2004; 109(suppl II):II-2–II-10.
14. Pradhan AD, Manson JE, Rifai N, Buring JE, Ridker PM. C-reactive protein, interleukin 6, and risk of developing type 2 diabetes mellitus. JAMA 2001; 286:327–334.
15. Haffner SM, Valdez RA, Hazuda HP, Mithcell BD, Morales PA, Stern MP. Prospective analysis of the insulin-resistance syndrome (syndrome X). Diabetes 1992; 41:715–722.
16. Isomma B, Almgren P, Tuomi T, et al. Cardiovascular morbidity and mortality associated with, the metabolic syndrome. Diab Care 2001; 24:683–689.
17. Trevisan M, Liu j, Bahsas FB, Menotti A. Syndrome X and mortality: a population-based study. Am J Epidemiol 1998; 148:958–966.

18. Lakka HM, Laaksonen DE, Lakka TA, et al. The metabolic syndrome and total and cardiovascular disease mortality in middle-aged men. JAMA 2002; 288:2709–2716.

19. Costa LA, Canani LH, Lisboa HR, Tres GS, Gross JL. Aggregation of features of the metabolic syndrome is associated with increased prevalence of chronic complications in type 2 diabetes. Diab Med 2004; 21:252–255.

20. Olijhoek JK, van der Graaf Y, Banga JD, Algra A, Rabelink TJ, Vissere FL. The SMART Study Group. The metabolic syndrome is associated with advanced vascular damage in patients with coronary heart disease, stroke, peripheral arterial disease or abdominal aortic aneurysm. Eur Heart J 2004; 25:342–348.

21. Karelis AD, St-Pierre DH, Conus F, Rabasa-Lhoret R, Poehlman ET. Metabolic and body composition factors in subgroups of obesity: what do we know? J Clin Endocrinol Metab 2004; 89(6):2569–2575.

22. Reilly MP, Rader DJ. The metabolic syndrome: more than the sum of its parts? Circulation 2003; 108(13):1546–1551.

23. Nieves DJ, Cnop M, Retzlaff B, et al. The atherogenic lipoprotein profile associated with obesity and insulin resistance is largely attributable to intra-abdominal fat. Diabetes 2003; 52(l):172–179.

24. Han TS, van Leer EM, Seidell JC, Lean ME. Waist circumference action levels in the identification of cardiovascular risk factors: prevalence study in a random sample. BMJ 1995; 311(7017):1401–1405.

25. Busetto L. Visceral obesity and the metabolic syndrome: effects of weight loss. Nutr Metab Cardiovasc Dis 2001; 11(3):195–204.

26. Abate N, Garg A, Peshock RM, Stray-Gundersen J, Grundy SM. Relationships of generalized and regional adiposity to insulin sensitivity in men. J Clin Invest 1995; 96(l):88–98.

27. Lebovitz HE. The relationship of obesity to the metabolic syndrome. Int J Clin Pract (suppl) 2003; (134):18–27.

28. Jensen MD, Haymond MW, Rizza RA, Cryer PE, Miles JM. Influence of body fat distribution on free fatty acid metabolism in obesity. J Clin Invest 1989; 83(4):1168–1173.

29. Grundy SM. What is the contribution of obesity to the metabolic syndrome? Endocrinol Metab Clin North Am 2004; 33(2):267–282.

30. Carr MC, Brunzell JD, Deeb SS. Ethnic differences in hepatic lipase and HDL in Japanese, black, and white Americans: role of central obesity and LIPC polymorphisms. J Lipid Res 2004; 45(3):466–473.

31. Stampfer MJ, Krauss RM, Ma J, Blanche PJ, Holl LG, Sacks FM, Hennekens CH. A prospective study of triglyceride level, low-density lipoprotein particle diameter, and risk of myocardial infarction. JAMA 1996; 276(11):882–888.

32. Gardner CD, Fortmann SP, Krauss RM. Association of small low-density lipoprotein particles with the incidence of coronary artery disease in men and women. JAMA 1996; 276(11):875–881.

33. Assman G, Schulte H. Relation of high-density lipoprotein cholesterol and triglycerides to incidence of atherosclerotic coronary disease (the PROCAM experience). Am J Cardiol 1992; 70:733–737.

34. Poli KA, Tofler GH, Larson MG, et al. Association of blood pressure with fibrinolytic potential in the Framingham offspring population. Circulation 2000; 101(3):264–269.
35. Kazumi T, Kawaguchi A, Sakai K, Hirano T, Yoshino G. Young men with high-normal blood pressure have lower serum adiponectin, smaller LDL size, and higher elevated heart rate than those with optimal blood pressure. Diab Care 2002; 25(6):971–976.
36. Manzella D, Barbieri M, Rizzo MR, et al. Role of free fatty acids on cardiac autonomic nervous system in noninsulin-dependent diabetic patients: effects of metabolic control. J Clin Endocrinol Metab 2001; 86:2769–2774.
37. Egan BM, Greene EL, Goodfriend TL. Nonesterified fatty acids in blood pressure control cardiovascular complications. Curr Hypertens Rep 2001; 3(2):107–1016.
38. National Institutes of Health. Clinical guidelines on the identification, evaluation, and treatment of overweight and obesity in adults: the evidence report. Obes Res 1998; 6(suppl 2):51S–209S.
39. Eckel RH, Krauss RM. American Heart Association call to action: obesity as a major risk factor for coronary heart disease: AHA nutrition committee. Circulation 1998; 97:2099–2100.
40. Kip KE, Marroquin OC, Kelley DE, et al. Clinical importance of obesity versus the metabolic syndrome in cardiovascular risk in women: a report from the Women's Ishemia Syndrome Evaluation (WISE) study. Circulation 2004; 109:706–713.
41. Arad Y, Newstein D, Cadet F, Roth M, Guerci AD. Association of multiple risk factors and insulin resistance with increased prevalence of asymptomatic coronary artery disease by an electron-beam computed tomographic study. Arterioscler Thromb Vasc Biol 2001; 21(12):2051–2058.
42. Morricone L, Donati C, Hassan T, Cioffi P, Caviezel F. Relationship of visceral fat distribution to angiographically assessed coronary artery disease: results in subjects with or without diabetes or impaired glucose tolerance. Nutr Metab Cardiovasc Dis 2002; 12(5):275–283.
43. Tirkes AT, Gottlieb RH, Voci SL, Waldman DL, Masetta J, Conover DL. Risk of significant coronary artery disease as determined by CT measurement of the distribution of abdominal adipose tissue. J Comput Assist Tomogr 2002; 26(2):210–215.
44. Schmitdt MI, Duncan BB, Watson RL, Sharrett AR, Brancati FL, Heiss G. A metabolic syndrome in whites and African-Americans: the Atherosclerosis Risk in Communities Baseline Study. Diab Care 1996; 19:414–418.
45. Meigs JB, D'Agostinio Sr. RB, Wilson PW, Cupples LA, Nathan DM, Singer DE. Risk variable clustering in the insulin resistance syndrome: the Framingham Offspring Study. Diabetes 1997; 46:1594–1600.
46. Ford ES, Giles WH, Dietz WH. Prevalence of the metabolic syndrome. Findings from the Third National Health and Nutrition Examination Survey. JAMA 2002; 287:356–359.
47. Cook S, Weitzman M, Auinger P, Nguyen M, Dietz WH. Prevalence of the metabolic syndrome in adolescents. Findings from the Third National Health and Nutrition Examination Survey, 1988–1994. Arch Pediatr Adolesc Med 2003; 157:821–827.

48. Laaksonen DE, Lakka HM, Niskanen LK, Kaplan GA, Salonen JT, Lakka TA. Metabolic syndrome and development of diabetes mellitus: application and validation of recently suggested definitions of the metabolic syndrome in a prospective cohort study. Am J Epidemiol 2002; 156:1070–1077.

49. Balkau B, Vernay M, Mhamdi L, et al. D. E. S. I. R. Study Group. The incidence and persistence of the NCEP (National Cholesterol Education Program) metabolic syndrome. The French D.E.S.I.R. study. Diab Metab 2003; 29(5):526–532.

50. Deepa R, Shanthirani CS, Premalatha G, Sastry NG, Mohan V. Prevanlence of insulin resistance syndrome in a selected south Indian population- the Chennai urban population study 7 (CUPS-7). Ind J Med Res 2002; 115:118–127.

51. Azizi F, Salehi P, Etemadi A, Zahedi-Asl S. Prevalence of metabolic syndrome in a urban population: Tehran Lipid and Glucose Study. Diab Res Clin Pract 2003; 61:29–37.

52. Aguilar-Salinas CA, Rojas R, Gomez-Perez FJ, et al. High prevalence of metabolic syndrome in Mexico. Arch Med Res.2004; 35(1):76–81.

53. Villegas R, Perry IJ, Creagh D, Hinchion R, O'Halloran D. Prevalence of the metabolic syndrome in middle-aged men and women. Diab Care 2003; 26:3198–3199.

54. Onat A, Ceyhan K, Basar O, Erer B, Toprak S, Sansoy V. Metabolic syndrome: major impact on coronary risk in a population with cholesterol levels- a prospective and cross-sectional evaluation. Atherosclerosis 2002; 165:285–292.

55. Balkau B, Charles MA, Drivsholm T, et al. Frequency of the WHO metabolic syndrome in European cohorts, and an alternative definition of an insulin resistance syndrome. Diab Metab 2002; 28:364–376.

56. Cameron AJ, Shaw JE, Zimmet PZ. The metabolic syndrome: prevalence in worldwide populations. Endocrinol Metab Clin 2004; 33:351–375.

57. Hekskanen T, Niskanen L, Lyytikainen R, et al. Metabolic syndrome in patients with schizophrenia. J Clin Psychiatry 2003; 64:575–579.

58. Basu R, Barr JS, Chengappa KNR et al. The prevalence of the metabolic syndrome in patients with schizoaffective disorder—bipolar subtype. Bipolar Disord 2004; 6:314–318.

59. Kato MM, Currier MB, Gomez CM, et al. Prevalence of metabolic syndrome in Hispanic and non-Hispanic patients with schizophrenia. Prim Care Companion J Clin Psychiatry 2004; 6:74–77.

60. Littrell KH, Petty R, Ortega T, et al. Insulin resistance and syndrome X among patients with schizophrenia, In: 156th Annual Meeting of the American Psychiatric Association, San Francisco, CA, 2003; May 17–22 (Abstract 550).

61. Kinder LS, Carnethon MR, Palaniappan LP, King AC, Fortmann SP. Depression and the metabolic syndrome in young adults: findings from the Third National Health and Nutrition Examination Survey. Psychosom Med 2004; 66:316–322.

62. McCaffery JM, Niaura R, Todaro JF, Swan GE, Carmell D. Depressive symptoms and metabolic risk in adult male twins enrolled in the National Heart, Lung, and Blood Institute Twin Study. Psychosom Med 2003; 65:490–497.

63. Raikkonen K, Matthews KA, Kuller LH. The relationship between psychological risk attributes and the metabolic syndrome in healthy women: antecedent or consequence? Metabolism 2002; 51:1573–1577.

64. Raikonen K, Matthews K, Salomon K. Hostility predicts metabolic syndrome risk factors in children and adolescents. Health Psychol 2003; 22:279–286.
65. Ravaja N, Keltikangas-Jarvinen L. Temperament and metabolic syndrome precursors in children: a three-year follow-up. Prevent Med 1995; 24:518–527.
66. Ravaja N, Keltikangas-Jarvinen L, Keskivaara P. Type A factors as predictors of changes in the metabolic syndrome precursors in adolescents and young adults- a 3- year follow-up study. Health Psychol 1996; 15:18–29.
67. Haupt DW, Newcomer JW. Abnormalities in glucose regulation associated with mental illness and treatment. J Psychosom Res 2002; 53:925–933.
68. Meduna LJ, Gerty FJ, Urse VG. Biochemical disturbances in mental disorders. Arch Neurol Psychiatry 1942; 47:38–52.
69. Dixon L, Weiden P, Delahanty P, et al. Prevalence and correlates of diabetes in nations schizophrenia samples. Schizophrenia Bull 2000; 26:903–912.
70. Ryan MC, Collins P, Thakore JH. Impaired fasting glucose tolerance in first-episode, drug-naïve patients with schizophrenia. Am J Psychiatry 2003; 160: 284–289.
71. Thakore JH, Mann JN, Vlahos I, et al. Increased visceral fat distribution in drug-naïve and drug-free patients with schizophrenia. Int J Obes 2002; 26:137–141.
72. Regenold WT, Thapar RK, Marano C, Gavirneni S, Kondapavuluru P. Increased prevalence of type 2 diabetes mellitus among psychiatric inpatients with biolor I affective and schizoaffective disorders independent of psychotropic drug use. J Affect Disord 2002; 70:19–26.
73. Shiloah E, Witz S, Abramovitch Y, et al. Effect of acute psychotic stress in nondiabetic subjects on B-cell function and insulin sensitivity. Diab Care 2003; 26:1462–1467.
74. Golden SH, Williams JE, Ford DE, et al. Depressive symptoms and the risk of type 2 diabetes. Diab Care 2004; 27:429–435.
75. Eaton WW, Armenian H, Gallo J, Pratt L, Ford DE. Depression and risk for onset of type II diabetes. A prospective population-based study. Diab Care 1996; 19:1097–1102.
76. Arroyo C, Hu FB, Ryan LM, Kawachi I, Colditz GA, Speizer FE, Manson J. Depressive symptoms and risk of type 2 diabetes in women. Diab Care 2004; 27:129–133.
77. Thakore JH, Richards PJ, Reznek RH, et al. Increased intra-abdominal fat deposition in patients with major depressive illness as measured by computed tomography. Biol Psychiatry 1997; 41:1140–1142.
78. Ford DE, Erlinger TP. Depression and C-reative protein in US adults data from the Third National Health and Nutrition Examination Survey. Arch Intern Med 2004; 164:1010–1014.
79. Penninx B, Kritchevsky SB, Yaffe K, et al. Inflammatory markers and depressed mood in older persons: results from the Health, Aging and Body Composition Study. Biol Psychiatry 2003; 54:566–572.
80. Panagiotakos DB, Pitsavos C, Chrysohoou C, et al. Inflammation, coagulation, and depressive symptomatology in cardiovascular disease- free people; the ATTICA study. Eur Heart J 2004; 25:492–499.
81. Danner M, Kasl SV, Abramson JL, Vaccarino V. Association between depression and elevated C-reactive protein. Psychosom Med 2003; 65:347–356.

82. Zhang Z, Yao Z, Liu W, Fang Q, Reynolds G. Effects of antipsychotics on fat deposition and changes in leptin and insulin levels. Brit J Psychiatry 2004; 184:58–62.
83. Ryan CM, Flanagan S, Kinsella U, Keeling F, Thakore JH. The effects of atypical antipsychotics on visceral fat distribution in first episode, drug-naïve vepatientswithschizophrenia.LifeSci2004; 74 : 1999–2008.
84. Wirshing DA, Wirshing WC, Kysar L, et al. Novel antipsychotics: comparison of weight gain liabilities. J Clin Psychiatry 1999; 60:358–363.
85. Wirshing DA, Boyd JA, Meng LR, Ballon JS, Marder S, Wirshing W. The effects of novel antipyshotics on glucose and lipid levels. J Clin Psychiatry 2002; 63:856–865.
86. Wirshing DA. Adverse effects of atypical antipsychotics. J Clin Psychiatry 2001; 62:7–10.
87. Newcomer JW, Haupt DW, Fucetola R, et al. Abnormalities in glucose regulation during antipsychotic treatment of schizophrenia. Arch Gen Psychiatry 2002; 59:337–345.
88. Caliero E, Borba CP, Hayden DL, Schoenfeld DA, Goff DG, Henderson DC. Clozapine and olanzapine induce insulin resistance in patients with schizophrenic disorders (Abstract). Diabetes 2001; 50(suppl 2):A91.
89. Lindenmayer J, Czobor P, Volavka J, et al. Changes in glucose and cholesterol levels in patients with schizophrenia treated with typical or atypical antipsychotics. Am J Psychiatry 2003; 160:290–296.
90. Garyfallos G, Dimelis D, Kouniakis P, et al. Olanzapine versus risperidone: weight gain and elevation of serum triglyceride levels. Eur Psychiatry 2003; 18:320–321.
91. Casey DE, Haupt DW, Newcomer JW, et al. Antipsychotic-induced weight gain and metabolic abnormalities: implications for increased mortality in patients with schizophrenia. J Clin Psychiatry 2004; 65 (suppl 7):4–18.
92. Koro CE, Fedder DO, L'Italien G, et al. An assessment of the independent effects of olanzapine and risperidone exposure on the risk of hyperlipidemia in schizophrenic patients. Arch Gen Psychiatry 2002; 59:1021–1026.
93. Marder SR, McQuade RD, Stock E, et al. Aripiprazole in the treatment of schizophrenia: safety and tolerability in short-term, placebo-controlled trials. Schizophrenia Res 2003; 61:123–136.
94. Daniel DG. Tolerablility of ziprasidone: an expanding perspective. J Clin Psychiatry 2003; 64(suppl 19):40–9.
95. Pfizer Inc. FDA Psychopharmacological Drugs Advisory Committee. Breifing document for Zeldox® capsules (ziprasidone HCL). New York, NY:Pfizer Inc; July 2002.
96. Glick ID, Romano SJ, Simpson G, et al. Insulin resistance in olanzapine- and ziprasidone- treated patients; results of a double-blind, controlled 6-week trial (poster). Presented at the 154th annual meeting of the American Psychiatric Association; New Orleans, LA. 2001:May 5–10.
97. Simpson GM, Weiden PJ, Pigott T, et al. Ziprasidone versus olanzapine in schizophrenia; 6-month blinded continuation study (poster). Presented at the 155th annual meeting of the American Psychiatric Association; Philadelphia, PA. May 2002:18–23.

98. Weiden PJ, Daniel DG, Simpson G, Romano SJ. Improvement in indices of health status in outpatients with schizophrenia switched to ziprasidone. J Clin Psychopharmacol 2003; 23:595–600.
99. Romano SJ, Cutler N, Weiden PJ, et al. Ziprasidone's effects on weight and lipids in patients with schizophrenia (poster). Presented at the 155th annual meeting of the American Psychiatric Association; Philadelphia, PA. May 2002:18–23.
100. Myer JM. Awareness of obesity and weight issues among chronically mentally ill inpatients: a pilot study. Ann Clin Psychiatry 2002; 14:39–45.
101. Tuomilehto J, Lindstorm J, Eriksson JG, et al. Prevention of type 2 diabetes mellitus by changes in lifestyle among subjects with impaired glucose tolerance. N Engl J Med 2001; 344:1343–1350.
102. Leon AS, Sanchez O. Meta-analysis of the effects of aerobic exercise training on blood lipids. Circulation 2001; 104(suppl II):414–415 (Abstract).
103. Fagard RH. Exercise characteristics and blood pressure response to dynamic physical training. Med Sci Sports Exerc 2001; 33(6 suppl):S484–S492.
104. Thompson PD, Crouse SF, Goodpaster B, Kelly D, Niall M, Pescatello L. The acute versus the chronic response to exercise. Med Sci Sports Exerc 2001; 33(6 suppl):S438–S445.
105. Katzmarzyk PT, Leon AS, Wilmore JH, et al. Targeting the metabolic syndrome with exercise: evidence from the HERITAGE Family Study. Med Sci Sports Exerc 2003; 35:1703–1709.
106. Sharman MJ, Gomez AL, Kraemer WJ, Volek JS. Very low-carbohydrate and low-fat diets affect fasting lipids and postprandial lipemia differently in overweight men. J Nutr 2004; 134:880–885.
107. Stern L, Iqbal N, Seshadri P, et al. The effects of low-carbohydrate versus conventional weight loss diets in severely obese adults: one-year follow-up of a randomized trial. Ann Intern Med 2004; 140:778–785.
108. Gaede P, Vedel P, Larsen N, Jensen GV, Parving HH, Pedersen O. Multifactorial intervention and cardiovascular disease in patients with type 2 diabetes. N Engl J Med 2003; 348:383–393.
109. Diabetes Prevention Program Research Group. Reduction in the incidence of type 2 diabetes with lifestyle intervention or metformin. N Engl J Med 2002; 346:393–403.
110. Einhorn D, Aroda VR, Henry RR. Glitazones and the management of insulin resistance: what they do and how might they be used. Endocrinol and Metab Clin 2004; 33:595–616.
111. Durbin RJ. Thiazolidinedione therapy in the prevention/delay of type 2 diabetes in patients with impaired glucose tolerance and insulin resistance. Diab Obes Metab 2004; 6:280–285.
112. Wong ND, Pio JR, Franklin SS, L'Italien GJ, Kamath TV, Williams GR. Preventing coronary events by optimal control of blood pressure and lipids in patients with the metabolic syndrome. Am J Cardiol 2003; 91:1421–1426.

9

Obesity, Polycystic Ovary Syndrome, and Mood Disorders

Margaret F. Reynolds

*Behavioral Neuroendocrinology Program, Stanford University
School of Medicine, Stanford, California, U.S.A.*

Natalie L. Rasgon

*Department of Psychiatry and Behavioral Science, Department of Obstetrics and
Gynecology, Stanford University School of Medicine,
Stanford, California, U.S.A.*

INTRODUCTION

Connections between obesity and psychiatric disorders have been noted as early as in the 1930s and 1940s, and have recently become a source of heightened interest and debate (1,2). As the prevalence and severity of obesity continue to rise, the question of how obesity intersects with psychiatric conditions, such as mood disorders, has become increasingly urgent. Like the endocrine system itself—marked by complexity and reflexivity of feed-forward and feedback pathways—the interplay of obesity and mood disorders is clearly multidimensional. Attending to the question of obesity, for example, also means addressing the effects of other conditions that fall under the metabolic syndrome, particularly those involving glucose regulation such as insulin resistance (IR), type-2 diabetes, glucose tolerance, and dyslipidemia. In addition, the discussion cannot ignore other intersecting topics such as the psychosocial aspects of obesity, chronic mental health problems, and the potential impact of medication use in mood disorders.

Unlike the delicate balancing act that is a normally functioning endocrine system, however, the interplay of obesity and psychiatric disorders appears to represent the unhinging of a finely tuned system of checks and balances. Understanding exactly where and why this dysregulation is taking place not only holds the promise of illuminating connections between the endocrine, nervous, cardiovascular, and immune systems, but is also a critical task for progress in clinical preventative and treatment measures.

This chapter focuses on an exploration of polycystic ovary syndrome (PCOS) as a particular disorder that is not only practically important to address—because many women with mood or metabolic disorders exhibit features of PCOS—but is also theoretically important, as PCOS may lend a unique perspective on the potential role of IR as an interface between obesity and mood disorders. PCOS, a common endocrine disorder of reproductive-age women, which is closely associated with obesity and IR, is increasingly at the center of the debate surrounding the connections between metabolic dysregulation and mood disorders. Rates of mood disorders may be higher in populations of women with PCOS; reciprocally, rates of reproductive dysfunction may be higher in populations of women with bipolar disorder. As is the case with other facets of this topic, medication use may also play into this equation. Thus, an exploration of PCOS in relation to metabolic and psychiatric disorders may shed light on the interconnectedness of the obesity and mood disorders, and provides practical information for clinical and research use.

THE METABOLIC SYNDROME: OBESITY AND IR

Obesity and Metabolic Syndrome: Definitions and Prevalence Rates

Obesity is operationalized by the measure of body mass index (BMI), which is calculated by dividing weight (in kilograms) by height (in meters) squared. Clinical guidelines by the National Heart, Lung, and Blood Institute define overweight as BMI between 25 and $29.9 \, kg/m^2$ and obesity as a BMI of $30 \, kg/m^2$ or greater (3). Obesity can be further divided into classes I, II, and III; class I obesity is defined as BMI between 30 and $34.9 \, kg/m^2$, class II as BMI between 35 and $39.9 \, kg/m^2$, and class III as a BMI greater than $40 \, kg/m^2$ (4).

This definition of overweight is based on epidemiological data showing increases in morbidity and mortality in BMI values above 25, and when applied to the U.S. population yields estimates that approximately 55% of adults in the United States are overweight. Roughly a half of this population (19.9% and 24.9% of the general population for men and women, respectively) is further considered obese, with more recent estimates showing almost one-third of the general population as obese (3,5). It is interesting to note that while the percentage of "overweight but not obese" individuals has remained relatively stable over the past three decades, the prevalence of obesity has increased steadily during this time, with the percentage of individuals registering as "normal weight" consequently diminishing (6).

The subject of obesity cannot easily be disentangled from the topics of IR, glucose tolerance, and dyslipidemia, among other metabolic and cardiovascular conditions. This is particularly true when discussing the relationship between obesity and psychiatric disorders. Obesity may be defined, in a general sense, as the excessive accumulation of body fat, and operationalized by specific parameters such as BMI, but the complexity of the condition is not adequately conveyed by these definitions. Obesity is a chronic multisystem disease that includes genetic, metabolic, hormonal, immunological, and behavioral aspects and that effects adipose, muscle, hepatic, nervous, adrenal, and vascular tissues (7).

The observation that a constellation of metabolic and cardiovascular conditions are often clustered together has resulted in what is now a common concept referred to as the "metabolic syndrome." Initially introduced by Reaven as "syndrome X" or the "insulin resistance syndrome," it functions as an overarching concept connecting a variety of abnormalities including, but not limited to, obesity, hypertension, dyslipidemia, abnormalities of glucose regulation (i.e., IR, glucose intolerance, hyperinsulinemia, and type-2 diabetes mellitus), and atherosclerosis (8–10). Metabolic syndrome has since been operationalized by the Expert Panel on Detection, Evaluation, and Treatment of High Cholesterol in Adults (referred to as the "Adult Treatment Panel III" or ATP III) as having three or more of the elements presented in Table 1. The metabolic syndrome has an estimated prevalence of more than 21% in the U.S. population, a number that will likely continue to rise Table 2.

Mood disorders have long been associated with obesity but have also been connected with abnormalities of glucose regulation such as IR, glucose intolerance, and type-2 diabetes (22). Thus, it is of particular importance to outline how obesity and abnormalities of glucose regulation are understood to be related. The role of the immune system via inflammatory mediators is also increasing the topic of research and debate in relation to mood disorders.

Table 1 Adult Treatment Panel III Guidelines for Diagnosis of Metabolic Syndrome. Patients Must Exhibit at Least Three of the Following Conditions

Measure	Definition
High blood pressure	$\geq 130/85$ mm Hg or antihypertensive medication use
High triglycerides	≥ 150 mg/dL
Low HDL cholesterol	< 40 mg/dL in men; < 50 mg/dL in women
High fasting glucose	≥ 110 mg/dL or antidiabetic medication use
Abdominal obesity	Waist circumference > 102 cm in men: > 88 cm in women

Table 2 Theoretical Relationships Between Mood Disorders and Weight Disorders

Mood disorder	Associated weight disorder
Major depressive disorder	Underweight, overweight, obesity
Atypical features	Overweight, obesity
Typical (melancholic) features	Underweight, abdomincal obesity
Juvenile onset	Overweight, obesity
Bipolar disorder	Abdominal obesity, overweight, obesity

Based on data from studies of obesity and related conditions in persons with syndromal mood disorders. *Source*: From Refs. 11–21.

Obesity and IR

As the prior nomenclature of "insulin resistance syndrome" suggests, impaired insulin responsiveness is thought to be central to the metabolic syndrome. The term "insulin resistance" refers to a resistance to the effects of insulin on glucose uptake, metabolism, or storage. Specifically, it is manifested by decreased insulin-stimulated glucose transport in adipocytes and skeletal muscle and by impaired suppression of hepatic glucose output, usually the result of impaired insulin signaling or downregulation of GLUT4, the major glucose transporter responsive to insulin (23). Although IR is known to occur in lean individuals, perhaps as the result of inherited insulin receptor and postreceptor defects, it is widely accepted that visceral obesity is the primary determinant of IR (23–25).

Skeletal muscle was originally thought to be the driving tissue behind systemic glucose homeostasis, but recent studies have suggested that adipose tissue plays a greater role than previously conjectured (23,26,27). Large epidemiological studies show that risk for diabetes increases with BMI, suggesting that the amount of adipose tissue exerts an effect on IR (28). One proposed explanation of this observation relates to the expansion of cell membrane surface area, which would lead to a decrease in insulin receptor density and/or proximity to insulin signaling molecules (7).

Another explanation, however, is rooted in the discovery of adipocytes as endocrine cells, which can express and secrete peptide and steroid hormones and cytokines such as tumor necrosis factor alpha (TNF-α), plasminogen-activator inhibitor-1, angiotensinogen, interleukon-6 (IL-6), leptin, cortisol, and estrogen. For example, it is hypothesized that excessive TNF-α secretion, possibly by adipocytes, impairs insulin signaling and reduces GLUT4 gene expression (29,30).

That these adipocytes can secrete hormones and cytokines clearly suggests adipose tissue as a source of paracrine effect on nearby tissues. It also suggests that adipocytes possess the capacity to affect metabolism at diverse systemic sites such as the brain, liver, gonads, and lymphoid organs (23).

The potential role of leptin provides one example of this possibility. Leptin is an adipocyte-derived hormone that can exert influence on satiety, energy expenditure, and neuroendocrine function (31). When administered to rodents, it demonstrates an acute as well as long-term insulin-sensitizing effect (32–34). It is thought to influence insulin through central actions within the hypothalamus [with effects transmitted to the periphery via alterations in appetite and possible suppression of the hypothalamic–pituitary–adrenal (HPA) axis or other neuroendocrine pathways] and/or through local effects on peripheral target cells. This latter influence may be driven by leptin's promotion of lipid oxidation and insulin sensitivity (23,35,36).

Free fatty acids (FFAs) may also play a role in the relationship between obesity and IR, further allowing adipose tissue to regulate glucose homeostasis. Heightened FFA levels are consistently associated with obesity and are likely due to release from expanded adipose tissue, as well as impaired hepatic metabolism. Elevated FFAs impact insulin sensitivity via a number of pathways. First, they impair insulin's ability to suppress hepatic glucose output; second, they impair the ability of insulin to stimulate glucose uptake into skeletal muscle; and third, they inhibit insulin secretion from pancreatic β-cells (23).

Thus, it is commonly understood that the increases in adipose tissue observed in obesity can engender other metabolic changes such as the development of IR, type-2 diabetes, and dyslipidemia. The question, and possibility, that IR may not only be caused by obesity but also contribute to obesity has also been raised, although the exact mechanisms of such a directional relationship remain unclear (23). Findings thus far support the observation that it is often difficult to separate the effects of obesity and IR, as they are closely tied phenomena.

Lastly, some researchers have pointed out that IR may occur independent of obesity and that the sensitivity of insulin is greatly impacted (perhaps, even more than loss of adipose tissue outright) by factors such as cardiovascular fitness (37). Indeed, it would be incomplete to ignore the impact of obesity on cardiovascular fitness, and in turn the impact of cardiovascular fitness on IR. Exercise—both low and high intensity—can positively impact immunological factors, lipid levels, and metabolism of glucose. Thus, obesity, with its propensity to further discourage individuals from vigorous exercise, may impact the metabolic syndrome via cardiovascular parameters.

OVERVIEW OF MOOD DISORDERS: BIPOLAR DISORDER AND MAJOR DEPRESSIVE DISORDER

"Mood disorders" have had a long and varied history within the field of medicine, but recent advances in the last 50 years have provided increasingly detailed information on such aspects as classification, clinical distinctions, genetics, neuropathophysiology, neurochemistry, and treatment. The major disorders that constitute this category, as recognized and described by the *Diagnostic and Statistical Manual of Mental Disorders, Fourth Edition* (DSM-IV), are bipolar I disorder and major depressive disorder. In addition, the DSM-IV has recognized a host of variants of these disorders characterized by less severe symptomatology. These include dysthymic and cyclothymic disorders; minor depressive, recurrent brief, and premenstrual dysphoric disorder; and bipolar II disorder (38). In addition to bipolar I and II, many studies include bipolar disorder not otherwise specified (NOS) in subject populations with bipolar disorder.

It is estimated that major depressive disorder has a lifetime prevalence rate of 10% to 25% for women and 5% to 12% for men. The gender differences in rates of depressive disorders are at the center of much debate, but it is generally recognized that both biological and social factors may play a role. Rates of prevalence for bipolar disorder are broken into subsets of bipolar I and bipolar II. The lifetime prevalence rate of bipolar I disorder is 0.4% to 1.6%, while that of bipolar II disorder is less than 1%. Additionally, it has been recognized that around 5% to 15% of individuals with bipolar disorder exhibit "rapid cycling" characteristics (39,40). While approximately equal numbers of men and women exhibit bipolar I, bipolar II is more prevalent in women, as are rapid cycling characteristics (41–44).

As a group, mood disorders are characterized by a number of biological characteristics. For example, data have consistently suggested that mood disorders are associated with heterogeneous dysregulations of biogenic monoamines such as the neurotransmitters norepinephrine (NE), serotonin (5-HT), dopamine, and acetylcholine. This concept is bolstered by evidence from treatment of mood disorders with pharmacological agents that affect neurotransmitter levels. Neuroendocrine axes—particularly, those implicating the thyroid, adrenal, and hypothalamus glands—also show dysregulation in patients with mood disorders. Particular abnormalities include the hypersecretion of cortisol, decreased basal levels of follicle-stimulating hormone (FSH) and luteinizing hormone (LH), and the prevalence of thyroid disorders (45).

In addition to the implication of the hypothalamus, neuroanatomical studies support the roles of the limbic system and basal ganglia in presentation of mood disorder characteristics, and a number of brain imagining studies have shown decreased blood flow in the frontal cortex. These findings make sense in light of the fact that monoaminergic systems are distributed throughout these areas (46).

Mood disorders share other characteristics, including genetic correlations; however, data suggest that there may be a stronger genetic component to bipolar I disorder than to major depressive disorder. Family studies have found that first-degree relatives of bipolar I disorder probands are 8 to 18 times more likely than similarly situated control subjects to have bipolar disorder. These first-degree relatives are also more likely to experience major depressive disorder. To a lesser extent, the same phenomenon is observed for first-degree relatives of individuals with major depressive disorder. Concordance rates in monozygotic and dyzogtic twins for bipolar I disorder and major depressive disorder indicate genetic components as well (47,48).

POLYCYSTIC OVARY SYNDROME: THE INTERFACE OF OBESITY, MOOD DISORDERS, AND IR

PCOS is an endocrine disorder at the center of much interest to date, due in part to the high rates of obesity and IR observed in populations of women with PCOS. In addition, our preliminary research has suggested that mood disorders occur at a higher rate in populations of women with PCOS, prompting a tentative theory that IR and other forms of metabolic dysregulation contribute to the pathophysiology of mood disorders. This section reviews the current understanding of PCOS as a disorder of endocrine dysregulation, and describes literature and hypotheses that place IR as a possible link between mood disorders and obesity. An important topic in this discussion is the potential role of pharmacological agents used to treat mood disorders, a number of which have been implicated in the development of PCOS and in negatively influencing various metabolic parameters. Lastly, we will address the clinical implications of these findings that clinicians face practically in the treatment of mood disorders and obesity.

PCOS: An Overview

Definition and Diagnosis

Polycystic ovary syndrome, as defined by the 1990 NICHD PCOS Conference, is an endocrine disorder characterized by chronic anovulation and hyperandrogenemia (evidenced either as clinical hyperandrogenism and/or biochemical evidence of elevated testosterone levels) in the absence of other endinocrinopathies such as congenital adrenal hyperplasia, hyperthyroidism, Cushing syndrome, or hyperprolactinemia (49,50). This is the currently accepted definition in the United States, although specific characteristics such as the levels of total or free testosterone that define biochemical hyperandrogenemism frequently vary.

In 2003, the Rotterdam Consensus supported the concept of PCOS as a syndrome of ovarian dysfunction, with the cardinal features of chronic anovulation (oligomenorrhea or amenorrhea), and hyperandrogenemia. In addition, the consensus agreed that polycystic ovary morphology (PCO), while not an essential component of PCOS, could be used as a factor in its diagnosis. The consensus also recognized the variability in presentation of this disorder; for example, it noted that some women may have regular cycles yet still be included in the syndrome. As a result, the consensus proposed that "two of the three" previously outlined symptoms (ovulatory dysfunction in the form of oligomenorrhea or amenorrhea, hyperandrogenism, and PCO) be present for diagnosis (51). However, this definition does not appear to be widely in use to date, as definitions across studies still vary, and its adoption in the research arena has yet to be broadly documented.

The name "polycystic ovary syndrome" suggests PCO to be an essential trait of PCOS, and in many countries outside the United States, presentation of PCO (as observed via ultrasound) is necessary for a diagnosis—a reality that complicates the comparison of international studies on PCOS (52). PCO morphology is indeed found at a higher rate in women with clinical and/or endocrine abnormalities consistent with PCOS (i.e., anovulation and hyperandrogenism). The genesis of the PCOS disorder reflects this grouping of symptoms; in 1935, Stein and Leventhal first identified what is now recognized as the constellation of conditions surrounding PCOS: hirsutism, anovulation, PCO, and obesity (53). However, up to one-quarter of the healthy female population exhibits PCO without any other symptoms of PCOS, and researchers have found that up to one-half of all women exhibiting the clinical symptoms of PCOS do not have PCO (52,54,55). For these and other reasons, most operational definitions of PCOS in the United States for research purposes have tended to exclude PCO as a defining criterion. Although the Rotterdam Consensus now includes PCO as one potential diagnostic criterion, it remains to be seen whether the option of including PCO as a diagnostic component of PCOS will be adopted by American researchers.

Anovulation is recognized in a variety of forms: ovulatory dysfunction, polymenorrhea, secondary amenorrhea, or oligomenorrhea (perhaps the most common symptom of anovulation, typically operationalized as eight or fewer menstrual cycles per year or cycle length of greater than 35 to 40 days). Hyperandrogenemia can be clinically evaluated (i.e., hyperandrogenism), through the presence of acne or hirsutism, the latter of which is usually evaluated by the Ferriman–Gallwey scale (56). It can also be biochemically evaluated through the measurement of serum levels of total or free testosterone.

Given the varying definitions of PCOS, incidence rates are wide ranging, from 3% to 52% depending on the definition used and the population studied (57–59). However, a widely acknowledged estimated incidence is between 4% and 6% (49,60).

Pathophysiology

Biochemical aspects of PCOS that have been identified highlight the concept of the "vicious circle" of endocrine dysregulation that appears to occur at the level of the hypothalamic–pituitary–gonadal (HPG) axis (Fig. 1). In this model, excess androgens, deranged GnRH release, elevated inhibin B levels, and IR/hyperinsulinemia coalesce to suppress FSH and increase LH-stimulated ovarian steroidogenesis. Specifically, insulin is known to

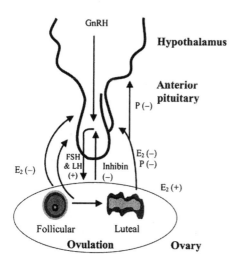

Figure 1 The hypothalamic-pituitary-ovarian axis. *Abbreviations*: GnRH, gonado-trophin releasing hormone; P, progesterone E_2, estradiol; FSH, follicle-stimulating hormone; LH, luteinizing hormone; (−), negative feedback; (+), positive feedback.

stimulate ovarian androgen production in women with PCOS via action on ovarian thecal cells (61–63). This prevents follicle maturation and leads to the development of small, immature follicles, and follicular cysts. Because immature ovarian follicles do not express aromatase, the enzyme that converts androgens to estrogens, the ovary secretes primarily androgens in response to LH. These androgens, in addition to those released from the adrenal gland, may contribute to the clinical and biochemical features of hyperandrogenemia. They also increase circulating estrogen levels, as excess androgens are peripherally aromatized to estrogens. These estrogens then feed back into the cycle to disrupt normal LH regulation and cyclicity.

Biochemical observations in women with PCOS have confirmed a number of endocrine theories of PCOS. LH levels are often high, perhaps due to an increased amplitude and frequency of LH pulses, and while FSH levels tend to stay within range, women with PCOS frequently exhibit high LH:FSH ratios (64–68). Heightened free or total testosterone levels are also common, but much variability in androgen levels has been observed (69,70). For example, hirsute women do not necessarily have higher concentrations of androgens but may simply exhibit greater sensitivity to androgen levels (71,72).

It has also been noted that obese subjects with marked hirsutism may exhibit normal serum concentrations of total testosterone but, because obesity has been known to suppress sex-hormone binding globulin (SHBG), experience an increased rate of androgen production (52). Low SHBG may also contribute to an increase in circulating estrogen. Although estrogen levels are often within normal range, the condition of anovulation means there is no midluteal increase in estradiol concentrations and as a result of the lack in cyclical progesterone secretion, these estrogen levels are generally unopposed (73). Because adipose tissue can convert androgens to estrone, obesity may also impact the estrogen levels (74,75).

Lastly, hyperprolactinemia has been noted in patients with PCOS. This biochemical feature has been reported in between 5% and 30% of women with PCO, with roughly 17% of women with PCOS exhibiting it (76–79). A recent study investigating hyperprolactinemia in nonobese PCOS subjects found higher mean insulin and HOMA levels in hyperprolactinemic versus normoprolactinemic subjects. The authors concluded that nonobese PCOS patients with hyperprolactinemia may be at greater risk for IR (80). A further study links the hyperprolactinemia insulin-resistant state to a number of conditions, including elevated FFAs, a decrease in the number of insulin receptors, or postreceptor binding defects in insulin action (81). As is the case with most aspects of PCOS, no clinical features have been discovered to be uniformly present in all cases of PCOS; thus, there is currently no "sine qua none" of PCOS to aid in the definitive diagnosis of the disorder.

Metabolic Aspects of PCOS

With the dramatic rise in rates of metabolic syndrome and the increased awareness about its serious cardiovascular health sequalae, the metabolic aspects of PCOS—including obesity and IR—have increasingly become the focus of discussion and research. PCOS is clearly associated with obesity, with some researchers estimating up to 50% of the PCOS population as obese, in contrast to recent estimates that one-third of the general population is obese (5,58). As Franks points out in his seminal paper on PCOS, it has long been recognized that syndromes characterized by extreme IR are associated with ovarian hyperandrogenism (52). In line with this observation, research has shown higher rates of IR in populations of women with PCOS, with findings that up to 40% of women with PCOS exhibit this abnormality (82,83).

Although the details of the interrelation of adipose tissue, IR, excess androgens, and HPA dysregulation have yet to be fully mapped, a number of observations provide important clues. IR in women with PCOS appears both in obese and nonobese women, and rates of IR in both of these groups are considered higher than the normal population (84). In vitro studies suggest that insulin augments the ovarian androgen response to LH (85,86). Insulin may also affect androgen levels by suppressing SHBG levels (87). As might be expected given the higher rates of IR, women with PCOS also show a higher prevalence of type-2 diabetes (estimated at 7.5% to 10%) and impaired glucose tolerance (estimated at 31% to 35%) (88). Significantly, women with PCOS also appear to have an increased risk of cardiovascular pathology that develops more precociously than the general female population (89–93). For example, it has been reported that the rate of conversion from impaired glucose tolerance to type-2 diabetes increases from 5 to 10-fold in PCOS populations (82,94,95).

Studies suggest that IR in PCOS may be at least partially independent of the effect of obesity. Higher rates of IR have been noted in both lean and obese subject populations with PCOS, although IR appears to be worse when there is an interaction between obesity and PCOS (96). Excess circulating androgens are one possible point of influence, but research suggests that insulin affects androgen secretion more than a relationship in the opposite direction (52). In addition, it has been noted that IR and diabetes are more likely to be seen in women with anovulatory features rather than in women who only exhibit clinical features of hyperandrogenism (52).

Treatment and Management

PCOS is recognized as the most common cause of infertility in women of reproductive age. Treatment of PCOS often reflects this deficit, with the goal of treatment being regular ovulation for fertility purposes. However, treatment for PCOS can also be directed at the clinical symptoms of hyperandrogenism (such as acne, hirsutism, or alopecia), or aimed at regulating metabolic parameters such as high IR or obesity. Generally, treatment for PCOS is tailored to address the particular problematic symptoms of that individual, but health care practitioners are increasingly aware of the need to prevent, treat, and manage the long-term health sequalae of the disorder.

The first line of treatment for PCOS has also changed dramatically over the past century. Around the time of Stein and Leventhal's original identification of the disorder, surgical management through what was known as "ovarian wedge resection" (a procedure that removed a portion of the ovarian capsule and that was shown to prompt normal ovulatory cycling) was a popular, yet invasive, form of treatment. However, wedge resection often failed to combat the excess androgen levels associated with the disorder. Although it fell heavily out of favor in the latter part of the 20th century, laparoscopic takes on the same procedure have been enjoying a small revival.

Instead, PCOS is now typically treated through the administration of hormones, such as estro-progestin oral contraceptives (OCPs), or pharmacological agents such as spironolactone or metformin. Use of OCPs is still a common method of inducing regular cycling. This method has the benefit of creating regular bleeding periods, reducing the risks of unopposed estrogen, and reducing the androgens produced by the ovary. OCPs are thought to reduce hyperandrogenic clinical features via the suppression of LH, an increase in SHBG, and the inhibition of 5α-reductase and androgen receptor binding (97,98). However, for women whose primary concern is the desire to become pregnant, OCP use is clearly contraindicated.

In these cases, methods of inducing ovulation are necessary. Anti-estrogens such as clomiphene citrate have historically been popular for this function. Suppressing the amount of estrogen early in the menstrual cycle often causes the hypothalamus and pituitary to increase production of FSH and LH, thereby promoting the development and release of a follicle. Although still utilized, this form of fertility treatment has fallen in popularity as of late. Instead, the use of insulin sensitizers has become prevalent as the first line of fertility treatment for anovulatory women with PCOS.

In the early 1990s, research started to indicate that IR showed an inverse correlation with menstrual disorders (99). It was consequently discovered that improvement of peripheral insulin sensitivity with insulin sensitizing agents such as metformin, a biguinide, could induce ovulation and normal cycling (100–103). In addition to ovulatory effects, administration of metformin has been shown to decrease levels of LH, the LH:FSH ratio, testosterone, androstenedione, DHEAS, and basal 17-OH-progesterone, and to increase levels of SHBG (104). Reductions in the Ferriman–Gallwey scores of women on metformin for six months indicate that effects on biochemical androgens are clinically exhibited as well (105).

Treatment options to combat excess androgens in relation to their clinical manifestations (acne, hirsutism, and alopecia) can be used alone or in conjunction with metformin. These consist of flutamide and spironolactone, androgen receptor agonists, and finasteride, a drug that inhibits type-2 5α-reductase. The former are both used mainly to combat hirsutism, but flutamide has been shown to have many positive metabolic effects (lowering insulin levels after administration of glucose and decrease in LDL levels) in addition to lowering androgen levels. Moreover, it has been shown to prompt a recovery of ovulatory cycles; however, administration must be carefully monitored given the possible hepatoxicity (104).

Prevalence of PCOS in Mood Disorder Populations

In 2000, we published a report on the prevalence of PCOS in a population of 22 women ages 18 to 45 with bipolar disorder (I, II, or NOS) and who were being treated with lithium and/or divalproex. None of these patients met criteria for PCOS as defined by the 1990 NIH consensus. However, all of the women receiving lithium reported some type of menstrual disturbance (amenorrhea, oligomenorrhea, menorrhagia, or dysmenorrhea) in their histories, while 67% of the women receiving valproate reported some type of menstrual disturbance in their histories. For the women receiving lithium, the most common menstrual disturbances were dysmenorrhea (60%) and oligomenorrhea (20%); all but one woman reported these symptoms to have started before treatment with lithium. In the valproate group, the most common menstrual disturbances were oligomenorrhea (30%) and menorrhagia (30%). Incidents of amenorrhea (four in total: one in the lithium group, two in the valproate group, and one in the mixed group) were reported to have commenced before treatment for bipolar disorder. Clinical evaluations did not reveal significant hirsutism in any groups, and while hormonal screenings showed that women receiving valproate exhibited elevated concentrations of total and bioavailable testosterone and DHEA when compared to women receiving lithium, these differences were not significant (106).

Thus, although this study showed no differences in rates of menstrual disturbances, hirsutism, or PCOS between medication groups (a claim that has been made and will be addressed shortly), it did provide preliminary data on the rates of menstrual dysfunction in a group of women treated for bipolar disorder, showing that experiences of menstrual dysfunction were relatively common among this population. Given the lack of a control group, the study could not comment on whether these rates were significantly higher than those of a normal, healthy population, but the high rates were certainly suggestive of such a difference. Another interesting finding of this study was that most menstrual abnormalities appeared to first emerge before pharmacological treatment for bipolar disorder was started, suggesting that high rates of menstrual abnormalities may be linked more to the etiology of bipolar disorder than its treatment.

Another study by our research group, albeit in a small sample, corroborated the finding that menstrual abnormalities, in particular long cycles, are common in women with bipolar disorder. In a study that evaluated mood over the menstrual cycle in 17 women between the ages of 18 and 45 with bipolar disorder, 11 women (59%) were found to have long cycles (greater than 29 days), with three of these women (18%) exhibiting oligomenorrhea (cycles greater than 35 days) (107). Similarly, a study analyzing the results of a county-wide survey among high-schoolers also found associations between menstrual abnormalities—particularly late menarche, secondary amenorrhea, and long cycles—and depressive disorder symptoms as measured by the Beck Depression Inventory. The latter two menstrual abnormalities were also associated with eating disorder symptoms (108). Such findings strengthen the observation that menstrual abnormalities are associated with mood disorders in a unique way.

Research has also investigated the biochemical and endocrinological aspects of mood disorders that may reflect PCOS. Matsunaga et al. (109) examined functioning of the HPG axis in 12 women with bipolar or psychotic symptoms which fluctuated with the menstrual cycle and found 67% of the women exhibited elevated basal LH concentrations, 50% exhibited decreased basal FSH, and 50% exhibited elevated serum testosterone, all of which are common biochemical features of PCOS. This evidence suggests that women experiencing mood disorder symptoms in close relation to their menstrual cycle may be more likely to exhibit or develop PCOS features. However, the majority (8 out of the 12, or 67%) of these women exhibited psychotic features, whereas only four exhibited strictly bipolar disorder features.

Similarly, Baischer et al. (110) studied the HPG axis in 20 premenopausal women with major depression according to the DSM-III-R and compared results of common reproductive hormone concentrations immediately before pharmacological treatment for depression was started, as well as one month into treatment with clomipramine, to a group of 10 healthy controls. The authors found significantly elevated levels of testosterone in the untreated depressed patients compared to the controls. However, while the testosterone levels of the depressed women after one month of clomipramine treatment remained higher than the controls, this difference was no longer statistically significant. In addition, treated patients showed higher levels of prolactin and lower levels of FSH compared to controls. These results again suggest that HPG and/or HPA axis dysregulation is common in female mood disorder populations, particularly related to excess androgens.

There is some confusion as to whether noted androgen excess is a result of HPA or HPG dysfunction. Weber et al. (111), in a study of androgen concentrations in women with major depressive disorder (as defined by the DSM-IV) compared to healthy controls, found that circulating levels of androstenedione, testosterone, and dihydrotestosterone to be elevated in depressed women, as were cortisol and DHEA concentrations. Given that the authors found no differences in LH or FSH between depressed women and controls, the authors concluded that elevated androgen levels are most likely of adrenal origin and thus linked to HPA axis dysregulation. However, the question of HPG axis influence has not yet been decided.

Clearly, although more studies have looked at individual endocrine or clinical characteristics in relation to mood disorders, few studies exist that examine the rate of PCOS in populations of women with mood disorders. Our own research projects represent the first attempts to describe and investigate the rate of menstrual abnormalities, and strictly-defined PCOS more specifically, in a bipolar population; however, the studies lack healthy control groups with which to compare data in the bipolar population, and additionally there was no control group of women with bipolar disorder who were not being treated. Despite the fact that many women reported the onset of menstrual abnormalities before medication use, data is retrospective, thus it is hard to know what role medication use may have played in the development or course of menstrual abnormalities. There have been no studies to date that investigate the rate of menstrual abnormalities in a depressed population. Endocrine studies, however, have shown profiles of HPA and HPG axis dysregulation similar to those seen in PCOS.

Prevalence of Mood Disorders in PCOS Populations

Women with PCOS or PCOS-like features experience both biochemical and psychosocial conditions that contribute to an elevated risk of depression. While hyperandrogenemia and IR—in addition to other endocrine and metabolic disorders common to PCOS—exhibit the potential to impact mood pathophysiologically, it is impossible to ignore the psychosocial aspects of PCOS that may also engender depressive symptoms. Women with PCOS experience obesity (particularly abdominal obesity), hirsutism, acne, menstrual abnormalities, and infertility at higher rates than the normal population. All these conditions can lead to social stigmatism, stress, low self-esteem, and other factors that negatively influence psychological well-being.

Few studies have addressed these psychosocial dimensions of PCOS, but those that have confirm the hypothesis that PCOS negatively impacts mental health and well-being via these routes. A qualitative paper reporting on the experiences of women with PCOS noted that women's sense of feminine identity is often fractured, and in adolescents with PCOS at least one study has shown that a diagnosis of PCOS has a negative impact on health-related quality of life measures such as physical functioning, general behavior, and family activities (112,113).

A study examining quality of life, psychosocial well-being, and sexual satisfaction measures in 50 women with PCOS compared to 50 age-matched healthy controls found that women with PCOS exhibited greater psychological disturbances, depression, and anxiety. Women with PCOS were found to have lower life satisfaction ratings and decreased scores for physical role function, bodily pain, social function, emotional role function, and mental health. Many of these measures remained significant even after controlling for BMI (114). In addition, informal data collected from women who attended the PCOS Society meetings and visited the National PCOS Association website—both populations with possible selection bias—indicated that 65% to 85% of women self-identified as having PCOS reported depression (115).

The pathophysiology of PCOS is also considered a potential influence on risk for mood disorders. Given the studies showing an association between elevated androgen levels and depression, it is not surprising some studies have shown that women with hyperandrogenic syndromes are at higher risk for mood disorders (110,111,116–118). The biochemical connections between depression and hyperandrogenemia may be rooted in HPA axis dysregulation (in particular the consequent elevated cortisol levels which are often observed in depressed populations) but may also be impacted by HPG dysregulation.

In a pilot study of 32 women diagnosed with PCOS, we found that 16 (50%) exhibited CES-D scores of greater than or equal to 16, indicating depression. An interesting finding of this study was that patients who were not being treated for their PCOS exhibited higher rates of depression than women receiving OCP treatment (66% vs. 29% of women exhibited depression respectively). However, there were no clinical or biochemical differences between these two groups. Furthermore, untreated depressed patients exhibited more PCOS functions, in particular significantly higher

BMI and IR values, than untreated nondepressed patients. Besides the striking observation that depression was more common in women with PCOS compared to the general population [50% compared to recent rates of 10% in the general population], these preliminary results suggest that aspects of the metabolic syndrome, such as IR, may be pathologically linked to depression (119). In addition, further research should investigate the possibility that oral contraceptives are uniquely protective against depression in this particular population (120).

A previously published case study by our group also suggests a pathological link between PCOS and depression via IR. We reported that a woman with diagnosed PCOS and treatment-resistant recurrent major depression was treated for PCOS with metformin, an insulin sensitizer, and spironolactone, a diuretic used to treat hyperandrogenemia. At baseline, the patient exhibited a high HOMA value of 3.9. Consistent with the diagnosis of treatment-resistant major depression, the patient was experiencing prominent depressive symptoms at the commencement of her PCOS treatment despite a treatment regime with a common antidepressant, and thus she agreed to taper off her antidepressant two weeks into her PCOS treatment. Consequently, at follow-up three months later the patient was euthymic, and remained so for one year. She had lost approximately 10 pounds, regained regular menstrual cycles, and her HOMA score, while still higher than what is considered normal, had dropped to 2.8 (121). Although limited to a single case study, such an observation provides further reason to investigate the role of IR as a central component of some mood disorders.

Taken together, these limited preliminary studies certainly implicate endocrine aspects of metabolic syndrome and hyperandrogenemia in the pathogenesis of mood disorders, and strongly suggest that IR and weight gain or obesity may mediate connections between PCOS and depression. Still, much research remains to be done in order to fully understand the mechanisms of these relationships. For example, it is clear that not all women with depression exhibit IR, nor do all women experiencing obesity exhibit IR or depression. Thus, future studies should target how to identify sub-populations whose obesity or IR, particularly in the context of PCOS, puts them at greater risk for mood disorders. It is possible that treatment of IR, in these cases, may successfully prevent or treat certain mood disorder symptoms. In this vein, we are currently launching a pilot study to examine this possibility.

Issues in Treatment of Mood Disorders with Antiepileptic Drugs: Is PCOS a Risk?

The associations between obesity and mood disorders have gained attention in part because of the observation that pharmacological treatment of mood disorders (particularly with antiepileptic and antipsychotic medications) may impact metabolic parameters. One of the critical questions appears to be: to what extent may medication use lead to a development of the metabolic syndrome? As has been explored in this chapter and others, associations between mood disorders and the metabolic syndrome are well documented, but it remains unclear what mechanisms, including those related to medication use, may connect these conditions.

We revisit the topic of medication use in mood disorders because of the recent arguments that some medications not only impact the metabolic system but also contribute to the development of PCOS or PCOS-like features such as menstrual abnormalities or hyperandrogenism. This section reviews the literature on this topic and discusses the ways in which research in this area has contributed to our understanding of the potential metabolic aspects of mood disorder.

The debate about the impact of pharmacological agents on reproductive function and PCOS started not in a mood disorder population but in an epileptic one, emerging out of clinical observations by Isojarvi et al. (122) that women with epilepsy who received the antiepileptic drug (AED) valproate experienced an increased rate of menstrual abnormalities. In this cross-sectional study, androgen levels were slightly elevated in women receiving valproate but were only significantly higher when compared with normal women.

However, studies have shown that rates of PCOS are consistently higher in epileptic populations compared to the general population (123–126). Some authors have argued that epileptic discharges from the amygdala to the hippocampus may affect the secretion of gonadotropin releasing hormone (GnRH), which would promote LH secretion over FSH secretion (126,127). Moreover, LH pulse frequencies were shown to be associated with left-sided (as opposed to right-sided) temporal foci and PCOS may be more common with left temporolimbic epileptiform discharges than with right ones (128,129). Thus, debate ensued about whether, and to what extent, increased risk for PCOS in epileptic populations reflected iatrogenic influences or the underlying etiology of epilepsy.

These and other observations contributed to the argument that higher rates of PCOS did not necessarily reflect sole iatrogenic influence. This debate was revived—in the new context of mood disorder populations—when the antiepileptic drugs valproate and carbamazepine attained widespread use for the treatment of bipolar disorder. A complicating factor in the determination of whether the etiology of bipolar disorder plays a role in the development of PCOS-like features (vs. iatrogenic causes) is the fact that studies examining untreated bipolar patients are few and far between. Thus, rates of menstrual abnormalities and clinical hyperandrogenism in the absence of medication use have not been adequately pinpointed. Few studies have examined these measures longitudinally, and even fewer have recorded these measures before starting pharmacological treatment.

Results of the limited studies that are focused on a population of women with bipolar disorder do not propose definitive answers. As mentioned earlier, one study described an association between endocrine abnormalities reminiscent of PCOS (e.g., elevated LH and decreased FSH concentrations) and bipolar or psychotic symptoms (109). However, it is unclear whether or how these women were being treated for their psychiatric symptoms. A number of our own studies have repeatedly suggested high rates of menstrual abnormalities in a bipolar population, but no studies examine rates of menstrual abnormalities before treatment or in comparison to an untreated bipolar group (106,107,130). However, our results did suggest that many cases of long menstrual cycles preceded the onset of bipolar disorder, which may mean that woman at risk for bipolar disorder also harbor an underlying predisposition to reproductive dysfunction. In addition, a study that compared menstrual disturbances between valproate-only, lithium-only, and valproate+lithium medication groups did not find significant differences in rates of menstrual disturbance, suggesting that valproate may not play such a central role as had been earlier conjectured.

A number of studies suggested that valproate use in women treated for bipolar disorder may be associated with menstrual abnormalities and elevated androgens. A study by O'Donovan et al. (131) found that out of 17 bipolar women receiving valproate, 15 bipolar women on non-valproate medications, and 22 control women with no psychiatric history, rates of menstrual disturbance were significantly higher in the valproate group. There were no significant differences in BMI between the groups. Similarly, a cross-sectional study by McIntyre et al. (132) compared 18 bipolar women receiving valproate and 20 bipolar women receiving lithium with regards to rates of menstrual irregularities and reproductive hormone levels. Menstrual irregularities were reported in 50% of the women receiving valproate, compared to 15% of the women receiving lithium. Free testosterone was significantly higher in the valproate group as well, but LH was elevated in both groups.

Lastly, Akdeniz et al. (133) explored similar parameters in 30 women with bipolar disorder who were receiving valproate monotherapy, lithium monotherapy, or valporate–lithium combination therapy, and compared this data to 15 women with IGE receiving valproate. The authors found that none of the bipolar patients receiving lithium reported experiencing menstrual disturbances, while 20% of bipolar women on valproate therapy did (compared to 47% of the women with IGE receiving valproate). No hormonal measures (including LH, FSH, total or free testosterone, and lipid levels) were different in the bipolar valproate group compared to the bipolar lithium group, except for fasting glucose levels, which were elevated in both bipolar and epileptic subjects receiving valproate.

The results of these studies do not paint a coherent picture of the relationship between AED treatment of bipolar disorder and the development of metabolic or reproductive dysfunction. It appears likely that both iatrogenic and etiological factors play a role in the development of PCOS-like features in a bipolar population. Lastly, medication use in major depressive disorder has not been shown to have a significant negative effect on reproductive or metabolic function. Thus higher rates of menstrual dysfunction in populations of women with depressive disorders may provide additional evidence that the underlying etiology of mood disorders contributes to the endocrine and metabolic features of PCOS.

Theoretical Implications of PCOS and Mood Disorders

Taken together, research on PCOS as an endocrine disorder with metabolic facets reveals insight into the commonalities of pathophysiology among obesity, PCOS, and mood disorders, and suggests that IR may be a common underlying factor. While obesity—particularly visceral obesity—is closely associated with IR, limited findings suggest that the mechanisms of IR in PCOS and mood disorder populations may operate in subtly distinct ways, i.e., be more primary rather than secondary in nature. As populations of women with mood disorders have been shown to exhibit higher rates of obesity and IR, possibly preceding pharmacotherapeutic treatment, the role of these factors in the development of menstrual abnormalities or PCOS features over the course of the mood disorder (particularly in relation to medication use) deserves further investigation.

Specifically, two important and related questions emerge as highly important sites of research and thinking. Clearly, it is important to understand how various medications used to treat mood disorders may affect the metabolic and reproductive systems of women. While literature on this topic is not abundant, a number of studies have provided a promising start; however, there is as always a need for more longitudinal, controlled studies evaluating metabolic and reproductive parameters of women *treated* for mood disorders. In particular, studies that track PCOS features specifically—such as strictly operationalized anovulation and hyperandrogenemia—will be welcome additions to the field.

However, research in this area must also tackle the important question of whether or not the underlying etiology of mood disorders influences the development of metabolic and/or reproductive dysfunction. Particularly, since studies suggest that IR and other forms of metabolic dysregulation may manifest in mood disorder populations separate from or *prior* to medication use, it is crucial to understand whether women with mood disorders are at elevated risk for reproductive dysfunction, and whether such a risk is tied to metabolic pathophysiology.

Such a research question will demand studies that establish reliable rates of reproductive and metabolic dysfunction in female bipolar populations before medication commencement and that compare these rates to control groups. While even cross-sectional studies of this nature are needed at this juncture, longitudinal studies that track metabolic and reproductive parameters from onset of mood disorder through treatment are ideal. Again, evaluating specific parameterizations of PCOS in these populations will be important. Lastly, research that examines the specificities of the relationship between obesity, IR, and other metabolic syndrome attributes such as dyslipidemia in a mood disorder population will be important in characterizing whether IR is predominantly primary or secondary in nature, particularly as IR in PCOS populations may not be limited to affects of obesity.

Practical Considerations Regarding PCOS and Mood Disorders

Given the rising rates of obesity and metabolic syndrome in our population as a whole, monitoring these parameters in a mood disorder population is clearly an important element of treatment and management. It is even more important given the potential metabolic effects (particularly related to weight gain, which appears not an uncommon experience among individuals treated for mood disorder) of medication use. As has been pointed out by a number of other authors, the development and implementation of healthy lifestyle patterns (such as healthy eating and exercising patterns) should be a primary starting point when formulating treatment and management guidelines. Weight loss is often cited as a target of intervention, but the beneficial effects of cardiovascular exercise should not be overlooked.

Preliminary studies also suggest that women with mood disorders and their clinicians may want to loosely "monitor" their reproductive functioning. Such monitoring does not necessarily demand a comprehensive endocrine evaluation, say, but might start with the simple administration of a reproductive/menstrual history questionnaire that ascertains to what extent a female patient has experienced menstrual abnormalities, difficulties conceiving, and/or clinical manifestations of hyperandrogenemia. This process would help to identify women at risk for reproductive dysfunction earlier, rather than later, and enable greater awareness of changes in reproductive functioning that may accompany medication use. While studies on the effects of specific medications on reproductive function remain inconclusive, literature has shown some increases in androgens associated with valproate use. Thus, monitoring of androgens and other reproductive hormones may be of interest to women who experience development of hyperandrogenemic symptoms and/or menstrual disturbances.

Perhaps of greatest importance in the clinical community is to recognize that reproductive dysfunction may be elevated in mood disorder populations; and indeed, the opposite may be true as well. This ensures that clinicians have their eyes open to the first signs of metabolic and reproductive dysfunction so that appropriate action may occur in a timely manner and with the least long-term effects. It may also have the added benefit of encouraging greater collaboration between researchers in the gynecological, endocrinological, metabolic, and psychiatry specialties, which can lead to further advances in the understanding of how IR plays into the pathophysiology of psychiatry and reproductive disorders.

REFERENCES

1. McCowen P, Quastel J. Blood sugar studies in abnormal mental states. J Ment Sci 1931; 77:525–548.
2. Richardson H. Obesity as a manifestation of neurosis. Med Clin North Am 1946; 30:1187–1202.
3. Clinical guidelines for the identification, evaluation, and treatment of overweight and obesity in adults: the evidence report. National Heart, Lung, and Blood Institute: Bethesda, MD, 1998.
4. Pi-Sunyer F. NHLBI obesity education initiative expert panel on the identification, evaluation, and treatment of overweight and obesity in adults—the evidence report. Obes Res 1998; 6(suppl 2):51S–209S.
5. Flegal KM, Carroll MD, Ogden CL, et al. Prevalence and trends in obesity among US adults, 1999–2000. JAMA 2002; 288(14):1723–1727.
6. Flegal KM, Carroll MD, Kuczmarski RJ, et al. Overweight and obesity in the United States: prevalence and trends, 1960–1994. Int J Obes Relat Metab Disord 1998; 22(1):39–47.
7. Campfield LA, Smith FJ. The pathogenesis of obesity. Best Practice Res Clin Endocrinol Metab 1999; 13(1):13–30.
8. Reaven GM. Banting lecture 1988. Role of insulin resistance in human disease. Diabetes 1988; 37(12):1595–1607.
9. Reaven GM. Syndrome X. Blood Press Suppl 1992; 4:13–16.
10. Reaven GM. Role of insulin resistance in human disease (syndrome X): an expanded definition. Annu Rev Med 1993; 44:121–131.
11. Elmslie JL, Mann JI, Silverstone JT, et al. Determinants of overweight and obesity in patients with bipolar disorder. J Clin Psychiatry 2001; 62(6):486–491.
12. Elmslie JL, Silverstone JT, Mann JI, et al. Prevalence of overweight and obesity in bipolar patients. J Clin Psychiatry 2000; 61(3):179–184.
13. Fagiolini A, Frank E, Houck PR, et al. Prevalence of obesity and weight change during treatment in patients with bipolar I disorder. J Clin Psychiatry 2002; 63(6):528–533.
14. Fagiolini A, Kupfer DJ, Houck PR, et al. Obesity as a correlate of outcome in patients with bipolar I disorder. Am J Psychiatry 2003; 160(1):112–117.
15. Hasler G, Merikangas K, Eich D, et al. Psychopathology as a risk factor for being overweight. Conference on New Research Abstracts of the 156th Annual Meeting of the American Psychiatric Association. San Francisco, California, May 17–22, 2003. NR106:39–40.
16. Kendler KS, Eaves LJ, Ealters EE, et al. The identification and validation of distinct depressive syndromes in a population-based sample of female twins. Arch Gen Psychiatry 1996; 53(5):391–399.

17. McElroy SL, Frye MA, Suppes T, et al. Correlates of overweight and obesity in 644 patients with bipolar disorder. J Clin Psychiatry 2002; 63(3):207–213.
18. Mueller-Oberlinghausen B, Passoth PM, Poser W, et al. Imparied glucose tolerance in long-term lithium-treated patients. Int Pharmacopsychiatry 1979; 14(6): 350–362.
19. Pine DS, Cohen P, Brook J, et al. Psychiatric symptoms in adolescence as predictors of obesity in early adulthood: a longitudinal study. Am J Public Health 1997; 87(8):1303–1310.
20. Pine DS, Goldstein RB, Wolk S, et al. The association between childhood depression and adulthood body mass index. Pediatrics 2001; 107(5):1049–1056.
21. Shioiri T, Kato T, Murashita J, et al. Changes in the frequency distribution pattern of body weight in patients with major depression. Acta Psychiatr Scand 1993; 88(5):356–360.
22. Ford ES, Giles WH, Dietz WH. Prevalence of the metabolic syndrome among US adults: findings from the third National Health and Nutrition Examination Survey. JAMA 2002; 287(3):356–359.
23. Kahn BB, Flier JS. Obesity and insulin resistance. J Clin Invest 2000; 106(4):473–481.
24. Hunter SJ, Garvey WT. Insulin action and insulin resistance: diseases involving defects in insulin receptors, signal transduction, and the glucose transport effector system. Am J Med 1998; 105(4):331–345.
25. Wajchenberg BL. Subcutaneous and visceral adipose tissue: their relation to the metabolic syndrome. Endocr Rev 2000; 21(6):697–738.
26. Shepherd PR, Gnudi L, Tozzo E, et al. Adipose cell hyperplasia and enhanced glucose disposal in transgenic mice overexpressing GLUT4 selectively in adipose tissue. J Biol Chem 1993; 268(30):22,243–22,246.
27. Tozzo E, Gnudi L, Kahn BB. Amelioration of insulin resistance in streptozotocin diabetic mice by transgenic overexpression of GLUT4 driven by an adipose-specific promoter. Endocrinology 1997; 138(4):1604–1611.
28. Colditz GA, Willett WC, Stampfer MJ, et al. Weight as a risk factor for clinical diabetes in women. Am J Epidemiol 1990; 132(3):501–513.
29. Peraldi P, Spiegelman B. TNF-alpha and insulin resistance: summary and future prospects. Mol Cell Biochem 1998; 182(1–2):169–175.
30. Hotamisligil GS. The role of TNF-alpha and TNF receptors in obesity and insulin resistance. J Intern Med 1999; 245(6):621–625.
31. Friedman JM. Obesity in the new millennium. Nature 2000; 404(6778):632–634.
32. Halaas JL, Gajiwala KS, Maffei M, et al. Weight-reducing effects of the plasma protein encoded by the obese gene. Science 1995; 269(5223):543–546.
33. Campfield LA, Smith FJ, Guisez Y, et al. Recombinant mouse OB protein: evidence for a peripheral signal linking adiposity and central neural networks. Science 1995; 269(5223):546–549.
34. Pelleymounter MA, Cullen MJ, Baker MB, et al. Effects of the obese gene product on body weight regulation in ob/ob mice. Science 1995; 269(5223): 540–543.
35. Muoio DM, Dohm GL, Fiedorek FT Jr, et al. Leptin directly alters lipid partitioning in skeletal muscle Diabetes 1997; 46(8):1360–1363.

36. Shimabukuro M, Koyama K, Lee Y, et al. Leptin- or troglitazone-induced lipopenia protects islets from interleukin Ibeta cytotoxicity. J Clin Invest 1997; 100(7):1750–1754.
37. Reaven GM. Role of insulin resistance in the pathophysiology of non-insulin dependent diabetes mellitus. Diab Metab Rev 1993; 9(suppl 1): 5S–12S.
38. Akiskal HS. Mood disorders introduction and overview. In: Sadock BK, Sadock VA, eds. Kaplan and Sadock's Comprehensive Textbook of Psychiatry. 7th ed. Baltimore: Williams & Wilkins, 2000.
39. Blazer DG, Kessler RC, McGonagle KA, et al. The prevalence and distribution of major depression in a national community sample: the National Comorbidity Survey. Am J Psychiatry 1994; 151(7):979–986.
40. Eaton WW, Kramer M, Anthony JC, et al. The incidence of specific DIS/DSM-III mental disorders: data from the NIMH Epidemiologic Catchment Area Program. Acta Psychiatr Scand 1989; 79(2):163–178.
41. Burt VK, Rasgon N. Special considerations in treating bipolar disorder in women. Bipolar Disord 2004; 6(1):2–13.
42. Parry BL. Reproductive factors affecting the course of affective illness in women. Psychiatr Clin North Am 1989; 12(1):207–220.
43. Robb JC, Young LT, Cooke RG, et al. Gender differences in patients with bipolar disorder influence outcome in the medical outcomes survey (SF-20) subscale scores. J Affect Disord 1998; 49(3):189–193.
44. Kilzieh N, Akiskal HS. Rapid-cycling bipolar disorder. An overview of research and clinical experience. Psychiatr Clin North Am 1999; 22(3):585–607.
45. Thase ME. Mood disorders: neurobiology. In: Sadock BK, Sadock VA, eds. Kaplan and Sadock's Comprehensive Textbook of Psychiatry. 7th ed. Baltimore: Williams & Wilkins, 2000.
46. Drevets WC. Functional anatomical abnormalities in limbic and prefrontal cortical structures in major depression. Prog Brain Res 2000; 126:413–431.
47. Kieseppa T, Partonen T, Haukka J, et al. High concordance of bipolar I disorder in a nationwide sample of twins. Am J Psychiatry 2004; 161(10):1814–1821.
48. Kendler KS, Pedersen N, Johnson L, et al. A pilot Swedish twin study of affective illness, including hospital-and population-ascertained subsamples. Arch Gen Psychiatry 1993; 50(9):699–700.
49. Dunaif A, Thomas A. Current concepts in the polycystic ovary syndrome. Annu Rev Med 2001; 52:401–419.
50. Dunaif A. Insulin resistance and the polycystic ovary syndrome: mechanism and implications for pathogenesis. Endocr Rev 1997; 18(6):774–800.
51. Revised 2003 consensus on diagnostic criteria and long-term health risks related to polycystic ovary syndrome (PCOS). Hum Reprod 2004; 19(1):41–47.
52. Franks S. Polycystic ovary syndrome. N Engl J Med 1995; 333(13):853–861.
53. Stein I, Leventhal I. Amenorrhea associated with bilateral polycystic ovaries. Am J Obstet Gynecol 1935; 29:181–191.
54. Swanson M, Sauerbrei EE, Cooperberg PL. Medical implications of ultrasonically detected polycystic ovaries. J Clin Ultrasound 1981; 9(5):219–222.
55. Rosenfield RL. Current concepts of polycystic ovary syndrome. Baillieres Clin Obstet Gynaecol 1997; 11(2):307–333.

56. Ferriman D, Gallwey JD. Clinical assessment of body hair growth in women. J Clin Endocrinol Metab 1961; 21:1440–1447.
57. Rodin DA, Bano G, Bland JM, et al. Polycystic ovaries and associated metabolic abnormalities in Indian subcontinent Asian women. Clin Endocrinol (Oxf) 1998; 49(1):91–99.
58. Lobo RA, Carmina E. The importance of diagnosing the polycystic ovary syndrome. Ann Intern Med 2000; 132(12):989–993.
59. Knochenhauer ES, Key TJ, Kahsar-Miller M, et al. Prevalence of the polycystic ovary syndrome in unselected black and white women of the southeastern United States: a prospective study. J Clin Endocrinol Metab 1998; 83(9): 3078–3082.
60. Herzog AG, Schachter SC. Valproate and the polycystic ovarian syndrome: final thoughts. Epilepsia 2001; 42(3):311–315.
61. Barbieri RL, Smith S, Ryan KJ. The role of hyperinsulinemia in the pathogenesis of ovarian hyperandrogenism. Fertil Steril 1988; 50(2):197–212.
62. Velazquez EM, Mendoza S, Hamer T, et al. Metformin therapy in polycystic ovary syndrome reduces hyperinsulinemia, insulin resistance, hyperandrogenemia, and systolic blood pressure, while facilitating normal menses and pregnancy. Metabolism 1994; 43(5):647–654.
63. Dunaif A, Finegood DT. Beta-cell dysfunction independent of obesity and glucose intolerance in the polycystic ovary syndrome. J Clin Endocrinol Metab 1996; 81(3):942–947.
64. Waldstreicher J, Santoro NF, Hall JE, et al. Hyperfunction of the hypothalamic-pituitary axis in women with polycystic ovarian disease: indirect evidence for partial gonadotroph desensitization. J Clin Endocrinol Metab 1988; 66(1):165–172.
65. van Santbrink EJ, Hop WC, Fauser BC. Classification of normogonadotropic infertility: polycystic ovaries diagnosed by ultrasound versus endocrine characteristics of polycystic ovary syndrome. Fertil Steril 1997; 67(3):452–458.
66. Laven JS, Imani B, Eijkemans MJ, et al. New approach to polycystic ovary syndrome and other forms of anovulatory infertility. Obstet Gynecol Surv 2002; 57(11):755–767.
67. Fauser BC, Pache TD, Lamberts SW, et al. Serum bioactive and immunoreactive luteinizing hormone and follicle-stimulating hormone levels in women with cycle abnormalities, with or without polycystic ovarian disease. J Clin Endocrinol Metab 1991; 73(4):811–817.
68. Taylor AE, McCourt B, Maltin KA, et al. Determinants of abnormal gonadotropin secretion in clinically defined women with polycystic ovary syndrome. J Clin Endocrinol Metab 1997; 82(7):2248–2256.
69. Yen SS, Vela P, Rankin J. Inappropriate secretion of follicle-stimulating hormone and luteinizing hormone inpolycystic ovarian disease. J Clin Endocrinol Metab 1970; 30(4):435–442.
70. Conway GS, Honour JW, Jacobs HS. Heterogeneity of the polycystic ovary syndrome: clinical, endocrine and ultrasound features in 556 patients. Clin Endocrinol (Oxf) 1989; 30(4):459–470.
71. Barth JH. Alopecia and hirsuties. Current concepts in pathogenesis and management. Drugs 1988; 35(1):83–91.

72. Lobo RA. Hirsutism inpolycystic ovary syndrome: current concepts. Clin Obstet Gynecol 1991; 34(4):817–826.
73. Yen SS. The polycystic ovary syndrome. Clin Endocrinol (Oxf) 1980; 12(2):177–207.
74. Polson DW, Adams J, Wadsworth J, et al. Polycystic ovaries—a common finding in normal women. Lancet 1988; 1(8590):870–872.
75. Polson DW, Franks S, Reed MJ, et al. The distribution of oestradiol in plasma in relation to uterine cross-sectional area in women with polycystic or multifollicular ovaries. Clin Endocrinol (Oxf) 1987; 26(5):581–588.
76. Franks S. Polycystic ovary syndrome: a changing perspective. Clin Endocrinol-(Oxf) 1989; 31(1):87–120.
77. Futterweit W. Pituitary tumors and polycystic ovarian disease. Obstet Gynecol 1983; 62(3 suppl):74s–79s.
78. Luciano AA, Chapler FK, Sherman BM. Hyperprolactinemia in polycystic ovary syndrome. Fertil Steril 1984; 41(5):719–725.
79. Murdoch AP, Dunlop W, Kendall-Taylor P. Studies of prolactin secretion in polycystic ovary syndrome. Clin Endocrinol (Oxf) 1986; 24(2):165–175.
80. Bahceci M, Tuzcu A, Bahceci S, et al. Is hyperprolactinemia associated with insulin resistance in non-obese patients with polycystic ovary syndrome? J Endocrinol Invest 2003; 26(7):655–659.
81. Tuzcu A, Bahceci M, Dursun M, et al. Insulin sensitivity and hyperprolactinemia. J Endocrinol Invest 2003; 26(4):341–346.
82. Ehrmann DA, Barnes RB, Rosenfield RL, et al. Prevalence of impaired glucose tolerance and diabetes in women with polycystic ovary syndrome. Diabetes Care 1999; 22(1):141–146.
83. Legro RS, Kunselman AR, Dodson WC, et al. Prevalence and predictors of risk for type 2 diabetes mellitus and impaired glucose tolerance in polycystic ovary syndrome: a prospective, controlled study in 254 affected women. J Clin Endocrinol Metab 1999; 84(1):165–169.
84. Dunaif A, Graf M, Mandeli J, et al. Characterization of groups of hyperandrogenic women with acanthosis nigricans, impaired glucose tolerance, and/or hyperinsulinemia. J Clin Endocrinol Metab 1987; 65(3):499–507.
85. Barbieri RL, Makris A, Ryan KJ. Insulin stimulates androgen accumulation in incubations of human ovarian stroma and theca. Obstet Gynecol 1984; 64(suppl 3):73S–80S.
86. Bergh C, Carlsson B, Olsson JH, et al. Regulation of androgen production in cultured human thecal cells by insulin-like growth factor I and insulin. Fertil Steril 1993; 59(2):323–331.
87. Peiris AN, Sothmann MS, Aiman EJ, et al. The relationship of insulin to sex hormone-binding globulin: role of adiposity. Fertil Steril 1989; 52(1):69–72.
88. Legro RS, Kunselman AR, Dunaif A. Prevalence and predictors of dyslipidemia in women with polycystic ovary syndrome. Am J Med 2001; 111(8):607–613.
89. Wild RA. Polycystic ovary syndrome: a risk for coronary artery disease? Am J Obstet Gynecol 2002; 186(1):35–43.
90. Paradisi G, Steinberg HO, Hempfling A, et al. Polycystic ovary syndrome is associated with endothelial dysfunction. Circulation 2001; 103(10):1410–1415.

91. Talbott, EO, Guzick DS, Sutton-Tyrrell K, et al. Evidence for association between polycystic ovary syndromeand premature carotid atherosclerosis in middle-aged women. Arterioscler Thromb Vase Biol 2000; 20(11):2414–2421.
92. Dahlgren E, Janson PO, Johansson S, et al. Polycystic ovary syndrome and risk for myocardial infarction. Evaluated from a risk factor model based on a prospective population study of women. Acta Obstet Gynecol Scand 1992; 71(8):599–604.
93. Talbott E, Clerici A, Berga SL, et al. Adverse lipid and coronary heart disease risk profiles in young women with polycystic ovary syndrome: results of a case-control study. J Clin Epidemiol 1998; 51(5):415–422.
94. Norman RJ, Masters L, Milner CR, et al. Relative risk of conversion from normoglycaemia to impaired glucose tolerance or non-insulin dependent diabetes mellitus in polycystic ovarian syndrome. Hum Reprod 2001; 16(9):1995–1998.
95. Solomon CG, Hu FB, Dunaif A, et al. Long or highly irregular menstrual cycles as a marker for risk of type 2 diabetes mellitus. JAMA 2001; 286(19): 2421–2426.
96. Robinson S, Chan SP, Spacey S, et al. Postprandial thermogenesis is reduced in polycystic ovary syndrome and is associated with increased insulin resistance. Clin Endocrinol (Oxf) 1992; 36(6):537–543.
97. Azziz R. Reproductive endocrinologic alterations in female asymptomatic obesity. Fertil Steril 1989; 52(5):703–725.
98. Burkman RT Jr. The role of oral contraceptives in the treatment of hyperandrogenic disorders. Am J Med 1995; 98(1A):130S–136S.
99. Robinson S, Kiddy D, Gelding SV, et al. The relationship of insulin insensitivity to menstrual pattern in women with hyperandrogenism and polycystic ovaries. Clin Endocrinol (Oxf) 1993; 39(3):351–355.
100. Morin-Papunen LC, Vauhkonen I, Koivunen RM, et al. Insulin sensitivity, insulin secretion, and metabolic and hormonal parameters in healthy women and women with polycystic ovarian syndrome. Hum Reprod 2000; 15(6):1266–1274.
101. Moghetti P, Castello R, Negri C, et al. Metformin effects on clinical features, endocrine and metabolic profiles, and insulin sensitivity in polycystic ovary syndrome: a randomized, double-blind, placebo-controlled 6-month trial, followed by open, long-term clinical evaluation. J Clin Endocrinol Metab 2000; 85(1):139–146.
102. Pasquali R, Gambineri A, Biscotti D, et al. Effect of long-term treatment with metformin added to hypocaloric diet on body composition, fat distribution, and androgen and insulin levels in abdominally obese women with and without the polycystic ovary syndrome. J Clin Endocrinol Metab 2000; 85(8): 2767–2774.
103. Ibanez L, Valls C, Potau N, et al. Sensitization to insulin in adolescent girls to normalize hirsutism, hyperandrogenism, oligomenorrhea, dyslipidemia, and hyperinsulinism after precocious pubarche. J Clin Endocrinol Metab 2000; 85(10):3526–3530.
104. Bruni V, Dei M, Pontello V, et al. The management of polycystic ovary syndrome. Ann N Y Acad Sci 2003; 997:307–321.

105. Kelly CJ, Gordon D. The effect of metformin on hirsutism in polycystic ovary syndrome. Eur J Endocrinol 2002; 147(2):217–221.
106. Rasgon NL, Altshuler LL, Fairbanks L, et al. Medication status and polycystic ovary syndrome in women with bipolar disorder: a preliminary report. J Clin Psychiatry 2000; 61(3):173–178.
107. Rasgon N, Bauer M, Glenn T, et al. Menstrual cycle related mood changes in women with bipolar disorder. Bipolar Disord 2003; 5(1):48–52.
108. Bisaga K, Petkova E, Cheng J, et al. Menstrual functioning and psychopathology in a county-wide population of high school girls. J Am Acad Child Adolesc Psychiatry 2002; 41(10):1197–1204.
109. Matsunaga H, Sarai M. Elevated serum LHand androgens in affective disorder related to the menstrual cycle: with reference topolycystic ovary syndrome. Jpn J Psychiatry Neurol 1993; 47(4):825–842.
110. Baischer W, Koining G, Hartmann B, et al. Hypothalamic-pituitary-gonadal axis in depressed premenopausal women: elevated blood testosterone concentrations compared to normal controls. Psychoneuroendocrinology 1995; 20(5):553–559.
111. Weber B, Lewicka S, Deuschle M, et al. Testosterone, androstenedione and dihydrotestosterone concentrations are elevated in female patients with major depression. Psychoneuroendocrinology 2000; 25(8):765–771.
112. Kitzinger C, Willmott J. The thief of womanhood': women's experience of polycystic ovarian syndrome. Soc Sci Med 2002; 54(3):349–361.
113. Trent ME, Rich M, Austin SB, et al. Quality of life in adolescent girls with polycystic ovary syndrome. Arch Pediatr Adolesc Med 2002; 156(6):556–560.
114. Elsenbruch S, Hahn S, Kowalsky D, et al. Quality of life, psychosocial well-being, and sexual satisfaction in women with polycystic ovary syndrome. J Clin Endocrinol Metab 2003; 88(12):5801–5807.
115. Rao RC, Rasgon N, Hwang JL, et al. Prevalence of depression in women with polycystic ovary syndrome in American Psychiatric Association. May, 2001. New Orleans, Louisiana.
116. Shulman LH, DeRogatis L, Spielvogel R, et al. Serum androgens and depression in women with facial hirsutism. J Am Acad Dermatol 1992; 27(2 Pt 1): 178–181.
117. Fava GA, Grandi S, Savron G, et al. Psychosomatic assessment of hirsute women. Psychother Psychosom 1989; 51(2):96–100.
118. Bruce-Jones W, Zolese G, White P. Polycystic ovary syndrome and psychiatric morbidity. J Psychosom Obstet Gynaecol 1993; 14(2):111–116.
119. Judd LL, Akiskal HS, Pauhis MP. The role and clinical significance of subsyndromal depressive symptoms (SSD) in unipolar major depressive disorder. J Affect Disord 1997; 45(1–2):5–17; discussion 17–18.
120. Rasgon NL, Rao RC, Hwang S, et al. Depression in women with polycystic ovary syndrome: clinical and biochemical correlates. J Affect Disord 2003; 74(3):299–304.
121. Rasgon NL, Carter MS, Elman S, et al. Common treatment of polycystic ovarian syndrome and major depressive disorder: case report and review. Curr Drug Targets Immune Endocr Metabol Disord 2002; 2(1):97–102.

122. Isojarvi JI, Laatikainen TJ, Pakarinen AJ, et al. Polycystic ovaries and hyperandrogenism in women taking valproate for epilepsy. N Engl J Med 1993; 329(19):1383–1388.
123. Bauer J, Jarre A, Klingmuller D, et al. Polycystic ovary syndrome in patients with focal epilepsy: a study in 93 women. Epilepsy Res 2000; 41(2):163–167.
124. Bilo L, Meo R, Valentino R, et al. Characterization of reproductive endocrine disorders in women with epilepsy. J Clin Endocrinol Metab 2001; 86(7): 2950–2956.
125. Bilo L, Meo R, Nappi C, et al. Reproductive endocrine disorders in women with primary generalized epilepsy. Epilepsia 1988; 29(5):612–619.
126. Herzog AG, Seibel MM, Schomer DL, et al. Reproductive endocrine disorders in women with partial seizures of temporal lobe origin. Arch Neurol 1986; 43(4):341–346.
127. Knobil E. The neuroendocrine control of the menstrual cycle. Recent Prog Horm Res 1980; 36:53–88.
128. Drislane FW, Coleman AE, Schomer DL, et al. Altered pulsatile secretion of luteinizing hormone in women with epilepsy. Neurology 1994; 44(2):306–310.
129. Herzog AG. A relationship between particular reproductive endocrine disorders and the laterality of epileptiform discharges in women with epilepsy. Neurology 1993; 43:1907–1910.
130. Rasgon NL, Altshuler LL, Fairbanks L, et al. Reproductive function and risk for PCOS in women treated for bipolar disorder. Bipolar Disord 2005; 7(3):246–259.
131. O'Donovan C, Kusumakar V, Graves GR, et al. Menstrual abnormalities and polycystic ovary syndrome in women taking valproate for bipolar mood disorder. J Clin Psychiatry 2002; 63(4):322–330.
132. McIntyre RS, Mancini DA, McCann S, et al. Valproate, bipolar disorder and polyeystic ovarian syndrome. Bipolar Disord 2003; 5(1):28–35.
133. Akdeniz F, Taneli F, Noyan A, et al. Valproate-associated reproductive and metabolic abnormalities: are epileptic women at greater risk than bipolar women? Prog Neuropsychopharmacol Biol Psychiatry 2003; 27(1):115–121.

10

Dietary Therapy of Obesity

Robert F. Kushner and Bethany Doerfler
*Department of Medicine, Northwestern University Feinberg School of Medicine
and Wellness Institute, Northwestern Memorial Hospital,
Chicago, Illinois, U.S.A.*

INTRODUCTION

It is generally accepted that the cause of obesity is multifactorial, brought
about by an interaction between predisposing genetic and metabolic factors
and a rapidly changing environment. Among the cultural and societal factors, unhealthy diets and sedentary behaviors have been identified as the
primary causes. This makes sense since by simple definition, obesity is a disorder of energy imbalance, where energy in exceeds energy out. The resulting weight gain is a function of time (months or years) × surplus energy
(kcal). Energy balance is critical as daily calorie mismatch of only +1%
would theoretically lead to a gain of approximately two pounds of fat per
year (1). Data from the National Health and Nutrition Examination Surveys (NHANES) shows that during 1971 to 2000, a significant increase in
average energy intake occurred—for men, average intake increased from
2450 to 2618 kcal, and for women, from 1542 to 1877 kcal (2). In contrast,
trends in physical activity have remained stable with only about one-quarter
of Americans engaging in recommended levels of activity between 1990 and
1998 (3). Due to this increasing "calorie gap" between intake and expenditure, the prevalence of obesity in the United States over the past 30 years has
doubled, increasing from 14.5% to 30.9%. These two principal factors,
overconsumption of calories and lack of engagement in physical activity,
overwhelm an individual's innate physiological adjustment to maintain

normal energy balance. Attention to these two behavioral factors forms the cornerstone for obesity treatment.

Dietary therapy, exercise counseling, and behavioral change are the principal interventions of lifestyle modification. The primary intent of lifestyle modification is to empower individuals with the knowledge, skills, strategies, resources, and support to choose dietary, physical activity, and coping patterns that are consistent with maintenance of health, prevention of disease, and improved disease management. These are essential features of obesity care as patient choice and ability to implement change will ultimately determine outcome. Provision of support for lifestyle modification is indicated for all patients who are overweight, obese, or those at risk for gaining weight. This is particularly pertinent for patients who have been prescribed weight gaining psychotropic medication regardless of their body mass index (BMI). This chapter deals with the interventions of lifestyle modification—dietary therapy for the management of obesity (4).

DIETARY ASSESSMENT

Assessing Motivation and Readiness

Dietary therapy begins by conducting a thorough dietary assessment of the patient starting with evaluation of readiness and motivation to make dietary changes. Although it is reasonable to ask patients if they are interested and ready to change their diets further inquiry about readiness should be explored by assessing the patient and his/her environment. The National Institutes of Health (NIH) practical guide to identification, evaluation, and treatment of overweight and obesity in adults recommends that providers assess patient motivation and support, stressful life events, psychiatric status, time availability and constraints, appropriateness of goals, and expectations to help establish the likelihood of lifestyle change (5). One helpful method to begin a readiness assessment is to "anchor" the patient's interest and confidence to change on a numerical scale. To measure this, simply ask the patient, "On a scale from 0 to 10, with 0 being not important and 10 being very important, how important is it for you to change your diet at this time?" and "Also on a scale from 0 to 10, with 0 being not confident and 10 being very confident, how confident are you that you can change your diet at this time?" (6). Answers to these two questions can be used to initiate further dialogue, such as, "I see you have ranked the importance of changing your diet at eight and your confidence at four. What should happen to raise your confidence of changing your diet to eight or nine?" This technique allows patients to articulate specific needs or concerns that can be addressed during counseling, such as nutrition knowledge, cooking skills, financial concerns, and fear of excessive hunger or deprivation, among others. Once motivation and readiness are assessed, the next step is to evaluate the patient's weight and dietary history.

Taking a Weight History

A weight history is best appreciated and understood by asking the patient to graph his or her weight as it relates to life events. We have found that this simple exercise can be one of the most revealing, reflective, and insightful activities performed during the evaluation process. Patients who feel that they have tried everything are often able to identify how and why previous attempts were unsuccessful. Typically, common weight change patterns emerge such as progressive weight gain, weight cycling, or long periods of weight stability followed by short bursts of weight gain. Engaging the patient to verbally review his or her weight chart should be part of the encounter. For example, if weight gain begins after childbirth, a discussion may reveal the inclusion of more fast food stops, or cleaning up and eating unfinished treats, or feeling too tired for exercise. Alternatively, an asthmatic who was placed on steroids for several months may report a rapid increase in appetite and cravings for sweetened foods. Asking the patient what triggered an intentional weight loss as well as what caused recidivism after a successful treatment is also useful. Figure 1 shows two examples of weight graphs from our patients. The provider should listen to themes that will help dictate the content and style of the nutrition intervention.

Dietary History and Food Logs

After discussing the weight history, the focus turns to the present by obtaining a diet recall. This may be achieved by asking the patient the following: "Can you take me through a typical day in terms of eating, starting with the first thing you had to eat or drink all the way through your day to the last thing you had to eat or drink?" By asking about a typical day instead of what was for breakfast, lunch, and dinner, patients are more likely to feel comfortable identifying routine patterns such as grabbing fast food for breakfast or skipping meals entirely. Be sure to ask about spreads, dressings, butter, oils, and margarines that can add extra calories. Also inquire about portion sizes and the timing and location of eating and snacking. During this entire process, it is extremely important that patients do not feel judged or graded for their dietary choices. Food is a very personal and intimate experience for many people and it is often hard for them to honestly and openly reveal this information. This perspective must be kept in mind throughout the evaluation and counseling session.

Although a diet recall provides a glimpse into a typical day, many patients consume majority of extra calories on weekends or during out of town trips. Keeping a food log or food journal for several days or weeks may uncover these sources of excessive calories. Emphasize the addition of key details such as time (*when*), place where meals and snacks are eaten (*where*), and estimated portion sizes (*how much*). The sample food log

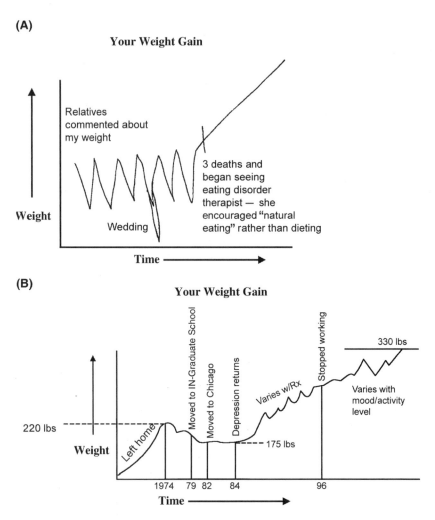

Figure 1 Weight graphs from two patients. (**A**) A 28-year-old woman with history of rapid weight cycling associated with mood disorder. (**B**) A 45-year-old man with history of depression and medication-induced weight gain. *Abbreviation*: IN: Indiana.

provided in Figure 2 depicts a typical patient struggling to make healthy choices. While the reported diet on the whole appears healthy, closer examination of this log identifies several barriers to success. First, the work place harbors various diet traps, such as catered meetings with unhealthy foods, and patient needs strategies to overcome the ease of making poor choices. Second, waiting for more than three to four hours to eat enhances cravings and sets the stage for eating larger portions and making poor choices. Finally, quick meals on the run are often accompanied by extra calories such

Date: *FRIDAY, October 29*

Time/Place	AMOUNT/FOOD SELECTION	TRIGGERS (Reason for eating)	THOUGHTS/FEELINGS (Before, during, after eating)
7:30 Car	Granola Bar - 2 Low fat Yogurt drink - 1, 12oz bottle Coffee w/ 3 creamers	time	Rushed getting to work
8:30 WORK	Glazed donut - 1	It was there	Angry at myself
3:00 Sub Shop	Turkey Sub - Sandwich Foot long Chips - 1.5 oz bag Diet Pop - 22 oz	hungry	Trying to be good
7:30 Kitchen with family	Pasta with tomato sauce - 3 cups Mixed green Salad w/ Low-fat dressing - 2 cups Diet Pop - 1 can	family eating	
10:00 Living Room TV	Low-fat microwave popcorn 1 whole bag	wanted something	too full

Figure 2 Food log depicting sample diet entries along with triggers and thoughts/feelings. Food logs are used as a tool to track dietary intake, increase awareness, understand eating behaviors, improve planning, and enhance restraint.

as chips; preplanning meals can reduce impulsive choices. Some clinicians will ask patients who identify themselves as *emotional eaters* to record triggers or antecedents to eating certain foods as well as thoughts and feelings after eating. Adding triggers to a food log may be helpful as counseling progresses. For many patients, beginning with the physical environment, food choices, and portion size is most useful.

Although both the dietary recall and food log methods for dietary assessment are biased by under-reporting (i.e., they should not be used to count calories), they are extremely useful for identifying diet and lifestyle patterns. The diet recall is an essential aspect of the initial assessment to shape the direction of the intervention. Food logs are useful for helping patients identify patterns that need to be changed, to provide accountability on newly established dietary goals, and to encourage meal planning and restraint. While almost all patients benefit from recording food logs, many of them express a love–hate relationship with the process. Patients often enjoy identifying key eating patterns, but dislike the constant accountability of recording every bite of food. Furthermore, patients may feel embarrassed if family or coworkers see them journaling or are able to read the contents. If this is the case, using a day planner, electronic personal digital assistant (PDA), or personal journal may help provide more anonymity. Also, reserving the use of a food log for problem times such as evenings or weekends may help reduce the perceived burden.

Food logs do not need to be kept forever. Outside of initially identifying patterns and providing accountability, they can be used to work through a plateau or other difficult times. Overall, explaining food logs as a tool to develop greater awareness of eating patterns may help convince skeptics.

THE DIETARY PRESCRIPTION

General Recommendations

As noted in the introduction, weight loss occurs when calories consumed are less than calories expended, producing a calorie deficit. Typically, a calorie restriction of 500 to 1000 kcal/day from the habitual diet is recommended to produce a weight loss of approximately 1 to 2 pounds/week. This often translates into a diet of 1000 to 1200 kcal/day for most women; and a diet between 1200 and 1600 kcal/day for men and heavier women (5). Although several energy expenditure equations are available to more accurately calculate caloric requirements (discussed further), there is little need to employ them in the early counseling process. Recommendations regarding the composition of calories has been addressed by the Institute of Medicine (IOM) report on macronutrients (7). These guidelines recommend an adult diet that has 45% to 65% of calories from carbohydrates, 20% to 35% from fat, and 10% to 35% from protein. The guidelines also recommend daily fiber intake of 38 g (men) and 25 g (women) for persons over 50, and 30 g (men) and 21 g (women) for those under 50. The IOM report highlights a very important point when it comes to macronutrients—rather than endorsing a fixed ratio of calories from carbohydrates, fat, and protein, we need to think in terms of safe and acceptable macronutrient ranges. Within these ranges, however, there is a large body of literature suggesting that reduction of fat is an effective approach for control of obesity (8,9).

In 2005, the USDA revised their Dietary Guidelines for Americans based on current evidence-based science (10). The guidelines, which focus on health promotion and risk reduction, can be applied to treatment of the overweight and obese patient as well as keeping in mind the need for total caloric reduction. The dietary recommendations include maintaining a diet rich in whole grains, fruits, vegetables, and dietary fiber; consuming two servings (8 oz) of fish high in omega three fatty acids per week; decreasing sodium to less than 2300 mg per day; consuming three cups of milk (or equivalent low-fat or fat-free dairy products) per day; limiting cholesterol to less than 300 mg per day, keeping total fat between 20% and 35% of daily calories, and keeping saturated fats to less than 10% of daily calories.

Disease-Specific Conditions

The primary goal of obesity treatment is to improve obesity-related comorbid conditions and to reduce the risk of developing future conditions. The decision as to what extent the patients can be treated aggressively and which dietary method is to be used is determined by the patient's risk status, their expectations, and the resources that are available. Intervention studies have repeatedly shown that a weight loss of 5% to 10% is clinically significant and leads to improvements in glycemic, lipemic, and hypertensive control. Beyond caloric restriction, the composition of the prescribed diet will vary slightly depending on the underlying comorbid condition. For example, the National Cholesterol Education Program (NCEP), Adult Treatment Panel (ATP III) and therapeutic lifestyle changes (TLC) diet that emphasizes restriction in total fat, saturated fat, and cholesterol would be prescribed for a patient with hyperlipidemia (11). The Dietary Approaches to Stop Hypertension (DASH) diet emphasizes that increased intake of fruits, low fat dairy products, nuts, seeds, and dry beans would be selected for patients with hypertension (12–14). Instruction on these dietary approaches should be accomplished by referral to a registered dietitian (discussed further).

STRATEGIES FOR DIETARY COUNSELING

Dietary Patterns Approach

While patients respond well to target calories needed for weight loss, calorie counting is purely quantitative and patients often benefit from qualitative information on the eating and lifestyle patterns that make it hard for them to control their weight. Although pattern identification is commonly used in other areas of medical therapeutics, for example, glucose levels in diabetics or wheezing in asthmatics, it has not been previously applied to the management of obesity. Using a qualitative lifestyle personality patterns approach, the initial emphasis of treatment is to identify and then provide targeted strategies to improve weight-gaining lifestyle patterns. To apply this method, information from the previously taken dietary history is used to define the patient's eating habits, attitudes, and behaviors into identifiable patterns.

For example, if a patient is presented with skipping meals earlier in the day and consumes the majority of calories at night in front of the television (nighttime nibbler), the initial intervention would focus on consuming regular meals, meal timing, and reducing distractions. Alternatively, if a patient frequents fast food restaurants because of a demanding work schedule (convenient diner), the initial intervention would focus on quick grab and go meals or healthy fast food choices. By tackling one pattern at a time, weight control is more manageable and remains patient-centered (15). Table 1 illustrates common dietary patterns and effective dietary strategies to resolve these patterns. The lifestyle personality approach has also been applied to common exercise and coping patterns.

Making Small Substitutions

An important point when counseling patients is to focus on eating favorite foods but reducing portion sizes or making substitutions where appropriate. Focus on changing the caloric density of foods as well as the portion size can reduce calories. Calorie dense foods are easy to overeat and their calories add up quickly. For example, a one-ounce bag of potato chips contains roughly double the calories of a piece of fruit, and chips are much easier to overeat than apples. A 500-kcal deficit can easily be achieved by reducing a 12-inch sub to a 6-inch sub and changing a 4-ounce bag of chips to a 1-ounce size. Ultimately, making small substitutions in the types of foods chosen and trimming portions helps shave calories and produce sustainable changes.

Meal Replacements

Portion sizes have increased by as much as 700% in America since the 1970s (16). Furthermore, Americans are eating more than ever; we now spend 40% of our food budget on dining out (17). Many patients admit that while they choose healthy foods, portion size is a problem and they are often unsure of what is a normal or reasonable portion size. An increase in meals away from home also increases calories. A turkey sandwich can vary from 250 to 750 kcal depending on the restaurant, the condiment additions, and the portion size. One of the most effective tools to achieve ideal portions and effectively produce a calorie deficit is incorporation of meal replacements. Meal replacements are foods that are designed to take the place of a meal while at the same time providing nutrients and good taste within a known caloric limit. Patients who replace one or two meals per day often lose more weight and are more likely to maintain that weight loss than patients who try to count calories on their own (18). In a meta-analysis of six studies with a study duration ranging from 3 to 51 months, use of partial meal replacements resulted in a 7% to 8% weight loss (19).

Meal replacements consist of shakes, meal bars, or frozen meals. These portion and calorie controlled foods typically provide between 200 and

Table 1 Patterns Approach to Weight Management

Pattern	Symptom	Behavioral strategies
Meal skipper	Grazing or no structure to meals	Establish regular meal and snack times to reduce overeating Use tools such as food logs to help identify hunger and fullness when eating Plan quick snacks such as meal replacement bars or shakes if short on time
Night-time nibbler	Consuming majority of calories late in the evening	Avoid skipping meals Planned afternoon snacks can reduce predinner hunger Add evening activities such as reading, books on tape, or knitting to substitute eating
Convenient diner	Majority of foods are quick, prepacked foods away from home	Eat out with a game plan Develop mental list of quick, healthy choices at each restaurant Healthy requests such as ordering appetizer portion, salads with dressing on the side or extra veggies keep calories in check
Fruitless feaster	Diet adequate with meat and starch, but low in fruits and vegetables	Plan to add either fruits or vegetables to each meal. Veggie soup, salads, and fruit cups are often available when eating out Availability is key; pay for precut, prewashed fruits and vegetables
Steady snacker	Constant munching, hungry or not	Designate snack times and preplan healthy snacks Identify behaviors or environments that foster mindless munching such as eating in front of TV or standing while eating Avoid eating out of the container
Hearty portioner	Healthy or not, portions are large and always finished	Slow down at meals to reduce amount consumed Become acquainted with proper portion size either through meal replacements, preportioned picnic plates or the diabetic exchange list Split or share entrees when eating out
Swing eater	The professional dieter who may eat "good" in public but "bad" in private	Reduce guilt of eating "bad" foods by planning small amounts of less healthy snacks 2 to 3 times/week

(Continued)

Table 1   Patterns Approach to Weight Management (*Continued*)

Pattern	Symptom	Behavioral strategies
		Always choose portion-controlled snacks such as ice cream cups or snack size bags of chips
		Focus on food satisfaction by adding heart healthy fats and fiber

Source: From Ref. 15.

400 kcal. Combined with a slice of vegetables and fruit, meal replacements help to provide a nutritionally balanced meal while reducing total daily calorie intake. Additional fruits and vegetables are essential to provide adequate fiber and antioxidants. Patients can select from canned vegetable soups, fresh or frozen vegetables, as well as fresh, frozen, or canned precut fruits. Overall, since meal replacements are convenient and reasonably priced, they provide an effective and healthy option for busy people who make poor food choices due to time constraints.

Calorie Counting

Many patients benefit from knowing the calorie level goal to consume at each meal or snack in order to lose weight. Calculating individual caloric needs and designating a calorie allotment for each meal and snack gives the patient-specific parameters. For example, a 1500 kcal diet may include the following distribution: breakfast: 300 kcal, lunch: 400 kcal, afternoon snack: 150 kcal, dinner: 500 kcal, and evening snack: 150 kcal. If a patient enjoys having a larger dinner, then adjustments can be made accordingly to stay within the total day's allowance such as eliminating the evening snack and redistributing those calories to dinner. If desired, several equations can be used to estimate specific calorie needs. These include the Harris Benedict equation, the Mifflin St. Jeor equation, and those of the Institute of Medicine and the World Health Organization. The equations use the patient's gender, age, height, and weight for calculation. To achieve weight loss, approximately 500 to 1000 kcal/day can be subtracted from the calculated energy requirements. Another rapid method used to approximate these formulas is simply to allow for 10-kcal/lb/body weight or 22-kcal/kg/body weight (20,21). For example, a 125-kg patient will need 2750 kcal to maintain weight and therefore would lose weight by consuming approximately 1750 to 2250 kcal/day.

Once a target calorie range has been established, the next step is recording the calorie content of foods consumed on a food log. The traditional method is to keep a food log with matching calorie values by hand, either in a journal or on paper. A variety of books, Internet sites, and computer software programs help to estimate calorie content of foods and track personal progress. Table 2 gives details on a few of the many Internet sites and software programs that are available for patients when counting calories.

Popular Diets

A current area of intense controversy is the use of low carbohydrate diets for weight loss. Although the public and media tend to lump all of the low carbohydrate popular diets into one category, they actually represent a continuum of carbohydrate percentage levels and differ slightly in theory. As previously discussed, the Institute of Medicine recommends a diet in which 45% to 65% of calories come from carbohydrates (8). In contrast, most of the popular lower carbohydrate diets (Southbeach, Zone, and Sugar Busters!) recommend a carbohydrate level of approximately 40% to 46%. The Atkins diet contains 5% to 15% carbohydrates depending on the phase of the diet. Whereas Atkins believes that all carbohydrates are the primary cause of obesity and insulin resistance, the other lower carbohydrate diets place a greater emphasis on choosing low glycemic index foods to reduce dietary insulin response.

Until recently, the theories and arguments of popular lower carbohydrate diet books have relied on poorly controlled, non-peer-reviewed studies and anecdotes (21). In recent years, several randomized, controlled trials have demonstrated greater weight loss at six months with improvement in coronary heart disease risk factors, including an increase in HDL cholesterol and a decrease in triglyceride levels (22–26). However, weight loss between groups did not remain statistically significant at one year (22,26). A study that enrolled patients with diabetes and the metabolic syndrome showed relative improvements in glycemic control, insulin sensitivity, and dyslipidemia in those subjects randomized to the lower carbohydrate diet (26). Since lower carbohydrate diets are just now being scrutinized with greater scientific vigor, it is premature to make definitive conclusions regarding their role in the treatment of obesity and/or the metabolic syndrome. However, conclusions from two comprehensive reviews are pertinent. The executive summary of a USDA conference on popular diets concluded that diets that reduce caloric intake result in weight loss regardless of macronutrient composition (27). And a systemic review by Bravata et al. (28) concluded that there is insufficient evidence to make recommendations for or against the use of low-carbohydrate diets and that participant weight loss was principally associated with decreased caloric intake and increased diet duration but not with reduced carbohydrate content.

Very Low Calorie Diets

Very low calorie diets (VLCD) are prescribed as a form of more aggressive dietary therapy. The primary purpose of prescribing a VLCD is to promote

Table 2 PC and Internet Resources for Calorie Management

Product	Web address	Equipment needed	Special features	$ or free
Personal tracking software				
Balance log	www.healthetech.com	Palm™ OS, PDA Home PC	Check calories consumed and calories burned through exercise and use 24 hr support	$
Calorie king	www.calorieking.com	Palm™ OS, PDA Home PC	Search calorie content of over 40,000 foods; track calorie needs and get maintenace advice	$
Fit day	www.fitday.com	Home PC	Look up calories and over 30 nutrients for foods consumed, record, and track progress for weight and measurements	$-internet use free
Nutrigenie software	www.nutrigenie.com	Palm™ OS, PDA Home PC	Software to track foods and monitor specific diets such as the DASH diet	$
United States department of agriculture nutrient database	www.nal.usda.gov/fnic/foodcomp/	Home PC	Search the USDA nutrient database for calories, fats, vitamins, and minerals	Free
E-diet manager	www.pilotgear.com/software/showsoftware.cfm?prodID=42865	Palm™ OS	Establish weight loss and exercise goals; monitor calories and fat of over 4000 foods	$

Diet and exercise assistant	www.keyoe.com	Palm™ OS, PDA, Home PC	Set personal nutrition and fitness goals and track progress; analyze calorie intake	$
Electronic comprehensive health programs				
Jenny Craig	www.JennyCraig.com	Home PC	Phone consultations, 24-hr support, on-line menu planner, and interactive journal to make program home-based	$
Weight watchers	www.weightwatchers.com	Home PC	Weight watchers at home. Monitor exercise and weight progress; use interactive restaurant guides, meal ideas, and on-line support	$
E-diets	www.ediets.com	Home PC	Customized exercise and meal plans from 19 popular diets with more than 2000 recipes to incorporate	$
WebMD	www.webmd.com	Home PC	Nutrition advice from RD along with customized diet analysis, eating plans, and RD feedback on food logs	$
Patterns approach to weight management	www.diet.com	Home PC	Interactive internet site with customized meal plans, group and buddy support, and professional advice from MD and RD	$
Shape magazine	www.ishape.com	Home PC	Individualized exercise plans and five-meals-a-day menu plans and recipes	$

Abbreviation: DASH, dietary approaches to stop hypertension.

a rapid and significant (13–23 kg) short-term weight loss over a three- to six-month period. These propriety formulas typically supply ≤ 800 kcal, 50 to 80 gm protein, and 100% of the RDI for vitamins and minerals. A meta-analysis found that after a weight loss of ≥ 20 kg, individuals significantly maintained more weight loss than after low calorie diets or weight loss of < 10 kg (29). In contrast, others studies have found no difference in long-term weight loss between VLCD and low calorie diets (30). According to a review by the National Task Force on the prevention and treatment of obesity, indications for initiating a VLCD include well-motivated individuals who are moderately to severely obese (BMI > 30), have failed at more conservative approaches to weight loss, and have a medical condition that would be immediately improved with rapid weight loss (31). Conditions include poorly controlled type 2 diabetes, hypertriglyceridemia, obstructive sleep apnea, and symptomatic peripheral edema. The risk for gallstone formation increases exponentially at rates of weight loss above 1.5 kg/week (32). Prophylaxis against gallstone formation with ursodeoxycholic acid, 600 mg/day, is effective in reducing this risk (33). Because of the need for close metabolic monitoring, these diets are usually prescribed by physicians specializing in obesity care.

TEAM APPROACH

Optimal treatment for the overweight and obese patient takes place under a multidisciplinary team of providers including physicians, registered dietitians, exercise physiologists, and health psychologists. Working together with the patient, each provider can individualize strategies and allow the patient to address all issues while maintaining focus on key goals. In the case of a patient with binge eating disorder, for example, the health psychologist may address antecedents to the binge, the dietitian may focus on adding scheduled meal and snack times to decrease the opportunity of a binge, the exercise physiologist may focus on increasing exercise to regulate mood, while the physician may explore pharmacotherapy to help regulate mood and food cravings. Providers can be in the same office or decentralized and still work as a team. Various modes of communication such as email, phone, or written correspondence can provide sufficient interaction. While all patients would benefit from a team approach not every provider has access to a multidisciplinary team. Referring to other health care providers can improve quality of care. Consideration for referral to a registered dietitian should be made if a patient needs specific strategies on how to eat healthy food or has a medical condition such as diabetes, hypertension, or dyslipidemia and would benefit from medical nutrition therapy (MNT). A registered dietitian in your area can be found by contacting the American Dietetic Association at www.eatright.org. Similarly, if a patient has physical pain or a medical condition that limits exercise, a referral to a physical therapist or exercise physiologist can improve motility without exacerbating the condition. A qualified exercise physiologist can be found by contacting the American College of Sports Medicine (ACSM) at www.ACSM.org.

CONCLUSION

Dietary therapy is a central component of lifestyle modification. It begins with a thorough dietary assessment that includes reviewing the weight history and associated life events, ascertaining the patient's current dietary patterns by using the typical day recall method or food diaries, and establishing motivation and readiness to make dietary changes. Several techniques can be used for dietary counseling including a qualitative lifestyle patterns approach, making small substitutions, calorie counting, use of meal replacements, or VLCDs. The primary goal is to reduce calorie intake and establish long-term healthy eating habits. The strategies and counseling methods used will vary depending on the patient's needs and abilities. Overall, the best diet is the one that can be followed for a lifetime.

REFERENCES

1. Hill JO, Wyatt HR, Reed GW, Peters JC. Obesity and the environment: where do we go from here? Science 2003; 299:853–855.
2. Trends in intake of energy and macronutrients—United States, 1971–2000. MMWR 2004; 53(4):80–86.
3. Physical activity trends—United States, 1990–1998. MMWR 2004; 50(9): 166–169.
4. American Diabetes Association, American Psychiatric Association, American Association of Clinical Endocrinologists, and North American Association for the Study of Obesity. Consensus development conference on antipsychotic drugs and obesity and diabetes. Obes Res 2004; 12:362–368.
5. National Heart, Lung, and Blood Institute (NHLBI) and North American Association for the Study of Obesity (NAASO). Practical guide to on the identification, evaluation, and treatment of overweight and obesity in adults. Bethesda, MD: National Institutes of Health, NTH Publ number 00–4084, 2000.
6. Rollnick S, Mason P, Butler C. Health Behavior Change: A Guide for Practitioners. London: Churchill Livingstone, 1999.
7. National Research Council. Dietary reference intakes for energy, carbohydrate, fiber, fat, fatty acids, cholesterol, protein, and amino acids. Washington, DC: National Academy Press, 2002; 1–936.
8. Bray GA, Popkin BM. Dietary fat intake does affect obesity. Am J Clin Nutr 1998; 68:1157–1173.
9. Astrup A, Grunwald GK, Melanson EL, Saris WH, Hill JO. The role of low-fat diets in body weight control: a meta-analysis of ad libitum dietary intervention studies. Int J Obes Relat Metab Disord 2000; 24:1545–1552.
10. U.S. Department of Health and Human Services and U.S. Department of Agriculture Dietary Guidelines for Americans, 2005. 6th ed. Washington, D.C.:U.S.

Government Printing Office, January 2005. (Available at www.health.gov/dietaryguidelines/dga2005/document/.)

11. Expert panel on detection, evaluation, and treatment of high blood cholesterol in adults. Executive summary of the third reports of the National Cholesterol Education Program (NCEP) expert panel on detection, evaluation, and treatment of high blood cholesterol in adults (Adult Treatment Panel III). JAMA 2001; 285:2486–2497.

12. Appel LJ, Moore TJ, Obarzanek E, et al. DASH Collaborative Research Group. A clinical trial of the effects of dietary patterns on blood pressure. N Engl J Med 1997; 336:1117–1124.

13. Sacks FM, Svetkey LP, Vollmer WM, et al. DASH-Sodium Collaborative Research Group. Effects on blood pressure of reduced dietary sodium and the dietary approaches to stop hypertension (DASH) diet. N Engl J Med 2001; 344:3–10.

14. Windhauser MM, Ernst DB, Karanja NM, et al. DASH Collaborative Research Group. Translating the dietary approaches to stop hypertension diet from research to practice: dietary and behavior change techniques. J Am Diet Assoc 1999; 99:S90–S95.

15. Kushner RF, Nancy N. Dr. Kushner's Personality Type Diet. New York, NY: St. Martin's Griffin Press, 2004.

16. Young LR, Nestle M. The contribution of expanding portion sizes to the US obesity epidemic. Am J Pub Health 2002; 92(2):246–249.

17. Putnam J, Gerrior S. Trends in the U.S. food supply, 1970–1997. USDA/ERS. Chapter 7:33–160. (http://www.ers.usda.gov.)

18. Ditschuneit HH, Flechtner-Mors M, Johnson TD, Adler G. Metabolic and weight loss effects of a long-term dietary intervention in obese patients. Am J Clin Nutr 1999; 69:198–204.

19. Heymsfield SB, van Mierlo CAJ, van der Knaap HCM, Frier HI. Weight management using meal replacement strategy: meta and pooling analysis from six studies. Int J Obes 2003; 27:537–549.

20. Bray GA. Contemporary Diagnosis and Management of Obesity. Pennsylvania: Handbooks in Healthcare Co, 1998.

21. Cheuvront SN. The zone diet phenomenon: a closer look at the science behind the claims. J Am Coll Nutr 2003; 22:9–17.

22. Foster FD, Wyatt HR, Hill JO, et al. A randomized trial of a low-carbohydrate diet for obesity. New Engl J Med 2003; 348:2082–2090.

23. Yancy WS, Olsen MK, Guyton JR, Bakst RP, Westman EC. A low-carbohydrate, ketogenic diet versus a low-fat diet to treat obesity and hyperlipidemia. Ann Intern Med 2004; 140:769–777.

24. Brehm BJ, Seeley RJ, Daniels SR, D'Alessio DA. A randomized trial comparing a very low carbohydrate diet and a calorie-restricted low fat diet on body weight and cardiovascular risk factors in healthy women. J Clin Endocrinol Metab 2003; 88:1617–1623.

25. Samaha FF, Iqbal N, Seshadri P, et al. A low-carbohydrate as compared with a low-fat diet in severe obesity. N Engl J Med 2003; 348:2074–2081.

26. Stern L, Iqbal N, Seshadri P, et al. The effects of low-carbohydrate versus conventional weight loss diets in severely obese adults: one-year follow-up of a randomized trial. Ann Intern Med 2004; 140:778–785.

27. Freedman MR, King J, Kennedy E. Popular diets: a scientific review. Obes Res 2001; 9(suppl 1):1S–40S.
28. Bravata DM, Sanders L, Huang J, et al. Efficacy and safety of low-carbohydrate diets. A scientific review. JAMA 2003; 289:1837–1850.
29. Anderson JW, Konz EC, Frederich RC, Wood CL. Long-term weight-loss maintenance: a meta-analysis of US studies. Am J Clin Nutr 2001; 74:579–584.
30. Wadden TA, Osei S. The treatment of obesity: an overview. In: Wadden TA, Stunkard AJ, eds. Handbook of Obesity Treatment. New York: The Guilford Press, 2002:229–248.
31. National task force on the prevention and treatment of obesity. Very low-calorie diets. JAMA 1993; 270:967–997.
32. Weinsier RL, Wilson LJ, Lee J. Medically safe rate of weight loss for the treatment of obesity: a guidelines based on risk of gallstone formation. Am J Med 1995; 98:115–117.
33. Shifman ML, Kaplan GD, Brinkman-Kaplan V, et al. Prophylaxis against gallstone formation with urodeoxycholic acid in patients participating in a very-low-calorie diet program. Ann Intern Med 1995; 122:899–905.

11

Behavioral Weight Management of Obese Patients with Mental Disorders

Susan L. McElroy and Renu Kotwal

Psychopharmacology Research Program, Department of Psychiatry, University of Cincinnati College of Medicine, Cincinnati, Ohio, U.S.A.

BEHAVIORAL WEIGHT MANAGEMENT IN THE TREATMENT OF OBESITY

Once viewed primarily as a cosmetic problem due to a personal choice or character flaw, obesity is now seen as a largely incurable, chronic medical disease with increased morbidity and mortality that results from a persistent imbalance between energy intake and energy expenditure and that requires long-term, if not life-long, management (1–7). In many instances, this imbalance is thought to be due to genetic factors (e.g., thrifty genes) adversely interacting with a "toxic" or "obesigenic" environment (e.g., increased access to highly palatable, energy dense food and/or reduced access to physical activity). Behavioral weight management addresses these "trait-environment mismatches" to bring about lifestyle changes aimed at decreasing energy intake through calorie reduction and increasing energy expenditure through enhancing physical activity. As such, behavioral weight management remains the cornerstone of obesity treatment (1,3,4,8–16).

GOALS OF BEHAVIORAL WEIGHT MANAGEMENT IN THE TREATMENT OF OBESITY

The traditional goal of the treatment of obesity was reduction to ideal body weight. This goal, however, has changed dramatically in the past decade, such that several scientific bodies now recommend a 5–15% reduction in initial body weight (1,2,17,18). This change occurred for several reasons. First, extensive research indicates that most patients with obesity typically lose only 10–15% of initial body weight with state-of-the-art behavioral treatment. After six months, weight loss slows down and plateaus. Second, even for patients who manage to lose a large amount of weight initially, most cannot maintain the loss over the long term. In one review, Sarwer and Wadden (9) found that most patients had regained 35–50% of their weight loss by one year after treatment, regardless of weight loss method used. Wing and Hill (19) thus proposed defining successful long-term weight loss maintenance as intentionally losing at least 10% of initial body weight and keeping it off for at least one year. By this definition, they estimated that 20% of overweight and obese persons who attempt to lose weight were successful. For patients who are unable to lose weight or maintain weight loss, prevention of further weight gain is an appropriate goal.

Third, considerable research shows that small weight losses, on the order of 5–10% of baseline body weight, are associated with significant health improvements, including in hypertension, lipoprotein profile, and type 2 diabetes (1,20). Many of these improvements persist with maintenance of weight loss, even if partial weight regain occurs. Moreover, although behavioral weight management has not yet been shown to reduce the increased morality associated with obesity, it has been shown to reduce by half the incidence of type 2 diabetes in persons at high risk (21–25). For example, in the Finnish Diabetes Prevention Study (DPS), 552 middle-aged, overweight subjects with impaired glucose tolerance were randomized to usual care or intensive lifestyle intervention (22,23,25). After a mean follow-up of 3.2 years, weight reduction was 3.5 kg in the intervention group compared with 0.9 kg in the usual care group. The risk of diabetes was reduced by 58% ($p < 0.001$) in the intervention group compared with the control group. In the Diabetes Prevention Program (DPP), 3234 nondiabetic persons with elevated fasting and postload plasma glucose concentrations were randomized to placebo, metformin (850 mg twice daily), or a lifestyle modification program with the goals of at least a 7% body weight loss and at least 150 minutes of physical activity per week (21,24,25). After a mean follow-up of 2.8 years, the incidence of diabetes was 11.0, 7.8, and 4.8 cases per 100 person-years in the placebo, metformin, and lifestyle groups, respectively. The average weight loss in the three groups were 0.1, 2.1, and 5.6 kg, respectively. Lifestyle and metformin were superior to placebo, and lifestyle was superior to metformin, in reducing diabetes in persons at high risk.

Behavioral weight management ideally has three goals: decrease in calorie intake, increase in physical activity, and learning of cognitive behavioral strategies to reinforce positive changes in dietary habits and physical activity. In this chapter, these three components of behavioral weight management in persons with obesity without mental illness will be briefly summarized. Then, research on the use of behavioral weight management in obese persons with psychotic, mood, and eating disorders will be reviewed.

Dietary Treatment

Calorie reduction is generally considered the most important component of dietary treatment for weight loss for obesity (1,26). Thus, dietary therapy for weight loss in obesity usually consists of instructing patients on how to modify their diet to achieve a decrease in calorie intake. In its 1998 review, the National Institutes of Health (NIH) found 25 randomized controlled trials of low calorie diets varying in duration from six months to one year (1). Compared with controls, low calorie diets produced a mean weight loss of about 8%. Four studies that included a long-term weight loss maintenance intervention (ranging 3–4.5 years) found an average weight loss of 4% over the period. Long-term diets may be more effective, especially if patients are able to adhere to them. In their 2000 review of the long-term outcome of the dietary treatment of obesity, Ayyad and Andersen (27) found a 15% success rate among 2131 individuals followed for a median of five years after dietary interventions that were ≥3 years in duration. In this review, success was defined as maintenance of all weight lost or of at least 9–11 kg of initial weight lost.

There is some controversy as to the nature of the calorie reduction that should occur in dietary therapy for obesity. For example, greater initial weight loss can be achieved with very low calorie diets (VLCD; <800 calories/day) as compared to low calorie diets (800–1500 calories/day). However, most studies have shown that at one year there is no difference in weight loss between the two strategies because of regain of lost weight. Thus, the NIH guidelines recommend that a moderate reduction in caloric intake be used to achieve a gradual weight loss (1).

There is also some controversy about the optimal macronutrient composition of the diet for weight loss and weight maintenance. A recent review of four randomized controlled trials of low fat diets versus calorie-restricted diets in overweight or obese subjects found no differences in weight loss between the two groups at six months, 12 months, or 18 months (28). The weighted sum of weight loss in the low fat group was 0.1 kg compared with 2.3 kg in the control group. Three recent randomized controlled trials in obese subjects found greater weight loss with a low carbohydrate diet compared with a calorie- and fat-restricted diet at six months, but not at one year in the two extended trials (29–33). Most recently, Dansinger et al. (34) compared four popular diets: 160 overweight or obese participants with known hypertension, dyslipidemia, or fasting hyperglycemia were randomized to Atkins, Ornish, Weight Watchers, or Zone Diets for one year (34). There was a nonsignificant trend toward a higher rate of discontinuation rate for the more extreme diets (48% for Atkins and 50% for Ornish) than for the moderate diets (35% for Zone and 35% for Weight Watchers). All four diets resulted in modest statistically significant weight loss at one year, with no statistically significant differences between groups. In contrast with the association between diet type and weight loss, a strong association was found between self-reported dietary adherence and weight loss that was almost identical for each diet. On average, participants in the top percentile of adherence lost 7% of body weight. Cardiac risk factor reductions were associated with weight loss regardless of diet type. The authors concluded that adherence level rather than diet type was the key determinant of clinical benefit.

The balance of evidence therefore suggests that macronutrient composition does not seem to play a major role regarding weight loss, as all low calorie diets (high protein, low carbohydrate, and low fat) produce weight loss. However, some data suggest diets high in fiber, calcium (especially from dairy sources), or fruits and vegetables might be associated with lower body weights (35–37). Also, there are concerns about the long term (>1 year) safety of low carbohydrate diets since they may be deficient in important nutrients and fiber and their high saturated fat content may be atherogenic (38,39). Moreover, an increasing number of studies have reported beneficial health effects beyond weight loss from long-term use of diets that are reduced in saturated fats or rich in fruits, vegetables, fish, legumes, and nuts. As noted earlier, the Finnish DPS Group and the DPP showed that a reduced fat diet in combination with physical activity in obese persons with impaired glucose tolerance delayed the onset of type 2 diabetes (25). The Dietary Approaches to Stop Hypertension (DASH) diet has been shown to reduce blood pressure in persons with and without hypertension and the Mediterranean diet has been shown to decrease cardiac mortality in patients with coronary heart disease (40–43). The DASH diet is high in fruits, vegetables, and low fat dairy products and reduced in fat; the Mediterranean diet is rich in fruits, vegetables, fish, legumes, and nuts.

Physical Activity

Physical activity is helpful for achieving weight loss, and may be especially important for long-term maintenance of weight loss (1,44–46). Correlational studies have consistently found an association between long-term weight loss and increased physical activity. In addition, physical activity improves cardiorespiratory fitness and reduces comorbidities associated with obesity (1). In a post hoc analysis of the Finnish DPS, participants in the upper third of change in total leisure time physical activity were 80% less likely to develop diabetes than those in the lower third (47).

However, controlled trials have shown the effect of prescribed exercise for maintenance of weight loss to be modest. Experts have attributed these disparate observations to poor adherence with prescribed exercise, inadequate duration of exercise, as well as the prescription of too little exercise (44–46). Indeed, a recent controlled study indicated that higher levels of physical activity are likely required for maintenance of weight loss for obesity. Jeffrey et al. (48) randomized 202 overweight men and women to either a standard behavior therapy (SBT) for obesity incorporating an energy expenditure goal of 1000 kcal/wk or to a high physical activity (HPA) treatment in which the energy expenditure goal was 2500 kcal/wk. To help HPA participants achieve this exercise goal, their treatment included encouragement to recruit one to three exercise partners into the study, personal counseling from an exercise coach, and small monetary incentives. HPA group reported obtaining significantly higher mean physical activity levels than the SBT group at 6, 12, and 18 months, and displayed significantly greater mean weight losses at 12 (8.5 kg vs. 6.1 kg) and 18 months (6.7 kg vs. 4.1 kg) (but not six months).

Of note, physical activity may be divided into two types: programmed and lifestyle. Programmed exercise consists of regularly scheduled periods of relatively high intensity activity (e.g., 20–40 minutes of walking, running, or swimming). Lifestyle activity involves increasing energy expenditure throughout the day by walking whenever possible instead of riding, taking elevators or escalators, and not using energy saving devices. Controlled studies have shown lifestyle activity to be just as effective as programmed activity in maintaining weight loss and in improving fitness, decreasing blood pressure, and reduced cholesterol (49,50). Thus, lifestyle activity provides an alternative for obese persons who do not like or are unable to participate in more strenuous exercise.

Most obesity treatment guidelines recommend that physical activity should be an integral part of behavioral treatment programs for weight loss and weight maintenance (1,17,18). Since many overweight and obese patients have low exercise tolerance, they should begin with short bouts of low intensity activity (e.g., walking at a slow pace 10 minutes three times per week) (1,3). NIH guidelines suggest most patients should be encouraged to gradually increase to 30–45 minutes of moderate physical activity 3–5 times per week (1). Progression to 30–60 minutes of moderate physical activity every day may enhance weight loss and weight maintenance (18).

Behavior Modification

The goal of behavioral treatment for obesity is to modify behaviors that adversely impact psychological and physical health and positively reinforce changes in diet and physical activity that can produce and maintain weight loss, or least prevent further weight gain. In addition to education about reducing calorie intake and increasing physical activity, cognitive-behavioral approaches include: self-monitoring of weight, eating habits, and physical activity; stimulus control training; problem solving; contingency management; cognitive restructuring; and enlisting social support. Cognitive-behavioral treatment can also be used to help obese and overweight individuals enhance their self-esteem, become more assertive in coping with the adverse effects of the stigma associated with obesity, and to reduce body image dissatisfaction (15). Behavioral treatments of obesity that have received systematic study have ranged from self-help and commercialized programs that provide some instruction about diet and physical activity to specialized cognitive behavioral therapies (CBT) targeted for weight loss and weight maintenance that incorporate dietary and physical activity components.

Behavioral weight loss programs directly available to consumers include commercial programs such as Weight Watchers, Jenny Craig, LA Weight Loss, Nutrisystem, Diet Smart, and eDiets.com, and self-help programs such as Take Off Pounds Sensibly (TOPS) and Overeaters Anonymous (OA). Weight Watchers, one of the less costly of these programs, has been shown to be superior to self-help and usual care in two randomized prospective trials. In the first study, Rippe et al. (51) randomized 80 women to attend Weight Watchers or usual care. At 12 weeks, attrition rates were 25% and 65%, and participants lost 7.5% and 1.6% of baseline weight, respectively. In the second trial, Heshka et al. (52) randomized 413 subjects without a history of psychiatric illness to receive free vouchers to attend weekly Weight Watchers sessions at a location of their choosing over 26 weeks (the intervention group, $n = 211$) or to receive two brief dietary consultations with a nutritionist and access to nutrition-oriented educational materials (the self-help group, $n = 212$). Intent-to-treat analysis showed that the Weight Watchers group lost significantly more of their initial weight than the self-help group at one year (5.3% vs. 1.5%), and maintained a significantly greater weight loss at two years (3.2% vs. 0%; $p < 0.001$ at both time points). The Heshka et al. (52) study and other data suggest that self-help programs (e.g., TOPS and OA) and commercial weight loss programs available over the internet (e.g., eDiets.com) produce minimal weight loss (53,54).

Comprehensive cognitive behavioral programs (CBPs) for obesity available to clinicians and patients include the Kelly Brownell LEARN Program for Weight Control and Cooper et al.'s (13) Cognitive Behavioral Treatment of Obesity (8,11). A review of 12 of the more recent largest and longest CBPs trials, most of which included dietary and/or exercise components, found that participants lost an average of 10.4 kg at 5.6 months, with an average weight loss of 8.1 kg at final follow-up at 17.6 months (16). Methods of strengthening the effectiveness of the behavioral component of obesity treatment include lengthening the duration of treatment, daily weight charting, and increasing the intensity of treatment. For example, a four-year continuing treatment program administered in Sweden has produced average weight loss maintenance results of 12.6 and 10.5 kg at four years and 10 years follow-up, respectively (55,56). This program included an initial six-week hospital day treatment that combined behavioral therapy with a VLCD and cooking and exercise training. The four-year maintenance program included weekly sessions with advice from dieticians and monitoring of body weight. Importantly, patients had the opportunity to re-enroll in hospital day treatment for two weeks for relapse at any time; 99% of participants used this option at least once.

Another means of enhancing the effectiveness of behavioral weight management may be by increasing its components. In its 1998 review, the NIH evaluated 15 studies that compared the combination of dietary therapy and physical activity with diet alone ($n = 15$) and/or physical activity alone ($n = 6$), and concluded that the combination produced greater weight loss than diet alone or physical therapy alone (1). In their 2000 review of 17 studies of long-term dietary treatment of obesity, Ayyad and Andersen (27) concluded that diet combined with group therapy produced better long-term success rates (median 27%) than did diet alone (median 15%) or diet combined with behavior modification (median 14%). Recent studies comparing multiple with single-component lifestyle behavioral interventions suggest that multiple-component interventions may be more effective for achieving health benefits. For example, the PREMIER clinical trial found that an "established" multicomponent intervention and the established intervention plus the DASH diet significantly reduced blood pressure and rates of hypertension as compared to "advice only" in a group of patients with above-optimal blood pressure (42). Interventions included weight loss, sodium reduction, increased physical activity, and limited alcohol intake. In another study, Djuric et al. (57) randomized 48 breast cancer survivors to Weight Watchers (subjects received free coupons to attend weekly meetings), individualized nutritional counseling with a dietician, comprehensive treatment (Weight Watchers and individualized nutritional counseling), or no intervention (control group). Subjects in all three intervention groups lost weight (control—1.1 kg, Weight Watchers—2.7 kg, individualized—8.0 kg, and comprehensive—9.5 kg), but only the individualized and comprehensive groups had significant losses. Also, subjects in the comprehensive group showed the most improvement in cholesterol levels and had decreased leptin levels.

Successful Weight Maintenance

Considerable research demonstrates that initial weight loss is much easier to achieve than is long-term maintenance of weight loss. Much of what is known about the correlates of successful weight maintenance comes from the National Weight Control Registry (NWCR), founded in 1994 to study individuals who have maintained a 30-lb weight loss for at least one year (19,58,59). As of 2001, the NWCR had over 3000 subjects; 80% were women and their average age was 45 years. Their average weight loss was 30 kg and their average duration of weight maintenance was 5.5 years.

Of the NWCR participants, 89% reported modifying both diet and exercise to achieve and maintain successful weight loss. Regarding diet, participants reported consuming 1381 kcal/day with 24% of calories from fat, 19% from protein, and 56% from carbohydrates. Only 7.6% of registrants reported eating <90 g of carbohydrate per day and <1% of registrants ate diets with <24% carbohydrates (1500 calories and ≤90 g of carbohydrate per day). Compared with participants with higher carbohydrate intake, those consuming diets with <24% carbohydrate maintained their weight loss for less time and were less physically active.

Regarding exercise, 91% reported engaging in regular physical activity (about 1 hr/day) to lose weight and to maintain weight loss. The most common physical activity was walking, reported by 76% of participants. Also, 44% weighed themselves at least once per day and 31% weighed themselves at least once per week. Thus, the three most common behavioral factors characteristic of NWCR participants were eating a low calorie and low fat diet, engaging in high levels of physical activity, and self-monitoring of bodyweight.

The psychological features of NWCR participants were notable for low depression scores and low rates of binge eating and vomiting (59). NWCR participants had an average Center for Epidemiologic Studies Depression Scale (CES-D) score of 9.2 (range 0–52), with 18% of participants scoring >16, the cutoff used to determine cases of depression. These findings are comparable to CES-D scores of 4.1 to 10.4 in nondepressed community control subjects, with 21% of individuals reporting scores >16. Eight percent of registrants reported four or more binges/month, and 1.8% reported any episodes of vomiting in the preceding month for weight loss purposes. Over 90% of participants reported improvement in their overall quality of life, level of energy, general mood, self-confidence, and mobility. However, 14% reported worsening in time spent thinking about food and 20% reported worsening in time spent thinking about weight.

BEHAVIORAL WEIGHT MANAGEMENT OF OBESITY WITH MENTAL DISORDERS

Although relatively few studies have evaluated behavioral weight treatments in obese patients with mental disorders, available controlled clinical trial data suggest such treatments are generally safe and may be effective (at least over the short term) in obese patients with psychotic and eating disorders. No controlled clinical trials, however, have yet assessed behavioral weight treatments in obese patients with mood disorders.

Psychotic Disorders

Increasing evidence indicates that patients with schizophrenia commonly have abdominal obesity, overweight, and obesity, as well as unhealthy lifestyle habits that contribute to weight gain, such as consuming high-fat diets and engaging in low levels of exercise (60–64). Moreover, many antipsychotics are associated with weight gain and metabolic abnormalities. Indeed, expert consensus guidelines aimed at improving the physical health of patients with schizophrenia have recently been published by the American Psychiatric Association (APA) and the American Diabetes Association (ADA) (65,66). For patients with psychotic disorders receiving second generation antipsychotics, these guidelines recommend regular monitoring of body mass index (BMI), plasma glucose level, and plasma lipid profile. Specific recommendations made by the APA guidelines include recording the patient's BMI before medication initiation or change and at every visit for the first six months thereafter. Subsequently, BMI can be determined quarterly as long as it remains stable. These guidelines also specify that, unless the patient is underweight, a weight gain of one BMI unit indicates the need for an intervention. Suggested interventions include closer monitoring of the patient's weight, a change in the patient's antipsychotic medication, the use of an adjunctive medication to reduce weight, and engagement of the patient in a weight management program.

Despite the recommendation that weight management programs be used, relatively few studies have tested such programs in patients with psychotic disorders (67,68). Indeed, dietary therapy has received little empirical study in psychotic disorders, despite growing evidence indicating that dietary composition may be important in the pathophysiology of these illnesses. Epidemiologic data has suggested that high dietary intake of refined sugar and saturated fat may be associated with a poor outcome for persons with schizophrenia, whereas high intake of fish and seafood may be associated with a better outcome (69–71). Decreased polyunsaturated fatty acid levels have been found in the brains and erythrocytes of patients with schizophrenia (70,71). Also, placebo-controlled trials have found supplemental eicosapentaenoic acid to be effective in reducing symptoms in patients with schizophrenia (70,71). Thus, the role of dietary composition in the treatment of psychosis is an area in great need of exploration.

There are also no controlled trials of exercise in schizophrenia. Preliminary studies conducted to date suggest exercise is safe, may improve mood, and may be associated with weight loss (72,73). However, these studies also suggest that adherence with exercise is poor among patients with schizophrenia unless there is substantial psychosocial support. In one pilot study, 10 of 20 stable patients with schizophrenia or schizoaffective disorder treated with olanzapine for at least four weeks were randomized to receive free access to a Young Men's Christian Association (YMCA) fitness facility for six months (73). Nine patients had dropped out at six months and all nine met criteria for poor attendance. The main reason given for poor attendance was lack of motivation. The mean weight change in the YMCA group was a gain 2 kg; mean weight change in the other group was not assessed. The one patient who completed the program and met criteria for full attendance lost 15 kg.

Because the core symptoms of schizophrenia—psychosis, apathy, and cognitive impairment—lead to problems in social and occupational functioning and in self-care, it might be predicted that patients with this illness and other psychotic disorders would be particularly unresponsive to behavioral weight management (74,75). However, a range of psychosocial treatments have been shown to be effective in patients with schizophrenia when added to antipsychotic medication. These strategies include CBT, family intervention, social skills training, teaching illness self-management skills, and integrated treatment for co-occurring substance misuse (74–78). It is thus notable that the five controlled trials published to date suggest behavioral weight management may be safe and effective in controlling weight gain and obesity in some patients psychotic disorders, particularly when administered in conjunction with some of these psychosocial treatment strategies.

In the first controlled study, Rotatori et al. (79) randomized 14 chronically ill psychiatric patients living in a "semi-independent" residential facility to a 14-week behavioral program that focused on techniques to reduce calorie intake ($n = 7$) or a waiting list control group ($n = 7$). Both individual and group reinforcement contingencies were used throughout the behavioral program. There were no drop outs and the seven patients randomized to behavioral treatment displayed a mean 7.3 lb weight loss, compared with a 5.6 lb mean gain in the control group.

Ball et al. (80) evaluated a Weight Watchers Program in 11 outpatients with schizophrenia or schizoaffective disorder and olanzapine-related weight gain (baseline mean BMI = 31.9). A comparison group of 11 patients matched on olanzapine use and weight gain continued their usual olanzapine treatment but did not participate in the program. The program consisted of 10 weekly Weight Watchers meetings held at an outpatient research program. In addition, exercise sessions (the primary mode was walking) were scheduled three times a week. A parent or caregiver was asked to supervise each patient's diet and exercise at home. Tokens were used to reinforce adherence to diet and exercise.

Participants who completed the Weight Watchers program ($n = 11$) lost more weight (mean = 5.1 lb) than comparison group participants (mean = 0.5 lb), but the difference was not statistically significant. However, there was a significant sex by group by time interaction for BMI ($p = 0.05$). All seven male participants lost weight (mean = 7.3 lb), whereas three of the four female participants gained weight (mean not reported). No significant correlation was found between exercise participation and weight loss. Psychiatric rating scales showed that patients remained clinically stable during the study. Importantly, no adverse events were observed with either the diet or the exercise program.

Menza et al. (81) evaluated a 52-week multimodal weight control program in 31 patients with schizophrenia ($n = 20$) or schizoaffective disorder ($n = 11$) receiving antipsychotic medication and participating in two day-treatment programs. Sixteen patients who were approached declined to participate. A comparison group consisted of 20 "usual care" patients who were contemporaneously treated in the same clinics. The weight control program encorporated nutritional counseling, exercise, and behavioral modification and consisted of four phases: (*i*) an assessment phase, (*ii*) an intensive 12-week weight control program with group meetings twice per week and one 15-minute individual session per week, (*iii*) a 12-week, step-down, less intensive weight control program with one group meeting per week and one 15-minute individual session per month, and (*iv*) a 6-month weight-maintenance extension program with a group meeting once per week and one 15-minute individual session per month. Behavioral strategies used included self-monitoring of eating and physical activity, stress management, stimulus control, problem solving, and social support. Techniques aimed at enhancing subjects' confidence in their ability to cope with obstacles and succeed in change were employed. Special teaching approaches for people with cognitive deficits, such as repetition, homework, and the use of visual materials, were also used throughout the program.

Twenty-seven (87.1%) of the 31 patients in the intervention group completed the 12-week intensive program and lost a mean of 2.7 kg and a mean of 1.0 BMI units, compared with a mean gain of 2.9 kg and 1.2 BMI units in the control group. Twenty (64.5%) patients completed the entire 52-week program. Statistically significant prepost improvements in weight, BMI, glycolated hemoglobin, diastolic and systolic blood pressure, exercise level, nutrition knowledge, and stages of change (for exercise and weight) were seen in the intervention group. Weight and BMI also decreased significantly in the intervention group compared with the "usual care" group, who gained weight. The authors concluded that individuals with schizophrenia and schizoaffective disorder were willing to attend, and benefited from, a weight control program that focused on nutrition, exercise, and behavioral modification.

Brar et al. (68) conducted a 14-week multicenter, open-label, randomized study comparing group-based behavioral therapy for weight loss with usual care in stable patients with schizophrenia or schizoaffective disorder. Patients had been treated with risperidone for six weeks after being switched from olanzapine and had BMIs >26. (After switching to risperidone, patients showed no weight loss.) Behavior therapy included 20 sessions over the 14-week period and focused on learning healthy eating habits. There was no exercise component. Members of the usual care group were encouraged to lose weight on their own only without specific instructions, but received monthly anthropometric assessments. Of 70 patients randomized, 50 (71.4%) completed the program. Both groups lost weight but the between group difference was not statistically significant (−2.0 kg vs. −1.1 kg for behavior therapy and usual care, respectively). However, there was a trend for more patients in the behavior therapy group than in the usual care group to have lost ≥5% of their body weight at endpoint (26.5% vs. 10.8%). Moreover, post hoc analysis of patients attending at least one behavior therapy session showed that significantly more patients in the behavior therapy than the usual care group had lost ≥5% of their body weight at endpoint (32.1% vs. 10.8%) and at week 14 (40.9% vs. 14.3%).

The fifth controlled trial was conducted to determine if behavioral weight management could prevent psychotropic-associated weight gain. Littrell et al. (82) randomized 70 patients with schizophrenia or schizoaffective disorder into an intervention group (22 males, 13 females) using Eli Lilly's "Solutions for Wellness" program or a standard of care control group. All patients began olanzapine at the onset of the study, and body weights were recorded monthly over six months. The intervention group received one-hour weekly seminars over 16 weeks related to dietary guidelines, developing support systems, and education about exercise. Patients in the intervention group showed no significant weight changes at four or six months (0.8 or −0.1 lb, respectively), whereas weight gain was seen in the control group (7.1 and 9.6 lb at four and six months, respectively). This study is important because behavioral weight management may be more effective for preventing psychotropic-associated weight gain than for reversing it once it has developed, though this has not yet been systematically shown.

Mood Disorders

Patients with mood disorders commonly have obesity, and obese patients seeking weight management commonly have mood disorders (83). However, as noted, we found no prospective study that evaluated behavioral weight management in obese patients with syndromal mood disorders, including in patients whose mood disorders were stabilized by antidepressants or mood stabilizers. Indeed, current obesity treatment guidelines generally recommend treating mood disorder before obesity when the two conditions co-occur, and do not provide recommendations regarding behavioral weight management for obese patients with treated mood disorders desiring weight loss (1). Early studies of weight-reduction interventions, in which patients generally were not screened for mental disorders, reported a relatively high rate of mood disturbances, ranging from mild depressive and anxiety symptoms to syndromal depression, completed suicides, and psychoses (84). By contrast, subsequent studies of behavioral weight loss therapy, in which patients with significant psychopathology were usually excluded but often had mild depressive symptoms, generally found that such treatments were associated with improvement in mood (usually assessed with self-report measures such as the Beck Depression Inventory) as patients lost weight (85,86).

Of note, many studies have examined the relationship between depressive symptoms (which have usually been mild) and adherence to behavioral weight treatment; the results of these studies have been mixed, with reports of either no relationship or a negative relationship (i.e., greater depressive symptoms were associated with less adherence) (85–89). We found only two studies that examined the effects of mood disorder diagnosis (as opposed to depressive symptoms) on weight loss treatment and maintenance. In the first study, Marcus et al. (90) evaluated 61 obese subjects with type 2 diabetes with the Inventory to Diagnose Depression—Lifetime Version before a 52-week behavioral weight-control program. Thirty-two percent of subjects reported a history of major depression. Subjects with and without a history of major depression showed comparable improvements in weight, glycemic control, and mood, but those with major depression showed a significantly higher rate of attrition (52.4% vs. 22.2%, $p = 0.03$). In the second study, Jenkins et al. (91) evaluated 39 obese breast cancer survivors during and six months after 24 months of individualized counseling for diet and exercise. Nine subjects had major depressive disorder and 10 had definable disorders of lesser severity (eight had adjustment disorders with depressive, anxious, or mixed depressive–anxious symptoms). Subjects with psychiatric disorders had significantly less weight loss at both the 12-month and the 6-month follow-up (30 month) time-points compared with subjects with no psychiatric disorders (6.3% vs. 12.6% and 1.2% vs. 7.8%, respectively). At the 6-month follow-up, women with major depression showed less weight loss (0.7%) than those with less severe definable disorders (3.7%). Moreover, the pattern of regain was different depending on presence of psychiatric diagnosis. The 10 women without diagnoses started regaining weight after 12 months, whereas the 19 women with any diagnoses started regaining weight after six months. Attrition rates were similar in subjects with and without diagnoses. Although further research is needed, these two studies suggest that obese patients with mood disorders may either adhere less well or respond less adequately to behavioral weight management than those without mood disorders.

Dietary therapy has also received very little study in mood disorders, despite preliminary data suggesting that dietary composition may affect mood (92). As with schizophrenia, polyunsaturated fats have been hypothesized to play an important role in the etiology of both depressive and bipolar disorders. Epidemiologic evidence suggests low fish consumption may be associated with increased risk of developing mood disorders and depressive symptoms (in some studies, this finding is evident in women but not men) (93,94). Cell membrane levels of $n-3$ polyunsaturated fats have been reported to be decreased in persons with major depression (70). Three double-blind, placebo-controlled studies showed omega-3 supplements to be effective adjunctive treatments for antidepressant-resistant major depression, and one double-blind, placebo-controlled trial showed such supplements improved depressive symptoms in treatment resistant bipolar disorder (70,95).

Moreover, dieting has been hypothesized to alter brain serotonin function by lowering plasma tryptophan levels. Thus, dieting has been shown to increase the prolactin response to tryptophan and D-fenfluramine in women, but not men, and to induce serotonin 2C receptor supersensitivity in women (96–99). In one of the few studies evaluating the effect of diet on persons with mood disorders that we were able to locate, Smith et al. (100) evaluated brain serotonin function and mood during short-term (three-week) dieting in women with a history of at least one episode of DSM-IV major depression who were fully recovered and medication free for at least six months. Specifically, 19 women with a past major depressive episode and 23 women with no history of major depression were placed on a daily 1000 kcal diet for three weeks. Fasting plasma tryptophan levels, prolactin response to an intravenous trytophan challenge, and mood ratings were evaluated before the diet and in the final week of the diet. A similar proportion of recovered (61%) and control (58%) subjects completed the three-week protocol; although the recovered subjects tended to weigh more, the two groups achieved similar weight loss. Plasma trytophan levels fell equivalently in both groups after dieting. Dieting increased the prolactin response to tryptophan in the women without a history of depression but this increase did not occur in the women with a history of depression. Mood ratings showed a significant reduction in happy scores in the recovered group relative to controls, though there were no differences on ratings of sad or irritable mood between the groups. The authors concluded that women with a history of major depression, but not those without depression, showed impaired regulation of brain serotonin function in response to dieting.

In contrast to behavioral weight management and dietary therapy, CBT and exercise have received more extensive study in patients with depressive disorders, but most studies did not use weight as an outcome (101–103). CBT, but not exercise, has also received some empirical study in bipolar disorder. In depressive disorders, CBT has been shown to be effective as monotherapy for mild-to-moderate depression and in combination with pharmacotherapy for moderate-to-severe depression (101,104). In bipolar disorder, CBT has been shown to enhance compliance with pharmacotherapy, to decrease interepisode depressive symptoms, and to reduce relapse (105,106).

Regarding exercise in depression, in 2001, Lawlor and Hopker (102) conducted a meta-analysis of 14 randomized controlled trials of exercise in clinically depressed patients and concluded that exercise was more effective than no treatment and comparable to CBT in reducing depressive symptoms. However, they noted that all 14 studies had important methodological weaknesses and, because of these weaknesses, also concluded that the effectiveness of exercise in depression could not be adequately determined. Dunn et al. (107) recently completed a study addressing many of the limitations of these earlier trials. They randomized 80 adults ages 20–45 years with mild to moderate major depressive disorder by DSM-IV criteria to one of four aerobic exercise groups or exercise placebo control (three days per week of flexibility exercise). The four exercise groups varied total energy expenditure (7.0 or 17.5 kcal/kg/wk) and exercise frequency (3 or 5 day/wk). The 17.5 kcal/kg/wk amount of exercise of week corresponded to the "public health dose," whereas the 7.0 kcal/kg/wk represented the "low dose." The primary outcome was change in depressive symptoms as determined by the Hamilton Rating Scale for Depression (Ham-D). Participants randomized to the public health dose (17.5 kcal/kg/wk), but not the low dose (7.0 kcal/kg/wk), of aerobic exercise showed a significant reduction in depressive symptoms as compared to the placebo group. Ham-D scores were decreased 47% from baseline for the public health dose compared with 30% for the low dose and 25% for placebo. There was no main effect of exercise frequency at 12 weeks. Thus, as with exercise for weight loss, exercise may also have a dose–response relationship for depressive symptoms for major depressive disorder.

In sum, the lack of studies of behavioral weight management in obese persons with mood disorders makes it difficult to provide specific guidelines for such treatment in such patients at this time. Research showing that CBT is effective for both depressive and bipolar disorders, along with findings that exercise may benefit major depression, suggests that incorporation of components of behavioral weight management into CBT for persons with depressive or bipolar disorders might prove an effective method for managing both the mood disorder and the associated problems with overeating, weight gain, inactivity, and obesity. However, these strategies need to be formally studied before specific recommendations can be made.

Eating Disorders with Obesity

It is increasingly apparent that certain eating disorders are associated with overweight and obesity. These include binge eating disorder (BED), bulimia nervosa (especially the nonpurging variant), subthreshold forms of these disorders (often called obesity with binge eating), and night eating syndrome (108–111). Although generally viewed as separate diagnostic entities, all of these syndromes are characterized by dyscontrol over eating. Because of early concerns that dieting (or restrictive eating) might induce eating disorders and even obesity in some persons by triggering disinhibition over eating, a comprehensive review evaluating the relationship among dieting, weight loss treatment, weight cycling, and eating disorders in overweight and obese adults was published in 2000 by the National Task Force on the Prevention and Treatment of Obesity (112). The review concluded that moderate calorie restriction in combination with behavioral weight loss treatment did not seem to cause binge eating in persons without pre-existing binge eating, and might ameliorate binge eating in those with binge eating before treatment.

A recent controlled study conducted by Wadden et al. (113) provided some support for these conclusions. They randomly assigned 123 obese women without eating or mood disorders to one of three diets for 40 weeks and prospectively assessed their eating behavior and mood. The three diets were: (*i*) a 1000 kcal/day diet that included four servings/day of a liquid meal replacement (MR), (*ii*) a 1200–1500 kcal/day balanced deficit diet (BDD) of conventional foods, or (*iii*) a nondieting (ND) approach that discouraged energy restriction. All women attended weekly group sessions for 20 weeks and biweekly sessions for 40 weeks. At week 20, participants in the MR, BDD, and ND groups lost 12.1%, 7.8%, and 0.1% of initial weight ($p < 0.001$). There were no significant differences among the groups in the number of persons who had objective binge eating episodes and symptoms of depression decreased more in the MR and BDD groups than in the ND group. At week 28, significantly more cases of binge eating were observed in the MR group than in the other two groups ($p < 0.003$). However, no differences were observed between groups at weeks 40 or 65, and no participant met criteria for BED at any time. In addition, women in all three groups displayed decreases in hunger and dietary disinhibition and women who received the MR and BDD reported significantly greater reductions in depressive symptoms than women in the ND group.

Moreover, emerging data suggests behavioral weight treatments may be helpful for weight loss in obese patients with binge eating or BED, at least over the short term. For example, at least seven studies have examined VLCDs in obese patients with and without binge eating behavior or BED (114). Taken together, these studies showed that the presence of binge eating did not reduce the effectiveness of VLCD programs for weight loss. Obese patients with and without binge eating lost approximately 20 kg during the dieting program and maintained the weight loss at six months. Most studies also found that BED patients were just as likely to adhere to VLCD programs as were non-BED patients. Two recent studies showed that VLCDs were also associated with significant reductions in binge eating (115,116). However, similar to non-BED subjects, BED subjects regained approximately three-fourths of lost weight at one-year follow-up.

No studies have examined the efficacy of a specialized diet (e.g., low carbohydrate) in obese patients with binge eating behavior or BED. Latner and Wilson (117) conducted a controlled two-week trial of dietary supplementation in 18 women with BED or bulimia nervosa (BN), and found that supplementation with protein was significantly more satiating and more effective in reducing binge eating than supplementation with carbohydrate. Weight gain occurred during both phases, but greater weight gain occurred with carbohydrate (1.1 kg) than protein supplementation (0.3 kg). Although the authors noted the preliminary nature of their findings and the need for further research, they suggested that increasing the level of protein in the diet of patients with BED and BN may help reduce their binge eating in particular and stabilize their eating patterns in general.

Specialized psychotherapies have received some empirical study in obese or overweight patients with BED or binge eating. The goal of CBT in BED is to modify binge-eating behavior with behavioral self-management strategies. The goal of interpersonal therapy (IPT) is to reduce binge eating by reducing interpersonal dysfunction and managing affective dysregulation. CBT and IPT have each been shown to be effective in reducing binge eating, both acutely and for up to 12 months (114,118,119). However, both modalities have been less effective for achieving and maintaining weight loss, although patients who achieve remission in binge eating may experience modest weight loss. For example, in a comparison study of CBT and IPT, after 20 weekly sessions, patients whose binge eating was in remission lost weight (mean BMI-0.5), whereas those who continued to binge gained weight (mean BMI $+0.4$). At 12-month follow-up, patients still in remission continued to lose weight (mean BMI-1.0), whereas those no longer in remission gained weight [mean BMI $+0.7$ ($p = 0.01$)]. Nonetheless, studies comparing CBT with behavioral weight loss treatment in obese patients with BED have generally found that behavioral weight loss is associated with greater weight loss whereas CBT is associated with greater reductions in binge eating (120,121).

Dialectical behavioral therapy (DBT) has also been reported to reduce binge eating in BED. As with CBT and IPT, it appears to be less effective for weight loss. In the only controlled study of DBT in BED, patients achieved an average 2.5-lb weight loss after 20 weeks, compared with an average 0.6-lb weight gain in the control group (122). This difference was not significant, and data on weight loss maintenance were not provided.

Several studies have evaluated combinations of components of behavioral weight management with specialized therapies in obese patients with BED. Two of three trials exploring exercise suggested it may be an effective adjunct for both weight loss and binge eating (123–125). In the first positive study, Pendleton et al. (124) randomized 114 obese women with BED to one of four groups: CBT with exercise and maintenance, CBT with exercise, CBT with maintenance, and CBT only. The CBT component consisted of weekly sessions for four months; the exercise condition included instruction and membership to a fitness center where attendance was recorded; and the maintenance component consisted of 12 biweekly meetings over six months that continued the initial treatment. Eighty-four (71.2%) women completed the study and were evaluated at 16-month follow-up. Subjects who received CBT with exercise showed significant reductions in BMI and binge eating frequency compared with subjects who received CBT only at four months and at the 16-month follow-up. The CBT with exercise and maintenance group had a 58% binge eating remission rate and an average reduction of 2.2 BMI units at the end of the study. BMI was also significantly reduced in the maintenance conditions. The authors concluded that adding exercise to CBT, and extending the duration of treatment, enhanced outcome by reducing both binge eating and BMI.

In the second positive study, Fossati et al. (125) compared CBT combined with a nutritional and physical activity program with CBT alone and CBT with a nutritional program for 12 weeks in 61 obese patients with BED. The nutritional program was focused primarily on fat restriction. The mean weight loss was greater after CBT with nutritional counseling and physical activity (2.8 kg; $p < 0.001$) than after CBT alone (0.3 kg) and after CBT plus nutritional counseling (1.5 kg; $p < 0.01$). There was no weight loss in the CBT alone group. Depression and eating disorder scores decreased in all three groups, but anxiety scores decreased only in the triple therapy group.

However, the combination of CBT and dietary therapy has not been shown to change the waist-to-hip (WHR) and hypothalamic pituitary adrenal axis abnormalities seen in BED with obesity. Gluck et al. (126) compared WHR and cortisol stress responsivity after a cold pressor test (CPT) in 22 obese (BMI > 27) women with and without BED. Although BMI and WHR did not differ between the groups, the BED group ($n = 11$) had higher morning basal cortisol and greater area-under-the-curve (AUC) cortisol after CPT, after controlling for insulin, than the non-BED group. In the BED group ($n = 11$), WHR was related to AUC cortisol and peak cortisol stress responsivity. Ten BED and 10 non-BED patients were randomized to six weeks of CBT and diet or a wait list control. There were no posttreatment differences in the BED group in WHR, morning basal cortisol, or AUC cortisol and the relationships between WHR and both AUC cortisol and peak cortisol stress responsivity remained significant. The authors concluded that BED was associated with HPA hyperactivity that might be related to abdominal obesity and was unresponsive to treatment with CBT and diet.

In sum, available research suggests behavioral weight management is as effective for obese persons with BED as it is for those without BED. There is no evidence binge eating is worsened with such treatment; if anything, binge eating tends to decrease. As with behavioral weight treatment in obese persons without binge eating, however, short-term weight loss is easier to achieve than is the maintenance of long-term weight loss. Exercise may be a promising adjunct for both weight loss and binge eating in obese patients with BED.

REFERENCES

1. National Institutes of Health (National Heart, Lung and Blood Institute). Clinical guidelines on the identification, evaluation and treatment of overweight and obesity in adults. The evidence report. Bethesda, Maryland: National Institutes of Health, 1998.
2. World Health Organization. Obesity: preventing and managing the global epidemic. Geneva: World Health Organization, 1998.
3. Anderson DA, Wadden TA. Treating the obese patient. Suggestions for primary care practice. Arch Fam Med 1999; 8:156–167.
4. Serdula MK, Khan LK, Dietz WH. Weight loss counseling revisited. JAMA 2003; 289:1747–1750.
5. Friedman JM. A war on obesity, not the obese. Science 2003; 299:856–858.
6. Friedman JM. Modern science versus the stigma of obesity. Nat Med 2004; 10:563–569.
7. Hu FB, Willet WC, Li T, et al. Adiposity as compared with physical activity in predicting mortality among women. N Engl J Med 2004; 351:2694–2703.
8. Brownell KD. The LEARN Program for Weight Control Dallas. Texas: American Healm Publishing, 1991.
9. Sarwer DB, Wadden TA. The treatment of obesity: what's new, what's recommended. J Women's Health Gender Based Med 1999; 8:483–493.
10. Wadden TA, Sarwer DB, Berkowitz RI. Behavioral treatment of the overweight patient. Balliére's Clin Endocrinol Metab 1999; 13:93–107.
11. Brownell KD. The LEARN Program for Weight Management 2000. Dallas, Texas: American Health Publishing, 2000.
12. Wadden TA, Foster GD. Behavioral treatment of obesity. Med Clin N Am 2000; 84:441–461.
13. Cooper Z, Fairburn CG, Hawker DM. Cognitive-Behavioral Treatment of Obesity. A Clinician's Guide. New York: The Guilford Press, 2003.
14. Wadden TA, Butryn ML. Behavioral treatment of obesity. Endocrinol Metab Clin N Am 2003; 32:981–1003.
15. Wistosky W, Swencionis C. Cognitive-behavioral approaches in the management of obesity. Adolesc Med 2003; 14:37–49.
16. Wing RR. Behavioral approaches to the treatment of obesity. In: Bray GA, Bouchard C, eds. Handbook of Obesity. Clinical Applications. 2nd ed. New York: Marcel Dekker, 2004:147–167.
17. Institute of Medicine. Weighing the Options: Criteria for Evaluating Weight Management Programs. Washington, DC: Government Printing Office, 1995.
18. Jackic JM, Clark K, Coleman E, et al. American College of Sports Medicine position stand on the appropriate intervention strategies for weight loss and prevention of weight regain for adults. Med Sci Sports Exerc 2001; 33:2145–2156.
19. Wing RR, Hill JO. Successful weight loss maintenance. Annu Rev Nutr 2001; 21:323–341.
20. Blackburn G. Effect of degree of weight loss on health benefits. Obes Res 1995; 3(suppl 2):211S–216S.
21. Tuomilehto J, Lindstrom J, Eriksson JG, et al. Prevention of type 2 diabetes mellitus by changes in lifestyle among subjects with impaired glucose tolerance. N Engl J Med 2001; 344:1343–1350.

22. Lindstrom J, Louheranta A, Mannelin M, et al. The Finnish Diabetes Prevention Study (DPS): Lifestyle intervention and 3-year results on diet and physical activity. Diabetes Care 2003; 26:3230–3236.
23. Lindstrom J, Eriksson JG, Valle TT, et al. Prevention of diabetes mellitus in subjects with impaired glucose tolerance in the Finnish Diabetes Prevention Study: results from a randomized clinical trial. J Am Soc Nephrol 2003; 14(suppl 2):S108–S113.
24. Knowler WC, Barrett-Connor E, Fowler SE, et al. Diabetes Prevention Program Research Group. Reduction in the incidence of type 2 diabetes with lifestyle intervention or metformin. N Engl J Med 2002; 346:393–403.
25. Tuomilehto J, Lindstrom J. The major diabetes prevention trials. Curr Diab Rep 2003; 3:115–122.
26. Freedman MR, King J, Kennedy E. Popular diets: a scientific review. Obesity Res 2001; 9(suppl 1):1S–40S.
27. Ayyad C, Andersen T. Long-term efficacy of dietary treatment of obesity: a systematic review of studies published between 1931 and 1999. Obes Rev 2000; 1:113–119.
28. Pirozzo S, Summerbell C, Cameron C, et al. Advice on Low Fat Diets for Obesity. (cochrane review). The Cochrane Library, Issue 1. Chichester: Wiley, 2004.
29. Foster GD, Wyatt HR, Hill JO, et al. A randomized trial of a low carbohydrate diet for obesity. N Engl J Med 2003; 348:2082–2090.
30. Samaha FF, Igbal N, Seshadri P, et al. A low carbohydrate as compared with a low fat diet in severe obesity. N Engl J Med 2003; 348:2074–2081.
31. Brehm BJ, Seeley RJ, Daniels SR, et al. A randomized trial comparing a very low carbohydrate diet and a caloric-restricted diet on body weight and cardiovascular risk factors in healthy women. J Clin Endocrinol Metab 2003; 88:1617–1623.
32. Stern L, Iqbal N, Seshadri P. The effects of low carbohydrate versus conventional weight loss diets in severely obese adults: one year follow-up of a randomized trial. Arch Intern Med 2004; 140:778–785.
33. Bravata DM, Sanders L, Huang J, et al. Efficacy and safety of low carbohydrate diets: a systematic review. JAMA 2003; 289:1837–1850.
34. Dansinger ML, Gleason JA, Griffith JL, et al. Comparison of the Atkins, Ornish, Weight Watchers, and Zone Diets for weight loss and heart disease reduction. A randomized trial. JAMA 2005; 293:43–53.
35. Howarth NC, Saltzman E, Roberts SB. Dietary fiber and weight regulation. Nutr Rev 2001; 59:129–139.
36. Zemel MB, Miller SL. Dietary calcium and dairy modulation of adiposity and obesity risk. Nutr Rev 2004; 62:125–131.
37. Rolls BJ, Ello-Martin JA, Tohill BC. What can intervention studies tell us about the relationship between fruit and vegetable consumption and weight management? Nutr Rev 2004; 62:1–17.
38. Astrup A, Larson TM, Harper A. Atkins and other low carbohydrate diets: hoax or an effective tool for weight loss? Lancet 2004; 364:897–899.
39. Lara-Castro C, Garvey WT. Diet, insulin resistance, and obesity: zoning in on data for Atkins dieters living in South Beach. J Clin Endocrinol Metab 2004; 89:4197–4205.

40. Harsha DW, Lin PH, Obarzanck E, et al. Dietary approaches to stop hypertension: a summary of study results. DASH collaborative research group. J Am Diet Assoc 1999; 99(suppl 8):535–539.
41. Appel LJ, Champagne CM, Harsha DW, et al. Effects of comprehensive lifestyle modification on blood pressure control: main results of the PREMIER Collaborative Research Group. JAMA 2003; 289:2083–2093.
42. de Lorgeril M, Salen P, Martin JL, et al. Mediterranean diet, traditional risk factors, and the rate of cardiovascular complications after myocardial infarction: final report of the Lyon Diet Heart Study. Circulation 1999; 99:779–785.
43. Singh RB, Dubnov G, Niaz MA, et al. Effect of an Indo-Mediterranean diet on progression of coronary artery disease in high risk patients (Indo-Mediterranean Diet Heart Study): a randomized single-blind trial. Lancet 2002; 360:455–1461.
44. Wing RR. Physical activity in the treatment of the adulthood overweight and obesity: current evidence and research issues. Med Sci Sports Exerc 1999; 31:S547–S552.
45. Fogelholm M, Kukkonen-Harjula K. Does physical activity prevent weight gain—a systematic review. Obes Rev 2000; 1:95–111.
46. Miller WC, Wadden TA. Exercise as a treatment for obesity. In: Bray GA, Bouchard C, eds. Handbook of Obesity. Clinical Applications. 2nd ed. New York: Marcel Dekker, 2004:169–183.
47. Laaksoner DE, Lindstrom J, Lakka TA, et al. Physical activity in the prevention of type 2 diabetes: the Finnish Diabetes Prevention Study. Diabetes 2005; 54:158–165.
48. Jeffrey RW, Wing RR, Sherwood NE, et al. Physical activity and weight loss: does prescribing higher physical activity goals improve outcome. Am J Clin Nutr 2003; 78:684–689.
49. Andersen RE, Wadden TA, Bartlett SJ, et al. Effects of lifestyle activity vs. structured aerobic exercise in obese women: a randomized trial. JAMA 1999; 281:335–340.
50. Dunn AL, Marcus BH, Kampert JB, et al. Comparison of lifestyle and structured interventions to increase physical activity and cardiorespiratory fitness: a randomized trial. JAMA 1999; 281:327–334.
51. Rippe JM, Price JM, Hess SA, et al. Improved psychological well-being, quality of life, and health practices in moderately overweight women participating in a 12-week structured weight loss program. Obes Res 1998; 6:208–218.
52. Heshka S, Anderson JW, Atkinson RL, et al. Weight loss with self help compared with a structured commercial program: a randomized trial. JAMA 2003; 289:1792–1798.
53. Womble LG, Wadden TA, McGuckin BG, et al. A randomized controlled trial of a commercial internet weight loss program. Obes Res 2004; 12: 1011–1018.
54. Tsai AG, Wadden TA. Systematic review: an evaluation of major commercial weight loss programs in the United States. Ann Intern Med 2005; 142:56–66.
55. Bjorvell H, Rossner S. Long term treatment of severe obesity: four year follow-up of results of combined behavioral modification programme. Br Med J 1985; 291:379–382.

56. Bjorvell H, Rossner S. A ten-year follow-up of weight change in severely obese subjects treated in a combined behavioral modification program. Int J Obes Relat Metab Disord 1992; 16:625–634.

57. Djuric Z, DiLaura NM, Jenkins I, et al. Combining weight loss counseling with weight watchers plan for obese breast cancer survivors. Obes Res 2002; 10:657–665.

58. McGuire MX, Wing RR, Klem ML, et al. Behavioral strategies of individuals who have maintained long-term weight losses. Obes Res 1999; 7:334–341.

59. Klem ML, Wing RR, McGuire MT, et al. Psychological symptoms in individuals successful at long-term maintenance of weight loss. Health Psychol 1998; 17:336–345.

60. Wallace B, Tennant C. Nutrition and obesity in the chronically mentally ill. Aust NZ J Psychiatry 1998; 32:82–85.

61. Allison DB, Fontaine KR, Heo M, et al. The distribution of body mass index among individuals with and without schizophrenia. J Clin Psychiatry 1999; 60:215–220.

62. Coodin S. Body mass index in persons with schizophrenia. Can J Psychiatry 2001; 46:549–555.

63. Daumit GL, Clark JM, Steinwachs DM, et al. Prevalence and correlates of obesity in a community sample of individuals with severe and persistent mental illness. J Nerv Men Dis 2003; 191:799–805.

64. Goff DC, Cather C, Evins AE, et al. Medical morbidity and mortality in schizophrenia: guidelines for psychiatrists. J Clin Psychiatry 2005; 66:183–194.

65. Marder SR, Essock SM, Miller AL, et al. Physical health monitoring of patients with schizophrenia. Am J Psychiatry 2004; 161:1334–1349.

66. Barrett E, Blonde L, Clement S, et al. Consensus development conference on antipsychotic drugs and obesity and diabetes. Diabetes Care 2004; 27:596–601.

67. Werneke V, Taylor D, Sanders TA, et al. Behavioral management of antipsychotic-induced weight gain: a review. Acta Psychiatr Scand 2003; 108:252–259.

68. Brar JS, Ganguli R, Pandina G, et al. Effects of behavioral therapy on weight loss in overweight and obese patients with schizophrenia or schizoaffective disorder. J Clin Psychiatry 2005; 66:205–212.

69. Peet M. International variation in the outcome of schizophrenia and the prevalence of depression in relation to national dietary practices: an ecological analysis. Br J Psychiatry 2004; 184:404–408.

70. Peet M. Eicosapentaenoic acid in the treatment of schizophrenia and depression: rationale and preliminary double-blind clinical trial results. Prostaglandins Leukot Essent Fatty Acids 2003; 69:477–485.

71. Peet M. Nutrition and schizophrenia: beyond omega-3 fatty acids. Prostaglandins Leukot Essent Fatty Acids 2004; 70:417–422.

72. Archie S, Wilson JH, Osbome S, et al. Pilot study: access to fitness facility and exercise levels in olanzapine-treated patients. Can J Psychiatry 2003; 48:628–632.

73. Fogarty M, Happell B, Pinikahana J. The benefits of an exercise program for people with schizophrenia: a pilot study. Psychiatr Rehabil J 2004; 28:173–176.

74. Mueser KT, McGurk SR. Schizophrenia. Lancet 2004; 363:2063–2072.

75. Knoblich G, Stottmeister F, Kircher T. Self monitoring in patients with schizophrenia. Psychol Med 2004; 34:1561–1569.

76. Eckman TA, Wirshing WC, Marder SR, et al. Technique for training schizophrenic patients in illness self-management: a controlled trial. Am J Psychiatry 1992; 149:1549–1555.
77. Mueser KT, Corrigan PW, Hilton DW, et al. Illness management and recovery: a review of the research. Psychiatr Serv 2002; 53:1272–1284.
78. Scott J, Kingdon D, Turkington D. Cognitive-behavior therapy for schizophrenia. In: Wright JA, ed. Cognitive-Behavior Therapy. Washington, DC: American Psychiatric Publishing, 2004:1–24.
79. Rotatori AF, Fox R, Wicks A. Weight loss with psychiatric residents in a behavioral self control program. Psychol Rep 1980; 46:483–486.
80. Ball MP, Coons VB, Buchanan RW. A program for treating olanzapine-related weight gain. Psychiatr Serv 2001; 52:967–969.
81. Menza M, Vreelaad B, Minsky S, et al. Managing atypical antipsychotic-associated weight gain: 12-month data on a multimodal weight control program. J Clin Psychiatry 2004; 65:471–477.
82. Littrell KH, Petty RG, Hilligross NM, et al. The effects of an educational intervention on antipsychotic-induced-weight gain. J Nur Scholarship 2003; 35:237–241.
83. McElroy SL, Kotwal R, Malhotra S, et al. Are mood disorders and obesity related? A review for the mental health professional. J Clin Psychiatry 2004; 65:634–651.
84. Stunkard AJ, Rush J. Dieting and depression reexamined. A critical review of reports of untoward responses during weight reduction for obesity. Ann Intern Med 1974; 81:526–533.
85. Wing RR, Epstein LH, Marcus MD, et al. Mood changes in behavioral weight loss programs. J Psychosom Res 1984; 25:189–196.
86. Smoller JW, Wadden TA, Stunkard AJ. Dieting and depression: a critical review. J Psychosom Res 1987; 31:429–440.
87. Clark MM, Maura R, King TK, et al. Depression, smoking, activity level, and health status: pretreatment predictors of attrition in obesity treatment. Addict Behav 1996; 21:509–513.
88. Linde JA, Jeffery RW, Levy RL, et al. Binge eating disorder, weight control self-efficacy and depression in overweight men and women. Int J Obes Relat Metab Disord 2004; 28:418–425.
89. Zeller M, Kirk S, Claytor R, et al. Predictors of attrition from a pediatric weight management program. J Pediatr 2004; 144:466–470.
90. Marcus MD, Wing RR, Guare J, et al. Lifetime prevalence of major depression and its effect on treatment outcome in obese type II diabetic patients. Diabetes Care 1992; 15:253–255.
91. Jenkins I, Djuric Z, Darga L, et al. Relationship of psychiatric diagnosis and weight loss maintenance in obese breast cancer survivors. Obes Res 2003; 11:1369–1375.
92. Casper RC. Nutrients, neurodevelopment, and mood. Cur Psychiatry Rep 2004; 6:425–429.
93. Hibbeln JR. Fish consumption and major depression. Lancet 1998; 351:1213.
94. Timonen M, Horrobin D, Jokelainen J, et al. Fish consumption and depression: the Northern Finland 1966 birth cohort study. J Affect Disord 2004; 82:447–452.

95. Su KP, Huang SY, Chiu CC, et al. Omega-3 fatty acids in major depressive disorder. A preliminary double-blind, placebo-controlled trial. Eur Neuropsychopharmacol 2003; 13:267–271.

96. Anderson IM, Parry-Billings M, Newsholme EA, et al. Dieting reduces plasma tryptophan and alters brain 5-HT function in women. Psychol Med 1990; 20:785–791.

97. Goodwin GM, Fairburn CG, Cowen PJ. Dieting changes serotonergic function in women, not men: implications for the etiology of anorexia nervosa? Psychol Med 1987; 17:839–842.

98. Walsh AES, Oldman AD, Franklin M, et al. Dieting decreases plasma tryptophan and increases prolactin response to D-fenfluramine in women but not men. J Affect Disord 1995; 33:89–97.

99. Cowen PJ, Clifford EM, Walsh AE, et al. Moderate dieting causes 5-HT$_{2C}$ receptor supersensitivity. Psychol Med 1996; 26:1155–1199.

100. Smith KA, Williams C, Cowen PJ. Impaired regulation of brain serotonin function during dieting in women recovered from depression. Br J Psychiatry 2000; 176:72–75.

101. Wright JH, Beck AT, Thase ME. Cognitive therapy. In: Hales RE, Yudofsky SC, Talbott JA, eds. The American Psychiatric Publishing Textbook of Clinical Psychiatry. 4th ed. Washington, DC: American Psychiatric Publishing, 2003:1245–1284.

102. Lawlor DA, Hopker SW. The effectiveness of exercise as an intervention in the management of depression: systematic review and meta-regression analysis of randomized controlled trials. BMJ 2001; 322:763–767.

103. Craft LL, Perna FM. The benefits of exercise for the clinically depressed. Prim Care Companion J Clin Psychiatry 2004; 6:104–111.

104. Hensley PL, Nadiga D, Uhylenhuth EH. Long-term effectiveness of cognitive therapy in major depressive disorder. Depress Anxiety 2004; 20:1–7.

105. Lam DH, Watkins ER, Hayward P, et al. A randomized controlled study of cognitive therapy for relapse prevention for bipolar affective disorder: outcome of the first year. Arch Gen Psychiatry 2003; 60:145–152.

106. Zaretsky A. Targeted psychosocial interventions for bipolar disorder. Bipolar Disord 2003; 5(suppl 2):80–87.

107. Dunn AL, Trivedi MH, Kampert JB, et al. Efficacy treatment for depression: efficacy and dose response. Am J Prev Med 2005; 28:1–8.

108. de Zwaan M. Binge eating disorder and obesity. Int J Obes Relat Metab Disord 2001; 25(suppl 1):S51–S55.

109. Dingemans AE, Bruna MJ, van Furth EF. Binge eating disorder: a review. Int J Obes Relat Metab Disord 2002; 26:299–307.

110. Devlin MJ, Goldfein JA, Dobrow I. What is this thing called BED? Current status of binge eating disorder nosology. Int J Eat Disord 2003; 34(suppl): S2–S18.

111. Srunkard AJ, Allison KC. Two forms of disordered eating in obesity: binge eating and night eating. Int J Obes 2003; 27:1–12.

112. National Task Force on the Prevention and Treatment of Obesity. Dieting and the development of eating disorders in overweight and obese adults. Arch Intern Med 2000; 160:2581–2589.

113. Wadden TA, Foster GA, Sarwer DB, et al. Dieting and development of eating disorders in women: results of a randomized controlled trial. Am J Clin Nutr 2004; 800:560–565.

114. Wonderlich SA, de Zwaan M, Mitchell JE, et al. Psychological and dietary treatments of binge eating disorder: conceptual implications. Int J Eat Disord 2003; 34(suppl):S58–S78.

115. Raymond NC, deZwaan M, Mitchell JE, et al. Effect of a very low calorie diet on the diagnostic category of individuals with binge eating disorder. Int J Eat Disord 2002; 31:49–56.

116. deZwaan M, Mitchell IE, Mussell MP, et al. Short-term cognitive behavioral treatment does not improve outcome on a comprehensive very low calorie diet program in obese women with binge eating disorder, cited in Wonderlich et al., Int J Eat Disord 2003; 34(suppl):S56–S78.

117. Latner ID, Wilson GT. Binge eating and satiety in bulimia nervosa and binge eating disorder: effects of macronutrient intake. Int J Eat Disord 2004; 36: 402–415.

118. Wilfley DE, Welch RR, Stein RI, et al. A randomized comparison of group cognitive-behavioral therapy and group interpersonal psychotherapy for the treatment of overweight individuals with binge eating disorder. Arch Gen Psychiatry 2002; 59:713–721.

119. Grilo CM, Masheb RM, Wilson GT. Efficacy of cognitive behavioral therapy and fluoxetine for the treatment of binge eating disorder: a randomized double-blind placebo controlled comparison. Biol Psychiatry 2005; 57:301–309.

120. Agras WS, Telch DF, Arnow B, et al. Weight loss, cognitive-behavioral, and desipramine treatments in binge eating disorder. An additive design. Behav Ther 1994; 25:225–238.

121. Nauta H, Hospers H, Kok G, et al. A comparison between a cognitive and a behavioral treatment for obese binge eaters and obese non-binge eaters. Behav Ther 2000; 31:441–461.

122. Telch CF, Agras WS, Linehan MM. Dialectical behavior therapy for binge eating disorder. J Consult Clin Psychol 2001; 69:1061–1065.

123. Levine MD, Marcus MD, Moulton P. Exercise in the treatment of binge eating disorder. Int J Eat Disord 1996; 19:171–177.

124. Pendleton VR, Goodrick GK, Poston WSC, et al. Exercise augments the effects of cognitive-behavioral therapy in the treatment of binge eating. Int J Eat Disord 2002; 31(2):172–184.

125. Fossati M, Amati F, Painot D, et al. Cognitive-behavioral therapy with simultaneous nutritional and physical activity education in obese patients with binge eating disorder. Eat Weight Disord 2004; 9:134–138.

126. Gluck ME, Geliebter A, Lorence M. Cortisol stress response is positively correlated with central obesity in obese women with binge eating disorder before and after cognitive-behavior treatment. Ann NY Acad Sci 2004; 1032:202–207.

12

Pharmacologic Agents in the Treatment of Obesity

Donna H. Ryan

*Pennington Biomedical Research Center, Louisiana State University,
Baton Rouge, Louisiana, U.S.A.*

INTRODUCTION

The purpose of this chapter is to review the data supporting the safety and efficacy of appetite suppressants, lipase inhibitors, anticonvulsants, antidepressants, and other agents in the treatment of obesity. There are currently two approved medications for long-term obesity management, although it is not unusual in clinical practice for medications to be prescribed "off label" to achieve weight loss. Furthermore, an intensive effort is underway by many pharmaceutical companies to bring more agents to market against a growing epidemic of obesity and its comorbidities, particularly type 2 diabetes. The noradrenergic drugs phentermine, diethylpropion, benzphetamine, and phendimetrazine are approved only for short-term use. Sibutramine, a norepinephrine–serotonin reuptake inhibitor, is approved for long-term use. Also approved for long-term use is orlistat, which inhibits pancreatic lipase and can block hydrolysis of 30% of the dietary triglyceride in subjects eating a 30% fat diet. A growing trend is the use of antidepressants and anticonvulsants (bupropion, topiramate, and zonisamide) for weight management and the review will cover the evidence supporting their weight loss effects. Several newer drugs (rimonibant, axokine) in clinical trials investigation will also be discussed. Despite limitations in the number and efficacy of current medications, the future prospects for obesity pharmacotherapy are optimistic.

Medicating for treatment of obesity can be a useful adjunct to diet and exercise and can help selected patients achieve and maintain meaningful weight loss. A report from the National Heart, Lung and Blood Institute of the NIH entitled *Clinical Guidelines on the Identification, Evaluation, and Treatment of Overweight and Obesity in Adult—The Evidence Report* emphasizes the need for physicians to address obesity in their patients (1). The *Guidelines* sanction the clinical use of weight loss drugs approved by the food and drug administration (FDA) for long-term use as part of a concomitant lifestyle modification program. Currently, this would include only sibutramine (trade-named Meridia or Reductil) or orlistat (Xenical). According to the *Guidelines*, medications are appropriate for those patients who have been unsuccessful in previous weight loss attempts and whose body mass index (BMI) exceeds $27 \, \text{kg/m}^2$ who have associated conditions such as diabetes, hypertension, or dyslipidemia, or whose BMI exceeds $30 \, \text{kg/m}^2$. Still, for many physicians, treatment of obesity is not a routine part of their clinical practices, and the majority of medications prescribed for weight loss are not those recommended as superior choices by the guidelines.

Drug treatment for obesity has been tarnished by a number of unfortunate problems (2). Since the introduction of thyroid hormone to treat obesity in 1893, almost every drug that has been tried in obese patients has led to undesirable outcomes that have resulted in their termination. Thus, caution must be used in accepting any new drugs for treatment of obesity, unless the safety profile would make it acceptable for almost everyone. The most recent medical disaster was the reports of valvular heart disease associated with the use of fenfluramine and dexfenfluramine (3–5). These drugs are potent releasers of serotonin and are associated with heart valve damage similar to that seen in carcinoid syndrome. Thankfully, the extent of the problem has not proven to be as great as first suspected (4,5). It is now recognized that risk for valvulopathy associated with fenfluramine is associated with duration of exposure to the medication and that the lesions are likely to remit off medication (4–7). The finding, however, will add caution when any future drugs are marketed to treat obesity and will provide support for those who believe drug treatment of obesity is inappropriate and risky.

Another issue to be considered is the way that all weight loss medications have been viewed as having the addictive properties of amphetamine (8). Abuse of either phentermine or diethylpropion is rare and sibutramine has evidence of abuse potential (2,9).

Another misconception about drug treatment of obesity is that the drugs are ineffective because weight regain occurs when drug treatment is stopped (10). Surgeries for obesity such as gastric bypass and gastric banding have been demonstrated in one large registry study to produce >16% weight loss from baseline that is sustained for up to 10 years from baseline (11,12). As long as the treatment is enforced (the surgical band in place and the restrictive and malabsorptive modifications to gastrointestinal architecture unchanged) weight loss will be maintained. If the surgery is reversed, weight regain occurs. As clinicians, we do not expect to cure such diseases as hypertension or hypercholesterolemia with medications. Rather, we expect to palliate them. When the medications for any of these diseases are discontinued, we expect the disease to recur. This means that medications only work when used. Of the currently available medications used for weight management, a chronic approach to treatment is required.

Two final misconceptions must be addressed regarding pharmacotherapy for obesity. A weight loss of less than 15% is considered unsatisfactory by most obese patients (12). Yet the reality is that *none* of our current treatment approaches, except gastric bypass, produce a consistent weight loss of >15% for the average patient (13). When weight loss plateaus at a level above their desired cosmetic goal, patients usually stop medications. Patients seem to want to take medications to lose weight, but do not seem willing to take medications to maintain modest weight losses.

Last to consider is the lack of appreciation for the meaningful health benefits produced by sustained weight loss, even though only 5% to 10% from baseline. Loss of 5% to 10% in the obese can translate into improvement in glycemic control, [important, considering the epidemic of diabetes (14)] improvement in blood pressure and hypertension control, and improvements in lipid profile, in symptoms of sleep apnea, arthritis, and other comorbid conditions (1). Furthermore, modest weight loss can translate into reduction in morbidity. Weight loss of 7% from baseline produced a 58% reduction in risk for developing type 2 diabetes over two to five years in individuals with impaired glucose tolerance (15). Similar diabetes risk reduction with modest weight loss has been demonstrated in the Finnish Diabetes Prevention Program (16).

Physicians must be cognizant of these misconceptions; they are barriers to success. It is against these limitations that the review examines medications currently in use for obesity management in primary care practice settings. Table 1 describes the medications that will be discussed.

DRUGS APPROVED BY THE FDA WITH AN INDICATION FOR WEIGHT MANAGEMENT

There are only two agents currently available with FDA approval and an obesity indication for long term use—orlistat and sibutramine. Some older agents are still available in the United States and approved for short-term use, i.e., "a few weeks." Those older agents include diethylpropion, phentermine, benzphetamine, and phendimetrizme.

Table 1 Drugs Approved by the FDA for Treatment of Obesity

Drug	Trade names	Dosage	DBA schedule
Pancreatic lipase inhibitor approved for long-term use			
Orlistat	Xenical	120 mg tid before meals	–
Norepinephrine serotonin reuptake inhibitor approved for long-term use			
Sibutramine	Meridia	5–15 mg/day	IV
	Reductil		
Noradrenergic drugs approved for short-term use			
Diethylpropion	Tenuate	25 mg tid	IV
Phentermine	Adipex-P	15–37.5 mg/day	IV
	Ionamin slow release	15–30 mg/day	
Benzphetamine	Didrex	25–50 mg tid	III
Phendimetrazine	Bontril	17.5–70 mg tid	III
	Prelu-2		
Medications used off-label for weight management			
Topiramate	Topamax	50–200 mg/day	–
Zonisamide	Zonegran	400–600 mg/day	–
Fluoxetine[a]	Prozac	60 mg/day	–
	Sarafem		
Bupropion	Wellbutrin	400 mg/day	–
Venlafaxine	Effexor	75–225 mg/day	–

[a]Weight loss efficacy is only demonstrated for a few weeks and then weight regain occurs on fluoxetine.
Abbreviation: FDA, food and drug administration.

Phentermine, Diethylpropion, Benzphetamine, Phendimetrazine, and Mazindol

This group of agents have been available in the U.S. market for more than 30 years. The published clinical data supporting their safety and efficacy consists of a few studies, each enrolling a few patients and most studies are of short duration. Only a handful of clinical trials for this group equals or exceeds 24 weeks duration. By far, phentermine is the most popular drug in this group and the others are not widely available. Phentermine is the most frequently prescribed weight loss agent in the United States, probably because it is inexpensive, since it is no longer protected by patent.

The best and one of the longest of the clinical trials reporting phentermine's weight loss efficacy lasted 36 weeks and compared placebo treatment against continuous phentermine or intermittent phentermine (Fig. 1) (17). The intermittent regimen was four weeks of phentermine 15 mg/day followed by four weeks of placebo. This was compared to continuous phentermine at 15 mg/day or placebo. Both continuous and intermittent phentermine therapy produced more weight loss than did placebo. In the drug-free

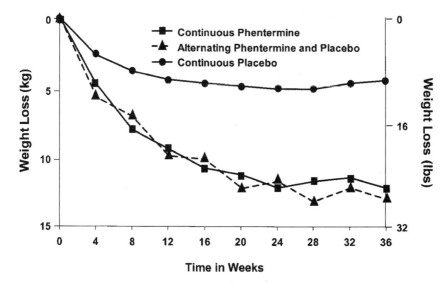

Figure 1 Comparison of weight loss with continuous and intermittent therapy using phentermine. Overweight patients were randomized to receive either placebo or one of two dosing-regimens with phentermine. One regimen provided 15 mg/day each morning for nine months and the other provided 15 mg/day for one month and then a month of no treatment. *Source*: From Ref. 17.

periods the patients treated intermittently slowed their weight loss only to lose more rapidly when the drug was reinstituted. As can be observed in Figure 1, intermittent phentermine produced comparable weight loss to continuous phentermine.

Phentermine and diethylpropion are classified by the U.S. Drug Enforcement Agency as schedule IV drugs, and benzphetamine and phendimetrazine as schedule III drugs, although states may schedule these agents differently. This regulatory classification indicates the government's belief that they have the potential for abuse, although this potential appears to be very low. Phentermine and diethylpropion are only approved for a "few weeks" use, which is usually interpreted as up to 12 weeks. Weight loss with phentermine and diethylpropion persists for the duration of treatment, suggesting that tolerance does not develop to these drugs. If tolerance were to develop, the drugs would be expected to lose their effectiveness or require increased amounts of drug for patients to maintain weight loss. This does not occur. Phentermine is not available in Europe. A review in a prestigious journal recommends obtaining written informed consent if phentermine is prescribed for longer than 12 weeks, because this is off-label usage and there are not sufficient published reports on the use of phentermine for long-term use (18).

The side effect profile for sympathomimetic drugs is similar (1). They produce insomnia, dry mouth, asthenia, and constipation. Sympathomimetic drugs can also increase blood pressure.

Sibutramine (Meridia®, Reductil in Europe)

In contrast to the older sympathomimetic drugs in Table 1, sibutramine has been extensively evaluated in several large-scale multicenter trials lasting 6 to 24 months conducted in men and women of all ethnic groups with ages ranging from 18 to 65 years and with a BMI between 27 and 40 kg/m^2. Sibutramine's clinical research history has been recently reviewed (19).

There is a dose–response effect with sibutramine. In a six-month dose-ranging study of 1047 patients, 67% of sibutramine treated patients achieved a 5% weight loss and 35% lost 10% or more. Data from this multicenter trial are shown in Figure 2 (20,21). There is a clear dose–response in this 24-week trial, and regain of weight occurred when the drug was stopped, indicating that the drug remained effective when used.

In another interesting study by virtue of the magnitude of weight lost, patients who initially lost weight eating a very low calorie diet were

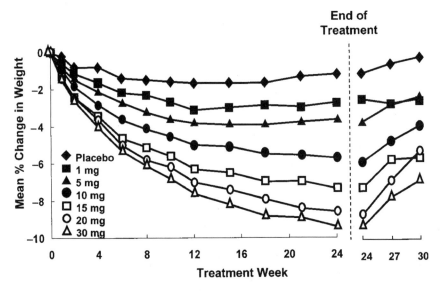

Figure 2 Dose-related weight loss with sibutramine. A total of 1047 patients were randomly assigned to receive placebo or one of six doses of sibutramine in a double-blind fashion for six months. By the end of the trial of sibutramine treated patients, weight loss had plateaued for most doses. When the drug was discontinued at six months, weight was regained, indicating that the drug remained effective during treatment. *Source*: From Ref. 35.

randomized to sibutramine 10 mg/day or placebo, and behavioral program. Sibutramine produced additional weight loss (−16% from baseline at 1 year), whereas the placebo-treated patients regained weight (22). These results indicate that the response to sibutramine is dependent on the intensity of the behavioral approaches that are used with sibutramine. By combining a very low calorie diet and intensive behavioral therapy along with sibutramine, the total weight loss at one year was quite impressive.

A number of observations about sibutramine can be drawn from the Sibutramine Trial of Obesity Reduction and Maintenance (STORM Trial), but the effects of sibutramine in aiding weight maintenance are the most persuasive aspect of the trial (23). Seven centers participated in this trial where 605 patients were initially enrolled in an open-label fashion and treated with 10 mg/day of sibutramine for six months (Fig. 3). Those patients who lost more than 5% (and 77% of enrolled patients met this goal) were then randomized, two-thirds to sibutramine and one-third to placebo. During the 18-month double-blind portion of the trial, the placebo-treated patients steadily regained weight, maintaining only 20% of their weight loss at the end of the trial. In contrast, the subjects treated with sibutramine maintained their weight for 12 months and then regained an average of only 2 kg, thus maintaining 80% of their initial weight loss after two years (24). In spite of the difference in weight at the end of the 18 months of controlled observation, the mean blood pressure of the sibutramine-treated patients

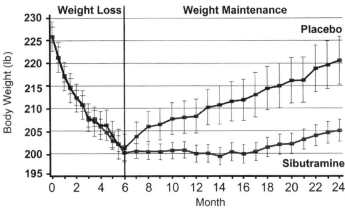

*Same diet, exercise for sibutramine, placebo;
$p \leq 0.001$, sibutramine vs. placebo for weight maintenance

Figure 3 The Sibutramine Trial of Obesity Reduction and Maintenance (STORM). In the six-month weight loss period, 605 patients received sibutramine 10 mg/day. At six months, 352 patients were randomized to receive placebo. Both groups received the same diet and exercise counseling. There was a dose titration allowed to a maximum of 20 mg/day sibutramine. *Source*: From Ref. 38.

was still higher than in the patients treated with placebo, even though they had a weight difference of several kilograms.

Sibutramine given continuously for one year has been compared to placebo and sibutramine given intermittently (25). In this study (Fig. 4), patients who had lost −2% or −2 kg after four weeks of treatment with sibutramine 15 mg/day were randomized to placebo as continued sibutramine versus sibutramine prescribed intermittently (weeks 1–12, 19–30, and 37–48). Both sibutramine treatment regimens gave equivalent results and were significantly better than placebo. As illustrated in Figure 4, the effect of stopping sibutramine results in small increases in weight, which is then reversed when the medication is restarted.

Four clinical trials document sibutramine use in patients with diabetes. One was for 12 weeks and the other three studies were for 24 weeks (24,26–28). In the 12-week trial, diabetic patients treated with sibutramine 15 mg/day lost −2.4 kg (2.8%) compared to −0.1 kg (0.12%) in the placebo group (29). In this study, Hemoglobin A1c (HbA1c) fell −0.3% in the drug-treated group and remained stable in the placebo-treated group. In the study by Gockel et al. (27)

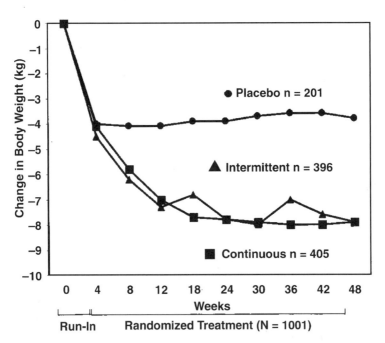

Figure 4 Sibutramine given intermittently or continuously compared to placebo. Mean (SE) change in body weight during the study period. Patients (*n* = 1102) received sibutramine 15 mg/day. Those who lost 2% or 2 kg in four weeks were randomized to placebo (*n* = 395) versus continued sibutramine (*n* = 405) versus intermittent sibutramine (weeks 1–12,19–30, and 37–48) (*n* = 395). *Source*: From Ref. 25.

60 female patients who had poorly controlled glucose levels (HbA1c > 8%) on maximal doses of sulfonylureas and metformin were randomly assigned to sibutramine 10 mg twice daily or placebo. The weight loss at 24 weeks was −9.6 kg in the sibutramine treated patients and −0.9 kg in those on placebo. The improvements in glycemic control were equally striking. In the sibutramine-treated patients, HbA1c fell −2.73% compared to −0.53% with the placebo. Insulin levels fell −5.66 U/mL compared to −0.68 U/mL for placebo and fasting glucose fell −124.88 mg/mL compared to −15.76 mg/mL for placebo. While the weight loss in most of the studies of patients with diabetes does not appear as great as in nondiabetic patients, in all of the studies the percentage of patients who achieved weight loss ≥5% from baseline was significantly greater than placebo. In all studies the degree of weight loss corresponds to the degree of improvement in glycemic control.

Two trials have been reported using sibutramine to treat hypertensive patients over one year, and two additional studies provide data on 12 weeks of treatment (21,30–32). In all instances, the weight loss pattern favors sibutramine. However, except for one study, mean weight loss, though favorable, was associated with small increases in mean blood pressure (31). In a three-month trial all patients were receiving β-blockers with or without thiazides for their hypertension (32). The sibutramine-treated patients lost −4.2 kg (4.5%) compared to a loss of −0.3 kg (0.3%) in the placebo-treated group. Mean supine and standing diastolic and systolic blood pressure were not significantly different between drug-treated and placebo-treated patients. Heart rate, however, increased +5.6 ± 8.25 (M ± SD) bpm in the sibutramine-treated patients as compared to an increase in heart rate of +2.2 ± 6.43 (M ± SD) bpm in the placebo group.

McMahon et al. (21) reported a 52-week trial in hypertensive patients whose blood pressure was controlled with calcium channel blockers with or without β-blockers or thiazides. Sibutramine doses were increased from 5 to 20 mg/day during the first six weeks. Weight loss was significantly greater in the sibutramine-treated patients, averaging −4.4 kg (4.7%) as compared to −0.5 kg (0.7%) in the placebo-treated group. Diastolic BP decreased −1.3 mmHg in the placebo-treated group and increased by +2.0 mmHg in the sibutramine-treated group. The SBP increased +1.5 mmHg in the placebo-treated group and by +2.7 in the sibutramine-treated group. Heart rate was unchanged in the placebo-treated patients, and increased +4.9 bpm in the sibutramine-treated patients (21). One small study in eight obese men demonstrated that an aerobic exercise program mitigated the adverse blood pressure effects of sibutramine (33).

Since the dose of sibutramine influences the amount of weight loss with the drug, the intensity of the behavioral component is also likely to have an effect (21,28). This is readily demonstrated in a study by Wadden (34). With minimal behavioral intervention, the weight loss in that study was about 5 kg over 12 months. When group counseling to produce behavior modification was added to sibutramine the weight loss increased to 10 kg, and when a structured meal plan using meal replacements was added to the medication and behavior plan, the weight loss increased further to −15 kg (34). This indicates that the amount of weight loss observed during pharmacotherapy is due in part to the intensity of the behavioral approach.

Sibutramine is available in 5, 10, and 15 mg pills; 10 mg/day as a single daily dose is the recommended starting level with titration up or down based on response. Doses above 15 mg/day are not recommended by the FDA. The chance of achieving meaningful weight loss can be determined by the response to treatment in the first four weeks. In one large trial, of the patients who lost −2 kg (−4 lb) in the first four weeks of treatment, 60% achieved a weight loss of more than 5%, compared to less than 10% of those who did not lose−2 kg (−4 lb) in four weeks (21,35). Except for blood pressure, weight loss with sibutramine is associated with improvement in profiles of cardiovascular risk factors. Combining data from the total of 11 studies on sibutramine showed a weight-related reduction in triglyceride, total cholesterol, and LDL cholesterol and a weight loss related rise in HDL cholesterol that was related to the magnitude of the weight loss (36).

Sibutramine should not be used in patients with a history of coronary artery disease, congestive heart failure, cardiac arrhythmias, or stroke. There should be a two-week interval between termination of monoamine oxidase inhibitors (MAOIs) and beginning sibutramine. Sibutramine should be used only with caution with selective serotonin reuptake inhibitors (SSRIs). Because sibutramine is metabolized by the cytochrome P_{450} enzyme system (isozyme CYP3A4) when drugs like erythromycin and ketoconazole are taken, there may be competition for this enzymatic pathway and prolonged metabolism can result.

There are two issues to consider regarding blood pressure management and sibutramine use. The first is the development of clinically significant blood pressure elevations. Individual blood pressure responses to sibutramine are quite variable. From the studies reviewed, withdrawals for clinically significant blood pressure increase are usually 2% to 5% of participants in the trial. Higher doses tend to produce higher withdrawal rates, thus lower doses are preferred (35). The other issue with blood pressure increases is the small mean increase of 2 to 4 mmHg in systolic and diastolic blood pressure that occurs in sibutramine treated patients versus controls. Weight loss is usually associated with improvement in risk factors for cardiovascular disease (blood pressure, lipids, measures of glycemic control). If sibutramine has mixed effects on risk factors, with improvement in some (lipids, glycemic control) but slight worsening of others, then the prescribing physician must use judgment in the decision to continue sibutramine.

Managing potential increases in blood pressure should be a part of the sibutramine treatment plan. Evaluation of blood pressure two to four weeks after starting sibutramine is recommended. The initial dose is usually 10 mg/day. About 5% of patients who take sibutramine will have unacceptable increases in blood pressure and for them, the medication should be stopped.

Orlistat (Xenical®)

Orlistat is a potent selective inhibitor of pancreatic lipase that reduces intestinal digestion of fat. The drug has a dose-dependent effect on fecal fat loss, increasing it to about 30% of ingested fat on a diet that has 30% of energy as fat (37). Orlistat has little effect in subjects eating a low-fat diet, as might be anticipated from the mechanism by which this drug works (37).

A number of long-term clinical trials with orlistat lasting six months to four years have been published, and these have been reviewed recently (38).

The results of one two-year trial are shown in Figure 5 (9). The trial consisted of two parts. In the first year patients received a hypocaloric diet calculated to be 500 kcal/day below the patient's requirements. During the second year the diet was calculated to maintain weight. By the end of year one the placebo-treated patients lost −6.1% of their initial body weight and

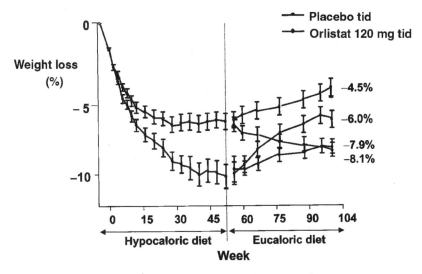

Figure 5 Orlistat and body weight change over two years of treatment. A total of 743 patients were randomized to receive either orlistat 120 mg three times daily or placebo for the first year and were then re-randomized to the same groups for a second year. Following the four-week single-blind (SB) run in, the first double-blind (DB) period utilized a diet that was calculated to be 600 kcal/day below maintenance, and the second DB period used a diet that was intended to maintain body weight. *Source*: From Ref. 39.

the drug-treated patients lost −10.2%. The patients were re-randomized at the end of year one. Those switched from orlistat to placebo gained weight from −10% to −6.0% below baseline. Those switched from placebo to orlistat lost from −6% to −8.1%, which was essentially identical to the −7.9% in the patients treated with orlistat for the full two years.

In a second two-year study, 892 patients were randomized (40). One group remained on placebo throughout the two years ($n = 97$ completers) and a second group remained on orlistat 120 mg three times a day for two years ($n = 109$ completers). At the end of one year, two-thirds of the group treated with orlistat for one year were changed to orlistat 60 mg three times a day ($n = 102$ completers) and the others to placebo ($n = 95$ completers) (40). After one year, the weight loss was −8.67 kg in the orlistat-treated group and −5.81 kg in the placebo group ($p < 0.001$). During the second year, those switched to placebo after one year reached the same weight as those treated with placebo for two years (−4.5% in those with placebo for two years and −4.2% in those switched from orlistat to placebo during year two).

In a third two-year study, 783 patients enrolled in a trial where, for two years, they remained in the placebo group or one of two orlistat-treated groups at 60 or 120 mg three times a day (40,41). After one year with a weight loss diet, the completers in the placebo group lost −7.0 kg, which was significantly less than the −9.6 kg in the completers treated with orlistat 60 mg thrice daily or −9.8 kg in the completers treated with orlistat 120 mg thrice daily. During the second year when the diet was liberalized to a "weight maintenance" diet, all three groups regained some weight. At the end of two years, the completers in the placebo group were −4.3 kg below baseline, the completers treated with orlistat 60 mg three times daily were −6.8 kg and the completers treated with orlistat 120 mg three times daily were −7.6 kg below baseline.

Another two-year trial that has been published was carried out on 796 subjects in a general practice setting (42). After one year of treatment with orlistat 120 mg/day, completers ($n = 117$) had lost −8.8 kg compared to −4.3 kg in the placebo completers ($n = 91$). During the second year when the diet was liberalized to "maintain body weight," both groups regained some weight. At the end of two years, the orlistat group receiving 120 mg three times daily was 5.2 kg below their baseline weight compared to −1.5 kg for the group treated with placebo. The percent change in body weight over two years of orlistat at 60 and 120 mg is depicted in Figure 6 which represents pooled data from multiple studies extracted from the integrated database of volunteers treated in a general practice setting.

Weight maintenance with orlistat was evaluated in a one-year study (43). Patients were enrolled who lost more than 8% of their body weight over six months eating a 1000 kcal/day (4180 kJ/day) diet. The 729 patients were one of four groups randomized to receive either placebo or 30, 60, or 120 mg of orlistat three times a day for 12 months. At the end of this time

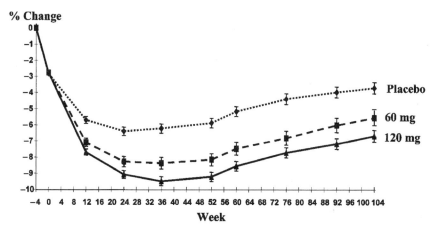

Figure 6 Orlistat in primary care practices. Percent change from initial body weight over two years of treatment. Data derived from an integrated data base. *Source*: From Ref. 37.

the placebo-treated patients had regained 56% of their body weight, compared to 32.4% in the group treated with orlistat, 120 mg three times a day. The other two doses of orlistat were not statistically different from placebo in preventing the regain of weight.

The modest weight reduction observed with orlistat treatment may have a beneficial effect on lipids and lipoproteins. Orlistat seems to have an independent effect on LDL cholesterol. From a meta-analysis of the data relating orlistat to lipids in five double-blind, randomized, placebo-controlled studies, orlistat-treated subjects had almost twice as much reduction in LDL cholesterol as their placebo-treated counterparts for the same weight loss category reached after one year (44).

One study is representative of the effects of orlistat on weight loss and on cardiovascular risk factors, particularly serum lipids, in obese patients with hypercholesterolemia (45). The main findings were that orlistat promoted clinically significant weight loss and reduced LDL-C in obese patients with elevated cholesterol levels more than could be attributed to weight loss alone. Another study, the ObelHyx study, demonstrates an additional 10% LDL-C lowering in obese subjects with baseline elevated LDL-C levels compared to placebo (46).

Orlistat's independent cholesterol-lowering effect probably reflects a reduction in intestinal absorption of cholesterol. Since lipase inhibition by orlistat prevents the absorption of approximately 30% of dietary fat, the prescribed diet of 30% of energy from fat would thus become in effect a 20% to 24% of available fat in the diet when associated with orlistat treatment. It has been hypothesized that inhibition of gastrointestinal lipase activity may lead to retention of cholesterol in the gut through a reduction in the amount of fatty acids and monoglycerides absorbed from the gut, and/or may lead to sequestration of cholesterol within a more persistent oil-phase in the intestine. Partial inhibition of intestinal fat and cholesterol absorption probably leads to decreased hepatic cholesterol and saturated fatty acid concentration, upregulation of hepatic LDL receptors, and decreased LDL-C levels.

The orlistat-treated subjects in trials lasting for at least one year were analyzed by Heymsfield et al. (47), who found that orlistat reduced the conversion of impaired glucose tolerance (IGT) to diabetes and that the transition from normal to impaired glucose tolerance was also reduced in subjects treated with orlistat for one year. In orlistat-treated subjects the conversion from normal glucose tolerance to diabetes occurred in 6.6% of patients, whereas approximately 11% of placebo-treated patients had a similar worsening of glucose tolerance. Conversion from IGT to diabetes was less frequent in orlistat-treated patients than in placebo-treated obese subjects, by 3.0% and 7.6%, respectively (47). Although these data are based on a retrospective analysis of one-year trials in which data on glucose tolerance was available, it shows that modest weight reduction—with pharmacotherapy—may lead to an important risk reduction for the development of type II diabetes.

One study randomized 550 insulin-treated patients to receive either placebo or orlistat 120 mg three times a day for one year (48). Weight loss in the orlistat-treated group was $-3.9 \pm 0.3\%$ compared to $-1.3 \pm .0.3\%$ in the placebo-treated group. Hemoglobin Alc was reduced -0.62% in the orlistat-treated group, but only -0.27% in the placebo group. The required dose of insulin decreased more in the orlistat group, as did plasma cholesterol (48).

Orlistat, in a study in patients with diabetes, improved metabolic control with a reduction of up to -0.53% in hemoglobin Alc (HbAlc) and a decrease in the concomitant ongoing antidiabetic therapy, despite limited weight loss (29). Independent effects of orlistat on lipids were also shown in this study (29). Orlistat also has an acute effect on postprandial lipemia in overweight patients with type 2 diabetes. By lowering both remnant-like particle cholesterol and free fatty acids in the postprandial period, orlistat may contribute to a reduction in atherogenic risk (49).

The longest clinical trial with orlistat is the Xenical Diabetes Outcome Study (XENDOS) (50). In this four-year randomized, placebo-controlled clinical trial 1640 patients were assigned to received orlistat 120 mg three times daily plus lifestyle and 1637 patients to receive matching placebos plus lifestyle. The study enrolled Swedish patients with a BMI $\geq 30\,\text{kg/m}^2$ with normal or impaired glucose tolerance (21%). More than 52% of the orlistat and 34% of the placebo-treated patients continued to adhere to the clinical protocol. The patients receiving orlistat were $-6.9\,\text{kg}$ below their baseline weight by the end of year 4 compared to -4.1 kg for the placebo-treated group ($p < 0.001$). Cumulative incidence of diabetes was 9.0% in the placebo group and 6.2% in the orlistat group, a 37% reduction in relative risk. Xendos provides evidence, not only of therapeutic benefit in terms of diabetes risk reduction, but also that long-term clinical trials of anti-obesity drugs can be successfully implemented.

Orlistat is not absorbed to any significant degree and its side effects are thus related to the blockade of triglyceride digestion in the intestine (37). Fecal fat loss and related GI symptoms are common initially, but subside as patients learn to use the drug (38,39). During treatment, small but significant decreases in fat-soluble vitamins can occur although these almost always remain within the normal range (51). However, a few patients may need supplementation with fat-soluble vitamins that can be lost in the stools. Since it is impossible to tell a priori which patients need vitamins, we routinely provide a multivitamin with instructions to take it before bedtime. Absorption of cyclosporin may also be significantly affected by orlistat.

Combining Orlistat and Sibutramine

Since orlistat works peripherally to reduce triglyceride digestion in the GI track and sibutramine works on noradrenergic and serotonergic reuptake mechanisms in the brain, their mechanisms do not overlap at all and combining them might provide additive weight loss. To test this possibility Wadden et al. (52) randomly assigned patients to orlistat or placebo in addition to sibutramine, following a year of treatment with sibutramine alone. During the additional four months of combination treatment there was no further weight loss. This result was a disappointment, but additional studies are obviously needed before firm conclusions can be made about combining therapies.

MEDICATIONS USED IN OBESITY MANAGEMENT, BUT WHICH DO NOT HAVE AN FDA-APPROVED INDICATION

Topiramate

Topiramate is a neuropsychiatric agent approved for treatment of certain forms of epilepsy, either as monotherapy and in combination with other antiepileptic drugs. Topiramate is a carbonic anhydrase inhibitor that also affects the $GABA_A$ receptor.

In a pooled analysis of a number of epilepsy trials, topiramate was shown to produce progressive weight loss over 18 months which was maintained for the 24 months of observation (53). Patients who had baseline weight exceeding 100 kg lost proportionally more weight compared to those with normal weight (53).

A prospective observational study of topiramate was performed in patients with epilepsy who were taking at least one antiepileptic medication, and provided an opportunity to observe weight effects of the drug (54). Of 49 patients who enrolled, 11 withdrew because of adverse events or because of subject choice (4,7). There were 38 who completed one year of topiramate exposure. The mean topiramate dose for completers was 129 mg/day. In those 38 subjects, there was -7.3% reduction in body weight at one year. The proportional weight loss was greater in the eight obese subjects (-11% from baseline). Patients lost more body fat than lean mass, as assessed by dual emission X-ray absorptiometry. In patients who lost weight, body fat mass was reduced -14.7% at one year, while lean body mass was only reduced -4.8%.

A number of clinical trials with topiramate were begun, but were stopped while in progress in order that the formulation of the drug could be reevaluated. To date, only one of these studies has been published (55). In that multicenter, placebo-controlled, dose-ranging study, topiramate was given for six months to 385 obese patients at doses of 64, 96, 192, or 384 mg daily. Figure 7 shows the weight loss results for completing subjects in this study. The mean percent weight loss in an intention to treat, last observation carried forward are more modest; at six months weight loss was -2.6% for placebo, -5.0%, -4.8%, -6.3%, and -6.3%, respectively, for

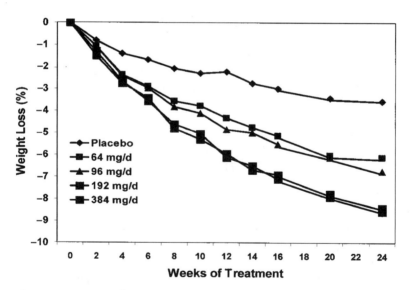

Figure 7 Topiramate dose-ranging study. Percent body weight change over time for subjects who completed the 24-week study. Topiramate produced significantly greater weight loss than placebo; the two higher doses were similar but significantly greater than the two lower doses. *Source*: From Ref. 55.

the 64, 96, 192, and 384 mg doses. While this weight loss pattern is relatively modest, the drug would be expected to show additional weight loss for up to 18 months, if the earlier clinical observation is correct (53).

While the clinical observations of weight loss with topiramate show promise, safety and tolerability are important. The chief safety issues with the medication are acute glaucoma, renal stones, and cognitive impairment (discussed below). Acute glaucoma is an extremely rare side-effect signaled by visual impairment and requires immediate cessation of the drug and opthalmalogical management for preservation of vision. Because topiramate is a carbonic anhydrous inhibitor, taste perversions (with carbonated drinks) are to be expected, as are paresthesias and increased risk for renal calculi.

Central nervous system symptoms are the most worrisome aspect of developing topiramate for an obesity indication. Cognitive impairment, described as mental slowing, somnolence or word-finding difficulty are reported with increased frequency on adverse event reporting forms. In the topiramate-treated patients in the published six month weight loss study, the adverse event (AE) reporting prevalence of difficulty with memory was 20% compared to 8% in placebo-treated patients (55). The AE prevalence of difficulty with concentration was 10% in those treated with topiramate compared to 5% of those treated with placebo. Overall in that study, 21% of topiramate-treated patients withdrew for adverse events compared to 11% of those on placebo. To improve tolerance, the manufacturers recommend slow dose titration. In the published weight loss six month trial, topiramate was started at 16 mg/day for one week, raised to 16 mg twice a day for week 2, and titrated upward in weekly increments of 32 mg/day until the target dose was reached (55).

Topiramate has been investigated and shown efficacy in migraine prevention, in bipolar disorder and in binge eating disorders (56–59). Its future development as an anti-obesity agent is uncertain, as additional longer term clinical trials have not been initiated.

Despite tolerability issues, interest in topiramate remains strong among obesity researchers, in part because of the prolonged weight loss effect of the drug, in part because of its uncertain mechanism of action, and in part because of its potential independent effect on glycemic control, which remains an unresolved issue.

Zonisamide

Zonisamide is marketed as an antiepileptic drug, is a sulfonamate derivative, and is a weak carbonic anhydrase inhibitor, all characteristics similar to topiramate. In clinical trials in epilepsy patients who took zonisamide in addition to other epilepsy medications, weight loss was observed as a side effect (60).

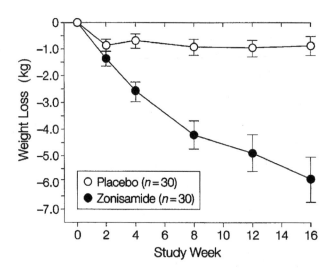

Figure 8 Zonisamide trial in 60 obese patients. Percent body weight changes from baseline to week 16 is depicted for obese patients randomized to either zonisamide or placebo. Data is from a last observation carried forward, intent-to-treat analysis shows statistically significant weight loss for the zonisamide group. Error bars indicate SE. *Source*: From Ref. 61.

In a 16-week double-blind randomized clinical trial, Gadde et al. (61) randomized 60 obese subjects to placebo or 600 mg/day of zonisamide. All patients were instructed in a 500 kcal/day deficit diet. Figure 8 demonstrates the weight loss pattern in this study of zonisamide and placebo-treated patients. During the 16-week double-blind period the zonisamide-treated patients lost −5.98%, compared to −1.09% in the placebo group. During the first 16 weeks of treatment, six zonisamide and three placebo subjects withdrew. Of the zonisamide-treated patients, 19 entered a 16-week single-blind extension and their mean weight loss was −9.4% at 32 weeks. In terms of safety, the chief issue was the adverse event reporting of fatigue by 10 in the zonisamide group and only one in the placebo group. There was also slight elevation of serum creatinine associated with zonisamide use, from 0.78 to 0.92 mg/dL. Zonisamide has been shown in epilepsy trials to be frequently associated with dizziness, cognitive impairment and somnolence and, rarely, with kidney stones and hematologic disease.

Antidepressants—Fluoxetine, Bupropion, and Venlafaxine

Most antidepressants are associated with weight gain (62). However, fluoxetine and bupropion have been evaluated in clinical trials for weight loss and venlafaxine has weight loss reported as a side effect in its prescribing information.

There was initial enthusiasm for fluoxetine as a weight loss agent when it was shown to produce dose-related weight loss in a small eight-week study of fluoxetine 10, 20, 40, and 60 mg and placebo (63). However, the weight loss efficacy was not replicated in a large (458 subject), 52-week, double-blind, 10-site trial (64). In that study, as shown in Figure 9, fluoxetine, 60 mg daily, was compared to placebo and did not produce a treatment difference at week 52. There was statistically significant greater mean weight loss compared to placebo early in the study, but after week 28 there is progressive weight regain despite continued treatment. While fluoxetine may play a role in management of depression in obese patients, it is an ineffective agent for long-term weight management.

Bupropion is a norepinephrine and dopamine reuptake inhibitor with FDA-approved indications for major depression and smoking cessation. Sustained-release bupropion has been shown to be associated with weight loss in overweight and obese subjects treated with the drug for depression (65).

Sustained-release bupropion was evaluated in a multi-center, double-blind, placebo-controlled randomized trial (66). In that study, there were 327 subjects randomized to placebo, or either 300 or 400 mg of daily bupropion SR. The results are shown in Figure 10. All subjects were randomly allocated to receive either placebo or active treatments (bupropion SR 300 mg/day or bupropion SR 400 mg/day) in a double-blind manner for 24 weeks. Then placebo-treated patients were randomized to either 300 or 400 mg of daily bupropion SR for 24 additional weeks. There was a dose–response relationship evident with mean weight loss of -7.2% and -10.1% for bupropion SR 300 and 400 mg, respectively, at 24 weeks. These were net

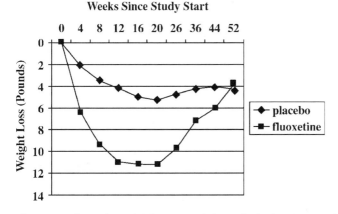

Figure 9 Fluoxetine trial for overweight and obesity. Percent body weight change over time for obese subjects randomized to daily fluoxetine 60 mg or placebo. After week 26, there are no statistically significant differences between the treatment groups. *Source*: From Ref. 64.

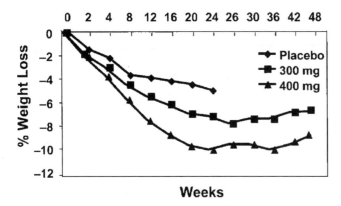

Figure 10 Bupropion SR and weight loss over 48 weeks. Percent weight loss from baseline over time is displayed as mean values with SEM. Bupropion SR 400 mg (▲) produced significantly greater weight loss than bupropion SR 300 mg (■) at weeks 24, 26, 30, 36, and 40 and greater weight loss than placebo () at weeks 12, 16, 20, and 24. *Source*: From Ref. 66.

−2.2% and −5.1% more than placebo. At 48 weeks, mean weight loss was −7.5% and −8.6% for bupropion SR 300 mg and 400 mg, respectively. The medication was well tolerated in this study with no significant difference in adverse events across treatment groups. Anxiety or insomnia led to withdrawal more often with bupropion SR treatment than with placebo, but these differences were not statistically significant.

Bupropion SR 300 mg/day has been evaluated in 422 obese patients with depression symptoms (Beck Depression Inventory Score of 10–30) in a randomized, double-blind, placebo-controlled study (67). Those patients on bupropion lost more weight at six months (−4.6% mean weight lost from baseline compared to −1.8% for the placebo group). However, there was no statistically significant difference between groups in prevalence of patients reporting ≥ 50% decrease in depressive symptoms. Improvement in depressive symptoms was related to weight loss ≥5%, regardless of treatment ($p < 0.0001$).

In summary, bupropion would seem a good choice for therapeutic trial in the depressed obese patient, since it has a favorable weight profile. For obese patients with depressive symptoms, bupropion might also be beneficial, provided there is a weight loss effect. The chief obstacle to recommending bupropion for the management of obesity in a general population would be the lack of an FDA-approved indication for weight management. Considering the large body of evidence documenting the safe use of the drug for depression, it is reasonable for clinicians to add it to the therapeutic tool-box for obesity. Bupropion seems to aid lifestyle approaches to produce weight loss roughly equivalent to sibutramine and orlistat. Clinicians should be familiar with its side effect profile and prescribe with care. Bupropion should not be given to patients with a history of epilepsy. Its side effect profile shows increased incidence of agitation, anxiety, and insomnia.

Venlafaxine (marketed as Effexor) is a reuptake inhibitor of serotonin and norepinephine, like sibutramine, and has a chemical structure similar to sibutramine. Venlafaxine is used for treatment of depression. Although there are no studies of this medication as a weight loss agent, the prescribing information documents treatment emergent anorexia reported in 11% of patients treated with venlafaxine and only 2% of those on placebo. A loss of 5% or more of body weight occurred in 6% of patients treated with venlafaxine and 1% on placebo. Venlafaxine has a side effect profile similar to sibutramine (68). Thus, venlafaxine would be among preferred choices for managing depression in obese patients.

FUTURE DIRECTIONS

Based on an explosion of knowledge regarding the biology of food intake and energy balance regulation, many pharmaceutical companies are searching for novel obesity drugs. The first of this new paradigm to developing obesity medications based on biologic advances—leptin—has thus far failed to produce meaningful weight loss in the healthy obese population. Leptin would seem to be a promising agent for obesity management. It is a peptide produced in adipose tissue. Leptin mutations result in obesity in animals and humans and treatment with recombinant leptin reverses obesity in these individuals (69,70). Leptin levels in the blood are highly correlated with the amount of body fat. A dose-ranging clinical trial of subcutaneously administered recombinant human leptin in obese individuals demonstrated only modest weight loss at 24 weeks and problems with reactions at the local injection site (71). The issue in human obesity may be resistance to leptin's action, suggesting that this may have limited usefulness in the general population of obese individuals.

Axokine is the trade name for a modified form of ciliary neurotrophic factor (CNTF). It acts through the same janus-kinase-signal for transduction and translation (JAK-STAT) system that leptin acts through. CNTF will reduce food intake in animals that lack leptin or the leptin receptors (72). In a clinical trial for amyotrophic lateral sclerosis, the drug was noted to reduce weight.

CNTF has been evaluated in a 12-week, double-blind, randomized, dose-ranging study at seven sites (73). There were 173 patients who received daily subcutaneous injections of placebo or one of three doses of CNTF (0.3, 1.0, or 2.0 µg/kg). All patients received instruction in a diet to reduce daily consumption by 500 kcal. Figure 11 depicts weight loss results. The mean weight loss over 12 weeks is modest, though statistically significant.

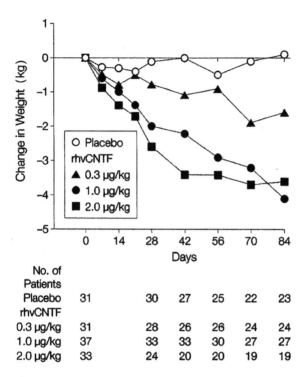

No. of Patients						
	0	14	28	42	56	70	84
Placebo	31		30	27	25	22	23
rhvCNTF							
0.3 µg/kg	31		28	26	26	24	24
1.0 µg/kg	37		33	33	30	27	27
2.0 µg/kg	33		24	20	20	19	19

Figure 11 CNTF treatment for obesity. Data shown are available data as observed at each time point. Beginning at week 2, the 1.0 mg/kg dosage group was statistically significantly different from placebo ($p = 0.02$). At day 84, all treatment groups show a statistically significant difference in weight compared with the placebo group ($p < 0.05$). *Abbreviation*: CNTF, ciliary neurotrophic factor. *Source*: From Ref. 73.

The chief issues with CNTF as a weight loss agent are that the parenteral medication invokes antibody formation (in 45–87% of patients in the cited study). Injection site reactions, nausea and cough, coupled with modest weight loss, limit the drug's usefulness in clinical practice.

The next medication expected to make it to market based on the "new biology" of food intake and energy balance regulations is rimonibant. Endocannabinoids may be involved in the regulation of food intake. Early results of two clinical trials of rimonibant have been posted on a website (74). Rimonibant is the first of a new class; CB1 blockers. This agent selectively blocks the CB1 receptor and is proposed to normalize the endocannabinoid system. The drug is being evaluated as an aid to both weight loss and smoking cessation.

The "new biology" of obesity has resulted in interest in other therapeutic targets. Several pharmaceutical companies are seeking to identify antagonists to the neuropeptide Y (NPY) receptor and agonists of cholecystokinin

(CCK). Peripheral peptides such as ghrelin and peptide yy (PPY) are other promising targets.

SUMMARY

At present only two drugs are approved for long-term treatment of obesity. Sibutramine inhibits the reuptake of serotonin and norepinephrine. In clinical trials it produces a dose-dependent 5% to 10% decrease in body weight. Its side effects include dry mouth, insomnia, asthenia, and constipation. In addition, in clinical trials, sibutramine produces a small mean increase in blood pressure and pulse that mandates attention to blood pressure monitoring on follow-up visits. Sibutramine is contraindicated in some individuals with heart disease. Orlistat is the other drug approved for long-term use in the treatment of obesity. It works by blocking pancreatic lipase and thus increasing the fecal loss of triglyceride. One valuable consequence of this mechanism of action is the reduction of serum cholesterol that averages about 5% more than can be accounted for by weight loss alone. In clinical trials, it too produces a 5% to 10% loss of weight. Its side effects are entirely due to undigested fat in the intestine (steatorrhea) that can lead to increased frequency and change in the character of stools. It can also lower fat-soluble vitamins. The ingestion of a vitamin supplement before bedtime is a reasonable treatment strategy when orlistat is prescribed.

Among the medications that have been on the market for more than 30 years, phentermine is still widely prescribed for obesity management, despite a lack of extensive clinical trial evidence supporting its use.

Several medications that are available and approved by the FDA for indications other than weight loss are also used in the clinic. Bupropion has been used widely for management of depression and smoking cessation when used with a lifestyle approach. It produces weight loss similar to that of orlistat and sibutramine. Its safety profile is relatively good with chief concern being its contraindication in seizure disorders.

Topiramate generates interest among clinicians who manage obesity because of the duration and amount of weight loss, although tolerability and safety profile limit its usefulness. Cognitive dysfunction, renal calculi, paresthesias, and acute glaucoma make this medication difficult to employ in the otherwise healthy obese population.

Other medications may play a role in managing the obese patient; zonisamide, fluoxetine, and venlafaxine, were also discussed in this review.

Finally, the future of obesity pharmacotherapy holds promise—and disappointments, too. While recombinant leptin has not shown efficacy in the general obese population, and recombinant ciliary neurotrophic factor shows efficacy only in a subgroup, early results with rimonibant are promising. Similar successes and failures are almost certainly in store in the development of additional drugs to treat obesity.

REFERENCES

1. National Institutes of Health, National Heart, Lung, and Blood Institute. Clinical guidelines on the identification, evaluation, and treatment of overweight and obesity inadults—the evidence report. Obes Res 1998; 6(suppl 2):51S–210S.
2. Bray GA, Greenway FL. Current and potential drugs for treatment of obesity [Review]. Endocr Rev 1999; 20:805–875.
3. Connolly HM, Crary JL, McGoon MD, et al. Valvular heart disease associated with fenfluramine–phentermine. N Engl J Med 1997; 337:581–588.
4. Ryan DH, Bray GA, Helmcke F, et al. Serial echocardiographic and clinical evaluation of valvular regurgitation before, during, and after treatment with fenfluramine or dexfenfluramine and mazindol or phentermine. Obes Res 1999; 7:313–322.
5. Jick H. Heart valve disorders and appetite-suppressant drugs. JAMA 2000; 283:1738–1740.
6. Hensrud DD, Connolly HM, Grogan M, Miller FA, Bailey KR, Jensen MD. Echocardiographic improvement over time after cessation of use of fenfluramine and phentermine. Mayo Clin Proc 1999; 74:1191–1197.
7. Mast ST, Jollis JG, Ryan T, Anstrom KJ, Crary JL. The progression of fenfluramine-associated valvular heart disease assessed by echocardiograpliy. Ann Intern Med 2001; 134:261–266.
8. Weintraub M, Bray GA. Drug treatment of obesity [Review]. Med Clin North Am 1989; 73:237–249.
9. Cole JO, Levin A, BeakeB, Kaiser PE, Scheinbaum ML. Sibutramine: a new weight loss agent without evidence of the abuse potential associated with amphetamines. J Clin Psychopharmacol 1998; 18(3):231–236.
10. Sjostrom CD, Peltonen M, Wedel H, Sjostrom L. Differentiated long-term effects of intentional weight loss on diabetes and hypertension. Hypertension 2000; 36:20–25.
11. Torgerson JS, Sjostrom L. The Swedish Obese Subjects (SOS) study—rationale and results. Int J Obes 2001; 25:S2–S4.
12. Foster GD, Wadden TA, Vogt RA, Brewer G. What is a reasonable weight loss? Patients expectations and evaluations of obesity treatment outcomes. J Consult Clin Psychol 1997; 65:79–85.
13. Sjostrom CD, Lissner L, Wedel H, Sjostrom L. Reduction in incidence of diabetes, hypertension and lipid disturbances after intentional weight loss induced by bariatric surgery: the SOS Intervention Study. Obes Res 1999; 7:477–484.
14. Bray GA. Obesity—A time-bomb to be defused. Lancet 1998; 352:160–161.
15. Knowler WC, Barrett-Connor E, Fowler SE, et al. Diabetes Prevention Program Research Group. Reduction in the incidence of type 2 diabetes with lifestyle intervention or metformin. N Engl J Med 2002; 346:393–403.
16. Tuomilehto J, Lindstrom J, Eriksson JG, et al. Finnish Diabetes Prevention Study Group. Prevention of type 2 diabetes mellitus by changes in lifestyle among subjects with impaired glucose tolerance. N Engl J Med 2001; 344:1343–1350.
17. Munro JF, MacCuish AC, Wilson EM, Duncan LJP. Comparison of continuous and intermittent anorectic therapy in obesity. Br Med J 1968; 1:352–354.
18. Yanovski SZ, Yanovski JA. Drug Obesity. New Engl J Med 2002; 346:591–602.

19. Ryan DH. The role of sibutramine in the clinical management of obesity. In: Proceedings of the 9th International Congress on Obesity, Sao Paulo. John Libbey Eurotext, 2002:127.

20. Cuellar GEM, Ruiz AM, Monsalve MCR, Berber A. Six-month treatment of obesity with sibutramine 15 mg a double-blind, placebo-controlled monocenter clinical trial in a Hispanic population. Obes Res 2000; 8(l):71–82.

21. McMahon FG, Fujioka K, Singh, BN, et al. Efficacy and safety of sibutramine in obese white and African–American patients with hypertension. Arch Int Med 2000; 160:2185–2191.

22. Apfelbaum M, Vague P, Ziegler O, Hanotin C, Thomas F, Leutenegger E. Long-term maintenance of weight loss after a very-low-calorie diet: A randomized blinded trial of the efficacy and tolerability of sibutramine. Am J Med 1999; 106:179–184.

23. James WPT, Astrup A, Finer N, et al. for the STORM study group. Effect of sibutramine on weight maintenance after weight loss: a randomized trial. Lancet 2000; 356:2119–2125.

24. Finer N, Bloom SR, Frost GS, Banks LM, Griffit J. Sibutramine is effective for weight loss and diabetic control in obesity with type 2 diabetes: a randomised, double-blind placebo-controlled study. Diabetes Obes Metab 2000; 2:105–112.

25. Wirth A, Krause J. Long-term weight loss with sibutramine. JAMA 2001; 286(11):1331–1339.

26. Fujioka K, Seaton TB, Rowe E, et al. the Sibutramine/Diabetes clinical study group. Weight loss with sibutramine improves glycemic control and other metabolic parameters in obese type 2 diabetes mellitus. Diabetes Obes Metab 2000; 2: 1–13.

27. Gockel A, Karakose H, Ertorer EM, Tanaci N, Tutuncu NB, Guvener N. Effects of sibutramine in obese female subjects with type 2 diabetes and poor blood glucose control. Diabetes Care 2001; 24:1957–1960.

28. Serrano-Rios M, Melchionda N, Moreno-Carretero E. Spanish Investigators. Role of sibutramine in the treatment of obese Type 2 diabetic patients receiving sulphonylurea therapy. Diabet Med 2002; 19(2):119–124.

29. Hollander P, Elbein SC, Hirsch IB, et al. Role of orlistat in the treatment of obese patients with type 2 diabetes. Diabetes Care 1998; 21:1288–1294.

30. McMahon FG, Weinstein SP, Rowe E, Ernst KR, Johnson F, Fujioka K. Sibutramine is safe and effective for weight loss in obese patients whose hypertension is well controlled with angiotensin-converting enzyme inhibitors. J Hum Hypertens 2002; 16:5–11.

31. Sramek, JJ, Seiowitz MT, Weinstein SP, et al. Efficacy and safety of sibutramine for weight loss in obese patients with hypertension well controlled by β-adrenergic blocking agents: a placebo-controlled, double-blind, randomized trial. Am J Hypertens 2002; 16:13–19.

32. Hazenberg BP. Randomized, double-blind, placebo-controlled, multicenter study of sibutramine in obese hypertensive patients. Cardiology 2000; 94:152–158.

33. Berube-Parent S, Prud-homme D, St-Pierre S, Doucet E, Tremblay A. Obesity treatment with a progressive clinical tri-therapy combining sibutramine and a supervised diet-exercise intervention. Int J Obes Relat Metab Disord 2001; 25(8):1144–1153.

34. Wadden RA, Berkowitz RI, Sarwer DB, Prus-Wisniewski R, Steinberg CM. Benefits of lifestyle modification in the pharmacologic treatment of obesity: a randomized trial. Arch Intern Med 2001; 161:218–227.

35. Bray GA, Blackburn GL, Ferguson JM, et al. Sibutramine produces dose-related weight loss. Obes Res 1999; 7:189–198.

36. Van Gaal LF, Wauters M, De Leeuw IH. The beneficial effects of modest weight loss on cardiovascular risk factors. Int J Obes 1997; 21(suppl 1):S5–S9.

37. Hauptman J. Orlistat: selective inhibition of caloric absorption can affect long-term body weight. Endocrine 2000; 13(2):201–206.

38. O'Meara S, Riemsma R, Shirran L, Mather L, ter Riet G. A systematic review of the clinical effectiveness of orlistat used for the management of obesity. Obes Rev 2004; 5:51–68.

39. Sjostrom L, Rissanen A, Andersen T, et al. Randomised placebo-controlled trial of orlistat for weight loss and prevention of weight regain in obese patients. European Multicentre Orlistat Study Group. Lancet 1998; 352:167–172.

40. Davidson MH, Hauptman J, DiGirolamo M, et al. Long-term weight control and risk factor reduction in obese subjects treated with orlistat, a lipase inhibitor. JAMA 1999; 281:235–242.

41. Rossner S, Sjostrom L, Noack R, Meinders AE, Noseda G, on behalf of the European Orlistat Obesity Study Group. Weight loss, weight maintenance, and improved cardiovascular risk factors after 2 years treatment with orlistat for obesity. Obes Res 2000; 8:49–61.

42. Hauptmann J, Lucas C, Boldrin MN, Collins H, Segal KR, for the Orlistat Primary Care Study Group. Orlistat in the long-term treatment of obesity in primary care settings. Arch Fam Med 2000; 9:160–167.

43. Hill JO, Hauptmann J, Anderson JW, et al. Orlistat, a lipase inhibitor, for weight maintenance after conventional dieting: a 1-y study. Am J Clin Nutr 1999; 69:1108–1116.

44. Zavoral JH. Treatment with orlistat reduces cardiovascular risk in obese patients. J Hypertens 1998; 16:2013–2017.

45. Muls E, Kolanowski J, Scheen A, Van Gaal LF. The effects of orlistat on weight and on serum lipids in obese patients with, hypercholesterolemia: a randomized, double-blind, placebo-controlled, multicenter study. Int J Obes Relat Metab Disord 2001; 25:1713–1721.

46. Tonstad S, Pometta D, Erkelens DW, et al. The effects of gastrointestinal lipase inhibitor, orlistat, on serum lipids and lipoproteins in patients with primary hyperlipidaemia. Eur J Clin Pharmacol 1994; 46:405–410.

47. Heymsfield SB, Segal KR, Hauptman J, et al. Effects of weight loss with orlistat on glucose tolerance and progression to type 2 diabetes in obese adults. Arch Intern Med 2000; 160:1321–1326.

48. Kelley D, Bray G, Pi-Sunyer FX, et al. Clinical efficacy of orlistat therapy in overweight and obese patients with insulin-treated type 2 diabetes mellitus: a one-year, randomized, controlled trial. Diabetes Care 2002; 25:1033–1041.

49. Ceriello A. The postprandial state and cardiovascular disease: relevance to diabetes mellitus. Diabetes Metab Res Rev 2000; 16:125–132.

50. Torgerson JS, Hauptman J, Boldrin MN, Sjostrom L. Xenical in the prevention of diabetes in obese subjects (XENDOS) study: a randomized study of orlistat

as an adjunct to lifestyle changes for the prevention of type 2 diabetes in obese patients. Diabetes Care 2004; 27:155–161.

51. Drent ML, van der Veen EA. First clinical studies with orlistat: a short review. Obes Res 1995; 3:S623–S625.

52. Wadden TA, Berkowitz RI, Womble LG, Sarwer DB, Arnold ME, Steinberg CM. Effects of sibutramine plus orlistat in obese women following 1 year of treatment by sibutramine alone: a placebo-controlled trial. Obes Res 2000; 8(6):431–437.

53. Reife R, Pledger G, Wu S. Topiramate as add-on therapy: pooled analysis of randomized controlled trials in adults. Epilepsia 2000; 41(suppl 1):S66–S71.

54. Ben-Menachem E, Axelsen M, Johanson EH, Stagge A, Smith U. Predictors of weight loss in adults with topiramate-treated epilepsy. Obes Res 2003; 11: 556–562.

55. Bray GA, Hollander P, Klein S, et al. for the U.S. Topiramate Research Group. A 6-month randomized, placebo-controlled, dose-ranging trial of topiramate for weight loss in obesity. Obes Res 2003; 11:722–733.

56. Storey JR, Calder CS, Hart E, Potter DL. Topiramate in migraine prevention: a double-blind, placebo-controlled study. Headache 2002; 41:968–975.

57. Chengappa KN, Rathore D, Levine J, et al. Topiramate as add-on treatment for patients with bipolar mania. Bipolar Disord 1999; 1:42–53.

58. McElroy SL, Suppes T, Keck PE, et al. Open-label adjunctive topiramate in the treatment of bipolar disorders. Biol Psychiatry 2000; 47:1025–1033.

59. Shapira NA, Goldsmith TD, McElroy SI. Treatment of binge-eating disorder with topiramate: clinical case series. J Clin Psychiatry 2000; 61:368–372.

60. Oommen KJ, Mathews S. Zonisamide: a new antiepileptic drug. Clin Neuropharmacol 1999; 22:192–200.

61. Gadde KM, Franciscy DM, Wagner HR III. Randomized trial of weight loss efficacy of zonisamide. Int J Obes 2002; 26(suppl 1):S81 (Abs).

62. Schwartz TL, Nihalani N, Jindal S, Virk S, Jones N. Psychiatric medication-induced obesity: a review. Obes Rev 2004; 5:115–121.

63. Levine LR, Enas GG, Thompson WL, et al. Use of fluoxetine, a selective serotonin-uptake inhibitor in the treatment of obesity: a dose–response study. Int J Obes 1989; 13:635–645.

64. Goldstein DJ, Rampey AH Jr, Enas GG, Potvin JH, Fludzinski LA, Levine LR. Fluoxetine: a randomized clinical trial in the treatment of obesity. Int J Obes Relat Metab Disord 1994; 18:129–135.

65. Settle E, Stahl S, Batey S, Johnson J, Ascher J. Safety profile of sustained-release bupropion in depression: results of three clinical trials. Clin Ther 1999; 21:455–463.

66. Anderson JW, Greenway FL, Fujioka K, Gadde KM, McKenney J, O'Neil PM. Bupropion SR enhances weight loss: a 48-week double-blind, placebo-controlled trial. Obes Res 2002; 10:633–641.

67. Jain AK, Kaplan RA, Gadde KM, et al. Bupropion SR vs. placebo for weight loss in obese patients with depressive symptoms. Obes Res 2002; 10:1049–1056.

68. Physicians Desk Reference, 58th ed, 2004:3413.

69. Montague CT, Farooqi IS, Whitehead JP, et al. Congenital leptin deficiency is associated with severe early-onset obesity in humans. Nature 1997; 387:903–908.

70. Farooqi IS, Jebb SA, Langmack G, et al. Effects of recombinant leptin therapy in a child with congenital leptin deficiency. N Engl J Med 1999; 341:913–915.

71. Heymsfield SB, Greenberg AS, Fujioka K, et al. Recombinant leptin for weight loss in obese and lean adults: a randomized, controlled, dose-escalation trial. JAMA 1999; 282:1568–1575.

72. Lambert PD, Anderson KD, Sleeman MW, et al. Ciliary neurotrophic factor activates leptin-like pathways and reduces body fat, without cachexia or rebound weight gain, even in leptin-resistant obesity. Proc Natl Acad Sci 2001; 98:4652–4657.

73. Ettinger MP, Littlejohn TW, Schwartz SL, et al. Recombinant variant of ciliary neurotrophic factor for weight loss in obese adults. JAMA 2003; 289:1826–1832.

74. http://en.sanofi-synthelabo.com/press/ppc_23804. Two pivotal studies indicate ACOMPLIA™ (rimonabant) offers a novel approach to cardiovascular risk management in overweight/obese people and smokers (accessed March 10,2004).

13

Overview of Agents with Efficacy in Binge Eating

Jose C. Appolinario

*Obesity and Eating Disorders Group, Institute of Psychiatry of
the Federal University of Rio de Janeiro and Institute of Endocrinology
and Diabetes of Rio de Janeiro, Rio de Janeiro, Brazil*

Josué Bacaltchuk

*Eating Disorders Program (PROATA), Federal University of São Paulo
and Janssen-Cilag Farmaceutica, São Paulo, Brazil*

INTRODUCTION

Binge eating, a hallmark of both bulimia nervosa (BN) and the new DSM-IV proposed diagnostic category binge eating disorder (BED), is a disturbed eating behavior defined as episodes of uncontrolled consumption of large amounts of food in a short period of time associated with a feeling of loss of control (1). BED is an example of an eating disorder not otherwise specified characterized by recurrent episodes of binge eating not being followed by inappropriate compensatory behaviors seen in BN (2).

Although weight is not a criterion for diagnosis, BED is more frequently observed in overweight and obese individuals. Fifteen to thirty percent of participants in weight loss programs and 70% in overeaters anonymous groups display this condition (3). These obese patients with BED present an earlier onset of obesity, begin dieting earlier, and have more weight fluctuations than obese patients without BED (4). Moreover, patients with BED usually exhibit higher than expected rates of eating related (body image distress) and general psychopathology (5). Studies have suggested an elevated prevalence of depressive disorders, anxiety disorders and substance use disorders (alcohol or drug abuse/dependence) in persons with BED compared to those without BED (6–8). In addition, epidemiological studies have found higher rates of binge eating among bipolar patients than in the general population (9). High levels of perfectionism and impulsivity as well as impulse control disorders (e.g., kleptomania) have also been found in patients with BED (10). As a clinical consequence, psychiatric comorbidity may render individuals more prone to developing binge eating and to have problems with weight control (11–13).

Considering the aforementioned characteristics, BED should be seen as a clinical condition characterized by symptoms on three domains (14). These domains may be represented behaviorally by the occurrence of binge eating without compensatory behavior; psychologically by body image disturbances and/or psychiatric comorbidity; and somatically by overweight or obesity. Thus, the treatment of BED should consider these three aspects of its clinical presentation (15).

Despite the fact that there is no established treatment for BED, medications are frequently part of a multi-modal approach that also includes psychological and nutritional interventions. The last decade has witnessed the development of promising pharmacological treatments for BED or similar conditions (16). Several classes of medications have been studied in the treatment of patients with BED including antidepressants, centrally acting anti-obesity agents, and anticonvulsants, and to a lesser extent, opioid antagonists (17–33).

Recent pharmacological studies conducted in BED have shown an increasing and progressive refinement. These methodological improvements could be observed in different aspects of the study design, such as the inclusion of subjects with BED diagnosed according to DSM-IV or DSM-IV-TR criteria, the introduction of a more equivalent primary outcome measures (reports of weekly binge eating frequency), the use of standardized instruments to evaluate eating-related and general psychopathology, and the assessment of anthropometric parameters.

However, apart from these advances, BED pharmacological trials still have important limitations. One important finding is the strong response to placebo reported in this group of patients (27). Of note, this high placebo response is not an exclusive BED phenomenon and has been found in other psychiatric conditions (34). In addition, the BED syndrome may have an intermittent course (with relapses and remissions) which may contribute to this high placebo response (35). Another important limitation of available controlled BED pharmacological studies is that all are short term. It is therefore unknown if their therapeutic effects would generalize to longer treatment periods. The next generation of pharmacotherapy studies will need to address several questions, such as the optimal medication, most appropriate dose regimen and treatment duration as well as effects of combined treatments (e.g., medication and psychotherapy, medication, and nutritional counseling, etc.).

This chapter summarizes the available information and future directions on the pharmacological treatment of BED. First, agents with efficacy in BED will be discussed and grouped by their pharmacological classes. Second, although still scarce, studies about combination and augmentation strategies will be analysed.

ANTIDEPRESSANTS

The use of antidepressants in the treatment of BED is supported by the following lines of evidence:

- antidepressants of several different classes have been shown to be effective in BN, which is closely related to BED,
- individuals with BED display a high prevalence of lifetime major depressive disorder,
- the use of certain antidepressants has been associated with some degree of weight loss (6,7,15,36,37).

Several classes of antidepressants have been studied in BED. Early investigations with tricyclics were followed by more recent trials with serotonin selective reuptake inhibitors (SSRIs) and other antidepressants.

Tricyclic Antidepressants

Initial studies were conducted before the publication of the provisional DSM-IV criteria for BED and employed tricyclic antidepressants in clinical conditions closely related to this diagnosis (17,18). In a first double-blind placebo-controlled study, McCaan et al. (17) noted that desipramine was significantly superior to placebo in reducing binge eating in 23 patients with non-purging BN. At the end of the trial, 60% of desipramine treated patients did not binge eat, compared with 15% of placebo-treated women. Additionally, patients quickly relapsed after the discontinuation of the medication. However, there were no differences between desipramine and placebo in change in weight, BMI, perception of body image, or depressive symptoms. These results lead to the hypothesis that antidepressants might also work in eating disorders by suppressing appetite rather than elevating mood, and that desipramine might also have a therapeutic effect in patients with BED. A second trial conducted by Alger et al. (18) compared imipramine 150–200 mg/day with placebo in obese binge eaters (individuals with a binge eating scale score $\geq$27) and normal weight BN patients. This study included an additional naltrexone group. A median reduction in binge eating frequency greater than 90% was observed, but there was no statistically significant difference between drug and placebo (due to an extremely high placebo response rate of 70%). This high placebo response along with the small sample size makes these results difficult to interpret. Adverse reactions for imipramine included drug rash and elevated liver enzymes; for naltrexone they included headache, nausea, agitation, diaphoresis, and elevated liver enzymes.

Serotonin Selective Reuptake Inhibitors

An open trial of fluvoxamine in 10 patients with binge eating without vomiting suggested SSRIs might be effective in BED (38). The five completer patients showed significant weight loss, as well as reduction in the number of binge episodes, anxiety, and clinical severity questionnaire scores. After these initial positive findings, Hudson et al. (19) assessed the efficacy of fluvoxamine in the treatment of BED in a three-center, nine-week, double-blind, placebo-controlled trial. Eighty-five overweight outpatients with BED were assigned to fluvoxamine or placebo. The authors found that, compared with placebo-fluvoxamine was associated with a significantly greater rate of reduction in binge frequency and body weight. However, they did not find a significant difference between active drug and placebo in terms of depressives symptoms. The estimated weight loss in the fluvoxamine group was 1.3 kg compared with 0.4 kg in the placebo group. A significant greater number of patients receiving fluvoxamine than placebo withdrew due to adverse events (insomnia and nausea). A second randomized controlled trial reported negative results relative to the efficacy of fluvoxamine in BED (23). In this study, 20 subjects with BED were randomly assigned to flexible-dose fluvoxamine or placebo for 12 weeks. A significant reduction in binge frequency, Beck Depression Inventory scores, and eating concern, shape concern and weight concern subscales of the Eating Disorder Examination were noted for both fluvoxamine ($n = 9$) and placebo ($n = 11$) groups. There were no significant differences between fluvoxamine and placebo for any treatment outcome variables. However, as the authors have pointed out, the results of this study are difficult to interpret because of several limitations, such as the very small sample size and the inclusion of potential confounding nonspecific treatment components, i.e., rigorous assessment and self-monitoring with very frequent clinical contact.

Sertraline was studied in the treatment of BED in a small controlled trial conducted by McElroy et al. (20). Thirty-four overweight patients with BED were randomly assigned to sertraline 50–200 mg/day or placebo (24). There was a significant reduction of binge frequency in the group treated with sertraline when compared to placebo (85% vs 46.5%), as well as a significant and a more marked weight loss (−5.4 kg). Again, the authors did not find statistical differences in depressive symptoms. Sertraline was safe and the only statistically significant adverse event observed in the sertraline group compared to placebo was insomnia.

The efficacy and tolerability of fluoxetine in BED was studied in a 6-week randomized controlled trial conducted by Arnold et al. (21) in 60 patients. Subjects receiving fluoxetine had a significantly greater reduction in frequency of binge eating, weight and a marginally significant reduction in HAM-D scores compared to placebo. Additionally, fluoxetine was considered well tolerated.

More recently, citalopram was also studied in a double-blind controlled trial with 38 overweight patients with BED (22). Compared to placebo, citalopram-treated individuals had a significant reduction in binge eating episodes and body weight. As observed in the fluoxetine study, the authors found a non-significant result in terms of associated depressive symptoms

In a recent review, Carter et al. (39) combined the data from the above 4 placebo-controlled clinical trials of SSRIs (19–22). Using a random regression method for a meta-analysis they estimated the effect of this class of drugs on binge eating frequency and other parameters. The combined estimate for difference between drug and placebo in percentage of subjects with a 50% or greater decrease in frequency of binges at endpoint was 23.0% (95% CI: 9.9, 36.2; $P = 0.001$), and for the difference in percentage of subjects with a cessation of binge eating at endpoint was 20.2 (95% CI: 7.5, 32.7; $P = 0.002$). The authors concluded that these effect sizes were clinically important and similar to those observed with SSRIs in major depressive disorder (40).

Other Antidepressants

Information about therapeutic effects of other classes of antidepressants in the treatment of BED has come from open reports. An open-label study evaluated venlafaxine, a serotonin noradrenaline reuptake inhibitor, in 35 overweight or obese patients with BED (41). There were significant decreases in weekly binge frequency, severity of binge eating and mood symptoms, weight, BMI, waist circumference, and diastolic blood pressure. Fifty percent of patients had at least a moderate response and 43% lost at least 5% of their baseline weight. Dry mouth, sexual dysfunction, insomnia, and nausea were the most common adverse events. A small open trial investigated the effectiveness and tolerability of reboxetine, a selective noradrenaline reuptake inhibitor in BED (42). In this study, nine patients with BED and obesity received reboxetine 8 mg/day for 12 weeks. The five completers showed a significant reduction in binge frequency (from 4.6 to 0.2 binge days/week at the end of the study) and in BMI. Of note, these authors included in the study designed an instrument to assess quality of life, an important aspect to evaluate the effectiveness of a intervention. Overall quality of life, assessed by World Health Organization Quality of Life Assessment Scale in pre- and post-treatment, was significantly improved as were general health ($p = 0.02$) and psychological domains ($p = 0.03$). No serious side effects were observed. Randomized, double-blind placebo-controlled trials are warranted to confirm these preliminary findings.

OPIOID ANTAGONISTS

The basis for the use of opioid antagonists such as naltrexone in BED includes the following lines of evidence:

- Animal studies have shown that these agents may help control food intake (43).
- Opioid antagonists interfere with food intake behavior and body weight in a biobehavioral model of obese binge eating (44).
- Opioid antagonists reduced food intake by up to 30% in normal weight, obese and bulimic patients (45).
- Individuals with BED display a high prevalence of alcohol use disorders (8).

Naltrexone is an opiate antagonist used to treat alcoholism. Despite the negative findings reported by Alger et al. (18) and discussed above, two case reports described potential benefits of naltrexone either alone or combined with fluoxetine and cognitive-behavioral therapy on binge eating behavior and weight in patients with BED unresponsive to antidepressants and psychotherapy (46,47). In addition, in an open label one-year trial of naloxone in 10 obese diabetic women with bulimia or binge eating resistant to antidepressants or psychotherapy, an early reduction in weekly binge eating episodes was sustained after one year of treatment (33). A significant and progressive reduction in body weight along with an improvement in glycemic control was also observed. Of note, no undesirable side effects were noted during the study. These positive findings need to be replicated in randomized controlled studies.

ANTI-OBESITY AGENTS

The use of anti-obesity agents in the treatment of BED is supported by a number of lines of evidence:

- Binge eating may be characterized by increased appetite and reduced satiety (48).
- BED is frequently associated with overweight or obesity and depression (3).
- Some antiobesity agents reduce appetite, increase satiety, induce weight loss, and may reduce depressive symptoms (49).

D-fenfluramine, currently withdrawn from the market because of its association with cardiac valve lesions and pulmonary hypertension, was the first antiobesity agent studied in BED. A positive placebo-controlled trial of d-fenfluramine was conducted by Stunkard et al. (24) in 28 obese subjects with BED. In this study, patients receiving d-fenfluramine showed a statistically significant reduction in binge eating behavior compared to placebo. Surprisingly, despite the anti-obesity action of d-fenfluramine, its therapeutic effect on binge eating was not associated with a reduction in body weight. In addition, the authors also reported a remarkable post-discontinuation relapse in binge eating.

The interest about the usefulness of anti-obesity agents in BED regained a renewed interest with the introduction of sibutramine to the obesity armamentarium. Sibutramine is a serotonin and noradrenaline reuptake inhibitor. Its efficacy for inducing initial weight-loss and subsequent weight maintenance is well proven in short- and long-term obesity clinical trials (50,51). Sibutramine induces weight loss mainly by enhancing satiety. As a secondary mechanism of action, sibutramine may prevent the decline in energy expenditure that usually follows weight loss (52). Side effects of sibutramine are usually mild and transient and include dry mouth, constipation, and insomnia. Small increases in blood pressure and heart rate have also been reported. Unlike fenfluramine and dexfenfluramine, sibutramine does not induce serotonin release, and has not been implicated in the development of valvular heart disease.

A small open study initially suggested the efficacy of sibutramine in BED (25). In this study, 10 obese patients with BED were treated with 15 mg/day of sibutramine for 12 weeks. Seven patients concluded the trial and evidenced a complete remission of binge eating as well as a reduction of body weight. These positive results led to a randomized controlled trial comparing sibutramine 15 mg/day with placebo in 60 obese patients with BED (26). The authors reported that sibutramine was more effective than placebo in primary and secondary outcome measures. The improvement in binge eating frequency was associated with a significant and important reduction in body weight as well as a concurrent decrease in depressive symptoms. The drug appeared safe in this population. The most common adverse effects (dry mouth and constipation) were mild and benign. The effects of sibutramine in BED addressed the three main aspects of the syndrome: disturbed eating behavior, body weight, and associated depressive symptoms.

It is important to mention that this drug may have a selective effect on binge eating behavior. Mitchell et al. (53) investigated the effects of sibutramine on binge eating behavior, hunger, and satiety in seven adult subjects who had problems with binge eating in a human feeding laboratory paradigm by using a randomized controlled cross-over study design. The authors found a significant difference in the number of kilocalories consumed between the sibutramine and placebo conditions, with a significant reduction of intake especially during binge eating episodes.

ANTICONVULSANTS

Several lines of evidence suggest that some anticonvulsants, such as topiramate and zonisamide, might be effective in BED:

- Some anticonvulsants have mood stabilizing properties (54). This action may have an important impact on the mood symptoms or impulsive features that may be associated with BED (55).
- Some anticonvulsants have been associated with anorexia and weight loss in epilepsy clinical trials (56–58).

- Some anticonvulsants have been investigated in obesity and BN (59–61).

Although phenythoyn and carbamazepine have been studied in binge eating syndromes (compulsive eating and BN), their adverse effects of weight gain have limited their use in obese binge eaters (62–64). Recently, there is an increasing interest about the usefulness of topiramate in BED. Topiramate is a broad spectrum neurotherapeutic agent that has been approved for use in many countries in epilepsy in children and adults and, in some countries, for the prophylaxis of migraine. Its mechanism of action is not fully understood, but the drug is known to enhance γ-amino butyric acid activity, block voltage-dependent Na^+ channels, antagonize kainate/AMPA glutamate receptors, and to inhibit carbonic anhydrase (65). Topiramate has shown positive results in BN and BED. Shapira et al. (27), in a clinical case series evaluated 13 patients with BED associated with mood disorders. The authors found that adjunctive topiramate was associated with a reduction in binge episodes and body weight. Evidence that topiramate could act in BED independently of its action in mood disorders came from a case report and an open study (28,29). In this study, eight obese women with BED without psychiatric comorbidity were treated with 150 mg/day of topiramate. Doses of topiramate were gradually increased in order to reduce central nervous system side effects. Four out of six patients who concluded the study obtained a complete remission of binge eating and the other two had an important reduction in binge eating associated with weight loss. The most frequent adverse effects (paresthesia, sleepiness, and fatigue) were transient and disappeared with the final dose. Mc Elroy et al. (30) confirmed these findings in a double-blind, placebo-controlled study in 61 obese patients with BED. Topiramate was associated with an important and significant decrease of binge eating, body weight, and related psychopathological symptoms. The average dose of topiramate was 213 mg/day. Topiramate in this study, however, was associated with a higher incidence of adverse effects, possibly due to the rapid dose escalation regimen and high dose used.

Considering the lack of data about long-term drug treatments in BED, a very welcome contribution in this area was recently presented. To assess the long-term usefulness of topiramate, McElroy et al. (31) conducted an open label extension of the above mentioned double-blind trial. In this extension study, 35 completers of the 61 patients from de double-blind phase entered in a 42-week open trial with topiramate (median dose of 250 mg/day). The authors reported that subjects who received topiramate during the double-blind and open extension showed a maintained reduction in binge eating frequency and weight. Likewise, subjects who received placebo during double-blind period showed a reduction of the same parameters in the open phase. In addition, the authors reported a high discontinuation rate with this agent. The most common reasons for topiramate discontinuation were protocol nonadherence, and adverse events.

Zonisamide is an anticonvulsant that has serotoninergic and dopaminergic activity in addition to its antagonistic effects on sodium and calcium channels. It has been associated with weight loss in clinical trials for seizure disorders (66). A preliminary, short-term, randomized double-blind, placebo-controlled study suggested its efficacy in promoting weight loss in obese individuals without comorbid neuropsychiatric conditions (60). In a 12-week, open trial of 15 patients with BED, zonisamide was effective in reducing binge eating frequency and body weight (32). Although it was generally well tolerated, one patient developed a serious renal adverse event (nephrolithiasis with hydronephrosis and pyelonephritis) during zonisamide treatment.

OTHER AGENTS

In general, one might expect that interventions specially designed for BN or obesity may have a therapeutic effect in binge eating syndromes. In line with this idea, agents such as ondansetron, bupropion, and inositol may be useful in the treatment of binge eaters. Although none of these drugs can be currently recommended for routine use without additional controlled studies, available data on their use in syndromes with binge eating and/or obesity are reviewed further.

A randomized controlled trial compared ondansetron—a peripheral inhibitor of 5-HT$_3$ receptors used for the treatment of nausea induced by antineoplastics—with placebo, during four weeks in 29 patients with BN (67). Patients treated with ondansetron showed a 50% reduction in binge frequency and a 33% increase in meals not followed by purging. The decrease in binge eating and vomiting with ondansetron was not associated with compensatory eating behaviors. Ondansetron appeared to normalize the physiological mechanisms controlling meal termination and satiation. Considering that binge eating and vomiting produce intense stimulation of vagal afferent fibers and that ondansetron and other 5-HT3 antagonists decrease afferent vagal activity, the authors hypothesized that the symptom improvement observed with ondansetron may have resulted from a pharmacological correction of abnormal vagal neurotransmission.

Bupropion is currently approved for the treatment of major depression and for smoking cessation (68). In general, it increases norepinephrine turnover and, to a lesser extent, blocks the reuptake of dopamine. Such effects on central nervous system norepinephrine and dopamine neurotransmission have hypothesized to contribute to the drug's weight loss properties (69). Two randomized controlled trials with bupropion have assessed its short- and long-term efficacy in obesity (70,71). Both studies showed that the use of bupropion in obese patients is associated with a moderate weight loss, which was maintained with treatment continuation. Additionally, in the field of eating disorders, bupropion was studied by Horne et al. (72) in a placebo-controlled, double-blind study in 81 patients with BN. The drug was significantly superior to placebo in reducing episodes of binge eating and purging. However, because there was a higher than expected frequency of seizures in the BN patients receiving bupropion, concerns persist about the safety profile of bupropion in patients with BN or anorexia nervosa.

Inositol is a precursor of the phosphatidylinositol system, an important intracellular secondary messenger system. There is some evidence suggesting its effectiveness in depression (73). The therapeutic value of inositol in patients with BN and BED was investigated by Gelber et al. (74) in a double-blind, cross-over, placebo-controlled trial with 20 patients. Results were based on 12 completers who showed significant effects of inositol in reducing severity of binge eating as assessed by a visual analog scale. However, the high dropout rate observed in this study and the small number of patients with BED in the completers, make these results difficult to interpret.

Lithium, a mood stabilizer used in the treatment of bipolar disorder, should also be mentioned. Bipolar disorder can be associated with BN and BED in some cases (75). Shisslak et al. (76) reported a case of a bulimic patient with manic symptoms who was successfully treated with lithium. In a randomized double-blind placebo-controlled study, lithium did not separate from placebo in BN, but this trial was difficult to interpret because of the high response to placebo (77).

COMBINED TREATMENT

Combining pharmacological agents with psychological and/or nutritional interventions is a strategy frequently used in treating patients with eating disorders. In theory, the use of a medication as an adjunct to psychotherapy may improve the efficacy of each single approach. In line with this, a recent meta analysis suggested that antidepressants plus cognitive-behavior therapy was superior to medication alone for patients with BN (78). Although combined treatment has also received increasing attention in BED, it has not yet been widely studied. Available clinical trials assessing the usefulness of combined treatment in BED suggest that combining medication does not necessarily add much to the effectiveness of CBT in reducing binge eating behavior. However, adding antidepressants appears to enhance weight loss beyond the effects of the psychotherapy (79).

An initial study investigated the usefulness of fluoxetine in the long-term treatment of obesity (with and without binge eating syndrome) (80). In this trial, 45 obese subjects received behavior modification strategies and were randomized to fluoxetine (60 mg/day) or placebo for 52 weeks. The authors reported that patients treated with fluoxetine plus behavior modification lost significantly more weight than those in the comparison group. However, the drug did not appear to bring any benefit for binge eaters. In another study, patients who had completed three months of group CBT received either desipramine openly plus weight loss management or weight management alone (81). Despite desipramine appearing to have no impact on binge eating during or after treatment, drug-treated patients showed greater weight loss at follow-up. Devlin et al. (82) studied the addition of fluoxetine and phentermine to individual CBT in an open trial of 16 obese women with BED. It was observed that at the end of 20 weeks of active treatment, patients showed a reduction in binge frequency, weight, and psychological distress, although they regained much of the lost weight within a year.

To assess whether adding imipramine to dietary counseling and psychological support had an effect on BED, Laederach-Hofmann et al. (83) randomized 31 obese binge eaters (mean BMI 39.5 kg/m^2) according to DSM-IV criteria to either adjunctive imipramine ($n = 15$) or placebo ($n = 16$) for eight weeks. Patients were followed during a six months medication-free period with diet counseling and support. Dietary counseling plus imipramine produced a decrease in binge frequency from approximately 7.1–2.8 binge episodes per week and a mean weight loss of 2.2 kg; dietary counseling plus placebo decreased binge frequency from 7.1 to 5.4 binges per week and induced a mean weight gain of 0.2 kg. Both treatments led to an improvement in depressive symptoms.

Rica et al. (84) found that the addition of fluoxetine to CBT does not seem to provide any clear advantages, while the addition of fluvoxamine could enhance the effects of CBT on eating behaviors. In addition, the modifications of eating behaviors were maintained at the one year follow-up, although the lost weight was partially regained.

AUGMENTATION STRATEGIES

Most clinicians have the general hope that their patients will respond to a single drug. However, for the majority of psychiatric diagnoses, response to monotherapy may be considered the exception and not the rule. Although polypharmacy should be used judiciously, some patients with BED may require combination treatment with different classes of agents. Unfortunately, there is a lack of information about combination pharmacotherapy in the treatment of BED. Indeed, only three open reports discuss this strategy in obese patients with disturbed eating behaviors (47,85,86). First, the addition of naltrexone to fluoxetine reduced binge eating frequency in an adolescent with BED associated with severe major depression (47). Subsequently, Schmidt do Prado-Lima et al. (85) reported remission of binge eating, decrease in BMI, and improvement in depression with the combination of venlafaxine and topiramate in an obese patient with BED, major depression, and borderline personality disorder. Lastly, an observational study conducted by Anghelescu et. al. (86) in five obese patients suggested that the combination of sibutramine, orlistat, and topiramate might have positive therapeutic effects. Patients showed a mean weight loss of 31.2 kg at the end of 96 weeks of treatment along with normalization of eating patterns, expressed as a reduction on the Three-Factor Eating Questionnaire.

COMMENTS

Evidence-based medicine implies that clinical practice should be grounded in rigorous scientific information. In terms of drug therapy, randomized placebo-controlled trials represent the top of a hierarchic classification of evidence, followed by open reports. When pharmacotherapy is selected for a patient with BED, the choice of which medication to use should consider such evidence-based principles.

A general overview of the response rates reported in controlled pharmacological studies of BED indicate that drug treatment is usually associated with positive effects on binge eating frequency and weight outcomes (Figs. 1 and 2) (19–22,24,26,30). Unfortunately, final conclusions about comparative effects of different drugs could only be estimated using more specific meta-analytical techniques. However, the similar methodology used in recent BED clinical trials facilitates comparisons across different studies.

As estimated by Carter et al. (39), the drug-placebo difference in percentage of patients with remission of binge eating at endpoint for SSRIs in BED was 20.2 % (19–22). In terms of body weight outcomes, the drug-placebo differences observed in weight change with SSRIs (Fig. 2) was −4.6 kg with fluoxetine, −1.7 kg with fluvoxamine, −4.4 kg with sertraline, and −2.3 with citalopram (19–22). As seen in Figure 1, the mean difference in the sibutramine study in the number of patients with remission from binge eating at the end of the trial was 20%, similar to that observed with SSRIs (26). In addition, the impressive amount of weight loss observed with this agent (drug-placebo difference of −8.8 kg) was higher than that reported in other BED pharmacological studies (Fig. 2). Regarding topiramate, its

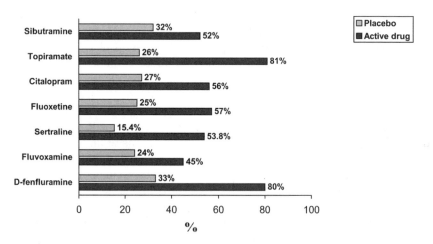

Figure 1 Remission rates of binge eating episodes (%) at the end of treatment in randomized controlled trials in BED. *Abbreviation*: BED, binge eating disorder. *Source*: From Refs. 19, 20, 21, 22, 24, 26, 30.

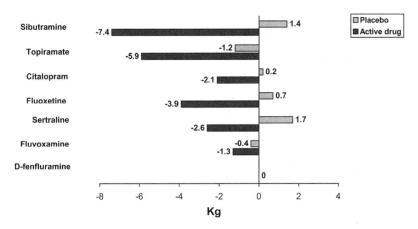

Figure 2 Weight change (kg) at the end of treatment in randomized controlled trials in BED. *Abbreviation*: BED, binge eating disorder. *Source*: From Refs. 19, 20, 21, 22, 24, 26, 30.

use was associated with a marked effect on binge eating behavior (30). A total of 64% of topiramate-treated patients had stopped bingeing compared with 30% of the placebo group (Fig. 1). Furthermore, the drug-placebo difference in weight change for topiramate was −4.7 kg (Fig. 2).

Initial evidences suggest that antidepressants, at least in the short term, do not add any positive impact to the efficacy of psychotherapy on binge eating frequency but may have a positive, although modest, impact on weight loss. Until now, the usefulness of combined treatments of psychotherapy with new agents, such as sibutramine and topiramate has not been adequately addressed. Since these agents have been associated with possibly greater effects on the behavioral and somatic domains of BED, the combination of sibutramine or topiramate with psychotherapeutic or nutritional treatments might improve the clinical benefits of these interventions. At last, the possible advantage of drug augmentation strategies for patients with BED has not been systematically investigated so far. Nevertheless, the association of fluoxetine and naltrexone, topiramate and venlafaxine, as well as orlistat plus sibutramine and topiramate have been described as useful pharmacological combinations to treat refractory BED patients, who often have complicating factors such as comorbid conditions.

CONCLUSIONS

In summary, the pharmacotherapy of binge eating is still at an early stage of development. Overall, the analysis of available evidences suggests that there are at least three classes of drugs with potential use in BED treatment: antidepressants, centrally-active antiobesity agents, and anticonvulsants with weight loss properties. SSRIs remains the best studied class of antidepressants in BED. The use of SSRIs in BED has been associated with a modest but clinically significant effect on binge eating behavior and a modest and variable weight loss. Sibutramine is an anti-obesity agent that has been shown efficacious in the treatment of BED. It reduces binge eating behavior, promotes a marked weight loss, and may reduce associated depressive symptoms. Topiramate is another promising agent in BED pharmacological treatment, with an important impact on eating related psychopathology and body weight. Further studies are needed to address several questions about the pharmacotherapy of BED, such as the optimal medication or medications, the most appropriate of dose and duration of treatment, as well as, the role and effect of combined treatments (medication plus psychotherapy, medication plus nutritional guidance, and combination pharmacotherapy).

REFERENCES

1. Stunkard AJ. Eating patterns and obesity. Psychiatr Q 1959; 33:284–295.
2. American Psychiatric Association. Diagnostic and Statistical Manual of Mental Disorders, Fourth Edition. Washington, DC: American Psychiatric Association, 1994.
3. de Zwaan M. Binge eating disorder and obesity. Int J Obes Relat Metab Disord 2001; 25(Suppl 1):S51–55.
4. de Zwaan M, Mitchell JE, Seim HC, et al. Eating related and general psychopathology in obese females with binge-eating disorder. Int J Eat Disord 1994; 15(1):43–52.
5. Eldredge KL, Agras WS. Weight and shape overconcern and emotional eating in binge-eating disorder. Int J Eat Disord 1996; 19(1):73–82.
6. Yanovski SZ, Nelson JE, Dubbert BK, et al. Association of binge-eating disorder and psychiatric comorbidity in obese subjects. Am J Psychiatry 1993; 150:1472–1479.
7. Fontenelle LF, Mendlowicz MV, de Menezes GB, et al. Psychiatric comorbidity in a Brazilian sample of patients with binge-eating disorder. Psychiatry Res 2003; 15:119(12):189–194.
8. Bulik CM, Sullivan PF, Kendler KS. Medical and psychiatric morbidity in obese women with and without binge-eating. Int J Eat Disord 2002; 32(1):72–78.
9. Angst J. The emerging epidemiology of hypomania and bipolar II disorder. J Affect Disord 1998; 50:143–151.
10. McElroy SL, Keck PE, Phillips KA. Kleptomania, compulsive buying, and binge-eating disorder. J Clin Psychiatry 1994; 56(Suppl 4):S14–S26.
11. Steiger H, Lehoux PM, Gauvin L. Impulsivity, dietary control and the urge to binge in bulimic syndromes. Int J Eat Disord 1999; 26(3):261–274.
12. Sansone RA, Wiederman MW, Sansone LA. The prevalence of borderline personality disorder among individuals with obesity: a critical review of the literature. Eat Behav 2000; 1(1):93–104.
13. Sansone RA, Wiederman MW, Monteith D. Obesity, borderline personality symptomatology, and body image among women in a psychiatric outpatient setting. Int J Eat Disord 200; 29(1):76–79.

14. Devlin MJ. binge-eating disorder and obesity. A combined treatment approach. Psychiatr Clin North Am 2001; 24:325–335.
15. Zhu AJ, Walsh BT. Pharmacologic treatment of eating disorders. Can J Psychiatry 2002; 47(3):227–234.
16. Appolinario JC, McElroy SL. Pharmacological approaches in the treatment of binge-eating disorder. Curr Drug Targets 2004; 5(3):301–307.
17. McCann UD, Agras WS. Successful treatment of nonpurging bulimia nervosa with desipramine: a double-blind, placebo-controlled study. Am J Psychiatry 1990; 147(ll):1509–1513.
18. Alger SA, Schwalberg MD, Bigaoueette JM, Michalek AV, Howard LJ. Effect of a tricyclic antidepressant and opiate antagonist on binge-eating behavior in normal weight bulimic and obese, binge-eating subjects. Am J Clin Nutr 1991; 53:865–867.
19. Hudson JI, McElroy SL, Raymond, NC. Fluvoxamine in the treatment of binge-eating disorder: a multicenter placebo-controlled double-blind trial. Am J Psychiatry 1998; 155:1756–1762.
20. McElroy SL, Casuto LS, et al. Placebo-controled trial of sertraline in the treatment of binge-eating disorder. Am J Psychiatry 2000; 157:1004–1006.
21. Arnold LM, McElroy SL, Hudson JI, Welge JA, Bennett AJ, Keck PE. A placebo-controlled, randomized trial of fluoxetine in the treatment of binge-eating disorder. J Clin Psychiatry 2002; 63:1028–1033.
22. McElroy SL, Hudson JI, Malhotra S, Welge JA, Nelson EB, Keck PE Jr. Citalopram in the treatment of binge-eating disorder: a placebo-controlled trial. J Clin Psychiatry 2003; 64(7):807–813.
23. Pearlstein T, Spurell E, Hohlstein LA, et al. A double-blind, placebo-controlled trial of fluvoxamine in binge-eating disorder: a high placebo response. Arch Women Ment Health 2003; 6(2):147–151.
24. Stunkard A, Berkowitz R, Tanrikut C, Reiss E, Young L. d-Fenfluramine treatment of binge-eating disorder. Am J Psychiatry 1996; 153:1455–1459.
25. Appolinario JC, Godoy-Matos A, Fontenelle LF, et al. An open-label trial of sibutramine in obese patients with binge-eating disorder. J Clin Psychiatry 2002; 63(l):28–30.
26. Appolinario JC, Bacaltchuk J, Sichieri R, et al. A randomized, double-blind, placebo-controlled study of sibutramine in the treatment of binge-eating disorder. Arch Gen Psychiatry 2003; 60(11):1109–1116.
27. Shapira NA, Goldsmith TD, McElroy SL. Treatment of binge-eating disorder with topiramate: a clinical case series. J Clin Psychiatry 2000; 61(5):368–372.
28. Appolinario JC, Coutinho W, Fontenelle L. Topiramate for binge-eating disorder. Am J Psychiatry 2001; 158(6):967–968.
29. Appolinario JC, Fontenelle LF, Papelbaum M, Bueno JR, Coutinho W. Topiramate use in obese patients with binge-eating disorder: an open study. Can J Psychiatry 2002; 47:271–273.
30. McElroy SL, Arnold LM, Shapira NA, et al. Topiramate in the treatment of binge-eating disorder associated with obesity: a randomized, placebo-controlled trial. Am J Psychiatry 2003; 160(2):255–261.
31. McElroy SL, Sapira NA, Arnold LM, et al. Topiramate in the long-term treatment of binge-eating disorder associated with obesity. Presented at 2004 International Conference on Eating Disorders, Orlando, Florida: April 30, 2004.

32. McElroy SL, Kotwal R, Hudson JI, Nelson EB, Keck PE. Jr. Zonisamide in the treatment of binge-eating disorder: an open-label, prospective trial. J Clin Psychiatry 2004; 65(1):50–56.

33. Raingeard I, Courtet P, Renard E, Bringer J. Naltrexone improves blood glucose control in type 1 diabetic women with severe and chronic eating disorders. Diabetes Care 2004; 27(3):847–848.

34. Versiani M. A review of 19 double-blind placebo-controlled studies in social anxiety disorder (social phobia). World J Biol Psychiatry 2000; 1(1):27–33.

35. Jacobs MJ, Wilfley DE, Gregory-Bills T, et al. Placebo response in pharmacotherapy for binge-eating disorder. Presented at 2003 International Conference on Eating Disorders, Denver, Colorado: May 29–31, 2003.

36. Williamson DA, Womble LG, Smeets MA, et al. Latent structure of eating disorder symptoms: a factor analytic and taxometric investigation. Am J Psychiatry 2002; 159(3):412–418.

37. Appolinario JC, Bueno JR, Coutinho W. Psychotropic drugs in the treatment of obesity: what promise? CNS Drugs 2004; 18(10):629–651.

38. Gardiner HM, Freeman CP, Jesinger DK, Collins SA. Fluvoxamine: an open pilot study in moderately obese female patients suffering from a typical eating disorders and episodes of bingeing. Int J Obes Relat Metab Disord 1993; 17(5):301–305.

39. Carter WP, Hudson JI, Lalonde JK, Pindyck L, McElroy SL, Pope HG Jr. Pharmacologic treatment of binge-eating disorder. Int J Eat Disord 2003; 34 (Suppl):S74–88.

40. Stahl SM, Entsuah R, Rudolph RL. Comparative efficacy between venlafaxine and SSRIs: a pooled analysis of patients with depression. Biol Psychiatry 2002; 52(12):1166–1174.

41. Malhotra S, King KH, Welge JA, Brusman-Lovins L, McElroy SL. Venlafaxine treatment of binge-eating disorder associated with obesity: a series of 35 patients. J Clin Psychiatry 2002; 63(9):802–826.

42. Silveira RO. Reboxetine in obese patients with binge-eating disorder. MSc dissertation, Federal University of Rio Grande do Sul, Porto Alegre, 2004.

43. Quinn JG, O'Hare E, Levine AS, Kim EM. Evidence for a mu-opioid-opioid connection between the paraventricular nucleus and ventral tegmental area in the rat. Brain Res 2003; 991(1–2):206–211.

44. Jarosz PA, Metzger BL. The effect of opioid antagonism on food intake behavior and body weight in a biobehavioral model of obese binge-eating. Biol Res Nurs 2002; 3(4):198–209.

45. de Zwaan M, Mitchell JE. Opiate antagonists and eating behavior in humans: a review. J Clin Pharmacol 1992; 32(12):1060–1072.

46. Marrazzi MA, Markham KM, Kinzie J, Luby ED. binge-eating disorder: response to naltrexone. Int J Obes Relat Metab Disord 1995; 19(2):143–145.

47. Neumeister A, Winkler A, Wober-Bingol C. Addition of naltrexone to fluoxetine in the treatment of binge-eating disorder. Am J Psychiatry 1999; 156(5):797.

48. Guss JL, Kissileff HR, Devlin MJ, Zimmerli E, Walsh BT. Binge size increases with body mass index in women with binge-eating disorder. Obes Res 2002; 10(10):1021–1029.

49. Rothman RB, Baumann MH. Therapeutic and adverse actions of serotonin transporter substrates. Pharmacol Ther 2002; 95(1):73–88.

50. Bray GA, Ryan DH, Gordon D, Heidingsfelder S, Cerise F, Wilson K. A double-blind randomized placebo-controlled trial of sibutramine. Obes Res 1996; 4(3):263–270.
51. James WP, Astrup A, Finer N, et al. Effect of sibutramine on weight maintenance after weight loss: a randomised trial. STORM Study Group. Sibutramine Trial of Obesity Reduction and Maintenance. Lancet 2000; 356(9248):2119–2125.
52. Ryan DH, Kaiser P, Bray GA. Sibutramine: a novel new agent for obesity treatment. Obes Res 1995; 3(Suppl 4):553S–559S.
53. Mitchell JE, Gosnell BA, Roerig JL, et al. Effects of sibutramine on binge eating, hunger, and fullness in a laboratory human feeding paradigm. Obes Res 2003; 11(5):599–602.
54. Ghaemi SN, Gaughan S. Novel anticonvulsants: a new generation of mood stabilizers? Harv Rev Psychiatry 2000; 8(1):1–7.
55. Hollander E, Allen A, Lopez RP, et al. A preliminary double-blind, placebo-controlled trial of divalproex sodium in borderline personality disorder. J Clin Psychiatry 2001; 62(3):199–203.
56. Bergen DC, Ristanovic RK, Waicosky K, Kanner A, Hoeppner TJ. Weight loss in patients taking felbamate. Clin Neuropharmacol 1995; 18(1):23–27.
57. French JA. The role of new antiepileptic drugs. Am J Manag Care 2001; 7(Suppl 7):S209–S214.
58. Pellock JM, Appleton R. Use of new antiepileptic drugs in the treatment of childhood epilepsy. Epilepsia 1999; 40(Suppl 6):S29–S38.
59. Bray GA, Hollander P, Klein S, et al. A 6-month randomized, placebo-controlled, dose-ranging trial of topiramate for weight loss in obesity. Obes Res 2003; ll(6):722–733.
60. Gadde KM, Franciscy DM, Wagner HR 2nd, Krishnan KR. Zonisamide for weight loss in obese adults: a randomized controlled trial. JAMA 2003; 289(14):1820–1825.
61. Hoopes SP, Reimherr FW, Hedges DW, et al. Treatment of bulimia nervosa with topiramate in a randomized, double-blind, placebo-controlled trial, part 1: improvement in binge and purge measures. J Clin Psychiatry 2003; 64(11):1335–1341.
62. Green RS, Rau JH. Treatment of compulsive eating disturbances with anticonvulsant medication. Am J Psychiatry 1974; 131(4):428–432.
63. Wermuth BM, Davis KL, Hollister LE, Stunkard AJ. Phenytoin treatment of the binge-eating syndrome. Am J Psychiatry 1977; 134(11):1249–1253.
64. Kaplan AS, Garfinkel PE, Darby PL, Garner DM. Carbamazepine in the treatment of bulimia. Am J Psychiatry 1983; 140(9):1225–1226.
65. Privitera MD. Topiramate: a new antiepileptic drug. Ann Pharmacother 1997; 31(10):1164–1173.
66. Oommen KJ, Mathews S. Zonisamide: a new antiepileptic drug. Clin Neuropharmacol 1999; 22:192–200.
67. Faris PL, Kim SW, Meller WH, et al. Effect of decreasing afferent vagal activity with ondansetron on symptoms of bulimia nervosa: a randomised, double-blind trial. Lancet 2000; 355(9206):792–797.
68. Schatzberg AF. New indications for antidepressants. J Clin Psychiatry 2000; 61(Suppl 11):9–17.
69. Zarrindast MR, Hosseini-Nia T. Anorectic and behavioural effects of bupropion. Gen Pharmacol 1988; 19(2):201–204.

70. Gadde KM, Parker CB, Maner LG, Wagner HR 2nd, Logue EJ, Drezner MK, Krishnan. Bupropion for weight loss: an investigation of efficacy and tolerability in overweight and obese women. Obes Res 2001; 9(9):544–551.
71. Anderson JW, Greenway FL, Fujioka K, Gadde KM, McKenney J, O'Neil PM. Bupropion SR enhances weight loss: a 48-week double-blind, placebo-controlled trial. Obes Res 2002; 10(7):633–641.
72. Horne RL, Ferguson JM, Pope HG, et al. Treatment of bulimia with bupropion: a multicenter controlled trial. J Clin Psychiatry 1988; 49(7):262–266.
73. Levine J, Barak Y, Gonzalves M, et al. Double-blind, controlled trial of inositol treatment of depression. Am J Psychiatry 1995; 152(5):792–794.
74. Gelber D, Levine J, Belmaker RH. Effect of inositol on bulimia nervosa and binge-eating. Int J Eat Disord 2001; 29(3):345–348.
75. Keck PE, McElroy SL. Bipolar disorder, obesity, and pharmacotherapy-associated weight gain. J Clin Psychiatry 2003; 64(12):1426–1435.
76. Shisslak CM, Perse T, Crago M. Coexistence of bulimia nervosa and mania: a literature review and case report. Compr Psychiatry 1991; 32(2):181–184.
77. Hsu LK, Clement L, Santhouse R, Ju ES. Treatment of bulimia nervosa with lithium carbonate. A controlled study. J Nerv Ment Dis 1991; 179(6):351–355.
78. Bacaltchuk J, Trefiglio RP, Oliveira IR, Hay P, Lima MS, Mari JJ. Combination of antidepressants and psychological treatments for bulimia nervosa: a systematic review. Acta Psychiatr Scand 2000; 101(4):256–264.
79. de Zwaan M, Roerig J. Pharmacological treatment of eating disorders: a review. In: Maj M, Halmi K, López-Ibor JJ, Sartorius N, eds. Eating Disorders: WPA Series—Evidence and Experience in Psychiatry. London: John Wiley & Sons Ltd, 2003.
80. Marcus MD, Wing RR, Ewing L, Kern E, McDermott M, Gooding W. A double-blind, placebo-controlled trial of fluoxetine plus behavior modification in the treatment of obese binge-eaters and non-binge-eaters. Am J Psychiatry 1990; 147(7):876–881.
81. Agras WS, Telch CF, Arnow B, et al. Weight loss, cognitive-behavioral, and desipramine treatments in binge-eating-disorder. An additive design. Behav Ther 1994; 25:225–238.
82. Devlin MJ, Goldfein JA, Carino JS, Wolk SL. Open treatment of overweight binge eaters with phentermine and fluoxetine as an adjunct to cognitive-behavioral therapy. Int J Eat Disord 2000; 28(3):325–332.
83. Laederach-Hofmann K, Graf C, Horber F, et al. Imipramine and diet counseling with psychological support in the treatment of obese binge eaters: a randomized, placebo-controlled double-blind study. Int J Eat Disord 1999; 26(3):231–244.
84. Ricca V, Mannucci E, Mezzani B, et al. Fluoxetine and fluvoxamine combined with individual cognitive-behaviour therapy in binge-eating disorder: a one-year follow-up study. Psychother Psychosom 2001; 70(6):298–306.
85. Schmidt do Prado-Lima PA, Bacaltchuk J. Topiramate in treatment-resistant depression and binge-eating disorder. Bipolar Disord 200; 4(4):271–273.
86. Anghelescu I, Klawe C, Szegedi A. Add-on combination and maintenance treatment: case series of five obese patients with different eating behavior. J Clin Psychopharmacol 2002; 22(5):52.

14

Psychotropic-Induced Weight Gain: Liability, Mechanisms and Treatment Approaches

Roger S. McIntyre

Department of Psychiatry, University of Toronto, Toronto, Ontario, Canada

Jakub Z. Konarski

Mood Disorder Psychopharmacology Unit, Institute of Medical Science, Toronto, Ontario, Canada

Paul E. Keck Jr.

Psychopharmacology Research Program, Department of Psychiatry, University of Cincinnati College of Medicine; General Clinical Research Center and Mental Health Care Line, Cincinnati Veterans Affairs Medical Center, Cincinnati, Ohio, U.S.A.

INTRODUCTION

Overweight and obesity are the most common nutritional disorders in the United States (1). Over the past two decades, there has been an epidemic rise in self-reported overweight (body mass index, BMI $>25 \, \text{kg/m}^2$) and obesity (BMI $>30 \, \text{kg/m}^2$) prevalence (2,3). Moreover, the prevalence of obesity in child and adolescent populations has almost tripled since 1970 (4). The medical complications of overweight and obesity are well established and include osteoarthritis, type II diabetes mellitus, cardiovascular disease, and some forms of cancer (5). Many of these foregoing maladies are relatively more common in some psychiatric populations (6–9). The etiology of overweight and obesity is multifactorial and includes many factors that are potentially modifiable with behavioral and preventative treatment strategies (10).

Investigations, both cross-sectional and longitudinal, describing body mass distribution and overweight trends in psychiatric populations indicate that subgroups of patients (e.g., schizophrenia, bipolar disorder) are at risk for overweight and associated morbidity (11,12). Preliminary results from body-composition studies further indicate that abdominal obesity, an independent risk factor for obesity-related morbidity, may also be more common in some psychiatric subgroups (13). Myriad etiological factors are unique to these persons including the frequent use of weight-gain promoting psychotropic medications (14).

Weight gain associated with a number of psychotropic medications is a serious problematic adverse event; it may predispose and portend iatrogenic morbidity (e.g., hypertension, type II diabetes mellitus), further belies medication acceptability, and it is axiomatic that it adversely affects self-esteem and overall quality of life (15).

Berken et al. (16) reported that concern about weight gain was a cited reason for noncompliance in up to 48% of patients receiving tricyclic antidepressants (TCAs) therapy. Weiden et al. (17) surveyed schizophrenic members of the National Alliance of the Mental III (NAMI) and National Mental Health Association (NMHA) ($n = 304$) regarding the impact of obesity and weight on compliance with medications. Respondents with BMI in the obese range were most likely to report stopping their medication; those in the overweight range had intermediate compliance rates, which were better than the obese respondents but poorer than the normal weight respondents ($p = 0.029$). It is unsurprising that weight gain was additionally associated with subjective distress taking medication.

The influence of weight gain on adherence is further underscored by results from a recent investigation of females with type I diabetes mellitus. The possibility of treatment-associated weight gain was a powerful detractor to treatment, accounting for more than half of the occasions in which insulin was deliberately omitted. The interruption of insulin treatment in these patients was associated with the progression of diabetic retinopathy and nephropathy (18).

This chapter will review extant published studies describing weight gain associated with three of the most commonly prescribed classes of psychotropic medications: conventional unimodal antidepressants, mood stabilizers/ AEDs, and antipsychotics. The absolute and relative weight-gain liability for each class of agents will be presented alongside a review of putative weight gain promoting mechanisms and possible avenues for prevention and treatment.

We conducted a MedLine search of all English language articles 1966–2004 using the keywords: overweight, obesity, body mass index, schizophrenia, psychosis, psychotic disorders, bipolar disorder, major depressive disorder, conventional antipsychotics (CAP), atypical antipsychotics (AAs), clozapine, olanzapine, risperidone, quetiapine, ziprasidone, aripiprazole, mood stabilizers, lithium, antiepileptic drugs (AEDs), lamotrigine, gabapentin, topiramate, zonisamide, levetiracetam, oxcarbazepine (OXC), carbamazepine (CBZ) divalproex, valproate, antidepressants selective serotonin reuptake inhibitors, (SSRIs), fluoxetine, paroxetine, fluvoxamine, sertraline, citalopram, escitalopram, venlafaxine, nefazodone, bupropion, duloxetine, mirtazapine, monoamine oxidase inhibitors (MAOIs), phenelzine, tranylcypromine, isocarboxazid, reversible inhibitors of monoamine (RIMA) oxidase, moclobemide, brofaromine, TCAs, desipramine, imiprarnine, nortriptyline, amitriptyline, diabetes mellitus, and glucose homeostasis. The search was supplemented with manual review of relevant references. Priority was given to randomized controlled data, when unavailable; studies of sufficient sample size are presented.

MEDICATION-ASSOCIATED WEIGHT GAIN: LIABILITY

Hitherto, psychotropic medication-associated weight gain has not been systematically investigated, monitored, or reported by clinician and/or researchers. The rigor in which much of the available weight-change data have been acquired and presented in psychiatric populations is paltry and consequently difficult to interpret. For example, rarely have investigations methodologically and statistically controlled for relevant sociodemography, dietary habits, comorbidity (e.g., binge eating disorder, hypothyroidism), patient behavior (e.g., inactivity, smoking), family history, premorbid weight status, illness-associated weight change, body composition, and concomitant treatment effects. Anthropometric indices most relevant to practitioners, the proportion of patients exhibiting categorical changes in body weight (e.g., >7–10%), premorbid-posttreatment, and pretreatment–posttreatment changes in BMI, waist-to-hip ratio (WHR), and body composition are less frequently reported. The translational value of psychotropic-associated weight change, presented as an isolated outcome variable, is thus limited and potentially misleading. With these limitations in mind, data from extant studies will be presented emphasizing results from controlled investigations when available.

Antidepressants

Antidepressant-associated weight gain is described with both acute and long-term treatment. Taken together, TCAs and nonselective irreversible MAOIs, are more likely to impart weight gain than the currently available contemporary antidepressants (i.e., SSRIs, venlafaxine, duloxetine, nefazodone, moclobemide, or bupropion) (19). It has been consistently reported that mirtazapine's weight-gain liability is approximately midway between the liability ascribed to the SSRIs and TCAs (Table 1).

Table 1 Short- and Long-Term Weight Gain Liability with Available
Antidepressants

Antidepressants	Weight gain liability
TCAs	++++
MAOIs	++++
RIMAs	0/−
SSRIs	+/−
Bupropion	0/−
Venlafaxine	0/−
Duloxetine	0/−
Nefazodone	0/−
Mirtazapine	++

Abbreviations: TCAs, tricyclic antidepressants; MAOIs, monoamine oxidase
inhibitors; SSRIs, selective serotonin reuptake inhibitors.

TCAs

TCAs exhibit multireceptor in vitro affinities and variably recruit and
engage serotonin and norepinephrine systems. Commonly reported adverse
events with TCAs (e.g., dry mouth, orthostatic hypotension, and weight
gain) are pharmacodynamically associated with their affinity for muscarinic
cholinergic, noradrenergic, and histaminergic receptors, respectively (20,21).

Weight gain is a frequently reported adverse event following short- and
long-term treatment with TCAs, with amitriptyline being the most notable
offender (22,23). Cumulative weight gain with maintenance TCA therapy
has been described with several agents. For example, Fernstrom et al. (24)
reported that up to 15% of imipramine-treated depressed patients had a
weight gain >10 lb after 16 weeks of treatment. It has been estimated that
up to 13% of patients treated with imipramine for an average of 33 weeks
had a 10% increase or more in overall bodyweight (25). Garland et al. (26)
further reported that TCA-treated patients can expect to gain approximately
0.5–1.4 kg/mo of maintenance TCA therapy (16).

MAOIs

MAOIs indirectly increase synaptic availability of monoamines by inhibiting
their catabolism. As a class of agents, they irreversibly inhibit both monoamine oxidase A and B. Commonly reported adverse events with MAOIs
are insomnia, headaches, nausea, and edema. Change in appetite, dietary
habits, and edema may be etiologically relevant to weight gain associated
with these agents (27).

It has been consistently reported that MAOI therapy is associated with
clinically significant weight gain with greater liability with phenelzine versus

other MAOIs (e.g., tranylcypromine, isocarboxazid). The RIMAs (e.g., moclobemide, brofaromine) are associated with less relative short-term weight gain than most TCAs and MAOIs (27,28). For example, in a six-week study of depressed patients, weight gain was observed in up to 2.6% of moclobemide-treated patients versus 21.6% of patients treated with maprotiline (29). In a larger maintenance study ($n = 1120$) in depressed patients, moclobemide treatment was associated with significant weight gain ($\geq 10\,$kg) in a relatively small percentage of patients (1.4%) (30).

SSRIs

The SSRIs have unequivocally advanced the pharmacotherapy of mood and anxiety disorders offering patients improved safety, tolerability, and simplicity of dosing when compared to their therapeutic predecessors (31). Although classified together, these agents are heterogeneous in their pharmacodynamic, tolerability, and safety profile (32). All SSRIs variably block the serotonin transporter, increasing the synaptic availability of the well-established satiety factor, serotonin (33). Serotonin and its multiple receptors comprise the most studied neurotransmitter system in appetite, feeding behavior, and metabolism (34).

Investigations examining the bariatric potential of fluoxetine in nondepressed obese patients have consistently reported a transient weight-reducing effect (35). Moreover, fluoxetine treatment (and some other SSRIs) has a favorable influence on abnormal eating patterns and associated psychopathology in patients with eating disorders, including binge eating disorder (36,37).

In samples of depressed patients, SSRI treatment is reported to be weight neutral or weight-loss promoting in short-term studies (≤ 8 weeks) (38–41). Longer term investigations (≥ 6 months) describing weight change with SSRI therapy are also available. Fava et al. (42) reported mean changes in body weight from baseline to endpoint for up to 26–32 weeks of treatment with sertraline, fluoxetine, and paroxetine. When weight gain was defined as $\geq 7\%$ increase in bodyweight, variable weight gain liability was reported (4.2% sertraline, 6.8% fluoxetine, and 25.5% paroxetine, $p = 0.016$). The interpretation of this investigation's results would have been benefited by the presence of a placebo-treated group.

Michelson et al. (41) described the weight gain trajectory in depressed patients receiving fluoxetine (20 mg/day) in a 50-week placebo-controlled study. A mean weight reduction of 0.4 kg/patient over the first four weeks of treatment was associated with fluoxetine treatment. Throughout this study until endpoint (week 50), an inexorable increase in weight was noted in both the intervention and the non-intervention group with no between group differences noted in study completers. Fluoxetine-associated weight gain in this study was associated with improvement in appetite in recovered depressed patients (43).

Novel Antidepressants

Nefazodone is a serotonin reuptake inhibitor and an antagonist at 5-HT_{2A} receptors. A metabolite of nefazodone, m-Chlorophenylpiperazine (m-CPP) is an agonist at the 5-HT_{2C} receptor, a pharmacodynamic profile predictive of anorexia and weight loss.

Nefazodone appears to be weight neutral in both short- and long-term treatment studies. For example, in a 36-week continuation study, nefazodone-treated patients exhibited weight gain comparable to placebo (7.6% vs. 8.6%, respectively, p = ns) (44). A retrospective analysis pooling data from six maintenance studies was completed comparing nefazodone with fluoxetine, sertraline, and paroxetine. Clinically significant weight gain ($\geq 7\%$ body weight increase) was reported in 9% of nefazodone-treated patients and 18% of the SSRI-treated patients, a trend that did not reach statistical significance (45).

Bupropion, pharmacodynamically similar to the appetite suppressant diethylpropion, blocks the reuptake of norepinephrine and, to a lesser extent, dopamine. Bupropion has consistently been described as weight neutral and/ or promoting weight loss in studies of variable duration. For example, an open-label eight-week study, followed by a 44-week placebo substitution phase reported significant weight loss with bupropion. Weight loss was observed after acute phase treatment (1.4 kg) with greater weight loss reported in patients with a higher baseline BMI (46). At the end of the double-blind phase, bupropion-treated patients experienced more absolute weight loss (1.7–2.4 kg) than did placebo-treated patients ($p < 0.001$).

Venlafaxine and duloxetine are inhibitors of both serotonin and norepinephrine reuptake transporters, pharmacological properties similar to the U.S. Food and Drug Administration (FDA)-approved bariatric treatment, sibutramine. Both agents are reported to be weight neutral in studies of varying duration (47–50). Goldstein et al. (48) evaluated duloxetine in a randomized, double-blind, four-arm study in which depressed out-patients were assigned to duloxetine 40, 80 mg/day, paroxetine 20 mg/day, or placebo. Duloxetine 80 mg/day resulted in a significant, albeit small, weight decrease compared with placebo (placebo +0.47 kg; duloxetine 40 mg/day +0.02 kg; duloxetine 80 mg/day −0.60 kg; paroxetine 20 mg/day +0.41 kg; duloxetine 80 mg/day vs. placebo, $p < 0.01$).

Mirtazapine's mechanism of action is related to the enhancement of noradrenergic and serotonergic neurotransmission primarily via $\alpha 2$ hetero-receptor (and autoreceptor) antagonism. Mirtazapine also exhibits high in vitro affinity for histaminergic (H1) receptor populations, which portends liability for treatment-associated sedation and weight gain.

Thase et al. (51) evaluated the antidepressant efficacy and tolerability of mirtazapine across 40 weeks of therapy in a double-blind, placebo-controlled trial in remitted depressed patients ($n = 156$). The mean increase in weight associated with mirtazapine during the lead-in open-label phase was 2.5 kg (5.6 lb). At the end of the double-blind phase, there was additional and clinically significant weight gain reported in the mirtazapine-treated group (1.4 kg, $p < 0.001$).

Taken together, the use of erstwhile antidepressants (i.e., TCAs, MAOIs) is associated with clinically significant weight gain. In groups of patients, SSRIs are on average weight neutral and may promote weight loss with short-term therapy. Notwithstanding, some patients may experience weight gain with acute SSRI therapy, and for others, short-term weight loss is obfuscated by an inexorable return to pretreatment weight status with maintenance treatment. The RIMAs, bupropion, venlafaxine, duloxetine, and nefazodone are not associated with weight gain (greater than placebo) in variable-length studies. Mirtazapine is the only recently introduced significant weight gain versus placebo in both acute and maintenance studies (19).

Antipsychotics

Reports of weight gain induced by CAPs began to appear soon after these agents became available (52,53). Doss (54) retrospectively described differential weight gain liability in 78 randomly assigned patients after 36 weeks of conventional antipsychotic (CAP) treatment. CAPs were similarly liable to induce weight gain in oral and depot formulations (55,56).

Allison et al. (57) meta-analyzed schizophrenia treatment trials ($n = 81$; 18 included placebo comparison) at least 10 weeks in duration comparing weight gain among patients using CAPs and newer AAs. A spectrum of weight gain liability was noted; clozapine 4.0 kg, olanzapine 3.5 kg, thioridazine 3.5 kg, sertindole 2.9 kg, chlorpromazine 2.1 kg, risperidone 2.0 kg, and ziprasidone 0.04 kg, while placebo was associated with weight loss (-0.44 kg). Although quetiapine was not included in this analysis, other study results indicate its short-term weight gain liability is similar to risperidone (58,59). Similarly, weight gain associated with aripiprazole was consistent with that reported for ziprasidone. A summary of information on weight gain reported in the prescribing information for each of the AAs is shown in Figure 1 and Table 2.

Short-term studies describing weight gain data supplied by manufacturers in U.S. package inserts indicate that all first-line AA (olanzapine, risperidone, quetiapine, ziprasidone, aripiprazole) medications cause substantially different rates of clinically significant weight gain (as defined by the U.S. FDA $\geq 7\%$ compared to placebo). Aripirazole, ziprasidone, and risperidone are associated with approximately two times the placebo incidence of weight gain in short-term clinical trials, with quetiapine approximately four times, and olanzapine approximately 10 times the placebo incidence of weight gain during short-term trials (Fig. 2) (60).

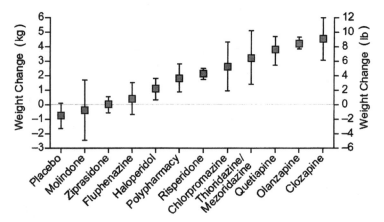

Figure 1 Ninety five percent confidence intervals for weight change after 10 weeks on standard drug doses, estimated from a random effects model.

Maintenance studies (i.e., one year) evaluating AAs weight gain liability in schizophrenic and bipolar populations have consistently reported a differential weight gain plateau with most overall weight gain accrued over the first two to six months of therapy (Table 1) (60–64).

The weight gain associated with AA drugs is associated with an increase in total body fat. Eder et al. (65) prospectively evaluated over an observation period of eight weeks, body weight, BMI, leptin, and body composition in schizophrenic patients ($n = 10$) treated with olanzapine and healthy comparison subjects ($n = 10$). Body composition was determined every four weeks by impedance analysis. The patients gained a mean of 3.3 kg (SD = 2.2, $p = 0.005$). This weight gain was mainly attributable to a

Table 2 Short- and Long-Term Weight Gain Liability with Available Antipsychotics

Antipsychotics	Weight gain liability
High potency CAPs	+/−
Low potency conventional antipsychotics	+++
Clozapine	++++
Olanzapine	+++
Risperidone	++
Quetiapine	++
Ziprasidone	+/−
Aripiprazole	+/−

Abbreviation: CAP, conventional antipsychotic.

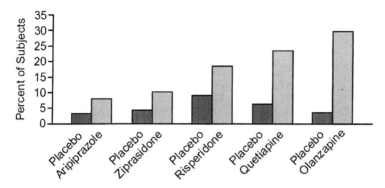

Figure 2 Incidence of weight gain (≥7%) reported in U.S. package inserts for short-term studies.

significant increase in body fat, with patients gaining an estimated mean of 2.2 kg of body fat (SD = 2.2, $p = 0.04$). Leptin serum levels increased significantly during olanzapine treatment but this was not correlated with body fat increases.

Zhang et al. (66) attempted to explore the effect of initial antipsychotic drug treatment on abdominal fat deposition and describe the increase in body fat in relation to circulating leptin, insulin, and lipids in persons with first-episode schizophrenia. Anthropometrics included both BMI and WHRs while subcutaneous abdominal fat and intra-abdominal fat (IAF) were measured with magnetic resonance imaging. Patients received treatment with chlorpromazine, risperidone, and quetiapine. Significant increases in SUB and IAF were identified after antipsychotic treatment ($p < 0.001$). The increase in fat was associated with a threefold increase in leptin secretion and an adverse lipid and nonfasting glucose profile.

Predicting which patients are at greater risk of weight gain with antipsychotic treatment would be instructive. Although many variables have been scrutinized, few (i.e., young age more at risk) are conclusive (Table 3). This is obviously a research vista for the future.

Taken together, a spectrum of weight gain liability is reported with antipsychotic treatment. Low potency CAPs, and several of the newer AA are the most notable offenders. This foregoing profile invites the need for practitioners to recognize and anticipate weight gain potential with these agents and incorporate this information into decisions regarding medication selection and patient monitoring.

Mood Stabilizers/AEDs

Although classified together, mood stabilizers and AEDs are a heterogeneous group of agents in their pharmacological and clinical profile. There

Table 3 Antipsychotic Correlates of Weight Gain

Variable	Findings	Study
Age	Younger more at risk	(67–70)
Sex	Females > males	(71)
	Males > females	(68)
	No difference in males and females	(70)
Ethnicity	Nonwhites gained more weight than whites	(70,72)
Environment	More weight gain in inpatients	(70)
Cigarette smoking	No association	(73)
Appetite increase	Positive association	(67,74)
Baseline weights	Normal or underweight at pretreatment baseline at higher risk	(68,70)
Previous treatment exposure	Antipsychotic naïve at higher risk	(69)
	Number or duration of prior hospitalizations: no association	(70)
Dose	Positive association	(70,75)
	No association	(76,77)
Duration	Risperidone weight gain 3.3 kg after one year	(78)

Finding	Reference
Risperidone (mean modal daily dose 4.9 mg) weight gain 2.3 kg after two years	(79)
Olanzapine (mean daily dose 15 mg, SD 2.5) weight gain 11.8 kg after one year	(80)
Olanzapine weight gain tapers between weeks 30 and 40	Eli Lilly (unpublished data)
Clozapine weight gain greatest during first year but continues up to 36 months and then plateaus	(81)
Plateaued at 20 weeks with olanzapine and clozapine versus 10 weeks with risperidone	(82)
Formulation Oral and depot equally likely	(68,70,76,77,83–88)
Clinical response Positive relation	(81,89)
No relation	(90)
Positive relationship with olanzapine and clozapine, no relationship with risperidone and haloperidol	(91)
Negative relationship with clozapine	(15,69)
Antipsychotic class Atypical > conventional	(15,69)

Source: From Ref. 92.

is increasing interest in the application of several newer generation AEDs for bipolar and other psychiatric disorders (e.g., bulimia nervosa, binge-eating disorder, alcohol dependence). Differential effects on appetite, eating behavior, and weight have been described with these agents in Table 4.

Lithium

Lithium, chemically isolated in 1817, is FDA-approved for the acute and maintenance treatment of bipolar disorder. Weight gain has been reported in up to two-thirds of patients receiving maintenance lithium therapy (93). An average weight gain of approximately 10 kg (22 lb) over 10 years has been described (94,95). Weight gain with lithium has been reported in maintenance placebo-controlled trials for bipolar disorder.

Bowden et al. (96) reported that an increase of ≥7% in body weight occurred in 4% of patients receiving placebo, and 16% of patients receiving lithium (23% of patients receiving divalproex).

In a 76-week maintenance study, primarily examining the efficacy of lamotrigine to placebo, lithium-treated patients (0.8–1.0 mEq/L; $n = 121$) gained 4.2 kg, (9.3 lb) while weight loss was noted in the placebo group [−2.2 kg (4.9 lb)]. Weight gain with lamotrigine [1.2 kg (7 lb)] was significantly less than lithium ($p = 0.01$) and not statistically different than placebo. The incidence of patients experiencing ≥7% increase in body weight, at the final double-blind study visit was 6, 10, and 7% for the placebo, lithium, lamotrigine groups, respectively (97). These results were replicated in a similar companion study (98).

Table 4 Short- and Long-Term Weight Gain Liability with Available Mood Stabilizers and AED

Mood stabilizer/AED	Weight gain liability
Lithium	+++
Divalproex	++++
CBZ	++
OXC	+/−
Lamotrigine	0/−
Pregabalin[a]	−
Gabapentm[a]	++
Topiramate	0/−
Levetiracetam	0/−
Zonisamide	0/−

[a]Dose dependent.
Abbreviations: AED, antiepileptic drug; CBZ, carbamazepine; OXC, oxcarbazepine.

Tohen et al. (99) compared weight gain in a lithium versus olanzapine one-year maintenance trial in bipolar I disorder ($n = 532$). Prior to randomization, patients were treated open-label with a combination of olanzapine and lithium for 6–12 weeks, and a mean weight gain of 3 kg. During the blinded monotherapy maintenance phase of the trial, patients assigned to the olanzapine arm experience statistically significant higher mean weight gain ($+2$ kg) compared with patients receiving lithium (-1 kg). In addition, a significantly larger proportion of patients receiving olanzapine (30%) gained $\geq 7\%$ of baseline body weight compared with patients receiving lithium (10%). Similarly, fewer patients receiving olanzapine (9%) experienced a weight loss of $\geq 7\%$ baseline body weight compared with patients receiving lithium (19%).

Lithium exerts an insulin-like activity on carbohydrate metabolism in some patients which may promote glucose absorption into the adipocytes. Moreover, lithium exerts a direct appetite and thirst stimulating effects, and is associated with both edema and hypothyroidism. One or more of these mechanisms may be salient to lithium-associated weight gain (100–102). Variables associated with lithium weight gain are concomitant medications, age, gender, adipocyte number, duration of treatment, dose, and thirst (103).

Valproic Acid

Valproate was first synthesized by the United States chemist Burton as an organic solvent in 1881 (104). Its simple short-chain branched fatty acid chemical structure differs significantly from other AEDs such as phenytoin, CBZ, and phenobarbital. Valproate affects cortical hyperexcitability by both increasing inhibition through raising the levels of γ-aminobutyric acid (GABA), the inhibitory neurotransmitter, and decreasing neuronal excitability by lowering the concentration of glutamate, the major excitatory neurotransmitter (105). Valproate has been shown to inhibit mitochondrial β-oxidation which could interfere with energy utilization (106).

Valproic acid is associated with clinically significant weight gain in both pediatric and adult populations. Moreover, valproic acid treatment may also be associated with changes in the metabolic and reproductive milieu in epileptic and bipolar populations (107–109). Valproic acid-associated weight gain of varying amounts (3–24 lb) over periods of up to one year have been described (110). It is further estimated that approximately 8.0–59% of patients receiving valproate can expect to gain between 8 and 14 kg (17.6–30.8 lb) up to 15–20 kg (33–44 lb) (95,103). Valproic acid-associated weight gain may be more common in men and with lengthier treatment exposure (11).

Bowden et al. (96) reported that a gain of $\geq 7\%$ body weight occurred in 4% of patients receiving placebo, 16% receiving lithium, and 23% treated with divalproex. Higher weight gain was associated with higher plasma levels of valproate. In this one-year study, higher serum levels of valproate, especially above 125 g/mL were associated with weight gain.

Tohen et al. (112) compared flexibly dosed olanzapine (5–20 mg/day) to divalproex (500–2500 mg/day) as prophylactic treatment for of bipolar patients ($N = 251$) in a randomized, double-blind trial. The patients in the olanzapine group had a significantly greater mean weight gain than those in the divalproex group 2.79 kg (SE = 0.32) versus 1.22 kg (SE = 0.32) ($p < 0.001$). Weight gain was significantly greater for the olanzapine patients from day 3 through week 15, inclusive; however, from weeks 19 through 47, there were no significant differences between groups in weight gain from baseline.

CBZ

CBZ has a tricyclic structure, with some GABAergic and antiglutamatergic effects that may not be as marked as some of its other multiple cellular and intracellular actions (4,5,33–35). CBZ has a "sedating" profile yielding somnolence, fatigue, and antimanic, and more modest antidepressant effects (36,37,113). CBZ has been associated with weight gain, perhaps by increasing appetite or by fluid retention from inappropriate secretion of antidiuretic hormone.

Randomized controlled trials (RCT) employing CBZ have confirmed its weight gain potential. Mattson et al. (114–116) reported weight gain (defined as > 5.5 kg) in up to 8% of epileptic patients receiving maintenance carbamazepme, compared with 20% of those receiving valproate. Joffe et al. (117) reported weight change in a small ($n = 24$) placebo-controlled study in patients with bipolar disorder. On average, CBZ-treated patients gained more weight (2 kg) than placebo-treated patients. The propensity for weight gain with CBZ was most notable in patients in the depressed phase.

Ketter et al. (118) evaluated patients with DSM-IV-defined bipolar disorder ($n = 94$), most recent episode manic/mixed, as part of an open-label extension phase of two double-blind placebo-controlled studies. Patients received beaded extended-release CBZ (200–1600 mg/day; mean dose 938 mg/day). No patient completing the study had clinically significant weight gain ($\geq 7\%$) and the mean percentage in weight change from day one to month six was minimal (0.7%) (118).

OXC is a 10-keto derivative of CBZ with an improved tolerability and safety profile compared to its congener (i.e., CBZ). Rattya et al. (119) evaluated 77 epileptic females (aged 8–18) receiving valproate ($n = 40$), CBZ ($n = 19$), and OXC ($n = 18$) and 49 healthy control girls examining longitudinal growth analysis from the age of one year. It was determined that no antiepileptic thwarted linear growth or pubertal development in girls with epilepsy. The weight of the girls receiving CBZ or OXC was similar to that of the control girls. However, the patients taking valproate gained significant weight, with a particular increase in those who started their medication before puberty.

At clinical examination, the BMI of valproate-treated girls ($19.8 \pm 4.8\,\mathrm{kg/m^2}$) was significantly higher than controls ($18.0 \pm 2.5\,\mathrm{kg/m^2}$) ($p < 0.03$).

Lamotrigine

Lamotrigine, derived from pyrimethamine, is a member of the phenyltriazine class of agents. Lamotrigine acts at voltage-sensitive sodium channels to stabilize neuronal membranes and inhibit transmitter release, principally glutamate. A recent review of published studies ($n = 32$) with lamotrigine confirm its weight neutrality (120). In this review most treated patients ($n = 463$) received lamotrigine as a concomitant therapy; the mean change in body weight was $0.4 \pm 5.0\,\mathrm{kg}$ ($0.9 \pm 11.1\,\mathrm{lb}$) in women and $0.6 \pm 5.0\,\mathrm{kg}$ ($1.3 \pm 11.1\,\mathrm{lb}$).

Biton et al. (121) compared the incidence and magnitude of change in body weight associated with lamotrigine ($n = 65$) or divalproex ($n = 68$) monotherapy in patients with epilepsy. Patients were treated in a randomized, double-blind study, with an eight-week escalation stage, followed by a 24-week maintenance phase. Weight remained stable among lamotrigine- treated patients, while significant weight gain was observed in valproate treated patients within 10 weeks of initiation with treatment. At the end of 32 weeks, the mean weight gain among valproate-treated patients ($12.8 \pm 9.3\,\mathrm{lb}$) was significantly higher than that for lamotrigine-treated patients ($1.3 \pm 11.9\,\mathrm{lb}$). Clinically relevant weight gain ($\geq 8.8\,\mathrm{lb}$ or $> 10\%$) compared with baseline weight, was more commonly observed in valproate-treated patients (28/45 62%) than lamotrigine-treated patients (6/50 12%). No significant predictors of weight gain were noticed.

In a six-month relapse prevention study in patients with rapid-cycling bipolar disorder ($n = 182$), there was no significant difference in mean weight change between patients completing the trial who received lamotrigine ($1.1\,\mathrm{kg}$) versus placebo ($-0.3\,\mathrm{kg}$) (122). Weight gain described with lamotrigine in two similarly designed 18-month maintenance studies in bipolar disorder was reported earlier (97,98).

Topiramate

Topiramate is a structurally and pharmacologically novel AED with proven anticonvulsant efficacy in refractory partial epilepsy (123). Mechanisms hypothesized to account for topiramate's antiepileptic properties include blockade of voltage-gated sodium channels, antagonism of the kainate/amino-3-hydroxy-5-methyl-4-isoxazole propionic acid (AMPA) subtype of glutamate receptor, enhancement of aminobutyric acid (GABA) activity at the GABA receptor via interaction with a nonbenzodiazepine receptor site, and carbonic anhydrase inhibition (124).

Weight loss and anorexia are frequently reported adverse events with topiramate. Data procured from epilepsy studies indicate that weight loss is typically observed in the first three months and continues for up to 18 months of treatment (125). Weight loss with topiramate is greater at higher doses in women and persons with high baseline BMI (126).

Similar weight loss data have been reported for topiramate-treated bipolar patients (127–129). McElroy et al. (130) explored the spectrum of effectiveness and tolerability of open-label naturalistic topiramate treatment in bipolar outpatients ($n = 56$) in the Stanley Foundation Bipolar Outcome Network. The average weight loss in the group was 1.5 lb at four weeks, 3.5 lb at 10 weeks, 10.3 lb at six months, and 13.6 lb at one year; an average decrease in BMI for the group was 0.9 at four weeks, 1.6 at six months, and 2.2 at one year. Several investigations demonstrated that topiramate reduced fat deposition in animals by reducing fat intake and stimulating energy expenditure (i.e., thermogenesis), perhaps via increased transcription of uncoupling proteins (UCPs) (131,132).

Gabapentin

Gabapentin is a novel anticonvulsant agent with multiple pharmacological actions including an interaction with the system 1-amino acid transporter, an increase of GABA synthesis and alteration of GABA release, high affinity binding to the [alpha]2 delta subunit of voltage-activated calcium channels, inhibition of voltage-activated sodium channels, alteration of monoamine neurotransmitter release, and blood serotonin levels (133–135).

DeToledo et al. (136) described weight changes associated with chronic, high-dose gabapentin therapy for seizure disorders. Patients ($n = 44$) received gabapentin (minimum dosage 1800 mg/day); 28 patients received more than 3000 mg/day. Overall 57% of patients gained more than 5% of their baseline bodyweight, with 10 (23%) patients gaining more than 10% of their baseline weight. Fifteen patients gained 5–10% of baseline, 16 patients had no change, and three patients lost 5–10% of their initial weight. Weight increase started between the second and the third months of gabapentin treatment in most patients and tended to stabilize after six to nine months of treatment, although the doses of gabapentin remained unchanged. Weight gain was described when gabapentin was prescribed as monotherapy or as adjunctive treatment. The mean weight gain with gabapentin therapy was reported as 1.9 kg (4.2 lb) at six months, and up to 2.9 kg (6.4 lb) after 12 months of therapy.

Frye et al. (137) reported on a comparative randomized, double-blind, crossover, six-week monotherapy study evaluating the effectiveness of lamotrigine (274 ± 128 mg) and gabapentin (3987 ± 856 mg) monotherapy versus placebo in refractory bipolar and unipolar mood disorders ($n = 31$). There was a standardized blinded titration to assess clinical efficacy or to determine the maximum tolerated daily dose (lamotrigine 500 mg or gabapentin 4800 mg). Weight change was significantly different between the lamotrigine (-0.96 ± 3.11 kg), gabapentin (1.83 ± 5.04 kg), and placebo (-0.40 ± 2.97 kg) phases (repeated measures analysis of variance, $F = 4.015, p = 0.024$). A pairwise contrast (lamotrigine vs. gabapentin, $F = 5.884, p = 0.021$) showed that patients lost weight when they received lamotrigine relative to the weight gained when they received gabapentin (138).

Pregabalin

Pregabalin was identified after an investigation into other three-substituted GABA analogs. It has since been shown to have a similar pharmacological profile to gabapentin with greater potency in preclinical models of pain and epilepsy (139). Pregabalin is a novel compound under active development for the treatment of several anxiety disorders.

The safety and efficacy of pregabalin for the treatment of social anxiety disorder was evaluated in a double-blind, multi-center clinical trial in which 135 patients were randomized to 10 weeks of double-blind treatment with either pregabalin 150 mg/day, pregabalin 600 mg/day, or placebo. Similar to gabapentin, pregabalin was associated with dose-dependent weight gain. Patients receiving pregabalin 600 mg/day experienced a mean weight gain of 1.7 kg at endpoint. By comparison, patients receiving pregabalin 150 mg/day had a mean weight gain of 0.6 kg, and patients receiving placebo had a mean weight loss of 0.1 kg (140).

Zonisamide

Zonisamide's anticonvulsant action is related to its sodium and calcium channel (T-type) blocking activity (141,142). Zonisamide also exhibits dose-dependent biphasic dopaminergic and serotonergic activity, a pharmacological profile which may bestow a weight loss effect.

Gadde et al. (143) tested zonisamide [mean dose (SE): 427 mg (29)] as a pharmacological treatment for obese adults (55 women, 5 men; BMI 36.3 $\pm$ 0.5; mean age 37) in a 16-week randomized, double-blind, placebo-controlled trial with optional single-blind extension for an additional 16 weeks. The mean (SE) absolute weight change for the zonisamide-treated group was 6.4 (0.8) kg versus 1.1 (0.4) kg for the placebo-treated group ($p < 0.001$). In the last observation carried forward (LOCF) population, 17/30 (57%), in the zonisamide-treated group, and 3/30 (10%), in the placebo group achieved a weight loss of $\geq 5\%$ by week 16. Mean (SE) waist circumference decreased more with zonisamide therapy over 16 weeks [103.5 (1.6) cm to 97.2 (1.8) cm vs. 103.2 (1.9) cm to 100.5 (2.0) cm, $p < 0.001$]. During the extension phase of the study, 10/19 of zonisamide patients, and none of the placebo patients, lost $\geq 3\%$ of body weight by week 32 ($p < 0.001$). The mean weight loss at week 32 for the zonisamide group was 9.2 (1.7) kg, compared with 1.5 (0.7) kg with placebo ($p < 0.001$).

McElroy et al. (144) conducted an open-label trail of zonisamide in 15 patients with DSM-IV-TR defined binge-eating disorder. Subjects were experiencing >3 binge eating episodes weekly, for at least the prior six months, and were between 18 and 65 years of age. The mean (SD) daily dose at endpoint evaluation was 513 (102.7) mg. Most patients achieved full remission of binge eating; the estimated weight loss at week 12 was 7.6 kg (16.8 lb) from the time trend analysis. The observed mean weight loss for completers at week 12 was 8.2 kg (18.1 lb).

Levetiracetam

Gidal et al. (106) analyzed the impact of adjunctive levetiracetam treatment on body weight in epileptic patients enrolled in four, prospective, randomized, placebo-controlled trials. Analysis of body weight was conducted on data pooled from these studies. Patients ($n = 970$) included in the present analysis were men and women greater than 16 years old, and who had levetiracetam (or placebo) exposure for at least four weeks. Mean levetiracetam dose and duration of treatment were 2053 mg/day (range of 167–4000 mg/day) and 125 days (range of 29–181 days), respectively. All patients received at least one concomitant AED including CBZ, gabapentin, lamotrigine, phenobarbital, phenytoin, vigabatrin, and valproate.

No significant change in body weight was observed within the levetiracetam treatment group, including those classified as either study completers, or those discontinued. In addition, changes in body weight were not cited as an adverse event requiring study withdrawal for any patient. A small, yet statistically significant increase in weight was observed for the placebo group. Clinically significant weight change as defined as $\geq 7\%$ change from baseline, occurred in approximately 9% of levetiracetam-treated patients (4.5% had increase in weight/4.5% decrease) versus 9.4% in placebo-treated patients (5.9% had increase/3.5% decrease). Weight changes were not significantly different between groups.

Summary

In aggregate, a spectrum of weight gain liability is reported with antidepressants, antipsychotics, mood stabilizers, and AEDs. This clinically significant weight gain associated with a number of these psychotropic medications has few conclusive predictors; a vista for future research. Weight gain associated with these treatments is obviously a salient issue to consider in medication selection and surveillance.

MEDICATION-ASSOCIATED WEIGHT GAIN: MECHANISMS

Body weight is the net balance between energy intake and energy expenditure (145). Energy expenditure can be further partitioned into resting energy expenditure and activity-related expenditure (146). Heritability studies indicate that up to 70% of body weight is genetically mediated; notwithstanding the obesity epidemic over the past two decades has underscored the etiological relevance of nongenetic factors (147). The regulation of energy and expenditure occurs centrally (e.g., increased appetite) and/or peripherally (e.g., taste aversion or heat dissipation) (148). Of the three classes of agents reviewed in this chapter, candidate mechanisms for AA mediated weight gain have been the most scrutinized.

Central Mechanisms

Catecholamines

It is hypothesized that established appetite suppressants (e.g., sibutramine) reduce weight by increasing the synaptic availability of several monoamines in the feeding center of the lateral hypothalamus (149,150).

Dopamine receptor blockade is a common feature of all effective antipsychotics. The associations of weight gain with D2 blocker suggests that dopamine neurotransmission may be of etiological relevance (151,152). For example, a recent positron emission tomography study noted a significant relationship between obesity and decreased availability of dopamine-D2 receptors in the striatum (153). Furthermore, centrally administered dopamine produces a robust decrease in feeding behavior in animal models (154).

Amphetamines and other agents which increase dopamine and norepinephrine neurotransmission have well-described appetite suppressant effects (155). It is conjectured that dopamine's effect on feeding behavior is via activation of brain reward pathways (156).

Serotonin

Serotonin is a satiety factor integral to eating behavior (157). Enhancing serotonin neurotransmission reduces food intake and increases energy expenditure in humans and animals by preferentially inhibiting the ingestion of carbohydrate versus protein or fat (158–160). The serotonin receptor 5-HT2C is a candidate receptor for medication-associated weight gain. Tecott et al. (161) bred a 5-HT2C knockout mouse which became obese later in life, developed laboratory evidence of the obesity syndrome (i.e., increased insulin and leptin), and had a propensity for seizures. Moreover, the anorexiants *m*-CPP and fenfluramine are nonspecific agonists for the 5-HT2C receptor (161–163).

Many psychotropic medications directly or indirectly modulate serotonin activity. Moreover, other biological systems that regulate energy intake and expenditure are in a delicate interplay with serotonin underscoring this monoamine as mechanistically relevant.

Histamine

Histamine has functional overlap with the adipocyte-derived hormone leptin. Histamine-receptor populations (H1, H2, H3) mediate feeding and drinking behavior in rats (65). It is postulated that histamine antagonism centrally stimulates energy intake by increasing appetite, with a resultant positive energy balance. Medications with high in vitro affinity for histamine receptors (e.g., low-potency CAPs, mirtazapine, TCAs, paroxetine) have well-established effects of weight gain. Cimetidine, an H2 antagonist, appears to reduce appetite and weight in overweight subjects and to improve glucose control in patients with type II diabetes (164).

Wirshing et al. (165) found a robust correlation between the affinity of AAs for the histamine receptor and antipsychotic-induced weight gain. Histamine receptor (H1) knock-out mice are less responsive to the anorectic affects of leptin and are prone to obesity (166). Kroeze et al. (150) screened 17 conventional and AA drugs for binding to 12 neurotransmitter receptors. Affinity for the H1-histamine receptor had the highest correlation with weight gain (Spearman $p = -0.72$; $p < 0.01$) followed by affinities for the α-1A adrenergic (Spearman $p = -0.54$; $p < -0.05$), 5-HT2C (Spearman $p = -0.49$; $p < 0.05$), and 5-HT6 receptors (Spearman $p = -0.52$; $p < 0.005$), whereas affinities for the eight other receptors that were screened for did not show any significant correlation with weight gain.

Muscarinic Cholinergic Receptors

Low-potency antipsychotics, TCAs, and paroxetine exhibit affinity for muscarinic cholinergic receptors. The absolute affinity for muscarinic receptors appears to have minimal correlation with antipsychotic-induced weight gain; however, it is possible that the ratio of muscarinic and dopaminergic affinity may predict weight gain with antipsychotic agents. For example, Yamada et al. (167) demonstrated that mice lacking M3 receptors showed decreased feeding behavior, had reduced weight and peripheral fat, and low levels of leptin and insulin.

Amino Acid Neurotransmitters

Agents that positively modulate GABA neurotransmission (e.g., divalproex) have been reported to promote weight gain, while other agents that decrease glutamatergic function (e.g., lamotrigine, topiramate, zonisamide) are associated with minimal weight gain or induce weight loss. For example, it has been noted that agonists at the glutamate N-methyl-D-aspartate (NMDA) receptor (e.g., glycine) stimulate feeding behavior in rats when infused in the hypothalamus. It has been hypothesized that some AAs enhance GABA function, which may alter the GABA-glutamate balance and thus foster weight gain (168–172). Functional overlaps between amino acid neurotransmitters and monoamines involved in appetite regulation (i.e., serotonin) are reported. For example, SSRIs have been shown to have regulatory effects on both glutamatergic and GABAergic functioning (173,174).

Reproductive Hormones

Obesity is associated with elevated levels of androgen in females and decreased levels in males. These changes (estrogen:androgen ratio) in hormonal levels may reduce the sensitivity of satiety neurons in the lateral hypothalamus. Baptista et al. (175,176) have reported on the diminution of plasma estradiol levels following acute and subacute antipsychotic administration in women receiving antipsychotics. This group has further conjectured that sustained hyperprolactnemia may be of etiological relevance in some case of antipsychotic-associated weight gain via changes in estrogen:androgen ratio. Parsing out the relevance of changes in the reproductive hormone milieu may illuminate efforts to understand weight-gain propensity differences between genders.

Cytokines

Proinflammatory cytokines [interleukin (IL), tumor necrosis factor alpha (TNF-α), interferon (INF)] and their soluble receptors mediate sickness behavior, play a critical role in various metabolic, immune, and appetitive behaviors, and further affect glucose, protein, and lipid metabolism (177). For example, circulating levels of TNF-α and its soluble receptors are increased in obese subjects compared with lean controls, and decrements in these levels are seen with weight loss. Moreover, patients who gain weight when treated with amitriptyline or nortriptyline exhibit elevations in soluble TNF-α receptor concentrations that precede the increase in BMI. Clozapine treatment has also been associated with changes in TNF-α, interleukin 2, and leptin concentration (178–188).

Leptin is an adipocyte-derived hormone integral to multiple physiological functions. Leptin acts to regulate energy intake and expenditure along with the modulation of the neuroendocrine axis. Leptin may signal the size of the peripheral fat storage and may trigger pubertal maturation. There is a positive correlation between plasma levels of leptin and weight gain, BMI and body fat percentage (189). McIntyre et al. (190) noted that plasma leptin levels were significantly increased in a cohort of patients with bipolar disorder who received olanzapine or risperidone for six months. Both AA agents imparted significant weight gain; significant increases in plasma leptin levels were also noted after the increase in weight was observed. The secondary rise in leptin levels following the observed weight gain suggests that leptin increases may not be integral to weight gain initiation, but might be relevant to further weight gain accrual (191).

Melkersson and Hulting (192,193) noted that clozapine and olanzapine produced predictable increases in leptin levels in persons who gained weight on these agents. However, the sexual dimorphism that is normally seen was not observed, mainly due to an increase of leptin levels in the men. These results were an extension of earlier work by the same group which determined that there was no correlation between leptin and BMI in patients treated with olanzapine (194).

Orexins

Orexins (hypocretins) are peptides that are expressed only in the lateral hypothalamus and perifornical area and mediate feeding behavior. Moreover, intraventricular administration of orexin increases dopaminergic activity and activates A10 dopamine neurons. A pilot study determined that the antipsychotics that induce the most weight gain (olanzapine, clozapine) produced a greater percentage of increase in orexin neurons expressing c-fos protein. Although it is unknown if orexin neurons increase dopamine release in the prefrontal cortex, it is possible that the neurobiological systems that mediate adverse events such as weight gain may also be relevant to therapeutic response (195–198).

Insulin

Valproic acid-associated weight gain is paralleled by an increase in fasting insulin and leptin levels and is known to be a possible associated adverse event (199–201). Luef et al. (202–204) recently demonstrated that postprandial insulin and proinsulin levels are increased in valproic acid-treated patients, suggesting a possible modulation of pancreatic insulin secretion by valproic acid.

Fatty acids are of central importance in the development of insulin resistance, also as signaling molecules to the nuclear peroxisome proliferator-activated receptors (PPARs). Stimulation of PPAR results in an increase in RNA expression for leptin and TNF-α, and both of these adipocyte products enhance insulin resistance by interfering with the insulin-receptor cascade (205). The effect of valproic acid on insulin is obviously in need of further study.

UCPs

UCPs regulate energy expenditure through peripheral mechanisms. UCP 1, 2, and 3 show tissue selectivity, with UCP 1 found in brown adipose tissue, UCP 2 ubiquitous in its distribution, with a preponderance in white adipose tissue, and UCP 3 found in skeletal muscle (206). UCPs reroute protons, the products of oxidative phosphorylation, either to storage or to be dissipated as heat. Although the effect of psychotropic medications on UCPs has not been delineated, some appetite suppressants and neurotherapeutic molecules have been shown to modulate uncoupling protein transcription (207–209).

For example, centrally, topiramate reduces the density of neuropeptide Yl and Y5 receptors (receptors for the orexigenic neuropeptide Y) while peripherally, topiramate has been shown to reduce leptin messenger RNA transcription in adipose tissue and significantly increases messenger RNA for UCP-2 in white adipose tissue. These central and peripheral affects were also noted with dexfenfluramine and it is hypothesized that these effects may contribute to increase thermogenesis and energy expenditure with these agents (210).

Peroxisome Proliferator-Activated Receptor

Energy storage in adipose tissue is in part mediated by receptors on preadipocytes that are called PPARs. These receptors promote the conversion of a nonlipid-storing preadipocyte to an adipocyte. Some psychotropic medications (e.g., antipsychotics) are associated with increased fat mass; however, it is not known if psychotropic medications have any effect on PPAR receptor expression or mRNA availability (189).

Pharmacogenetics

Polymorphisms are variations of the DNA sequence located in regulatory, noncoding or coding regions. Polymorphisms may affect the activity or conformation of the encoded protein, which may be relevant to psychotropic-associated weight gain. Pharmacogenetic studies in this area are scrutinizing both pharmacodynamic and pharmacokinetic factors salient to weight-gain mechanisms (211).

Pooley et al. (212) investigated the prevalence of the 5HT2C 759C/T polymorphism in a cohort of obese women ($n = 120$) undergoing a psychological treatment for weight loss. The investigators noted that the C allele was statistically more common in the obese group ($p = 0.008$), and that heterozygotes lost statistically less weight than did homozygotes after 6 and 12 months ($p = 0.006, 0.009$, respectively).

Rietschel et al. (213) evaluated four polymorphisms for the DRD_4 gene and its relationship to response and weight gain with clozapine in German patients with DSM-IV-defmed schizophrenia ($n = 149$). No association was detected between clozapine-associated weight gain (or any adverse events) and DRD_4 polymorphisms.

Basile et al. (211) investigated and failed to find any statistically significant correlation between clozapine-induced weight gain in persons with chronic schizophrenia and the 5HT2C:Cys23Ser polymorphism, and the G1018A polymorphism of the histamine receptor *H2* gene. This group further failed to find any association between the beta-3 adrenergic receptor polymorphism Trp64Arg and weight change. These foregoing negative findings are inconclusive as the sample size may be too small for a genetic study.

Reynolds et al. (214) studied first-episode schizophrenic patients ($n = 123$) of Chinese Han ethnicity. Most patients were treated with chlorpromazine ($n = 69$) or risperidone ($n = 46$). They noted significantly less ($p = 0.0003$) weight gain in patients with the -759C/T polymorphism of the 5HT2C receptor gene regulatory region.

This finding was further corroborated in a smaller group of first episode schizophrenic patients ($N = 32$) also of Han Chinese ethnicity. It was determined that the -759C/T polymorphism may account for up to

18% of the variance in clozapine-associated weight gain. When results were subsequently adjusted for gender, the -759C/T polymorphism could explain up to 32% of the weight gain in male patients (215).

Tsai et al. (216) investigated the relationship between the 5HT2C-759C/T polymorphism and clozapine-induced weight gain also in Han Chinese patients with a diagnosis of schizophrenia or schizoaffective disorder (53 men, 28 women). After four months of clozapine therapy, patients gained a mean (SD) of 2.1 kg (4.7 kg). These researchers did not find any association between change in BMI and the 5HT2C -759C/T genotype.

Theisen et al. (217) investigated the association between 5HT2C-759C/T polymorphism and changes in BMI induced by clozapine treatment in schizophrenic patients ($n = 97$). After 12 weeks of clozapine treatment, weight gain in patients with the CC genotype was greater when compared with those harboring a T allele, however this result did not reach statistical significance.

Zhang et al. (218) investigated and failed to find an association between antipsychotic-induced weight gain, the Taq1 A polymorphism of the dopamine D2 receptor (DRD_2) gene, and therapeutic response to antipsychotic treatment in first-episode Chinese Han patients (58 males, 59 females). Moreover, Hong et al. (219) failed to find any association between clozapine-induced weight gain and the Glu349Asp variant of the H-1 receptor in patients with schizophrenia ($N = 88$).

Fewer pharmacogenetic studies have evaluated polymorphisms in genes that encode for proteins involved in the metabolism of psychotropic agents. In a preliminary study, Ellingrod et al. (220) examined the relationship between CYP2D6 genotype and AA weight gain in DSM-III-R and DSM-IV-defined schizophrenia ($n = 11$). It was determined that genotype was significant ($p < 0.0097$) for those with a *1/*3 or *4 genotype experiencing a larger percent BMI change than those with a *1/*1 genotype. The authors hypothesize that this may be due to increased olanzapine concentrations leading to increased exposure, which may trigger AAP weight gain.

Basile et al. (211) evaluated the role of the C/A polymorphism in the first intron of the CYP1A2 gene. They genotyped 70 patients, 12 patients were homozygous for the C allele, 35 were homozygous for the A allele, and 23 were heterozygous. The C homozygotes gained an average of 5.1 ± 4.1 kg, the A homozygote gained 3.3 ± 4.4 kg, while the heterozygotes gained 2.9 ± 4.2 kg ($p = $ ns).

Genetic mechanisms which presage interindividual variation and propensity to psychotropic medication associated weight gain are recondite and possibly associated with polymorphisms at susceptibility loci salient to medication pharmacodynamics and pharmacokinetics. Available genetic results examining correlation with weight gain must be regarded as preliminary and inconclusive. Further studies of adequate sample size are overdue.

Further advances in molecular biology and high throughput DNA screening hold promise to elucidate genetic loci relevant to weight gain liability with psychotropic agents.

PREVENTION AND TREATMENT OF MEDICATION-ASSOCIATED WEIGHT GAIN

General Management

The National Institute of Health evidence-based guidelines invite the need for weight loss in obese persons and in overweight persons with >2 risk factors for obesity-related diseases. The foundation of any successful weight loss program according to the National Heart Lung Blood Institute/National Institute of Health (NIH) is a low calorie diet along with increased amount of physical activity in combination with behavioral strategies under the supervision of a health care professional. Medications for the treatment of obesity are approved for use in adults who have a BMI $\geq$27 plus obesity-related medical conditions, or a BMI $\geq$30 in the absence of any conditions (221).

Weight-reducing diets are estimated at approximately 500–1000 kcal/day less than the patient requires to maintain current body weight (1000–1200 kcal/day for women, 1200–1500 kcal/day for men) (222). Physical activity is sine que non and offers additional benefit on metabolic parameters, subjective energy, mood state, and cognitive functioning (223). Beneficial behavioral modifications include stress management, reward systems, self-monitoring of caloric intake, and involvement in client-centered support groups (224).

It is estimated that approximately 10% of body weight may be lost over six months with successful implementation of dietary, exercise, and behavioral modification techniques. This foregoing weight loss may appear modest, but is sufficient to improve obesity-associated morbidity (225). For most patients, sustaining weight loss is an insurmountable objective that contributes to patient and health care provider disappointment and nihilism (226,227). Pharmacotherapy has been recommended if behavioral strategies are insufficient in achieving therapeutic objectives after six months (221).

Management of Psychiatric Populations

The principles of preventing and treating excess weight in psychiatric populations are not dissimilar from the general population. Variables which cluster in this population include disease related phenomenology (e.g., appetite increase, cognitive impairment) comorbidity (binge-eating disorder, alcohol abuse), adverse health behaviors (e.g., smoking), disability, low socioeconomic status, sedentary lifestyle, consumption of high liquid carbohydrate diet, and insufficient access to primary and preventative health care.

The therapeutic objectives when treating medication-associated weight gain are to minimize and further prevent weight gain, and reduce and sustain weight loss in those who are categorically obese and overweight. It has been well established that decreases of 5–10% of body weight may reduce risk for cardiovascular disease, diabetes mellitus, and dyslipidemia.

Using the Behavioral Risk Factor Surveillance System (BRFSS), Mokdad et al. (228) in all U.S. states in 2000 surveyed adults 18 years or older ($n = 184,550$), revealing that only 43% of noninstitutionalized obese persons in the general population who had received routine primary care in the past year had been advised by health care professionals to lose weight. It has been established that counseling patients on the topic of weight management is an effective and obviously inexpensive intervention (229).

Psychiatric patients are less likely to receive primary and preventative health care when compared to the general population (8,230). Patient dietary habits, eating behaviors, concomitant drug and alcohol use, and opportunistic screening for obesity-associated morbidity and family medical history are integral components of patient evaluation and monitoring (231). Patients should be informed of the importance of drinking no- or low-caloric beverages, smoking cessation, avoiding alcohol, moderating carbohydrate consumption, and increasing the consumption of fresh, non-starchy fruits and vegetables (232). The need for exercise, several days per week, should be emphasized, and resources with discounted physical fitness centers should be considered when available. The salutary effects of healthy exercise on mood, motivation, body image, social and cognitive functioning, sleep, and overall quality of life should be emphasized (225,92,233). Patient body weight BMI, and WHR should be measured and monitored on a routine basis (i.e., baseline and minimum semi-annually; with more frequent monitoring with the substantial weight gain).

The 1998 National Institute of Health Evidence Report and other studies confirm how difficult it is for people to lose weight (secondary prevention) inviting the need for primary prevention of medication-associated weight gain if possible (234,235).

Several multi-disciplinary weight-management programs have provided promising results. Wirshing et al. (165) conducted a retrospective analysis of eight controlled trials with antipsychotics (risperidone, clozapine, olanzapine, sertindole, and haloperidol) in patients with schizophrenia. Patients received a step-wise weight treatment program that included dietary monitoring, weight monitoring, dietary counseling, exercise, and if necessary, consultation with a nutritionist. Weight gain from risperidone and olanzapine was favorably influenced by this multifaceted intervention.

Holt et al. (236) attempted to prevent lithium-induced weight gain in patients ($n = 25$) DSM-III-R defined bipolar disorder through evaluation and modification of diet in accordance with the British Dietetic Association. Patients' weights and BMI were evaluated prospectively for six months while receiving lithium maintenance therapy. The control group consisted of patients ($n = 25$) who started lithium therapy but were not given dietary advice. After six months of therapy, 14/25 patients in the control group gained weight; 5/25 gained >5kg, while 9/25 of the treatment group gained weight, and only 1/25 gained >5 kg. There was a significant difference in the BMI change [mean (SD)] between the two groups [control +0.8 ± (2.1), treatment −0.5 (1.8), $p < 0.05$]. No relationship was found between initial body weight, age, lithium dose, serum lithium level, or other medications and weight gain.

Littrell et al. (237) randomized a group of patients ($n = 70$) with schizophrenia or schizoaffective disorder to receive an intense educational program or standard care in conjunction with olanzapine therapy. The program was an hour in duration weekly for a period of four months initiated with olanzapine. At the end of six months treatment, the intervention group lost weight (−0.06 lbs), while the nonintervention group gained weight (9.57 lb, $p = 0.0007$).

Vreeland et al. (238) examined the effectiveness of an intensive weight management program in schizophrenia or schizoaffective disorder in patients ($n = 31$) who had experienced weight gain (BMI > 26) while receiving atypical antipsychotics over a period of at least six months. Patients in the treatment group received nutrition, exercise, and behavioral interventions, delivered during two group session, and one 15-minute individual section weekly for a total of 25 visits over a two-week period. Patients in the intervention group lost on average 2.7 kg (6 lb) or 2.7% of bodyweight, and those on the control group gained on average 2.9 kg (6.4 lb) or 3.1% of bodyweight. The difference between the two groups was significant ($p < 0.04$). The corresponding mean change in BMI was a drop from 34.32 to 33.34 (0.98 points, or 2.8%) in the intervention group and an increase from 33.4 to 34.6 (1.2 points or 3.6%) in the control group ($p < 0.03$).

Ball et al. (239) combined an exercise regimen with the Weight-Watchers program for 21 patients with schizophrenia who gained significant weight gain after beginning olanzapine treatment compared with a demographically and symptom-matched control group. The intervention group received 10 weekly Weight Watchers meeting and exercise sessions three times per week. Approximately half of the patients (11/21, 52%) completed the study. There were no differences in mean BMI from baseline to endpoint in patients who completed the study, although weight loss was observed in the male patients ($n = 7$).

Taken together, the evidentiary base supporting nonpharmacological approaches for medication-associated weight gain in psychiatric populations is sparse and obviously an area that requires further research. Available data suggest that dietary counseling, behavioral modification, and exercise regimens are beneficial in psychiatric patients and should be offered as both primary prevention and a treatment strategy.

Pharmacological Strategies

Medication for the treatment of obesity in the general population is approved for use in adults who have a BMI ≥ 27, plus obesity related medical conditions, or BMI ≥ 30 in the absence of such conditions (240). Medications approved for weight loss fall into two broad categories: medications that decrease food intake by decreasing appetite or increasing satiety (by increasing availability of anorexigenic neurotransmitter—serotonin, norepinephrine), and those that reduce nutrient absorption (e.g., orlistat). It is possible that increased energy expenditure seen with some medications (e.g., topiramate) may also be a relevant mechanism. The safety and efficacy for any bariatric treatment is not yet established in any psychiatric population for the treatment of primary or medication-associated obesity (241,242).

Appetite Suppressant Medications

There are several small studies with the use of appetite suppressants to control weight gain, largely in schizophrenic populations. Studies with D-fenfluramine, fenfluramine, bromocriptine, and phenylpropanolamine have produced equivocal results. These agents are associated with the induction of psychiatric symptoms and their coadministration with several psychotropic agents (e.g., MAOIs) is perilous.

Sibutramine treatment has been demonstrated to achieve and maintain weight loss over a period of 18 months (243). Henderson et al. conducted a 12-week double-blind placebo controlled trial with adjunctive sibutramine (10–15 mg) in olanzapine-treated schizophrenic and schizoaffective patients ($n = 37$). All patients were previously stabilized on olanzapine, reported a history of weight gain, and had a BMI $> 30 \, \text{kg/m}^2$ or BMI $27 \, \text{kg/m}^2$ plus another cardiovascular risk factor. In addition, all patients were offered group support and behavioral interventions (244).

At the completion of the study, the sibutramine-treated patients exhibited a significant reduction in weight relative to the placebo group (8.3 lbs vs. 1.8 lbs). A small increase in systolic blood pressure was reported as well as common sibutramine associated adverse events (e.g., dry mouth, constipation, blurred vision). Although sibutramine abuse liability is minimal, it may be associated with hypomanic induction and its use with serotonin-reuptake inhibiting antidepressants is contraindicated (245).

Topiramate has been proven to favorably influence abnormal and chaotic eating behavior, weight, and associated psychopathology, in patients with bulimia nervosa, binge-eating disorder, and obesity (246–249). McElroy et al. reported a net loss of 6 kg and mean decrease in BMI of 6% from baseline in bipolar patients ($n = 37$) treated adjunctively (antipsychotics, antidepressants, and mood stabilizers) with topiramate (mean dose = 420 mg) for one year. This described weight loss is commensurate with results from several other studies in bipolar disorder (128,129,169,250).

Van Ameringen et al. (251) evaluated the effectiveness of open-label topiramate 100–250 mg daily [mean week 10 (endpoint) dose 135 ± 44.1 mg/day] for SSRI associated weight gain ($n = 7$ paroxetine, $n = 4$ citalopram, $n = 2$ fluvoxamine, $n = 1$ sertraline, $n = 1$ fluoxetine). The sample ($n = 15$) met criteria for a DSM-IV-anxiety disorder, i.e., panic disorder with and without agoraphobia, social phobia, obsessive compulsive disorder PTSD, or generalized anxiety disorder. Patients had originally gained on average 13 ± 8.4 kg, with SSRI therapy. After 10 weeks of topiramate treatment, the mean weight loss was 4.2 ± 6.0 kg (9.3 ± 13.2 lb). Patients also exhibited significant change in BMI from week 10 to endpoint (mean baseline BMI 32.6 ± 9.3, mean endpoint BMI 31.0 ± 8.9, $p < 0.01$). Topiramate was generally well tolerated, with no worsening of the index psychiatric disorder.

Amantadine is indicated for the prevention and treatment of influenza and improves symptoms of Parkinson's disease likely through enhancing dopamine neurotransmission. Floris et al. (252) reported that significant weight loss was associated with the adjunctive administration of amantadine (100–300 mg/day) in a small, open-label study ($n = 12$). Eleven of 12 patients experience an average weight loss of 3.5 kg over 21 weeks.

Bahk et al. (253) evaluated the efficacy of amantadine in patients 18–65 who had gained >3 kg with olanzapine therapy. Subjects had various DSM-IV diagnoses (schizophrenia $n = 15$, bipolar disorder $n = 3$, major depressive disorder $n = 1$, psychotic disorder $n = 6$). Patients received amantadine [mean dose (SD) 160.1 (57.7) mg] for an average of 111.5 ± 76.7 days. Subjects receiving amantadine exhibited average weight loss of 1.07 ± 3.19 kg and the average BMI decreases by 0.84 ± 2.5 kg/m^2 which did not reach statistical significance.

Histamine antagonists have been employed as an antidote to medication-associated weight gain. Cimetidine has been reported to reduce appetite and weight via activation of the satiety peptide cholecystokinin (CCK) (254,255). Atmaca et al. (256) evaluated nizatidine as an antidote for olanzapine associated weight gain in patients with DSM-IV schizophrenia or related psychoses ($n = 132$). Patients were randomly assigned to receive olanzapine, 5–20 mg/dL, in combination with nizatidine (150 mg BID, 300 mg BID, or placebo). Patients received prospective repeated observations over 16 weeks. Statistically significant weight loss was noticed in the higher dose nizatidine group, compared with placebo, at week 3 and week 4 ($p < 0.05$). At 16 weeks, however, there were no significant differences between groups, albeit there was less overall weight gain in the 300 mg nizatidine group (3.9 kg vs. 4.8 kg). In two subsequent smaller double-blind studies, nizatidine treatment (150 mg BID) was associated with significant weight loss in olanzapine-treated patients and reduction in weight gain accrual in quetiapine-treated patients (257).

Metformin is an insulin-sensitizing agent that has been shown to have weight-reducing effects in nondiabetic subjects (258,259). The effectiveness of metformin was preliminarily evaluated in a small, open-label study in adolescent patients ($n = 19$) who experienced greater than 10% weight gain over baseline while receiving olanzapine, risperidone, quetiapine, or valproic acid (260). Metformin 500 TID was adjunctively administered for up to 12 weeks with diet and physical activity kept consistent. After 12 weeks of treatment, statistically significant differences in BMI ($2.22 \, kg/m^2$, $p = 0.003$) and weight ($2.93 \, kg$, $p = 0.008$) were noted. A small RCT, indicated that metformin may offer weight reduction for medication associated weight gain (261). Metformin is, however, associated with numerous GI adverse events, lactic acidosis, and drug interactions, and its use cannot be generally recommended for psychiatric populations.

Poyurovsky et al. (262) evaluated the efficacy of adjunctive fluoxetine ($20 \, mg/day$) to olanzapine ($10 \, mg/day$) in 30 first-episode patients with DSM-IV schizophrenia in a randomized, placebo-controlled trial. Both groups demonstrated increases in body weight over the study period. The ANCOVA with repeated measurement for weight and BMI revealed significant time effects ($p < 0.001$) for both, and lack of a group effect, or group by time interaction. The mean weight gain at week 8 was $7.9 \, kg$ (SD 4.6) in the group receiving olanzapine plus fluoxetine, and $6.0 \, kg$ (SD 4.2) in the group receiving olanzapine plus placebo ($p = 0.44$). Nine patients in each group gained at least 7% of their initial weight ($p = $ ns).

Poyurovsky et al. (263) subsequently evaluated six weeks of adjunctive reboxetine ($4 \, mg/day$) in 26 patients hospitalized for first-episode DSM-IV schizophrenia in another placebo-controlled RCT. Reboxetine is a selective norepinephrine reuptake inhibitor approved for usage in some European countries. Patients in both groups gained weight; at the end of the study completers in the olanzapine/reboxetine group gained significantly less weight ($2.5 \, kg \pm 2.7$) than the olanzapine/placebo group ($5.5 \pm 3.1 \, kg$, $p = 0.04$). Changes in BMI were also less in the combination group ($0.86 \pm 0.88 \, kg/m^2$) than in the olanzapine monotherapy group ($1.84 \pm 0.99 \, kg/m^2$, $p < 0.04$). Fewer patients in the combination group ($2/10$) than in the olanzapine monotherapy group ($7/10$) had an increase in weight $\geq 7\%$ ($p = 0.03$). The improvement in Hamilton Depression Rating scores was also significantly greater in the reboxetine group ($p = 0.03$).

Nutrient Absorption Reducers

Orlistat is currently approved by the U.S. FDA as a weight loss agent. Orlistat is an ex vivo agent with minimal systemic absorption and central nervous system (CNS) effects. It reduces energy absorption by blocking pancreatic and gastric lipases. Predictably, orlistat is associated with several uncomfortable gastrointestinal side effects: increased fecal urgency, defecation, and oily spotting (264).

Placebo-controlled trials have demonstrated sustained weight loss and reduced rate of regain of weight in overweight adults treated with orlistat. Furthermore, orlistat has also been demonstrated to improve glycated hemoglobin values, and decrease requirement for insulin sensitizing agents in type II diabetics.

Hilger (265) examined the effect of orlistat administration on plasma levels of psychotropic agents in a small ($n = 8$) outpatient study (major depressive disorder $n = 2$, bipolar disorder $n = 2$, schizophrenia $n = 2$) of patients tretaed with clozapine, haloperidol, clomipramine, desipramine, and CBZ. Orlistat was administered at 120 mg, three times per day for eight weeks in addition to dietary counseling. Weight loss was noted in all patients (0.5–13 kg) representing a mean drop in bodyweight of 6.1% $\pm$ 2.4, and a mean BMI reduction of 2.1 $\pm$ 1.2 kg/m^2 from baseline. There were no detectable changes in plasma levels in any of the psychotropic drugs administered.

SUMMARY

Overall, the management of medication-associated weight gain begins with surveillance, opportunistic screening, education, and baseline measurements. A multicomponent approach to the prevention and management of weight gain provides for patients the best chances for success. Psychiatric patients are less likely, than persons in the general population, to receive primary and preventative health care, and are particularly unlikely to have medical morbidity diagnosed and treated. Tacitly implied is the need for the role of the mental health care provider to broaden, with greater attention given to somatic health matters.

Recognizing and anticipating the clinical significance of medication-associated weight gain in a sine que non. In the interim, research attempting to parse out neurobiological mechanism which portend weight gain is under way, as are rigorously awaited psychosocial, behavioral, and pharmacological primary and preventative treatment approaches.

REFERENCES

1. Speakman JR. Obesity: the integrated roles of environment and genetics. J Nutr 2004; 134(suppl 8):2090S–2105S.
2. Flegal KM, Carroll MD, Ogden CL, Johnson CL. Prevalence and trends in obesity among US adults, 1999–2000. JAMA 2002; 288(14):1723–1727.
3. Hedley AA, Ogden CL, Johnson CL, Carroll MD, Curtin LR, Flegal KM. Prevalence of overweight and obesity among US children, adolescents, and adults, 1999–2002. JAMA 2004; 291(23):2847–2850.

4. Ogden CL, Flegal KM, Carroll MD, Johnson CL. Prevalence and trends in overweight among US children and adolescents, 1999–2000. JAMA 2002; 288(14):1728–1732.

5. Must A, Spadano J, Coakley EH, Field AE, Colditz G, Dietz WH. The disease burden associated with overweight and obesity. JAMA 1999; 282(16):1523–1529.

6. Osby U, Brandt L, Correia N, Ekbom A, Sparen P. Excess mortality in bipolar and unipolar disorder in Sweden. Arch Gen Psychiatry 2001; 58(9):844–850.

7. Lambert TJ, Velakoulis D, Pantelis C. Medical comorbidity in schizophrenia. Med J Aust 2003; 178(suppl):S67–S70.

8. Evans DL, Charney DS. Mood disorders and medical illness: a major public health problem. Biol Psychiatry 2003; 54(3):177–180.

9. Osby U, Correia N, Brandt L, Ekbom A, Sparen P. Mortality and causes of death in schizophrenia in stockholm county, Sweden. Schizophr Res 2000; 45(1–2):21–28.

10. Slyper AH. The pediatric obesity epidemic: causes and controversies. J Clin Endocrinol Metab 2004; 89(6):2540–2547.

11. Thakore JH, Mann JN, Vlahos I, Martin A, Reznek R. Increased visceral fat distribution in drug-naive and drug-free patients with schizopnrenia. Int J Obes Relat Metab Disord 2002; 26(1):137–141.

12. McElroy SL, Kotwal R, Malhotra S, Nelson EB, Keck PE, Nemeroff CB. Are mood disorders and obesity related, a review for the mental health professional. J Clin Psychiatry 2004; 65(5):634–651.

13. Ryan MC, Flanagan S, Kinsella U, Keeling F, Thakore JH. The effects of atypical antipsychotics on visceral fat distribution in first episode, drug-naive patients with schizophrenia. Life Sci 2004; 74(16):1999–2008.

14. Zimmermann U, Kraus T, Himmerich H, Schuld A, Pollmacher T. Epidemiology, implications and mechanisms underlying drug-induced weight gain in psychiatric patients. J Psychiatr Res 2003; 37(3):193–220.

15. Allison DB, Mackell JA, McDonnell DD. The impact of weight gain on quality of life among persons with schizophrenzia. Psychiatr Serv 2003; 54(4):565–567.

16. Berken GH, Weinstein DO, Stern WC. Weight gain. A side-effect of tricyclic antidepressants. J Affect Disord 1984; 7(2):133–138.

17. Weiden PJ, Mackell JA, McDonnell DD. Obesity as a risk factor for antipsychotic noncompliance. Schizophr Res 2004; 66(1):51–57.

18. Biggs MM, Basco MR, Patterson G, Raskin P. Insulin withholding for weight control in women with diabetes. Diabetes Care 1994; 17(10):1186–1189.

19. Schwartz TL, Nihalani N, Jindal S, Virk S, Jones N. Psychiatric medication-induced obesity: a review. Obes Rev 2004; 5(2):115–121.

20. Hall H, Ogren SO. Effects of antidepressant drugs on different receptors in the brain. Eur J Pharmacol 1981; 70(3):393–407.

21. Fuller RW, Wong DT. Effects of antidepressants on uptake arid receptor systems in the brain. Prog Neuropsychopharmacol Biol Psychiatry 1985; 9(5–6):485–490.

22. Ansseau M, von Frenckell R, Mertens C, et al. Controlled comparison of two doses of milnacipran (F 2207) and amitriptyline in major depressive inpatients. Psychopharmacology (Berl) 1989; 98(2):163–168.

23. Fava M. Weight gain and antidepressants. J Clin Psychiatry 2000; 61(Suppl): 37–41.
24. Fernstrom MH, Krowinski RL, Kupfer DJ. Chronic imipramine treatment and weight gain. Psychiatry Res 1986; 17(4):269–273.
25. Frank E, Kupfer DJ, Bulik CM, Levenson JA. Imipramine and weight gain during the treatment of recurrent depression. J Affect Disord 1990; 20(3):165–172.
26. Garland EJ, Remick RA, Zis AP. Weight gain with antidepressants and lithium. J Clin Psychopharmacol 1988; 8(5):323–330.
27. Cantu TG, Korek JS. Monoamine oxidase inhibitors and weight gain. Drug Intel Clin Pharm 1988; 22(10):755–759.
28. Rabkin L, Quitkin F, Harrison W, Tricamo E, McGrath P. Adverse reactions to monoamine oxidase inhibitors. Part I. A comparative study. J Clin Psychopharmacol 1984; 4(5):270–278.
29. Vaz-Serra A, Figueira ML, Firmino H, Albuquerque AL, Jara JM, Pestana LC. Multicenter double-blind study of moclobemide and maprotiline. Clin Neuropharmacol 1994; 17(suppl 1):S38–S49.
30. Moll E, Neumann K, Schmid-Burgk W, Stabl M, Amrein R. Safety and efficacy during long-term treatment with moclobemide. Clin Neuropharmacol 1994; 17(suppl 1):S74–S87.
31. Vaswani M, Linda FK, Ramesh S. Role of selective serotonin reuptake inhibitors in psychiatric disorders: a comprehensive review. Prog Neuropsychopharmacol Biol Psychiatry 2003; 27(1):85–102.
32. Goldstein BJ, Goodnick PJ. Selective serotonin reuptake inhibitors in the treatment of affective disorders III. Tolerability, safety and pharmacoeconomics. J Psychopharmacol 1998; 12(3 suppl B):S55–S87.
33. Leonard BE. Pharmacological differences of serotonin reuptake inhibitors and possible clinical relevance. Drugs 1992; 43(suppl 2):3–9.
34. Blundell JE, Lawton CL, Halford JC. Serotonin, eating behavior, and fat intake. Obes Res 1995; 3(suppl 4):471S–476S.
35. Ward AS, Comer SD, Haney M, Fischman MW, Foltin RW. Fluoxetine-maintained obese humans: effect on food intake and body weight. Physiol Behav 1999; 66(5):815–821.
36. Romano SJ, Halmi KA, Sarkar NP, Koke SC, Lee JS. A placebo-controlled study of fluoxetine in continued treatment of bulimia nervosa after successful acute fluoxetine treatment. Am J Psychiatry 2002; 159(1):96–102.
37. Arnold LM, McElroy SL, Hudson JI, Welge JA, Bennett AJ, Keck PE. A placebo-controlled, randomized trial of fluoxetine in the treatment of binge-eating disorder. J Clin Psychiatry 2002; 63(11):1028–1033.
38. de Jonghe F, Ravelli DP, Tuynman-Qua H. A randomized, double-blind study of fluoxetine and maprotiline in the treatment of major depression. Pharmacopsychiatry 1991; 24(2):62–67.
39. Croft H, Settle E Jr, Houser T, Batey SR, Donahue RM, Ascher JA. A placebo-controlled comparison of the antidepressant efficacy and effects on sexual functioning of sustained-release bupropion and sertraline. Clin Ther 1999; 21(4):643–658.

40. Moon CA, Jesinger DK. The effects of psychomotor performance of fluvoxamine versus mianserin in depressed patients in general practice. Br J Clin Pract 1991; 45(4):259–262.
41. Michelson D, Amsterdam JD, Quitkin FM, et al. Changes in weight during a 1-year trial of fluoxetine. Am J Psychiatry 1999; 156(8):1170–1176.
42. Fava M, Judge R, Hoog SL, Nilsson ME, Koke SC. Fluoxetine versus sertraline and paroxetine in major depressive disorder: changes in weight with long-term treatment. J Clin Psychiatry 2000; 61(11):863–867.
43. Mackle M, Kocsis J. Effects on body weight of the SSRI citalopram. 1998; Unpublished work.
44. Feiger AD, Bielski RJ, Bremner J, et al. Double-blind, placebo-substitution study of nefazodone in the prevention of relapse during continuation treatment of outpatients with major depression. Int Clin Psychopharmacol 1999; 14(1):19–28.
45. Sussman N, Ginsberg DL, Bikoff J. Effects of nefazodone on body weight: a pooled analysis of selective serotonin reuptake inhibitor- and Imipramine-controlled trials. J Clin Psychiatry 2001; 62(4):256–260.
46. Croft H, Houser TL, Jamerson BD, et al. Effect on body weight of bupropion sustained-release in patients with major depression treated for 52 weeks. Clin Ther 2002; 24(4):662–672.
47. Rudolph RL, Fabre LF, Feighner JP, Rickels K, Entsuah R, Derivan AT. A randomized, placebo-controlled, dose–response trial of venlafaxine hydrochloride in the treatment of major depression. J Clin Psychiatry 1998; 59(3):116–122.
48. Goldstein DJ, Mallinckrodt C, Lu Y, Demitrack MA. Duloxetine in the treatment of major depressive disorder: a double-blind clinical trial. J Clin Psychiatry 2002; 63(3):225–231.
49. Raskin J, Goldstein DJ, Mallinckrodt CH, Ferguson MB. Duloxetine in the long-term treatment of major depressive disorder. J Clin Psychiatry 2003; 64(10):1237–1244.
50. Montgomery SA, Entsuah R, Hackett D, Kunz NR, Rudolph RL. Venlafaxine versus placebo in the preventive treatment of recurrent major depression. J Clin Psychiatry 2004; 65(3):328–336.
51. Thase ME, Nierenberg AA, Keller MB, Panagides J. Efficacy of mirtazapine for prevention of depressive relapse: a placebo-controlled double-blind trial of recently remitted high-risk patients. J Clin Psychiatry 2001; 62(10):782–788.
52. Klett CJ, Caffey EM Jr. Weight changes during treatment with phenothiazine derivatives. J Neuropsychiatry 1960; 2:102–108.
53. Holden JMC, Holden UP. Weight changes with schizophrenic psychosis and psychotropic drug therapy. Psychosomatics 1970; 11:551–561.
54. Doss FW. The effect of antipsychotic drugs on body weight: a retrospective review. J Clin Psychiatry 1979; 40:52S–30S.
55. Johnson DAW, Breen M. Weight changes with depot neuroleptic maintenance therapy. Acta Psychiatr Scand 1979; 59:525–528.
56. Ganguli R. Weight gain associated with antipsychotic drugs. J Clin Psychiatry 1999; 60(suppl 21):20–24.

57. Allison DB, Mentore JL, Heo M, et al. Antipsychotic-induced weight gain: a comprehensive research synthesis. Am J Psychiatry 1999; 156(11):1686–1696.
58. Borison RL, Arvanitis LA, Miller BG. ICI 204,636, an atypical antipsychotic: efficacy and safety in a multicenter, placebo-controlled trial in patients with schizophrenia U.S. SEROQUEL Study Group. J Clin Psychopharmacol 1996; 16(2):158–169.
59. Peuskens J, Link CG. A comparison of quetiapine and chlorpromazine in the treatment of schizophrenia. Acta Psychiatr Scand 1997; 96(4):265–273.
60. Casey DE, Haupt DW, Newcomer JW, et al. Antipsychotic-induced weight gain and metabolic abnormalities: implications for increased mortality in patients with schizophrenia. J Clin Psychiatry 2004; 65(suppl 7):4–18.
61. Tran PV, Hamilton SH, Kuntz AJ, et al. Double-blind comparison of olanzapme versus risperidone in the treatment of schizophrenia and other psychotic disorders. J Clin Psychopharmacol 1997; 17(5):407–418.
62. Tohen M, Zarate CA, Jr. Antipsychotic agents and bipolar disorder. J Clin Psychiatry 1998; 59(suppl 1):38–48.
63. Guille C, Sachs GS, Ghaemi SN. A naturalistic comparison of clozapine, risperidone, and olanzapine in the treatment of bipolar disorder. J Clin Psychiatry 2000; 61(9):638–642.
64. Keck PE, Buse JB, Dagogo-Jack S, et al. Managing metabolic concerns in patients with severe mental illness. Minneapolis: Healthcare Information Programs, McGraw-Hill Healthcare Information Group; 2003.
65. Eder U, Mangweth B, Ebenbichler C, et al. Association of olanzapine-induced weight gain with an increase in body fat. Am J Psychiatry 2001; 158(10): 1719–1722.
66. Zhang ZJ, Yao ZJ, Liu W, Fang Q, Reynolds GP. Effects of antipsychotics on fat deposition and changes in leptin and insulin levels. Magnetic resonance imaging study of previously untreated people with schizophrenia. Br J Psychiatry 2004; 184:58–62.
67. Kelly DL, Conley RR, Love RC, Horn DS, Ushchak CM. Weight gain in adolescents treated with risperidone and conventional antipsychotics over six months. J Child Adolescent Psychopharmacology 1998; 8:151–159.
68. Kinon BJ, Basson B, Szynanski KA, Tollefson G. Factors associated with weight gain during olanzapine treatment. Poster Session No. 10 presented at the 38 Annual Meeting for NCDEU (New Clinical Drug Evaluation Unit Program); 1998 10–13; Boca Raton, FL.
69. Wetter ling T, Mubigbrodt HE. Weight gain: side effect of atypical neuroleptics? J Clin Psychopharmacology 1999; 19:316–321.
70. Lane HY, Chang YC, Cheng YC, Liu GC, Lin XR, Chang WH. Effects of patient demographics, risperidone dosage, and clinical outcome on body weight in acutely exacerbated schizophrenia. J Clin Psychiatry 2003; 64(3):316–320.
71. Gopalaswamy AK, Morgan R. Too many chronic men tally disabled patients are too fat. Acta Psychiatr Scand 1985; 72:254–258.
72. Basson BR, Kinon BJ, Taylor CC, Szymanski KA, Gilmore JA, Tollefson GD. Factors influencing acute weight change in patients with schizophrenia treated with olanzapine, haloperidol, or risperidone. J Clin Psychiatry 2001; 62(4):231–238.

73. Ellingrod VL, Miller D, Schultz SK, Wehring H, Arndt S. CYP2D6 polymorphisms and atypical antipsychotic weight gain. Psychiatr Genet 2002; 12(1):55–58.
74. Brady KT. Weight gain associated with psychotropic drugs. South Med J 1989; 82(5):611–617.
75. Nemeroff CB. Safety of available agents used to treat bipolar disorder: focus on weight gain. J Clin Psychiatry 2003; 64(5):532–539.
76. Johnson DA, Breen M. Weight changes with depot neuroleptic maintenance therapy. Acta Psychiatr Scand 1979; 59(5):525–528.
77. Ganguli R. Weight gain associated with antipsychotic drugs. J Clin Psychiatry 1999; 60(Suppl 21):20–24.
78. Amery W, Zuiderwijk P, Lemmens P. Safety profile of risperidone. Presented at the 10th European College of Neuropsychopharmacology Congress; 1997: 13–17; Vienna, Austria.
79. Csernansky J, Okamato A, Brecher M. Risperidone versus haloperidol for prevention of relapse in schizophrenia and schizoaffective disorders [abstract]. Biol Psychiatry 1999; 45(Suppl 8):S1–S7.
80. Beasley CM, Tollefson GD, Tran P. Safety of olanzapine. J Clin Psychiatry 1997; 58(Suppl 10):13–17.
81. Umbricht D, Kane JM. Medical complications of new antipsychotic drugs. Schizophr Bull 1996; 22(3):475–483. Review.
82. Wirshing DA, Wirshing WC, Kysar L, Berisford MA, Goldstein D, Pashdag J, Mintz J, Marder SR. Novel antipsychotics: comparison of weight gain liabilities. J Clin Psychiatry 1999; 60(6):358–363.
83. Leadbetter R, Shutty M, Pavalonis D, Vieweg V, Higgins P, Downs M. Clozapine-induced weight gain: prevalence and clinical relevance. Am J Psychiatry 1992; 149(1):68–72.
84. Bustillo JR, Buchanan RW, Irish D, Breier A. Related Articles, Links Differential effect of clozapine on weight: a controlled study. Am J Psychiatry 1996; 153(6):817–819.
85. Kryspin-Exener W. Beiträge zum Ver auf des Körpergewichts bei Psychosen. Wien Klin Wschr 1947; 59:531–534.
86. Planasky K, Heilizer F. Weight changes in relation to the characteristics of patients on chlorpromazine. J Clin Exp Psycho path 1959; 20:53–59.
87. Jalenques I, Tauveron I, Albuisson E, Audy V. [Weight gain and clozapine] Encephale 1996; 22 Spec No 3:77–79.
88. Gupta S, Droney T, Al-Samarrai S, Keller P, Frank B. Olanzapine-induced weight gain. Ann Clin Psychiatry 1998; 10(1):39.
89. Lamberti JS. Is antipsychotic drug—induced weight gain associated with a favorable clinical response? J Clin Psychiatry 2000; 61(9):678.
90. Czobor P, Volavka J, Sheitman B, Lindenmayer JP, Citrome L, McEvoy J, Cooper TB, Chakos M, Lieberman JA. Antipsychotic-induced weight gain and therapeutic response: a differential association. J Clin Psychopharmacol 2002; 22(3):244–251.
91. Zhang ZJ, Yao ZJ, Liu W, Fang Q, Reynolds GP. Effects of antipsychotics on fat deposition and changes in leptin and insulin levels. Magnetic resonance

imaging study of previously untreated people with schizophrenia. Br J Psychiatry 2004; 184:58–62.

92. Keck PE, Buse JB, Dagogo-Jack S, et al. Metabolic disease and severe mental illness. Postgrad Med Special Rep, 2003.
93. Baptista T, Teneud L, Contreras Q, et al. Lithium and body weight gain. Pharmacopsychiatry 1995; 28(2):35–44.
94. Kerry RJ, Liebling LI, Owen G. Weight changes in lithium responders. Acta Psychiatr Scand 1970; 46(3):238–243.
95. Sachs GS, Guille C. Weight gain associated with use of psychotropic medications. J Clin Psychiatry 1999; 60(suppl 21):16–19.
96. Bowden CL, Calabrese JR, McElroy SL, et al. A randomized, placebo-controlled 12-month trial of divalproex and lithium in treatment of outpatients with bipolar I disorder. divalproex maintenance study group. Arch Gen Psychiatry 2000; 57(5):481–489.
97. Calabrese JR, Bowden CL, Sachs G, et al. A placebo-controlled 18-month trial of lamotrigine and lithium maintenance treatment in recently depressed patients with bipolar I disorder. J Clin Psychiatry 2003; 64(9):1013–1024.
98. Bowden CL, Calabrese JR, Sachs G, et al. A placebo-controlled 18-month trial of lamotrigine and lithium maintenance treatment in recently manic or hypomanic patients with bipolar I disorder. Arch Gen Psychiatry 2003; 60(4):392–400.
99. Tohen M, Chengappa KN, Suppes T, et al. Relapse prevention in bipolar I disorder: 18-month comparison of olanzapme plus mood stabiliser V. Mood stabiliser alone. Br J Psychiatry 2004; 184:337–345.
100. Plenge P, Mellerup ET, Rafaelsen OJ. Lithium action on glycogen synthesis in rat brain, liver, and diaphragm. J Psychiatr Res 1970; 8(1):29–36.
101. Mellerup ET, Thomsen HG, Plenge P, Rafaelsen OJ. Lithium effect on plasma glucagon, liver phosphorylase-alpha and liver glycogen in rats. J Psychiatr Res 1970; 8(1):37–42.
102. Mellerup ET, Thomsen HG, Bjorum N, Rafaelsen O. Lithium, weight gain, and serum insulin in manic-depressive patients. Acta Psychiatr Scand 1972; 48(4):332–336.
103. Pijl H, Meinders AE. Bodyweight change as an adverse effect of drug treatment. Mechanisms and Management. Drug Saf 1996; 14(5):329–342.
104. Bowden CL. valproate. Bipolar Disord 2003; 5(3):189–202.
105. Smith MC. The efficacy of divalproex for partial epilepsies. Psychopharmacol Bull 2003; 37(suppl 2):54–66.
106. Gidal BE, Sheth RD, Magnus L, Herbeuval AF. Levetiracetam does not alter body weight: analysis of randomized, controlled clinical trials. Epilepsy Res 2003; 56(2–3):121–126.
107. O'Donovan C, Kusumakar V, Graves GR, Bird DC. Menstrual abnormalities and polycystic ovary syndrome in women taking valproate for bipolar mood disorder. J Clin Psychiatry 2002; 63(4):322–330.
108. McIntyre RS, Mancini DA, McCann S, Srinivasan J, Kennedy SH. Valproate, bipolar disorder and polycystic ovarian syndrome. Bipolar Disord 2003; 5(1):28–35.

109. Joffe H, Cohen LS, Stuppes T, et al. Polycystic ovarian syndrome is associated with valproate use in bipolar women. American Psychiatric Association 154th Annual Conference, New York, NY, May 1–6, 2004; 2004. Report No.: N54.

110. Hassan MN, Laljee HC, Parsonage MJ. Sodium valproate in the treatment of resistant epilepsy. Acta Neurol Scand 1976; 54(3):209–218.

111. Dinesen H, Gram L, Andersen T, Dam M. Weight gain during treatment with valproate. Acta Neurol Scand 1984; 70(2):65–69.

112. Tohen M, Ketter TA, Zarate CA, et al. Olanzapine versus divalproex sodium for the treatment of acute mania and maintenance of remission: a 47-week study. Am J Psychiatry 2003; 160(7): 1263–1271.

113. Ketter TA, Wang PW, Becker OV, Nowakowska C, Yang YS. The diverse roles of anticonvulsants in bipolar disorders. Ann Clin Psychiatry 2003; 15(2):95–108.

114. Mattson RH, Cramer JA, Collins JF. A comparison of valproate with carbamazepine for the treatment of complex partial seizures and secondarily generalized tonic-clonic seizures in adults. The Department of Veterans Affairs Epilepsy Cooperative Study No. 264 Group. N Engl J Med 1992; 327(11): 765–771.

115. Chadwick D. Safety and efficacy of vigabatrin and carbamazepine in newly diagnosed epilepsy: a multicentre randomised double-blind study. Vigabatrin European Monotherapy Study Group. Lancet 1999; 354(9172):13–19.

116. Hogan RE, Bertrand ME, Deaton RL, Sommerville KW. Total percentage body weight changes during add-on therapy with tiagabine, carbamazepine and phenytoin. Epilepsy Res 2000; 41(1):23–28.

117. Joffe RT, Post RM, Uhde TW. Effect of carbamazepine on body weight in affectively ill patients. J Clin Psychiatry 1986; 47(6):313–314.

118. Ketter TA, Kalali AH, Weisler RH. A 6-month, multicenter, open-label evaluation of beaded, extended-release carbamazepine capsule monotherapy in bipolar disorder patients with manic or mixed episodes. J Clin Psychiatry 2004; 65(5):668–673.

119. Rattya J, Vainionpaa L, Knip M, Lanning P, Isojarvi JI. The effects of valproate, carbamazepine, and oxcarbazepine on growth and sexual maturation in girls with epilepsy. Pediatrics 1999; 103(3):588–593.

120. Devinsky O, Vuong A, Hammer A, Barrett PS. Stable weight during lamotrigine therapy: a review of 32 studies. Neurology 2000; 54(4):973–975.

121. Biton V, Levisohn P, Hoyler S, Vuong A, Hammer AE. Lamotrigine versus valproate monotherapy-associated weight change in adolescents with epilepsy: results from a post hoc analysis of a randomized, double-blind clinical trial. J Child Neural 2003; 18(2):133–139.

122. Calabrese JR, Suppes T, Bowden CL, et al. A double-blind, placebo-controlled, prophylaxis study of lamotrigine in rapid-cycling bipolar disorder. lamictal 614 study group. J Clin Psychiatry 2000; 61(11):841–850.

123. Ben Menachem E, Henriksen O, Dam M, et al. Double-blind, placebo-controlled trial of topiramate as add-on therapy in patients with refractory partial seizures. Epilepsia 1996; 37(6):539–543.

124. Meldrum BS. Update on the mechanism of action of antiepileptic drugs. Epilepsia 1996; 37(suppl 6):S4–S11.

125. Shorvon SD. Safety of topiramate: adverse events and relationships to dosing. Epilepsia 1996; 37(suppl 2):S18–S22.
126. Chengappa KN, Gershon S, Levine J. The evolving role of topiramate among other mood stabilizers in the management of bipolar disorder. Bipolar Disord 2001; 3(5):215 232.
127. Calabrese JR, Bowden CL, Sachs GS, Ascher JA, Monaghan E, Rudd GD. A double-blind placebo-controlled study of lamotrigine monotherapy in outpatients with bipolar I depression. Lamictal 602 Study Group. J Clin Psychiatry 1999; 60(2):79–88.
128. Chengappa KN, Rathore D, Levine J, et al. Topiramate as add-on treatment for patients with bipolar mania. Bipolar Disord 1999; 1(1):42–53.
129. McIntyre RS, Mancini DA, McCann S, Srinivasan J, Sagman D, Kennedy SH. Topiramate versus bupropion SR when added to mood stabilizer therapy for the depressive phase of bipolar disorder: a preliminary single-blind study. Bipolar Disord 2002; 4(3):207–213.
130. McElroy SL, Suppes T, Keck PE, et al. Open-label adjunctive topiramate in the treatment of bipolar disorders. Biol Psychiatry 2000; 47[12]:1025–1033.
131. Richard D, Ferland I, Lalonde J, Samson P, Deshaies Y. Influence of topiramate in the regulation of energy balance. Nutrition 2000; 16(10):961–966.
132. York DA, Singer L, Thomas S, Bray GA. Effect of topiramate on body weight and body composition of osborne-mendel rats fed a high-fat diet: alterations in hormones, neuropeptide, and uncoupling-protein MRNAs. Nutrition 2000; 16(10):967–975.
133. Taylor CP. Mechanisms of action of gabapentin. Rev Neurol (Paris) 1997; 153(suppl 1):S39–S45.
134. Taylor CP, Gee NS, Su TZ, et al. A summary of mechanistic hypotheses of gabapentin pharmacology. Epilepsy Res 1998; 29(3):233–249.
135. Pande AC, Pollack MH, Crockatt I, et al. Placebo-controlled study of gabapentin treatment of panic disorder. J Clin Psychopharmacol 2000; 20(4):467–471.
136. DeToledo JC, Toledo C, DeCerce J, Ramsay RE. Changes in body weight with chronic, high-dose gabapentin therapy. Ther Drug Monit 1997; 19(4):394–396.
137. Frye MA, Ketter TA, Kimbrell TA, et al. A placebo-controlled study of lamotrigme and gabapentin monotherapy in refractory mood disorders. J Clin Psychopharmacol 2000; 20(6):607–614.
138. Beydoun A, Fischer J, Labar DR, et al. Gabapentin monotherapy: II. A 26-week, double-blind, dose-controlled, multicenter study of conversion from polytherapy in outpatients with refractory complex partial or secondarily generalized seizures. The US Gabapentin Study Group 82/83. Neurology 1997; 49(3):746–752.
139. Bryans JS, Wustrow DJ. 3-substituted GABA analogs with central nervous system activity: a review. Med Res Rev 1999; 19(2):149–177.
140. Pande AC, Feltner DE, Jefferson JW, et al. Efficacy of the novel anxiolytic pregabalin in social anxiety disorder: a placebo-controlled, multicenter study. J Clin Psychopharmacol 2004; 24(2):141–149.

141. Takano K, Tanaka T, Fujita T, Nakai H, Yonemasu Y. Zonisamide: electrophysiological and metabolic changes in kainic acid-induced limbic seizures in rats. Epilepsia 1995; 36(7):644–648.
142. Okada M, Kawata Y, Mizuno K, Wada K, Kondo T, Kaneko S. Interaction between Ca2+, K+, carbamazepine and zonisamide on hippocampal extracellular glutamate monitored with a microdialysis electrode. Br J Pharmacol 1998; 124(6):1277–1285.
143. Gadde KM, Franciscy DM, Wagner HR, Krishnan KR. Zonisamide for weight loss in obese adults: a randomized controlled trial. JAMA 2003; 289(14):1820–1825.
144. McElroy SL, Kotwal R, Hudson JI, Nelson EB, Keck PE. Zonisamide in the treatment of binge-eating disorder: an open-label, prospective trial. J Clin Psychiatry 2004; 65(1):50–56.
145. Tappy L, Binnert C, Schneiter P. Energy expenditure, physical activity and body-weight control. Proc Nutr Soc 2003; 62(3):663–666.
146. Speakman JR, Selman C. Physical activity and resting metabolic rate. Proc Nutr Soc 2003; 62(3):621–634.
147. Hebebrand J, Sommerlad C, Geller F, Gorg T, Hinney A. The genetics of obesity: practical implications. Int J Obes Relat Metab Disord 2001; 25(suppl 1):S10–S18.
148. Gale SM, Castracane VD, Mantzoros CS. Energy homeostasis, obesity and eating disorders: recent advances in endocrinology. J Nutr 2004; 134(2):295–298.
149. Jackson HC, Needham AM, Hutchins LJ, Mazurkiewicz SE, Heal DJ. Comparison of the effects of sibutramine and other monoamine reuptake inhibitors on food intake in the rat. Br J Pharmacol 1997; 121(8):1758–1762.
150. Kroeze WK, Hufeisen SI, Popadak BA, et al. H1-histamine receptor affinity predicts short-term weight gain for typical and atypical antipsychotic drugs. Neuropsychopharmacology 2003; 28(3):519–526.
151. Parada MA, Hernandez L, Paez X, Baptista T, de Parada P, de Quijada M. Mechanism of the body weight increase induced by systemic sulphide. Pharmacol Biochem Behav 1989; 33(1):45–50.
152. Parada MA, de Parada P, Hernandez L, Murzi E. Ventromedial hypothalamus vs. lateral hypothalamic D2 satiety receptors in the body weight increase induced by systemic sulpiride. Physiol Behav 1991; 50(6):1161–1165.
153. Wang GJ, Volkow ND, Logan J, et al. Brain dopamine and obesity. Lancet 2001; 357(9253):354–357.
154. Terry P, Gilbert DB, Cooper SJ. Dopamine receptor subtype agonists and feeding behavior. Obes Res 1995; 3(suppl 4):515S–523S.
155. Chen TY, Duh SL, Huang CC, Lin TB, Kuo DY. Evidence for the involvement of dopamine d(1) and d(2) receptors in mediating the decrease of food intake during repeated treatment with amphetamine. J Biomed Sci 2001; 8(6):462–466.
156. Beninger RJ, Miller R. Dopamine D1-like receptors and reward-related incentive learning. Neurosci Biobehav Rev 1998; 22(2):335–345.
157. Wirtshafter D. The control of ingestive behavior by the median raphe nucleus. Appetite 2001; 36(1):99–105.

158. Meguid MM, Fetissov SO, Varma M, et al. Hypothalamic dopamine and serotonin in the regulation of food intake. Nutrition 2000; 16(10):843–857.
159. De Vry J, Schreiber R. Effects of selected serotonin 5-HT(l) and 5-HT(2) receptor agonists on feeding behavior: possible mechanisms of action. Neurosci Biobehav Rev 2000; 24(3):341–353.
160. Harvey BH, Bouwer CD. Neuropharmacology of paradoxic weight gain with selective serotonin reuptake inhibitors. Clin Neuropharmacol 2000; 23(2): 90–97.
161. Tecott LH, Sun LM, Akana SF, et al. Eating disorder and epilepsy in mice lacking 5-HT2c serotonin receptors. Nature 1995; 374(6522):542–546.
162. Goodall E, Oxtoby C, Richards R, Watkinson G, Brown D, Silverstone T. A clinical trial of the efficacy and acceptability of d-fenfluramine in the treatment of neuroleptic-induced obesity. Br J Psychiatry 1988; 153:208–213.
163. Vickers SP, Benwell KR, Porter RH, Bickerdike MJ, Kennett GA, Dourish CT. Comparative effects of continuous infusion of MCPP, RO 60–0175 and D-fenfluramine on food intake, water intake, body weight and locomotor activity in rats. Br J Pharmacol 2000; 130(6):1305–14.
164. Sussman N, Ginsberg DL. Atypical neuroleptics and glucose regulation. Primary Psychiatry 1999; 6:38–40.
165. Wirshing DA, Wirshing WC, Kysar L, et al. Novel antipsychotics: comparison of weight gain liabilities. J Clin Psychiatry 1999; 60(6):358–363.
166. Masaki T, Yoshimatsu H, Chiba S, Watanabe T, Sakata T. Central infusion of histamine reduces fat accumulation and upregulates UCP family in leptin-resistant obese mice. Diabetes 2001; 50(2):376–384.
167. Yamada M, Miyakawa T, Duttaroy A, et al. Mice lacking the M3 Muscarinic acetylcholine receptor are hypophagic and lean. Nature 2001; 410(6825): 207–212.
168. Baptista T, Lacruz A, de Mendoza S, et al. Body weight gain after administration of antipsychotic drugs: correlation with leptin; insulin and reproductive hormones. Pharmacopsychiatry 2000; 33(3):81–88.
169. Gordon A, Price LH. Mood stabilization and weight loss with topiramate. Am J Psychiatry 1999; 156(6):968–969.
170. Ketter TA, Post RM, Theodore WH. Positive and negative psychiatric effects of antiepileptic drugs in patients with seizure disorders. Neurology 1999; 53(5 suppl 2):S53–S67.
171. Picard F, Deshaies Y, Lalonde J, Samson P, Richard D. Topiramate reduces energy and fat gains in lean (FA/?) and obese (FA/FA) zucker rats. Obes Res 2000; 8(9):656–663.
172. Stanley BG, Butterfield BS, Grewal RS. NMDA receptor coagonist glycine site: evidence for a role in lateral hypothalamic stimulation of feeding. Am J Physiol 1997; 273(2 Pt 2):R790–R796.
173. Paul IA, Nowak G, Layer RT, Popik P, Skolnick P. Adaptation of the N-methyl-D-aspartate receptor complex following chronic antidepressant treatments. J Pharmacol Exp Ther 1994; 269(1):95–102.
174. Bouwer CD, Harvey BH. Phasic craving for carbohydrate observed with citalopram. Int Clin Psychopharmacol 1996; 11(4):273–278.

175. Baptista T, Molina MG, Martinez JL, et al. Effects of the antipsychotic drug sulpiride on reproductive hormones in healthy premenopausal women: relationship with body weight regulation. Pharmacopsychiatry 1997; 30(6):256–262.
176. Baptista T. Body weight gain induced by antipsychotic drugs: mechanisms and management. Acta Psychiatr Scand 1999; 100(1):3–16.
177. Musselman, DL, Betan E, Larsen H, Phillips LS. Relationship of Depression to Diabetes Types 1 and 2: Epidemiology, Biology, and Treatment. Biol Psychiatry 2003; 54(3):317–329.
178. Kraus T, Haack M, Schuld A, Hinze-Selch D, Koethe D, Pollmacher T. Body weight, the tumor necrosis factor system, and leptin production during treatment with mirtazapine or venlafaxine. Pharmacopsychiatry 2002; 35(6):220–225.
179. Haack M, Hinze-Selch D, Fenzel T, et al. Plasma levels of cytokines and soluble cytokine receptors in psychiatric patients upon hospital admission: effects of confounding factors and diagnosis. J Psychiatr Res 1999; 33(5):407–418.
180. Argiles JM, Lopez-Soriano J, Busquets S, Lopez-Soriano FJ. Journey from cachexia to obesity by TNF. FASEB J 1997; 11(10):743–751.
181. Auwerx J, Staels B. Leptin. Lancet 1998; 351(9104):737–742.
182. Bromel T, Blum WF, Ziegler A, et al. Serum leptin levels increase rapidly after initiation of clozapine therapy. Mol Psychiatry 1998; 3(1):76–80.
183. Dandona P, Weinstock R, Thusu K, Abdel-Rahman E, Aljada A, Wadden T. Tumor necrosis factor-alpha in sera of obese patients: fall with weight loss. J Clin Endocrinol Metab 1998; 83(8):2907–2910.
184. Hauner H, Bender M, Haastert B, Hube F. Plasma concentrations of soluble TNF-alpha receptors in obese subjects. Int J Obes Relat Metab Disord 1998; 22(12):1239–1243.
185. Hinze-Selch D, Schuld A, Kraus T, et al. Effects of antidepressants on weight and on the plasma levels of leptin, TNF-alpha and soluble TNF receptors: a longitudinal study in patients treated with amitriptyline or paroxetine. Neuropsychopharmacology 2000; 23(1):13–9.
186. Old LJ. Tumor necrosis factor (TNF). Science 1985; 230(4726):630–632.
187. Uysal KT, Wiesbrock SM, Marino MW, Hotamisligil GS. Protection from obesity-induced insulin resistance in mice lacking TNF-alpha function. Nature 1997; 389(6651):610–614.
188. Wang KY, Arima N, Higuchi S, et al. Switch of histamine receptor expression from H2 to H1 during differentiation of monocytes into macrophages. FEBS Lett 2000; 473(3):345–348.
189. Yanovski JA, Yanovski SZ. Recent advances in basic obesity research. JAMA 1999; 282(16):1504–1506.
190. McIntyre RS, Mancini DA, Basile VS, Srinivasan J, Kennedy SH. Antipsychotic-induced weight gain: bipolar disorder and leptin. J Clin Psychopharmacol 2003; 23(4):323–327.
191. Hagg S, Soderberg S, Ahren B, Olsson T, Mjomdal T. Leptin concentrations are increased in subjects treated with clozapine or conventional antipsychotics. J Clin Psychiatry 2001; 62(11):843–848.
192. Melkersson KI, Hulting AL. Insulin and leptin levels in patients with schizophrenia or related psychoses—a comparison between different antipsychotic agents. Psychopharmacology (Berl) 2001; 154(2):205–212.

193. Melkersson KI, Hulting AL, Brismar KE. Elevated levels of insulin, leptin, and blood lipids in olanzapine-treated patients with schizophrenia or related psychoses. J Clin Psychiatry 2000; 61(10):742–749.
194. Herran A, Garcia-Unzueta MT, Amado JA, de La Maza MT, Alvarez C, Vazquez-Barquero JL. Effects of long-term treatment with antipsychotics on serum leptin levels. Br J Psychiatry 2001; 179:59–62.
195. Fadel J, Bubser M, Deutch AY. Differential activation of orexin neurons by antipsychotic drugs associated with weight gain. J Neurosci 2002; 22(15): 6742–6746.
196. Nakamura T, Uramura K, Nambu T, et al. Orexin-induced hyperlocomotion and stereotypy are mediated by the dopaminergic system. Brain Res 2000; 873(1):181–187.
197. Sakurai T, Amemiya A, Ishii M, et al. Orexins and orexin receptors: a family of hypothalamic neuropeptides and G protein-coupled receptors that regulate feeding behavior. Cell 1998; 92(4):573–585.
198. Uramura K, Funahashi H, Muroya S, Shioda S, Takigawa M, Yada T. Orexin-a activates phospholipase C- and protein kinase c-mediated Ca2+ signaling in dopamine neurons of the ventral tegmental area. Neuroreport 2001; 12(9):1885–1889.
199. Isojarvi JI, Laatikainen TJ, Knip M, Pakarinen AJ, Juntunen KT, Myllyla VV. Obesity and endocrine disorders in women taking valproate for epilepsy. Ann Neurol 1996; 39(5):579–584.
200. Isojarvi JI, Rattya J, Myllyla VV, et al. Valproate, lamotrigine, and insulin-mediated risks in women with epilepsy. Ann Neurol 1998; 43(4):446–451.
201. Pylvanen V, Knip M, Pakarinen A, Kotila M, Turkka J, Isojarvi JI. Serum insulin and leptin levels in valproate-associated obesity. Epilepsia 2002; 43(5):514–517.
202. Luef G, Abraham I, Hoppichler F. Increase in postprandial serum insulin levels in epileptic patients with valproic acid therapy. Metabolism 2002; 51(10):1274–1278.
203. Luef G, Abraham I, Haslinger M, et al. Polycystic ovaries, obesity and insulin resistance in women with epilepsy. A comparative study of carbamazepine and valproic acid in 105 women. J Neurol 2002; 249(7):835–841.
204. Luef G, Abraham I, Trinka E, et al. Hyperandrogenism, postprandial hyper-insulinism and the risk of pcos in a cross sectional study of women with epilepsy treated with valproate. Epilepsy Res 2002; 48(1–2):91–102.
205. Yoshikawa H, Tajiri Y, Sako Y, Hashimoto T, Umeda F, Nawata H. Effects of free fatty acids on beta-cell functions: a possible involvement of peroxisome proliferator-activated receptors alpha or pancreatic/duodenal homeobox. Metabolism 2001; 50(5):613–618.
206. Hesselink MK, Mensink M, Schrauwen P. Human uncoupling protein-3 and obesity: an update. Obes Res 2003; 11(12):1429–1443.
207. Berraondo B, Marti A, Duncan JS, Trayhum P, Martinez JA. Up-regulation of muscle ucp2 gene expression by a new beta3-adrenoceptor agonist, treca-drine, in obese (cafeteria) rodents, but down-regulation in lean animals. Int J Obes Relat Metab Disord 2000; 24(2):156–163.

208. Tai TA, Jennermann C, Brown KK, et al. Activation of the nuclear receptor peroxisome proliferator-activated receptor gamma promotes brown adipocyte differentiation. J Biol Chem 1996; 271(47):29,909–29,914.

209. Nagase I, Yoshida T, Saito M. Up-regulation of uncoupling proteins by beta-adrenergic stimulation in L6 myotubes. FEBS Lett 2001; 494(3): 175–180.

210. Shank RP, Gardocki JF, Streeter AJ, Maryanoff BE. An overview of the pre-clinical aspects of topiramate: pharmacology, phaimacokinetics, and mechanism of action. Epilepsia 2000; 41(suppl 1):S3–S9.

211. Basile VS, Masellis M, McIntyre RS, Meltzer HY, Lieberman JA, Kennedy JL. Genetic dissection of atypical antipsychotic-induced weight gain: novel preliminary data on the pharmacogenetic puzzle. J Clin Psychiatry 2001; 62(suppl 23):45–66.

212. Pooley EC, Fairhurn CG, Cooper Z, Sodhi MS, Cowen PJ, Harrison PJ. A 5-HT2C receptor promoter polymorphism (HT. Am J Med Genet 2004; 126B(1):124–127.

213. Rietschel M, Naber D, Oberlander H, et al. Efficacy and side-effects of clozapine: testing for association with allelic variation in the dopamine d4 receptor gene. Neuropsychopharmacology 1996; 15(5):491–496.

214. Reynolds GP, Zhang ZJ, Zhang XB. Association of antipsychotic drug-induced weight gain with a 5-HT2C receptor gene polymorphism. Lancet 2002; 359(9323):2086–2087.

215. Reynolds GP, Zhang Z, Zhang X. Polymorphism of the promoter region of the serotonin 5-HT[2C] receptor gene and clozapine-induced weight gain. Am J Psychiatry 2003; 160(4):677–679.

216. Tsai SJ, Hong CJ, Yu YW, Lin CH. -759C/T Genetic variation of 5HT(2C) receptor clozapine-induced weight gain. Lancet 2002; 360(9347):1790.

217. Theisen FM, Hinney A, Bromel T, et al. Lack of association between the -759C/T polymorphism of the 5-HT2C receptor gene and clozapine-induced weight gain among german schizophrenic individuals. Psychiatr Genet 2004; 14(3):139–142.

218. Zhang ZJ, Yao ZJ, Zhang XB, et al. No association of antipsychotic agent-induced weight gain with a DA receptor gene polymorphism and therapeutic response. Acta Pharmacol Sin 2003; 24(3):235–240.

219. Hong CJ, Lin CH, Yu YW, Chang SC, Wang SY, Tsai SJ. Genetic variant of the histamine-1 receptor (Glu349asp) and body weight change during clozapine treatment. Psychiatr Genet 2002; 12(3):169–171.

220. Ellingrod VL, Miller D, Schultz SK, Wehring H, Arndt S. CYP2D6 polymorphisms and atypical antipsychotic weight gain. Psychiatr Genet 2002; 12(l):55–58.

221. American Dietetic Association. Position of the American Dietetic Association: Integration of medical nutrition therapy and pharmacotherapy. J Am Diet Assoc 2003; 103(10):1363–1370.

222. Astrup A. Dietary approaches to reducing body weight. Baillieres Best Pract Res Clin Endocrinol Metab l999; 13(l):109–120.

223. Centers for Disease Control, National Center for Chronic Disease Prevention and Health Promotion. Physical activity and good nutrition: essential elements to prevent chronic diseases and obesity 2003. Nutr Clin Care 2003; 6(3):135–138.

224. Klein S, Sheard NE, Pi-Sunyer X, et al. Weight management through lifestyle modification for the prevention and management of type 2 diabetes: rationale and strategies. A Statement of the American Diabetes Association, the North American Association for the Study of Obesity, and the American Society for Clinical Nutrition. Am J Clin Nutr 2004; 80(2):257–263.

225. Avenell A, Broom L, Brown TJ, et al. Systematic review of the long-term effects and economic consequences of treatments for obesity and implications for health improvement. Health Technol Assess 2004; 8(21):111–182.

226. Hensrud DD, Weinsier RL, Darnell BE, Hunter GR. A prospective study of weight maintenance in obese subjects reduced to normal body weight without weight-loss training. Am J Clin Nutr 1994; 60(5):688–694.

227. Brownell KD, Rodin J. The dieting maelstrom. Is it possible and advisable to lose weight? Am Psychol 1994; 49(9):781–791.

228. Mokdad AH, Bowman BA, Ford ES, Vinicor, F, Marks JS, Koplan JP. The continuing epidemics of obesity and diabetes in the United States. JAMA 2001; 286(10):1195–1200.

229. Werneke U, Taylor D, Sanders TA, Wessley S. Behavioural management of antipsychotic-induced weight gain: a review. Acta Psychiatr Scand 2003; 108(4):252–259.

230. Druss BG, Bradford WD, Rosenheck RA, Radford MJ, Krumholz HM. Quality of medical care and excess mortality in older patients with mental disorders. Arch Gen Psychiatry 2001; 58(6):565–572.

231. McIntyre RS, Konarski JZ, Yatham LM. Comorbidity in bipolar disorder: a framework for rational treatment selection. Hum Psychopharmacology 2004; 19(6):369–386.

232. Schulze MB, Manson LE, Ludwig DS, et al. Sugar-sweetened beverages, weight gain, and incidence of type 2 diabetes in young and middle-aged women. JAMA 2004; 292(8):927–934.

233. Fontaine KR, Barofsky I, Bartlett SJ, Franckowiak SC, Andersen R. Weight loss and health-related quality of life: results at 1-year follow-up. Eat Behav 2004; 5(1):85–88.

234. Cleland R, Graybill DC, Hubbard V, et al. Commercial weight loss products and programs: what consumers stand to gain and lose. A public conference on the information consumers need to evaluate weight loss products and programs. Crit Rev Food Sci Nutr 2001; 41(1):45–70.

235. Serdula MK, Mokdad AH, Williamson DF, Galuska DA, Mendlein JM, Health GW. Prevalence of attempting weight loss and strategies for controlling weight. JAMA 1999; 282(14):1353–1358.

236. Holt RA, Maunder EM. Is lithium-induced weight gain prevented by providing healthy eating advice at the commencement of lithium therapy? J Hum Nutr Diet 1996; 9:127–133.

237. Littrell KH, Hilligoss NM, Kirshner CD, Petty RG, Johnson CG. The effects of an educational intervention on antipsychotic-induced weight gain. J Nurs Scholarsh 2003; 35(3):237–241.

238. Vreeland B, Minsky S, Menza M, et al. A program for managing weight gain associated with atypical antipsychotics. Psychiatr Serv 2003; 54(8):1155–1157.

239. Ball MP, Coons VB, Buchaman RW. A program for treating olanzapine-related weight gain. Psychiatr Serv 2001; 52(7):967–969.
240. Yanovski SZ, Yanovski JA. Obesity. N Engl J Med 2002; 346(8):591–602.
241. Raison CL, Klein HM. Psychotic mania associated with fenfluramine and phentermine use. Am J Psychiatry 1997; 154(5):711.
242. Khan SA, Spiegel DA, Jobe PC. Psychotomimetic effects of anorectic drugs. Am Fam Physician 1987; 36(2):107–112.
243. James WP, Astrup A, Finer N, et al. Effect of sibutramine on weight maintenance after weight loss: a randomised trial. STORM study group. Sibutramine trial of obesity reduction and maintenance. Lancet 2000; 356(9248):2119–2125.
244. Henderson DC, Copeland PM, Daley TB, Borba CP, Cather C, Nguyen DD, Louie PM, Evins AE, Freudenreich O, Hayden D, Goff DC. A Double-Blind, Placebo-Controlled Trial of Sibutramine for Olanzapine-Associated Weight Gain. Am J Psychiatry 2005; 162(5):954–962.
245. Benazzi F. Organic hypomania secondary to sibutramine-citalopram interaction. J Clin Psychiatry 2002; 63(2):165.
246. Hedges DW, Reimherr FW, Hoopes SP, et al. Treatment of bulimia nervosa with topiramate in a randomized, double-blind, placebo-controlled trial, part 2: improvement in psychiatric measures. J Clin Psychiatry 2003; 64(12):1449–1454.
247. Bray GA, Hollander P, Klein S, et al. A 6-month randomized, placebo-controlled, dose-ranging trial of topiramate for weight loss in obesity. Obes Res 2003; 11(6):722–733.
248. Hoopes SP, Reimherr FW, Hedges DW, et al. Treatment of bulimia nervosa with topiramate in a randomized, double-blind, placebo-controlled trial, part 1: improvement in binge and purge measures. J Clin Psychiatry 2003; 64(11):1335–1341.
249. McElroy SL, Arnold LM, Shapira NA, et al. Topiramate in the treatment of binge eating disorder associated with obesity: a randomized, placebo-controlled trial. Am J Psychiatry 2003; 160(2):255–261.
250. Chengappa KN, Chalasani L, Brar JS, Parepally H, Houck P, Levine J. Changes in body weight and body mass index among psychiatric patients receiving lithium, valproate, or topiramate: an open-label, nonrandomized chart review. Clin Ther 2002; 24(10):1576–1584.
251. Van Ameringen M, Mancini C, Pipe B, Campbell M, Oakman J. topiramate treatment for SSRI-induced weight gain in anxiety disorders. J Clin Psychiatry 2002; 63(11):981–984.
252. Floris M, Lejeune J, Deberdt W. Effect of amantadine on weight gain during olanzapine treatment. Eur Neuropsychopharmacol 2001; 11(2):181–182.
253. Bank WM, Lee KU, Chae JH, Pae CU, Jun T, Kim KS. Open label study of the effect of amantadine on weight gain induced by olanzapine. Psychiatry Clin Neurosci 2004; 58(2):163–167.
254. Stoa-Birketvedt G, Lovhaug N, Vonen B, Florholmen J. H2-receptor antagonist reduces food latake and weight gain in rats by non-gastric acid secretory mechanisms. Acta Physiol Scand 1997; 161(4):489–494.
255. Stoa-Birketvedt G, Waldum HL, Vonen B, Florholmen J. Effect of cimetidine on basal and postprandial plasma concentrations of cholecystokinin and gastrin in humans. Acta Physiol Scand 1997; 159(4):321–325.

256. Atmaca M, Kuloglu M, Tezcan E, Ustundag B. Nizatidine treatment and its relationship with leptin levels in patients with olanzapine-induced weight gain. Hum Psychopharmacol 2003; 18(6):457–461.

257. Atmaca M, Kuloglu M, Tezcan E, Ustundag B, Kilic N. Nizatidine for the treatment of patients with quetiapine-induced weight gain. Hum Psychopharmacol 2004; 19(1):37–40.

258. Fontbonne A, Charles MA, Juhan-Vague I, et al. The effect of metformin on the metabolic abnonnalities associated with upper-body fat distribution. BIGPRO Study Group. Diabetes Care 1996; 19(9):920–926.

259. Diabetes Prevention Trial—Type1 Diabetes Study group. Effects of insulin in relatives of patients with type 1 diabetes mellitus. N Eng J Med 2002; 346(22):1685–1691.

260. Morrison JA, Cottingham EM, Barton BA. Metformin for weight loss in pediatric patients taking psychotropic drugs. Am J Psychiatry 2002; 159(4):655–657.

261. Baptista T, Hernandez L, Prieto LA, Boyero EC, de Mendoza S. Metformin in obesity associated with antipsychotic drug administration: a pilot study. J Clin Psychiatry 2001; 62(8):653–655.

262. Poyurovsky M, Pashinian A, Gil-Ad I, et al. Olanzapine-induced weight gain in patients with first-episode schizophrenia: a double-blind, placebo-controlled study of fluoxetine addition. Am J Psychiatry 2002; 159(6):1058–1060.

263. Poyurovsky M, Isaacs I, Fuchs C, et al. Attenuation of olanzapme-induced weight gain with reboxetine in patients with schizophrenia: a double-blind, placebo-controlled study. Am J Psychiatry 2003; 160(2):297–302.

264. Heck AM, Yanovski JA, Calis KA. Orlistat, a new lipase inhibitor for the management of obesity. Pharmacotherapy 2000; 20(3):270–279.

265. Hilger E, Quiner S, Ginzel I, Walter H, Saria L, Barnas C. The effect of orlistat on plasma levels of psychotropic drugs in patients with long-term psychopharmacotherapy. J Clin Psychopharmacol 2002; 22(1):68–70.

15

Medical Management of Uncomplicated Obesity

Jonathan A. Waitman and Louis J. Aronne

Department of Medicine, Weill-Cornell University Medical College, New York, New York, U.S.A.

INTRODUCTION

Obesity is rapidly becoming the single greatest health threat facing our society. The age-adjusted prevalence of obesity, defined as a [body mass index (BMI) ≥ 30 kg/m^2], has increased from 22.9% in NHANES III (1988–1994; $p < 0.001$) to 30.5% in the most recent data from 1999 to 2000 (1). Poor diet and physical inactivity account for 400,000 deaths per year in the United States, second only to tobacco in preventable causes of death (2). As the number of overweight and obese patients has increased, so too have those who suffer from weight-related comorbid conditions such as diabetes, hypertension, heart disease, hyperlipidemia, osteoarthritis, and a multitude of malignancies. It is impossible to find an organ system that is not deleteriously affected by the burden of obesity. It is for this reason that weight loss has become a primary treatment objective for all physicians.

The ultimate goal of obesity treatment is to improve the comorbid conditions associated with obesity. Patients need to appreciate the concept that obesity is a chronic disease like diabetes or hypertension that will require long-term treatment. They should also understand that the efficacy of nonsurgical interventions is limited to a 5% to 15% body weight loss in the majority of successful patients, but that this weight loss is enough to induce better health. The foundation of obesity treatment is lifestyle modification including a healthy diet and physical activity.

Medications should be viewed as a potentially valuable adjunct to diet and exercise, rather than a substitute. Medications are currently indicated in the treatment of obesity for patients with $BMI > 30\,kg/m^2$ or $>27\,kg/m^2$ in the presence of other risk factors or diseases if diet and exercise are not successful. Sibutramine and orlistat are the only medications currently approved for the long-term treatment of obesity (3). Both these medications have proven efficacy in inducing and maintaining weight loss.

Lifestyle modification includes eating a healthy diet and incorporating physical activity into daily life. The goal of behavioral change therapy is to overcome barriers to compliance with such a regimen. Behavior therapy assumes that learned patterns of eating and physical activity can be changed, and that to change these patterns over the long term, the environment must be modified. In some cases behavioral therapy is administered on an individual basis, in other cases as group sessions. Professionals with training in psychology or a related area who can engage a group in a cohesive manner are optimal for leading such groups. More than 100 controlled trials have been published demonstrating the effectiveness of behavioral techniques, which have become more sophisticated over time (4).

Although dozens of behavioral techniques are used as part of the behavioral treatment of obesity, several have been shown to enhance compliance with a program of diet and exercise. These include self-monitoring, stimulus control, stress management, reinforcement, cognitive change, relapse prevention, and crisis intervention.

A summary of studies combining behavioral treatment with moderate dietary restriction and exercise as part of a comprehensive program showed 8.5 kg average weight loss from an initial average weight of 91.9 kg over 21 weeks of treatment with a 22% rate of attrition (4). A 5.6 kg loss was maintained after one year of follow-up. Longer periods of treatment yield better results, and long-term intermittent treatment is recommended.

In general, the goal of dietary interventions has been to induce a caloric deficit of 500 to 1000 kcal/day resulting in a weight loss of 0.5 to 0.9 kg/week. Diets containing 1000 to 1200 kcal/day for women and 1200 to 1600 kcal/day for men are commonly used to induce a caloric deficit. Very low calorie diets (<800 kcal/day) have not been found to be more effective than low calorie diets in achieving a sustainable weight loss in the long term, but could play a role when acute weight loss is indicated. Liquid meal replacements have been shown to enhance weight loss efficacy and, if used regularly, maintenance.

No single approach to diet works for everyone; in our opinion, the best approach is to customize diet to the individual patient. The best diet is the one with which the patient will comply. Recent findings suggest that foods with a lower glycemic index (blood glucose rise per ounce of food) may reduce food consumption (5). Diets with a lower caloric density (number of calories per ounce), such as vegetables, appear to be more filling and may also reduce overall food consumption. As a result, we recommend diets with a higher percentage of carbohydrate from vegetables and legumes and less from starch and sugar. In general, we recommend an adequate amount of lean protein and large quantities of vegetables as the mainstay of the diet with smaller amounts of whole grains and healthy oil sources.

Liquid meal replacements can be of value in certain individuals who prefer this mode of therapy. Use of these diets to substitute for a meal has been shown to reduce body weight and assist with weight maintenance (6).

Until recently there has been a paucity of scientific data regarding the low-carbohydrate diet. Several recent randomized-controlled trials examined the efficacy of the low-carbohydrate diet. Samaha et al. (7) compared the efficacy of a carbohydrate-restricted diet with a calorie- and fat-restricted diet in 132 severely obese subjects over a six-month period. Subjects assigned to the low-carbohydrate group lost more weight (mean, 5.7 ± 8.6 vs. 1.9 ± 4.2 kg; $p = 0.002$), had greater improvements in triglycerides ($p = 0.001$), insulin sensitivities ($p = 0.01$), and glycemic control ($p = 0.02$). Foster et al. (8) published a one-year trial comparing the use of a low-carbohydrate, high-protein, high-fat diet with a low calorie, high-carbohydrate, low-fat diet in 63 obese subjects. This study failed to show any significant difference in weight loss between the two groups after one year (4.4 ± 6.7 vs. 2.5 ± 6.3 percent body weight, $p = 0.26$). However, it should be pointed out that both groups showed improvements over baseline in diastolic blood pressure, triglycerides, and insulin sensitivity. These studies illustrate that in obese patients, a modest weight loss with dietary intervention alone conveys significant health benefits.

Exercise plays a major role in assisting with weight maintenance, and there is mounting evidence that increased physical activity plays a crucial role in the prevention and management of many chronic diseases even in the absence of weight loss (9). Aerobic exercise is usually recommended for weight management because of the large number of calories burned as well as the health benefits achieved. Strength training may also be of benefit to build lean body mass and improve body composition. Regular adherence to an exercise program is associated with better outcome because it may also improve dietary compliance or be a marker of better dietary compliance. Exercise further improves quality of life by enhancing self-esteem, reducing stress, and relieving depression.

Any physical activity that the patient enjoys and is willing to perform is recommended. For the completely sedentary patient, walking is often the best way to get started. Patients with physical limitations secondary to arthritis or size may start with water exercises, bedside stretching, seated activities, or a program designed by an exercise physiologist or physical therapist. In general, 30 to 45 minutes of exercise 3 to 5 day/wk is recommended, although more is better, and greater intensity may be better. Three 10-minute periods of activity yield about the same benefit as a single

30-minute period, and compliance with such a program is better. Increasing physical activity during daily life such as climbing stairs instead of taking an elevator, walking or cycling rather than taking a car, and parking further away from the entrance to the mall can be simple ways to add small periods of physical activity to a busy lifestyle.

SIBUTRAMINE (MERIDIA)

Sibutramine enhances satiety by blocking the reuptake of norepinephrine and serotonin in the central nervous system. It may also increase metabolic rate by activating the β3-adrenergic receptor peripherally.

Bray and Blackburn (10) conducted a placebo-controlled trial to evaluate different doses of sibutramine over a 24-week period. They found a statistically significant weight loss at all doses (1, 5, 10, 15, 20, and 30 mg) as compared to placebo. Wirth and Krause (11) showed that intermittent sibutramine was as effective as continuous sibutramine over a 44-week period. Apfelbaum et al. (12) took obese patients (BMI > 30) and gave them very low calorie diets for four weeks (12). This was followed by one year of sibutramine versus placebo. After 12 months, 75% of subjects in the sibutramine group maintained at least 100% of the weight loss achieved with a very low calorie diet, compared with 42% in the placebo group ($p < 0.01$) (12).

Berkowitz et al. (13) conducted the first randomized, placebo-controlled study examining the utility of a medication (sibutramine) in obese adolescents. All subjects were advised to reduce caloric intake and increase aerobic activity. At the end of six months, the sibutramine group had lost significantly more weight (mean weight loss -7.8 ± 6.3 vs. -3.2 ± 6.1 kg; $p = 0.001$). Nineteen of 43 participants experienced elevations in blood pressure and pulse rate requiring reductions in the dose of sibutramine. These studies illustrate sibutramine's efficacy as a weight loss and weight-maintenance agent, and that the majority of weight loss will take place during the first six months of treatment.

A recent study examined the utility of sibutramine in the treatment of binge eating disorder (BED). Sixty obese subjects with BED were randomized to receive sibutramine (15 mg/day) or placebo for 12 weeks. Subjects receiving sibutramine lost more weight (-7.4 vs. $+1.4$ kg; $p < 0.001$), and binged less frequently (66 vs. 41% reduction from baseline; $p = 0.03$) (14).

McMahon (15) and Sramek (16) each demonstrated the safety of sibutramine in the treatment of obese patients with well-controlled hypertension. These studies found statistically significant increases in pulse rate, but not blood pressure in the sibutramine groups. Sibutramine has been proven safe in patients being treated with angiotensin-converting enzyme (ACE) inhibitors (15), beta blockers (16), and calcium channel blockers (17).

Gokcel et al. (18) compared the effects of three different medications used in the management of obesity; sibutramine (10 mg twice daily), Orlistat

Table 1 Randomized Controlled Trials of Sibutramine

Study	Subjects	Study period	Dose (mg)	Placebo weight loss	Sibutramine weight loss	p
Bray	1463	24 wk	5	1.20%	3.90%	<0.05
			10		6.10%	
			15		7.40%	
			20		8.80%	
Wirth and Kraus	1102	44 wk	15	+0.2%		<0.05
Apfelbaum	160	1 yr	10	+0.5 kg	5.2 kg	<0.04
Cuellar	69	6 mo	15	1.26 kg	10.27 kg	0.001
Gockel	54	6 mo	20	0.91 kg	9.61 kg	0.0001
McMahon	220	1 yr	20	0.4 kg	4.5 kg	<0.05
McMahon	124	1 yr	20	0.70%	4.70%	<0.05

(150 mg three times per day), and metformin (850 mg twice daily). All subjects were females with BMI > 30. After six months of treatment all three groups showed improvements in lipid profiles, insulin resistance, glucose, and blood pressure. The sibutramine group displayed a statistically significant ($p < 0.0001$) greater reduction in BMI (13.57%) when compared to orlistat (9.06%) and metformin (9.9%).

The cardiac effects of the combination of other anorexigenic agents dexfenfluramine and fenfluramine led to the withdrawal of these drugs from the market in 1997. Zannad et al. (19) demonstrated that six months of sibutramine had no significant impact on cardiac dimension, valve function, or electrocardiograms.

The most frequent side effects associated with sibutramine are dry mouth, anorexia, and insomnia. Patients may experience an increase in blood pressure and pulse, and monitoring of these vital signs should be performed on a monthly basis initially, and every three months once the patient's weight has stabilized (Table 1).

ORLISTAT (XENICAL)

Orlistat promotes weight loss by inhibiting gastrointestinal lipases, thereby decreasing the absorption of fat from the gastrointestinal tract. On average, 120 mg of orlistat taken three times per day will decrease fat absorption by 30% (20). Orlistat has been found to be more effective in inhibiting the digestion of solid foods, as opposed to liquids (21).

Rossner et al. (22) found that subjects receiving orlistat lost significantly more weight in the first year of treatment, and fewer regained weight during the second year of treatment than those taking placebo. The orlistat group also had greater improvement in total and low-density lipoprotein (LDL) cholesterol. Subjects taking orlistat had lower serum levels of vitamins D, E, and β-carotene. However, these nutritional deficiencies are easily treated with oral multivitamin supplementation. Sjostrom et al. (23) demonstrated similar results over a two-year period. Subjects in the orlistat group lost significantly more weight in the first year (10.2 vs. 6.1%) and regained half as much weight during the second year.

Davidson et al. (24) showed in another two-year study that there was less weight regain in patients maintained on the 360 mg/day dose of orlistat, as opposed to a 60 mg/day dose or placebo. Subjects in the Orlistat group also had lower levels of serum glucose and insulin.

The recent XENical in the prevention of diabetes in obese objects trial was a four-year long placebo-controlled trial of orlistat for the prevention of type 2 diabetes (25). Subjects at risk for type 2 diabetes were treated with a diet and lifestyle program with the addition of orlistat 120 mg TID or placebo. Weight loss in the orlistat treated group was significantly better at both one and four years. The four-year incidence of type 2 diabetes was reduced from 9% in the placebo group to 6.2% in the orlistat group, a 37% reduction.

Hollander et al. (26) studied the effects of orlistat in obese patients with type 2 diabetes. Orlistat resulted in improved glycemic control (reduced blood glucose and HbAlC), and reductions in total cholesterol, LDL, triglycerides, and apo-lipoprotein B. Kelley (27) showed similar benefits in obese insulin-requiring diabetics.

Lindgarde (28) examined the impact of orlistat on cardiovascular profiles in obese subjects with at least one of the following: type 2 diabetes, hypercholesterolemia, and hypertension. Orlistat use was associated with greater weight loss and reductions in HbAlc, LDL, and total cholesterol.

The gastrointestinal side effects of orlistat, including fatty/oily stool, fecal urgency, oily spotting, increased defecation, fecal incontinence, flatus with discharge, and oily evacuation, are the main reason for discontinuation of therapy. These symptoms are usually mild to moderate and decrease in frequency the longer the medication is continued. Cavaliere (29) conducted a study to see if concomitant use of natural fibers (psyllium mucilloid) would ameliorate the adverse gastrointestinal events. Subjects who received the psyllium experienced far fewer symptoms. Only 29% of those taking psyllium with orlistat taken as 120 mg tid had GI events compared to 71% of the patients on placebo (Table 2).

PHENTERMINE

Phentermine (Fastin) is a sympathomimetic anorexigenic agent. A study from 1968 is the only longer term controlled trial of phentermine (30). In this study, 64 patients completed 36 weeks of placebo, phentermine, or

Table 2 Randomized Controlled Trials of Orlistat

Study	N	Study period	Dose (mg/day)	Weight loss placebo	Weight loss Orlistat	p
Rossner	729	1 yr	360	6.60%	8.60%	< 0.001
			180	6.60%	9.70%	< 0.001
Sjostrom	743	1 yr	360	6.10%	10.20%	< 0.001
Davidson	892	2 yr	360	5.81 kg	8.76 kg	< 0.001
Finer	228	1 yr	360	8.50%	5.40%	< 0.016
Hauptman	796	1 yr	360	4.14 kg	7.94 kg	< 0.01
			180	4.14 kg	7.08 kg	< 0.01
Hollander	391	57 wk	360	4.30%	6.40%	< 0.001
Lindgarde	382	1 yr	360	4.60%	5.90%	< 0.05
Kelley	550	1 yr	360	+1.27%	3.89%	< 0.001
Sjostrom	3304	1 yr	360	6.8%	11.4%	< 0.001
		4 yr	360	3.7%	6.25%	< 0.001

placebo and phentermine on alternating days. Both phentermine groups lost approximately 13% of their initial weight, while the placebo group lost only 5%. Despite the paucity of research to support its use, phentermine is the most commonly prescribed weight-loss medication in the United States representing 31% of drug-treated obese patients (31). Phentermine's main side effects are related to its sympathomimetic properties and include insomnia, constipation, and dry mouth. Phentermine and other sympatho-mimetics such as diethylpropion and phendimetrazine have not been studied for long-term safety and efficacy and their use beyond three months is considered "off-label."

AVAILABLE DRUGS THAT CAUSE WEIGHT LOSS

Bupropion (Wellbutrin)

Bupropion is an atypical antidepressant that is reported to induce weight loss. While the mean weight loss seen with bupropion is small, in some patients bupropion is preferable to the many other antidepressants which may induce weight gain.

Anderson et al. (32) conducted a 48 week randomized placebo-controlled trial of the weight loss effects of bupropion. There were three study arms: placebo, 300 mg and 400 mg of bupropion sustained release. Using a last observation carried forward (LOCF) analysis the weight loss for subjects was 4.0, 5.7, and 7.7% for placebo, bupropion SR 300 and 400 mg/day, respectively. In another study from 2002, obese adults with depressive symptoms were treated with bupropion SR or placebo for 26 weeks in addition to a 500 kcal/day-deficit diet. The bupropion SR group

($n = 193$) lost an average of 4.4 kg (4.6% of baseline weight) versus 1.7 kg (1.8% of baseline weight) on placebo ($n = 191$, $p < 0.001$, LOCF analysis) (33). Bupropion is contraindicated in patients with epilepsy and may cause anxiety and, rarely, seizures.

Metformin (Glucophage)

Metformin is a drug used in the treatment of type 2 diabetes that decreases hepatic gluconeogenesis and increases insulin sensitivity. Gokcel et al. (34) demonstrated that metformin achieved similar weight loss to orlistat over a six-month period. Kay et al. (35) studied the effects of metformin on obese, hyperinsulinemic, and nondiabetic subjects. When compared to placebo the metformin group achieved significantly greater weight loss (6.5 ± 0.8 vs. $3.8 \pm 0.4\%$, $p < 0.01$) and improvement in their hyperinsulinemia. In patients with fasting hyperglycemia, metformin accounted for greater weight loss than placebo, but less than life-style changes alone. The average weight loss was 0.1, 2.1, and 5.6 kg in the placebo, metformin, and lifestyle-intervention groups, respectively ($p < 0.001$) (36).

On the basis of this evidence metformin should be the first line drug in obese diabetic patients. There is also good evidence to endorse the use of metformin in obese patients with polycystic ovarian syndrome or nonalcoholic steatohepatitis. The most common side effects of metformin are nausea, flatulence, diarrhea, and bloating. The most serious side effect is lactic acidosis, but this is uncommon.

Topiramate (Topamax)

Topiramate is an antiepileptic agent that has been found to reduce body weight in patients with a variety of disorders including epilepsy, migraine headaches, bipolar disorder, and binge eating disorder (37,38). McElroy et al. (39) conducted the first randomized, placebo-controlled trial of topiramate in the treatment of obese binge eaters. After 14 weeks of treatment the subjects who received topiramate lost significantly more weight than the control group (mean weight loss 5.9 vs. 1.2 kg: $p = 0.005$). On a median dose of 212 mg/day, 64% of the topiramate-treated group had a complete remission of bingeing compared to 30% of those on placebo. A 94% reduction in binge frequency was observed in topiramate treated completers compared to a 46% reduction in the placebo group. In 2003, Bray et al. (40) studied the utility of topiramate in the treatment of obesity. A randomized, double-blind, placebo-controlled, dose-ranging trial was conducted on obese adults. Mean percent weight loss from baseline to week 24 was -2.6% in placebo-treated patients versus -5.0%, -4.8%, -6.3%, and -6.3% in the 64, 96, 192, and 384 mg/day topiramate groups, respectively. All doses of topiramate resulted in statistically significant greater weight loss than placebo. The most common side effects of topiramate are paresthesias, dry mouth somnolence, headache, difficulty with memory, concentration, and attention. These side effects are dose related and typically resolve spontaneously. Topiramate is also being studied for the treatment of migraine headaches, neuropathic pain, and alcoholism. Other side effects of topiramate include cognitive impairment, renal stones, and, rarely, acute angle glaucoma.

Zonisamide

Zonisamide is a second novel antiepileptic drug that has been found to induce weight loss. It exerts both serotonergic and dopaminergic activity. Gadde et al. (41) compared 16 weeks of zonisamide to a placebo in conjunction with a dietitian supervised diet and lifestyle in 60 obese subjects. Dose titration to a >5% weight loss effect was utilized and the mean dose of zonisamide taken by subjects was 427 mg/day. The zonisamide group lost significantly more weight [mean weight loss 5.8 ± 0.8 (6.0%) vs. 0.9 ± 0.4 kg (1.0%); $p < 0.001$]. Fifty-seven percent of the zonisamide group and 10% of the placebo group achieved a 5% reduction in body weight by week 16 ($p < 0.001$). A single blind extension for an additional 16 weeks yielded a total weight loss of 9 kg in the zonisamide group compared to 1.5 kg in the placebo group. Although fatigue was the only side effect that occurred with significantly higher frequency in the treatment group, other cognitive side effects and, rarely, kidney stones have been described in epilepsy trials.

DRUGS CURRENTLY IN CLINICAL TRIALS

Axokine

Axokine, an analog of ciliary neutrophic factor, appears to activate leptin-like pathways. The first randomized, placebo-controlled trial of Axokine was published by Ettinger et al. (42). Using an intent to treat analysis the study found that the subjects randomized to receive 1 µg/kg of axokine for 12 weeks lost significantly more weight (3.2 ± 0.4 vs. 0.2 ± 0.4 kg; $p < 0.001$). It appears that this medication has a prolonged effect following cessation, because six months after the conclusion of the dosing, patients who had received Axokine regained 0.1 versus 1.6 kg in the placebo group. However, one year follow-up was only available for 42% to 44% of subjects. The most common adverse effect was an injection site reaction.

Rimonabant

Rimonabant is a cannabinoid receptor antagonist which has shown promise in phase 2 trials and is now in phase 3 trials. No trial data has thus far been published on the use of rimonabant. However, unpublished data from the Rimonabant in Obesity (RIO) Lipids trial was presented in 2004 (43). This one-year placebo-controlled trial of 1036 subjects with dyslipidemia and a BMI of 27 to 40 showed that 20 mg of rimonobant produced greater weight loss than placebo. Perhaps more importantly, subjects who received rimonobant also showed significant improvements in high-density lipoprotein, triglycerides, and C-reactive protein.

MEDICATION-INDUCED OBESITY

The role of medications as a factor that can induce weight gain is often overlooked. Some commonly prescribed medications are associated with significant weight gain. This list includes medications used to treat diabetes, depression, schizophrenia, and hypertension. When evaluating an obese patient for the first time, the clinician should do a thorough review of all current prescription and over-the-counter medications to look for weight gaining medications and consider alternatives.

CONCLUSION

The obesity epidemic continues to grow at an alarming rate. Dietary changes, physical activity, and pharmacotherapy have been proven effective in weight reduction and improvement of comorbid conditions. As our understanding of obesity grows, so too will our armamentarium to combat this disease. There are several promising medications currently in clinical trials that induce weight loss through unique mechanisms. Ultimately obesity will most likely be treated with combinations of medications, in a manner similar to the treatment of other chronic diseases such as diabetes, hypertension, hyperlipidemia, and heart failure.

REFERENCES

1. Flegal KM, Carroll MD, Ogden C, Johnson CL. Prevalence and trends in obesity among US adults, 1999–2000. JAMA 2002; 288(14):1723–1727.
2. Mokdad AH, Marks JS, Stroup DF, Gerberding JL. Actual causes of death in the United States, 2000. JAMA 2004; 291(10):1238–1245.
3. National Institutes of Health, National Heart, Lung, and Blood Institute. The Practical Guide: Identification, Evaluation, and Treatment of Overweight and Obesity in Adults. NTH publication number 02–4084. Reprinted January 2002.
4. Wadden TA. Treatment of obesity by moderate and severe caloric restriction: results of clinical research trials. Ann Intern Med 1993; 119:688–693.
5. Pawlak DB, Ebbeling CB, Ludwig DS. Should obese patients be counseled to follow a low-glycaemic index diet? Yes. Obes Rev 2002; 3(4):235–243 [review].
6. Heymsfield SB, van Mierlo CA, van der Knaap HC, Heo M, Frier HI. Weight management using a meal replacement strategy: meta and pooling analysis from six studies. Int J Obes Relat Metab Disord 2003; 27(5):537–549.
7. Samaha F, et al. A low-carbohydrate as compared with a low-fat diet in severe obesity. NEJM 2003; 348(21):2074–2081.

8. Foster GD, et al. A randomized trial of a low-carbohydrate diet for obesity. NEJM 2003; 348(21):2082–2090.
9. Clinical Guidelines on the Identification, Evaluation, and Treatment of Overweight and Obesity in Adults: the Evidence Report. Bethesda, MD: National Institutes of Health, National Heart, Lung, and Blood Institute, 1998.
10. Bray GA, Blackburn GL, Ferguson JM, Greenway FL, Jain AK, Mendel CM, Mendels J, Ryan DH, Schwartz SL, Scheinbaum ML, Seaton TB. Sibutramine produces dose-related weight loss. Obes Res 1999; 7(2):189–198.
11. Wirth A, Krause J. Long-term weight loss with sibutramine: a randomized controlled trial. JAMA 2001; 286(11):1331–1339.
12. Apfelbaum M, Vague P, Ziegler O, Hanotin C, Thomas F, Leutenegger E. Long-term maintenance of weight loss after a very-low-calorie diet: a randomized blinded trial of the efficacy and tolerability of sibutramine. Am J Med 1999; 106(2):179–184.
13. Berkowitz RI, Wadden TA, Tershakovec AM, Cronquist JL. Behavior therapy and sibutramine for the treatment of adolescent obesity: a randomized-controlled trial. JAMA 2003; 289(14):1805–1812.
14. Appolinario JC, Bacaltchuk J, Sichieri R, Claudino AM, Godoy-Matos A, Morgan C, Zanella MT, Coutinho W. A randomized, double-blind, placebo-controlled study of sibutramine in the treatment of binge-eating disorder. Arch Gen Psychiatry 2003; 60(11):1109–1116.
15. McMahon FG, Weinstein SP, Rowe E, Ernst KR, Johnson F, Fujioka K. Sibutramine is safe and effective for weight loss in obese patients whose hypertension is well controlled with angiotensin-converting enzyme inhibitors. J Hum Hypertens 2002; 16(l):5–11.
16. Sramek JJ, Leibowitz MT, Weinstein SP, Rowe ED, Mendel CM, Levy B, McMahon FG, Mullican WS, Toth PD, Cutler NR. Efficacy and safety of sibutramine for weight loss in obese patients with hypertension well controlled by beta-adrenergic blocking agents: a placebo-controlled, double-blind, randomised trial. J Hum Hypertens 2002; 16(l):13–19.
17. McMahon FG, Fujioka K, Singh BN, et al. Efficacy and safety of sibutramine in obese white and African American patients with hypertension: a 1-year, double-blind, placebo-controlled, multicenter trial. Arch Intern Med 2000; 160(14):2185–2191.
18. Gokcel A, Gumurdulu Y, Karakose H, et al. Evaluation of the safety and efficacy of sibutramine, orlistat and metformin in the treatment of obesity. Diabetes Obes Metab 2002; 4(l):49–55.
19. Zannad F, Gille B, Grentzinger A, et al. Effects of sibutramine on ventricular dimensions and heart valves in obese patients during weight reduction. Am Heart J 2002; 144(3):508–515.
20. Zhi J, Melia AT, Guerciolini R, Chung J, Kinberg J, Hauptman JB, Patel IH. Retrospective population-based analysis of the dose–response (fecal fat excretion) relationship of orlistat in normal and obese volunteers. Clin Pharmacol Ther 1994; 56(l):82–85.
21. Carriere F, Renou C, Ransac S, et al. Inhibition of gastrointestinal lipolysis by Orlistat during digestion of test meals in healthy volunteers. Am J Physiol Gastrointest Liver Physiol 2001; 281(l):G16–G28.

22. Rossner S, Sjostrom L, Noack R, Meinders AE, Noseda G. Weight loss, weight maintenance, and improved cardiovascular risk factors after 2 years treatment with orlistat for obesity. European Orlistat Obesity Study Group. Obes Res 2000; 8(1):49–61.

23. Sjostrom L, Rissanen A, Andersen T, et al. Randomised placebo-controlled trial of orlistat for weight loss and prevention of weight regain in obese patients. European Multicentre Orlistat Study Group. Lancet 1998; 352(9123):167–172.

24. Davidson MH, Hauptman J, DiGirolamo M, et al. Weight control and risk factor reduction in obese subjects treated for 2 years with orlistat: a randomized controlled trial. JAMA 1999; 281(3):235–242.

25. Torgerson JS, Hauptman J, Boldrin MN, Sjostrom L. XENical in the prevention of diabetes in obese subjects (XENDOS) study: a randomized study of orlistat as an adjunct to lifestyle changes for the prevention of type 2 diabetes in obese patients. Diabetes Care 2004; 27(1):155–161.

26. Hollander PA, Elbein SC, Hirsch IB, et al. Role of orlistat in the treatment of obese patients with type 2 diabetes. A 1-year randomized double-blind study. Diabetes Care 1998; 21(8):1288–1294.

27. Kelley DE, Bray GA, Pi-Sunyer FX, et al. Clinical efficacy of orlistat therapy in overweight and obese patients with insulin-treated type 2 diabetes: a 1-year randomized controlled trial. Diabetes Care 2002; 25(6):1033–1041.

28. Lindgarde F. The effect of orlistat on body weight and coronary heart disease risk profile in obese patients: the Swedish Multimorbidity Study. J Intern Med 2000; 248(3):245–254.

29. Cavaliere H, Floriano I, Medeiros-Neto G. Gastrointestinal side effects of orlistat may be prevented by concomitant prescription of natural fibers (psyllium mucilloid). Int J Obes Relat Metab Disord 2001; 25(7):1095–1099.

30. Munro JF, MacCuish AC, Wilson EM, Duncan LJP. Comparison of continuous and intermittent anorectic therapy in Obesity. BMJ 1968:352–354.

31. Stafford RS, Radley DC. National trends in antiobesity medication use. Arch Intern Med 2003; 163(9):1046–1050.

32. Anderson JW, Greenway FL, Fujioka K, et al. Enhances weight loss: a 48-week double-blind, placebo-controlled trial. Obes Res 2002; 10(7):633–641.

33. Jain AK, Kaplan RA, Gadde KM, et al. Bupro pion SR vs. placebo for weight loss in obese patients with depressive symptoms. Obes Res 2002; 10(10):1049–1056.

34. Gokcel A, Gumurdulu Y, Karakose H, et al. Evaluation of the safety and efficacy of sibutramine, orlistat and metformin in the treatment of obesity. Diabetes Obes Metab 2002; 4(1):49–55.

35. Kay JP, Alemzadeh R, Langley G, D'Angelo L, Smith P, Holshouser S. Beneficial effects of metformin in normoglycemic morbidly obese adolescents. Metabolism 2001; 50(12):1457–1461.

36. Knowler WC, Barrett-Connor E, Fowler SE, et al. Reduction in the incidence of type 2 diabetes with lifestyle intervention or metformin. N Engl J Med 2002; 346(6):393–403.

37. Ben-Menachem E, Axelsen M, Johanson EH, Stagge A, Smith U. Predictors of weight loss in adults with topiramate-treated epilepsy. Obes Res 2003; 11(4):556–562.

38. Appolinario JC, Fontenelle LF, Papelbaum M, Bueno JR, Coutinho W. Topiramate use in obese patients with binge eating disorder: an open study. Can J Psychiatry 2002; 47(3):271–273.
39. McElroy SL, Arnold LM, Shapira NA, et al. Topiramate in the treatment of binge eating disorder associated with obesity: a randomized, placebo-controlled trial. Am J Psychiatry 2003; 160(2):255–261.
40. Bray GA, Hollander P, Klein S, et al. A 6-month randomized, placebo-controlled, dose-ranging trial of topiramate for weight loss in obesity. Obes Res 2003; 11(6):722–733.
41. Gadde KM, Franciscy DM, Wagner HR II, Ranga K, Krishnan R. Zonisamide for weight loss in obese adults: a randomized controlled trial. JAMA 2003; 289:1820–1825.
42. Ettinger MP, Littlejohn TW, Schwartz SL, et al. Recombinant variant of ciliary neurotrophic factor for weight loss in obese adults: a randomized, dose-ranging study. JAMA 2003; 289:1826–1832.
43. Presented by Jean-Pierre Desprès, PhD at the American College of Cardiology Annual Scietific Session New Orleans, LA, March 10, 2004. www.sanofiaventis.com.

16

Medical Management of Obesity Associated with Mood Disorders

Susan L. McElroy and Renu Kotwal

Psychopharmacology Research Program, Department of Psychiatry, University of Cincinnati College of Medicine, Cincinnati, Ohio, U.S.A.

Paul E. Keck Jr.

Psychopharmacology Research Program, Department of Psychiatry, University of Cincinnati College of Medicine; General Clinical Research Center and Mental Health Care Line, Cincinnati Veterans Affairs Medical Center, Cincinnati, Ohio, U.S.A.

INTRODUCTION

Obesity and mood disorders are each important public health problems that overlap to a considerable degree, especially in clinical populations (1–10). Thus, depressive symptoms and syndromal mood disorders are common in persons of all ages presenting for different weight loss treatments (1,3,9–16). Conversely, weight gain, overweight, and obesity are common among patients with mood disorders, including adults, adolescents, and children (10,17–26). In addition, depressive psychopathology is strongly associated with appetite-suppressant medication use in the community (27).

However, the medical management of patients with co-occurring obesity and mood disorders has received very little empirical study. There are no controlled pharmacotherapy trials in patients with comorbid obesity and a current mood disorder. Anti-obesity agents as a class have received little systematic study in mood disorders, and psychotropics have received little systematic study in obesity (28). This dearth of research exists despite the fact that most available anti-obesity agents act on the central nervous system and thus may affect mood, while many psychotropics have effects on appetite, eating behavior, and body weight (29–34). Indeed, many of the pharmacologic agents used to treat mood disorders, including some antidepressants, many mood stabilizers, and most antipsychotics, cause weight gain whereas some anti-obesity drugs (e.g., noradrenergic agents and sibutramine) may be mood destabilizing or "psychotogenic" for some mood disorder patients, especially those with bipolar disorders (26,32–45). Moreover, available authoritative texts and treatment guidelines for obesity generally do not address the management of obesity with comorbid mood disorders, whereas those for mood disorders do not address the management of mood disorders with comorbid obesity or obesity-related conditions (31,46–68).

In this chapter, we briefly review the relationship between obesity and mood disorders; the general medical and psychiatric comorbidity patterns of mood disorders; the therapeutic profiles of psychotropics commonly used in the treatment of mood disorders as well as their effects on appetite, eating behavior, and body weight; and the effects of anti-obesity agents on mood and related disorders. We conclude by presenting preliminary suggestions for the medical management of obesity associated with depressive and bipolar disorders.

OBESITY AND MOOD DISORDERS: A BRIEF OVERVIEW

Available clinical and epidemiological research regarding the relationship between obesity and mood disorders is somewhat inconsistent, due in large part to the heterogeneity among studies (2,5,7). Nonetheless, several conclusions from these studies can be made. First, studies using operationalized diagnostic criteria and structured clinical interviews have consistently found high rates of depressive and bipolar disorders in persons of all ages and both genders seeking treatment for obesity, especially severe obesity (10). For example, using the diagnostic interview schedule (DIS), Black et al. (1) found significantly higher rates of DSM-III major depression (19% vs. 5%) and any mood disorder (31% vs. 9%) in 88 consecutive morbidly obese adult patients seeking bariatric surgery compared with 76 normal weight controls. Similarly, using the Composite International Diagnostic Interview (CIDI), Britz et al. (3) found significantly higher rates of DSM-IV mood disorders in 47 adolescents and young adults receiving inpatient treatment for extreme obesity than both obese and nonobese general population controls. Specifically, 20 (43%) of the obese adolescents [mean body mass index (BMI) = 42.4] and young adult patients had a mood disorder, compared with 8 (17%) of 47 obese controls (mean BMI = 29.8) and 247 (15%) of 1608 general population controls.

Second, community studies using operationalized diagnostic criteria and structured assessments to diagnose mood disorders also suggest an association between obesity and major depressive episodes, although this association appears to be affected by various factors, including gender, definition of obesity, and possibly age (4–8,10,69,70). Thus, in a survey of 41,086 respondents aged 18 years and older, Carpenter et al. (4) found a positive association between obesity (BMI $\geq$ 30) and past-year major depressive episodes in women, but a negative association in men. In a survey of 1886 individuals aged 50 to 95 years, Roberts et al. (6) found a positive association between obesity (BMI $\geq$ 30) and current DSM-IV major depressive episodes that was evident in men and women. Onyike et al. (8) found a positive association between obesity (BMI $\geq$ 30) and past-month DSM-III major depressive episodes in women, but not men, in a group of respondents aged 15 to 39 years from the Third National Health and Nutrition Examination Survey (NHANES III). When obesity was stratified by severity, class 3 (severe) obesity (BMI $\geq$ 40) was associated with past-month major depression in women and men combined. Mustillo et al. (69) identified four developmental trajectories of obesity among 991 rural white children ages 9 to 16 years who were evaluated annually over an eight year period: no history of obesity (73%), chronic obesity (15%), childhood obesity (5%), and adolescent obesity (7%). Those with childhood obesity and chronic obesity were significantly more likely than those with no history of obesity to have DSM-IV depression. Kinder et al. (70) found that women, but not men, with a history of a major depressive episode were twice as likely to have the metabolic syndrome compared with those with no history of depression in a group of respondents' aged 17 to 39 years from the NHANES III.

In contrast, as mentioned earlier, Britz et al. (3) found no relationship between obesity and lifetime DSM-IV depressive or bipolar disorders in 1608 adolescents and young adults from the community. Also noted earlier, rates of DSM-IV mood disorders in a group of 47 adolescents and young adults receiving treatment for severe obesity in the same study were significantly higher than those in the obese and population control groups. However, the mean BMI of this group (42.4) was significantly higher than that of the obese control group (mean BMI = 29.8), further supporting a link between mood disorder and severe obesity.

A third conclusion is that studies of body weight in mood disorders have found associations with obesity and overweight on the one hand and underweight on the other (10). Thus, clinical studies have found bipolar disorder to be associated with obesity and abdominal obesity; juvenile major depression to be prospectively associated with overweight; and melancholic depression to be associated with underweight and, in normal weight women, hypercortisolemia and visceral fat deposition (21–24,71–74). Of eight studies assessing obesity-related conditions in community samples of persons with syndromal mood disorders (including the Roberts et al. study noted above), six found a positive association between a mood disorder or a mood disorder subtype (e.g., atypical depression) and obesity or overweight (6,75–81). Four of these studies were prospective, and all four found relationships between depression and obesity (6,76,80,81). In three studies, obesity developed after the onset of mood disorder in female or female and male adolescents and young adults (76,80,81). In another, major depression developed after the onset of obesity in men and women aged 50 years or older (6).

In sum, available research indicates that obesity (BMI ≥ 30) is associated with major depressive episodes in women and that severe obesity (BMI ≥ 40) is associated with major depressive episodes in men and women (1,3,4,6,8). Also, metabolic syndrome is associated with major depressive episodes in women (70). Conversely, major depressive disorder with atypical features, juvenile-onset major depressive disorder, and bipolar disorder may be associated with overweight or obesity, whereas major depressive disorder with melancholic features may be associated with underweight (21–24,71,75,76,81). Also, melancholic major depressive disorder with hypercortisolemia may be associated with visceral fat deposition (73,74). Moreover, mood disorder may precede development of overweight or obesity in some persons, especially patients with juvenile-onset major depression and young females in the community with major depression, and obesity may precede development of major depressive episodes in others, especially older adults (6,22,76,80,81).

In short, the relationship between obesity and mood disorders is likely to be complex, in part because obesity and mood disorders are themselves heterogeneous conditions (77,82–89). Indeed, emerging family history, twin, and molecular genetic research indicates that both obesity and mood disorders are complex genetic illnesses with various contributing environmental factors (90–100). Thus, some forms of obesity may be associated with mood disorders whereas other forms may not be. Similarly, some forms of mood disorder may be associated with obesity whereas other forms may be associated with underweight. Thus, comorbid obesity and a mood disorder may represent the co-occurrence of two related conditions with overlapping but distinct pathophysiologies in some cases, one condition with a single pathophysiology in other cases, and the chance co-occurrence of two unrelated conditions with independent pathophysiologies in yet other cases (10). These different comorbidity patterns would likely have different treatment implications.

COMORBIDITY AS A MARKER FOR MOOD DISORDER

The diagnosis of obesity is generally much easier to make than that of a mood disorder. Obesity is usually apparent whereas the clinician often has to actively elicit the signs and symptoms of depression and hypomania—particularly if they are not the presenting chief complaint or if they are in remission. Moreover, while depressive and manic symptoms can be denied or concealed, obesity is difficult, if not impossible, to hide. Thus, a mood disorder is much more likely than obesity to be an occult diagnosis.

It is well known that comorbidity—broadly defined as the co-occurrence of lifetime diseases or disorders—is common in individuals with obesity (31,50,56,82,83,101,102). Comorbidity with both general medical and mental disorders is also common in persons with mood disorders (103,104). Moreover, since mood disorders, unlike obesity, can be occult, their presence can be masked by their comorbid conditions. It is therefore imperative that the clinician be aware of the particular comorbidity patterns associated with mood disorders because such patterns can be markers for underlying mood disorders, including in obese patients. In addition, just as the general medical comorbidity pattern of an obese patient has implications for his or her medical treatment, the comorbidity pattern of a particular mood disorder patient has treatment implications for that patient. Thus, knowledge of the complete general medical and psychiatric comorbidity profile is especially important in the assessment and treatment of patients with both obesity and a mood disorder.

Regarding the specific general medical comorbidity profile of mood disorders, it is noteworthy that many of the general medical disorders that are associated with obesity are also associated with mood disorders. These include type 2 diabetes, hypertension, cardiovascular disease, the metabolic syndrome, asthma, breathing-related sleep disorders, and chronic pain (71,105–119,121–124). Indeed, epidemiologic studies have shown that, similar to obesity, depressive symptoms and/or major depressive disorder are independent risk factors for type 2 diabetes, hypertension, carotid atherosclerosis, coronary heart disease, and stroke, and that both major depressive disorder and bipolar disorder are associated with increased mortality from cardiovascular disease and some cancers (104,105,109–120,125–127). In contrast, medical disorders associated with bipolar and depressive disorders in community and clinical studies that have not been associated with obesity include migraine, Tourettes Syndrome, and multiple sclerosis (128–130).

Mental disorders that frequently co-occur with mood disorders are anxiety, substance use, eating, impulse control, attention deficit-hyperactivity, and conduct disorders (103,104,131–135). As discussed in other chapters, some of these disorders, particularly eating, substance use, and conduct disorders, are also associated with obesity. Comorbidity with mental disorders is especially common for bipolar disorder (131,132,136–141). In three major psychiatric epidemiologic studies (the Epidemiologic Catchment Area study, the National Comorbidity Survey, and the Zurich Cohort study), persons with bipolar disorder, defined narrowly or broadly, had higher rates of anxiety and substance use disorders than those with depressive disorders, even though persons with depressive disorders had higher rates of anxiety and substance use disorders than those in the general population (131,136–141). Thus, psychiatric comorbidity, especially complex combinations of mental disorders (sometimes called multimorbidity or complicated comorbidity), is a marker for mood pathology in general and bipolarity in particular.

Regarding the overlap among obesity, mood disorders, and comorbid mental disorders, many studies have shown that persons presenting for weight management often have eating, anxiety, and/or substance use symptoms or disorders as well as mood symptoms or disorders. For example, in addition to an elevated rate of lifetime mood disorders, the 88 morbidly obese adult patients seeking bariatric surgery evaluated by Black et al. (1) were also more likely to have lifetime anxiety disorders, bulimia, and tobacco dependence than the comparison group. Similarly, the 47 extremely obese adolescents and adults receiving inpatient treatment evaluated by Britz et al. (3) also demonstrated high lifetime prevalence rates of anxiety (47.5%), somatoform (15%), and eating (17%) disorders. Furthermore, 57% and 35% of female and male patients, respectively, described eating binges with lack of control. Indeed, an important finding in studies comparing obese persons with and without binge eating behavior or binge eating disorder (BED) is the higher rates of mood disorders, as well as anxiety and substance use disorders, in the obese persons with binge eating or BED (142–144). For example, in a study of 89 obese women and 39 obese men, subjects with BED have significantly higher lifetime rates of major depression, panic disorder, and bulimia nervosa (BN) than subjects without BED (142). Similarly, in a community study of 166 nonbulimic obese women, those with binge eating behavior had significantly higher rates of major depression, panic disorder, phobias, and alcohol dependence than those without binge eating behavior (144). Bingers also had increased overall rates of medical comorbidity compared with nonbingers. Thus, a particularly important subtype of obesity may be that associated with a mood disorder and an eating disorder with binge eating (BED or BN), or more broadly, mood and eating dysregulation. Conversely, an important subtype of depression may be that characterized by overeating and overweight (10).

Comorbid disorders may have a significant impact on the presentation, course, and outcome of mood disorders (104,132,133,145,146). Co-occurring substance use and anxiety disorders in particular, and comorbidity in general, have been associated with an earlier age of onset of affective symptoms, greater suicidality, less favorable response to pharmacological and psychological treatments, and reduced levels of medication adherence in patients with depressive and bipolar disorders (132,136,141,146).

Indeed, preliminary research suggests obesity in particular in patients with bipolar disorder is associated with more severe illness and poorer outcome (25,147). In one group of 175 patients with bipolar I disorder, greater BMI was correlated with more severe illness and a history of a suicide attempt (147). In addition, obese patients (35% of the group) had more depressive and manic episodes, higher baseline Hamilton depression rating scale (HAM-D) scores, and required more time receiving lithium-based treatment to achieve acute remission compared with non-obese patients (25). During maintenance treatment, significantly more obese patients experienced a recurrence ($N = 25$, 54%) compared with those who were not obese ($N = 28$, 35%). Also, the time to recurrence was significantly shorter for patients who were obese at baseline. When recurrence type was examined, the percentage of patients experiencing depressive recurrences was significantly greater for obese patients ($N = 15$, 33%) than for non-obese patients ($N = 11$, 14%).

Conversely, co-occurring depressive symptoms and mood disorders may complicate the course and treatment of many general medical disorders, including those that co-occur with obesity. Thus, depressive symptoms and major depression impair the functional recovery and increase the mortality from coronary heart disease and stroke (116,148,149). Regarding treatment adherence, a review of 12 studies found that depressed patients had three times greater odds of being noncompliant with medical treatment recommendations compared with nondepressed patients (150). Treatment modalities and diseases studied included dietary therapy in end stage renal disease, medication in angina and cancer, and health behavior recommendations in cancer, renal transplantation, and rheumatoid arthritis. Depression has also been associated with nonadherence with treatment in patients with diabetes, especially with exercise and diet recommendations (151–153).

Much less is known about the impact of mood disorders on the course and treatment of obesity. No controlled prospective study, to our knowledge, has evaluated the impact of a comorbid mood disorder on the long-term course or treatment of obesity. Early studies of weight-reduction interventions, in which patients generally were not screened for mental disorders, reported a relatively high rate of mood disturbances, ranging from mild depressive and anxiety symptoms to syndromal depression, completed suicides, and psychoses (154). Subsequent studies of behavioral weight loss therapy and bariatric surgery, in which patients with significant psychopathology were usually excluded, generally found that such treatments were associated with improvement in mood as patients lost weight (155–157). However, the psychiatric status of patients was usually not well characterized beyond ratings on depressive symptom scales, which, when reported, often suggested mild levels of symptoms (i.e., whether or not patients had syndromal mood disorders was not documented). Also, several groups have reported return of patients' depressive symptoms approximately two years post-surgery, when weight loss plateaued or weight gain occurred (158,159). Moreover, several studies have shown that depressive symptoms are associated with nonadherence with behavioral weight loss therapy of obesity (160–163). In one of the few studies of its type, Jenkins et al. (163) examined the relationship of psychiatric diagnosis on weight loss maintenance during and six months after 24 months of individualized counseling for diet and exercise in 39 obese breast cancer survivors. Nine subjects had major depressive disorder and 10 had definable disorders of lesser severity. Subjects with psychiatric disorders had significantly less weight loss at both the 12 month time-point and the 6-month follow-up period compared with subjects with no psychiatric disorders (6.3% vs. 12.6% and 1.2% vs. 7.8%, respectively).

Conversely, available research suggests successful weight loss mainte- nance is associated with a low level of depressive symptoms. In an ongoing study of a registry of 784 successful weight loss maintainers (629 women), individuals who had lost at least 13.6 kg (mean loss = 30 ± 15 kg) and main- tained the loss for at least one year (mean duration = 5.5 ± 6.8 years) had a level of depressive symptoms that resembled those in community samples and was lower than those in psychiatric samples (164). Moreover, evaluation of participants who recovered from weight regain showed that they had smaller increases in depressive symptoms than those who did not (165).

Taken together, these data suggest that short-term weight loss may have beneficial effects on mood in persons with mild depressive symptoms, but that stable mood may be important for long-term maintenance of weight loss. The effects of weight loss on mood in persons with acute mood syndromes, however, remains unknown. In treating a patient with obesity and a mood disorder, therefore, it is important to fully characterize the patient's obesity and mood disorder, as well as their general medical and psychiatric comorbidity profiles, before embarking on a treatment program. It is also crucial to monitor weight, mood symptoms, any associated general medical and psychiatric conditions, and adherence with treatment recom- mendations as treatment progresses.

THERAPEUTIC PROFILES OF PSYCHOTROPIC AND ANTI-OBESITY DRUGS

A growing number of psychotropic drugs are being used in the treatment of per- sons with mood disorders (59–68,166). These include antidepressants and mood stabilizers, as well as first and second generation (or typical and atypical) anti- psychotics, older and newer anticonvulsants, and anxiolytics, among others. Many of these medications have been classified or indicated for use in one mental disorder, but in fact been shown effective in other psychiatric or gen- eral medical disorders. Also, many of these medications are used in combina- tion to treat mood disorders, many have effects on appetite and body weight, and some have been evaluated in obesity (10,27–29,32–34,58,167).

Similarly, a growing number of anti-obesity drugs are available for the management of persons with obesity (29–31,49,58,168–171). These drugs can be broadly categorized into agents that reduce food intake by acting on the central nervous system (appetite suppressants) and those that modify fat absorption or otherwise alter metabolism (metabolic agents). Several drugs with documented efficacy in obesity have received some study in mood and related disorders (e.g., psychostimulants, topiramate, and sibu- tramine) (10).

However, to date, there have been no double-blind, placebo-controlled pharmacotherapy studies in patients with concurrent obesity and acute syndromal mood disorders. In managing the obese person with a mood disorder, therefore, it is imperative to know the complete therapeutic profile of available psychotropic and anti-obesity agents, including the potential effects of psychotropics on appetite, body weight, and metabolic parameters, and the potential effects of anti-obesity agents on both depressive and bipolar mood symptoms.

THERAPEUTIC AND APPETITE/WEIGHT PROFILES OF PSYCHOTROPICS USED IN MOOD DISORDER

Antidepressants

Antidepressants as a class are generally considered first line agents in the acute, continuation, and maintenance psychopharmacologic treatment of depressive disorders in adults (59,63,64,67,166,172). Although different antidepressants and antidepressant classes are comparably effective in major depressive disorder, some depressive subtypes may respond preferentially to certain antidepressant classes. Thus, atypical major depression may respond better to monoamine oxidase inhibitors (MAOIs) than to tricyclic antidepressants (TCAs) (173). Women with major depression may respond better to serotonin selective reuptake inhibitors (SSRIs) than to TCAs, whereas men appear to respond equally well to both classes (174,175). Pediatric major depression may respond better to SSRIs than to TCAs (176,177). In addition, psychotic depression may respond better to antidepressant–antipsychotic combinations or to electroconvulsive therapy than to single-drug treatments (178). These differential response patterns reinforce the concept that depressive illness is a heterogeneous condition, and should be considered when treating mood disorder patients with obesity and related conditions.

Presently, fluoxetine is the only drug approved by the U.S. Food and Drug Administration (FDA) for the treatment of depression in children and adolescents (age eight years and older) (179,180). It is also the only antidepressant approved by the FDA for the treatment of bipolar disorder, where it is approved for use in combination with olanzapine (as Symbyax) for the treatment of depressive episodes (181). The use of antidepressants in pediatric depressive disorders and bipolar disorders, however, is somewhat controversial (60,65,68,179–186). This is due to a relative lack of positive efficacy data with antidepressants as monotherapy agents from double-blind, placebo-controlled clinical trials along with reports suggesting that these agents may be associated with untoward psychological effects in both patient groups. Thus, for pediatric depression, TCAs have consistently failed to separate from placebo in clinical trials in depressed children (177). In a meta-analysis of published ($N = 5$) and unpublished ($N = 6$) controlled trials of SSRIs in pediatric depression, only two studies of fluoxetine showed unequivocal positive results (179). For bipolar depression, not one single antidepressant drug or antidepressant class has been shown to be effective as monotherapy in at least two adequately powered, placebo-controlled clinical trials (68). Untoward psychological effects associated with antidepressants in children and adolescents have been broadly described as behavioral disinhibition or activation, and include suicidal and impulsive aggressive behavior; hypomanic, manic or mixed symptoms; and rapid mood cycling (179,180). Use of antidepressants in patients with bipolar disorders has been associated with induction of manic and mixed states and rapid mood cycling, which can be associated with suicidality and aggression (182,184). One study found that antidepressant treatment of bipolar depression was more likely to be characterized by short-term nonresponse and loss of response, as well as manic switching and cycle acceleration, compared with that of unipolar depression (184). Of note, how often antidepressant-associated behavioral disinhibition in children represents prodromal or early-onset bipolar disorder is not yet known, but antidepressant treatment may be more likely to unmask an underlying bipolar disorder in children and adolescents than in adults (186). Also, emerging data indicate that some antidepressants (particularly, "single action" agents such as SSRIs and bupropion) may be less likely to induce manic switching and cycle acceleration than others (such as "multiple action" agents like TCAs and venlafaxine) (184,186). In addition, when administered with mood stabilizers or atypical antipsychotics, antidepressants may be effective in the short-term treatment of bipolar depression with a low rate of switching (181,185).

In short, some children with depressive disorders will require acute and maintenance treatment with antidepressants for optimal response, whereas others may develop behavioral disinhibition. Similarly, some bipolar patients will require acute and maintenance treatment with antidepressants (usually in combination with mood stabilizers) for optimal response, whereas others will destabilize upon antidepressant exposure. Importantly, for any patient who worsens on an antidepressant, it is crucial to determine whether or not the drug has induced manic symptoms or mood cycling. In our experience, affective dysregulation, including that induced by antidepressants, may be associated with increased appetite, hyperphagia, weight gain, and exacerbation of comorbid conditions, including eating disorders with binge eating (187). Indeed, it is our opinion that antidepressant-induced affective dysregulation may be one cause of weight gain in bipolar patients, including those with occult or soft spectrum forms of the disorder.

Just as antidepressants have varied effects in different mood disorder subtypes, they also have different effects on appetite and body weight. Agents that stimulate appetite or cause weight gain include TCAs (tertiary amines more so than secondary amines), monoamine uptake inhibitors (MAOIs), and the novel antidepressant mirtazipine (32–34,188,189). Agents that are weight neutral or may even suppress appetite or reduce body weight, at least over the short term, include some SSRIs (especially fluoxetine), the novel noradrenergic agent bupropion, and the serotonin–norepinephrine selective reuptake inhibitor (SNRI) venlafaxine (190–200). For SSRIs, controlled data indicate that this weight loss may not be sustained over the long term, but data are mixed as to whether there is weight gain above baseline weight (20,188,189). Paroxetine, though, may be more likely than other SSRIs to be associated with weight gain (188,193,201,202). The precise mechanism(s) of appetite suppression and weight loss of these agents are unknown, but they enhance serotonergic or noradrenergic function without antagonizing serotonin, histamine, and/or dopamine receptors (203–206). [Of note, the antiobesity agent sibutramine is a serotonin–norepinephrine selective reuptake inhibitor similar to venlafaxine (29–31,169).]

Several antidepressants associated with appetite suppression and weight loss have received empirical study in obesity and related conditions (28). In a series of double-blind, placebo-controlled trials, the SSRI fluoxetine, usually at a dose of 60 mg/day, was shown to have dose-related, modest, short-term (e.g., from six weeks to six months) weight loss effects in obese patients that were also associated with improvement in obesity-related cardiovascular risk factors such as hyperglycemia and hypercholesterolemia (31,207–212). However, in subsequent long-term studies, most of the lost weight was regained by one year despite continued drug therapy (31,209,211). An important exception is a meta-analysis of the six randomized controlled trials of fluoxetine in adults with type 2 diabetes which showed that modest weight loss persisted at 52 weeks (213). Specifically, mean weight reductions were 3.4 kg (95% CI, 1.7–5.2 kg) at 8–16 weeks of treatment; 5.1 kg (95% CI, 3.3–6.9 kg) at 24–30 weeks; and 5.8 kg (95% CI, 0.8–10.8 kg) at 52 weeks. Glycolated hemoglobin was also modestly reduced [1.0% (95% CI, 0.4–1.5%) at 8–16 weeks; 1.0% 95% CI, 0.6–1.4% at 24–30 weeks; and 1.8% (95% CI, −0.2–3.8%) at 52 weeks].

Regarding other SSRIs in the treatment of obesity, a 16-week trial of femoxetine 600 mg/day in 73 obese patients in general practice showed similar weight loss in patients receiving active drug (median = 8.3 kg) compared with patients receiving placebo (median = 6.2 kg) (214). However, there was a trend for greater weight loss in those patients with obesity for more than 20 years and in those patients receiving previous anorectic treatments. Two studies of citalopram in obesity were negative (215,216). The first was a 12-week trial of 60 mg/day in 65 patients with severe obesity and the second was a 6-month, cross-over trial of 40 mg/day in 16 men with abdominal obesity. Two short-term studies (12 and 13 weeks, respectively) of fluvoxamine in patients with obesity were also negative but both studies were small (40 subjects in each) (217,218). Nonetheless, in one study, subjects receiving fluvoxamine achieved a greater mean weight loss than those receiving placebo (217). In an uncontrolled comparison of two consecutive series of obese patients (BMI ≥ 30) with similar characteristics receiving six months of cognitive behavioral therapy (CBT) for weight loss, patients receiving sertraline 150 mg/day plus CBT ($N = 65$) lost significantly more weight than patients receiving CBT alone ($N = 60$; 6.5% vs. 3.0 %; $p < 0.01$) (219). In the only controlled study of sertraline in obesity, sertraline 200 mg/day was not different from placebo in preventing regain of weight in 30 obese women who completed 54 weeks of relapse prevention training following a very low calorie diet, even though active drug was initially associated with greater weight loss (220).

In short, of the SSRIs, only fluoxetine has been adequately studied in obesity, where its modest short term (from six weeks to six months) weight loss effects were shown not to persist at one year, except perhaps in diabetics, at a dose of 60 mg/day. The basis for the loss of fluoxetine's weight loss effect is unknown. [By comparison, in the long-term treatment studies of dexfenfluramine, sibutramine, and orlistat, the majority of the weight loss occurred in the first six months of treatment with a plateauing or partial but incomplete weight increase occurring in the following six months (58,168–170).]

Of note, SSRIs have been reported to improve metabolic and/or neuroendocrine parameters in the absence of weight loss (218,221,222). In one of the studies of fluvoxamine in obesity, post-treatment cholesterol levels were significantly lower in the fluvoxamine group than in the placebo group (218). Breum et al. (221) randomized 40 obese patients with type 2 diabetes or impaired glucose tolerance (IGT) to fluoxetine 60 mg/day or placebo in conjunction with diet. Both groups displayed similar significant weight loss with a nadir at six months and no differences at 12 months. Glycemic regulation improved in the 29 patients who completed the 12 months trial, but patients receiving fluoxetine ($N = 15$) showed a greater decline in fasting glucose and C-reactive protein levels. Maheux et al. (222) treated 12 obese type 2 diabetic patients with fluoxetine or placebo for four weeks and assessed insulin-mediated glucose disposal by the euglycemic hyperinsulinemic clamp technique. Compared to placebo-treated patients, fluoxetine-treated patients showed increased glucose disposal, an increased insulin sensitivity index, and an increased glucose metabolic clearance rate, despite no changes in weight. As noted earlier, Ljung et al. (216) treated 16 nondepressed abdominally obese men with citalopram or placebo for six months using a double-blind, cross-over design with a 2-month wash-out period between treatment periods. Although there were no changes in BMI and WHR with citalopram, patients showed improvement in neuroendocrine and metabolic parameters, such as normalization of abnormally low morning cortisol levels, a tendency for oral glucose tolerance test glucose concentrations to be decreased, and a tendency for diurnal urinary methoxycatecholamine excretion to decrease.

In contrast, successful sertraline and paroxetine treatment has been associated with statistically and clinically significant increases in low-density lipoprotein (LDL) cholesterol in panic disorder patients (223). Indeed, paroxetine administration in healthy male volunteers has been shown to induce an 11.5% increase in LDL cholesterol without associated changes in physical activity, weight, or diet (224). This increase in LDL cholesterol normalized after drug discontinuation. To complicate matters further, preliminary clinical data suggest that antidepressant-resistant depression may be associated with cholesterol levels greater than 200 mg/dL as well as higher triglyceride levels (225). Further research on the metabolic profiles of antidepressant agents and different mood disorder subtypes is greatly needed (226,227).

The SSRIs do not appear to be effective in olanzapine-induced weight gain. In an eight-week clinical trial comparing olanzapine monotherapy with the combination of olanzapine and fluoxetine in patients with bipolar depression, both groups showed comparable weight gain that was significantly greater than placebo (180). In addition, a small double-blind, placebo-controlled study showed that coadministration of fluoxetine (20 mg/day) with olanzapine (10 mg/day) for eight weeks was ineffective in preventing weight gain in 30 first-episode hospitalized patients with schizophrenia (228). The group receiving fluoxetine also showed significantly less improvement in positive and disorganized symptom dimensions. In contrast, fluoxetine has been reported to be effective clinically for excessive weight gain in postpartum women without depression and for steroid-induced obesity in patients with myasthenia gravis (229,230).

Bupropion has been shown superior to placebo in inducing modest weight loss in overweight or obesity in three double-blind, controlled trials, including one long-term (48-week) trial (231–233). In the first study, bupropion (mean dose 352 mg/day) was superior to placebo over eight weeks of treatment in inducing weight loss in 50 overweight or obese women (BMI 28.0–52.6 kg/m^2) without "serious/unstable psychiatric illness" (231). In the intent-to-treat analysis, bupropion subjects ($n = 25$) lost an average 4.9% of body weight compared with 1.3% in placebo subjects ($n = 25$; $p = 0.0001$). Importantly, subjects receiving bupropion showed significantly better compliance with dietary recommendations.

In the second study, which was 26 weeks in duration, bupropion sustained release (SR) (300 mg/day) was superior to placebo in inducing weight loss in obese patients who had depressive symptoms [Beck Depression Inventory (BDI) scores of 10–30] but who did not meet DSM-IV criteria for major depression (232). Mean baseline BMIs were 36.0 and 35.6 and mean BDIs were 15.2 and 15.1, respectively, in the bupropion and placebo groups. After six months, the patients receiving bupropion ($n = 195$) lost a mean of 4.4 kg compared with a mean of 1.7 kg in patients receiving placebo ($n = 191$). Of note, the mean decrease in BDI scores significantly favored bupropion only in the subgroup of patients with a past history of major depression.

In the third study, 327 subjects with obesity were randomized to bupropion SR 300 mg/day ($n = 110$), bupropion SR 400 mg/day ($n =105$), or placebo ($n=1$ 12) for 24 weeks (placebo) or 48 weeks (bupropion) (233). Subjects receiving bupropion 300 mg/day had significantly greater weight loss than placebo-treated subjects at 20 weeks. Subjects receiving bupropion 400 mg/day had significantly greater weight loss than placebo-treated patients at weeks 12,16, 20, and 24 and bupropion 300 mg/day-treated patients at weeks 24, 26, 30, 36, and 42. After 24 weeks of treatment, placebo-treated subjects were randomized to bupropion 300 mg/day or 400 mg/day and displayed additional weight loss. Patients receiving bupropion for 48 weeks showed a nadir in their weight loss at 32 or 36 weeks, and then showed a nonsignificant weight increase during subsequent weeks. Weight losses as the percentage of initial body weight at 48 weeks were 7.5% and 8.5% for bupropion 300 and 400 mg/day, respectively, in the completers' analyses. These data suggest bupropion's weight loss effects, unlike those of the SSRIs, may persist for up to one year.

Bupropion has also been shown to mitigate the weight gain associated with smoking cessation (234). There are no controlled studies of bupropion in psychotropic-induced weight gain. However, the selective norepinephrine reuptake inhibitor antidepressant reboxetine, which promotes noradrenergic neurotransmission as bupropion is thought to do, has been shown to reduce olanzapine-induced weight gain in a controlled study of 26 patients with schizophrenia (235). Patients receiving olanzapine with reboxetine 4 mg/day displayed a statistically significant lower increase in body weight (mean = 2.5 kg) than those receiving olanzapine with placebo (mean = 5.5 kg) after six weeks of treatment. Significantly fewer patients in the olanzapine/reboxetine group (20%) gained at least 7% of their initial weight than in the olanzapine/placebo group (70%). The reboxetine-treated patients also showed a statistically significantly greater reduction in depressive symptoms (as measured by the HAM-D).

Of note is a growing literature on the concurrent use of antidepressants with noradrenergic and serotonergic mechanisms, including those agents associated with weight loss, in patients with treatment-resistant mood disorders (236–239). Preliminary controlled data suggest such combination treatments may be more likely to result in remission than treatment with selective agents for some patients with depression. Thus, the combination of SSRIs with bupropion or desipramine has been reported to successfully treat depressed patients inadequately responsive to monotherapy with these medications. Comparable reports, however, have not appeared for obese patients or for mood disorder patients with obesity. Thus, no controlled trials have yet assessed combination treatment with serotonergic and noradrenergic antidepressants in patients with depressive syndromes and obesity. Nonetheless, in our clinical experience, such pharmacotherapy combinations can be particularly useful for some obese patients with depressive disorders.

As noted earlier, no controlled study has yet evaluated an antidepressant in patients with concurrent major depressive disorder and obesity. However, antidepressants have been shown to be effective in major depression when it co-occurs with some of the general medical disorders that frequently complicate obesity. Thus, SSRIs have been shown to be effective in major depression in patients with type 2 diabetes, recent stroke, and acute myocardial infarction or unstable angina, and bupropion has been shown effective in elderly depressed patients with various comorbid medical disorders (106,240–243). There is also preliminary evidence that antidepressants may reduce mortality after postroke depression, and that SSRIs may decrease the risk of myocardial infarction (244,245).

Antidepressants have also been shown to be effective in some of the mental and general medical conditions that co-occur with major depression, including those that may also co-occur with obesity. Regarding the comorbidity among depressive disorders, obesity, and binge eating, several antidepressant classes have been shown to be effective in BN, BED, or their variants (e.g., non-purging bulimia or obesity with binge eating) (246–249). Thus, the binge eating and purging of BN have been shown to respond to the TCAs imipramine, desipramine, and amitriptyline; the SSRI fluoxetine; the MAOIs phenelzine, isocarboxazid, and brofaromine; and the novel agents bupropion and trazodone in double-blind, placebo-controlled trials. Fluoxetine is approved by the FDA for the treatment of BN. In the fluoxetine trials of BN, 60 mg was superior to 20 mg in reducing binge eating (and purging), and the drug was shown to have long-term (up to 52-week) efficacy (246–248). The binge eating of BED has been shown to respond to the TCAs desipramine and imipramine and the SSRIs fluoxetine, fluvoxamine, citalopram, and sertraline (249). Moderate weight loss occurred with the SSRIs, but not with the TCAs. Since the SSRI trials in BED were short term (from six to nine weeks), it is unknown if the anti-bingeing and weight loss effects of these agents persist over longer treatment periods in this disorder.

TCAs, MAOIs, SSRIs, and SNRIs have all been shown to be effective in the treatment of many of the anxiety disorders (166,250). Several SSRIs and venlafaxine are approved by the FDA for the treatment of panic disorder (fluoxetine, paroxetine, and sertraline), generalized anxiety disorder (GAD) (venlafaxine), social anxiety disorder (paroxetine, sertraline, and venlafaxine), and/or post-traumatic stress disorder (PTSD) (fluoxetine, paroxetine, and sertraline). The TCA clomipramine and the SSRIs fluoxetine, fluvoxamine, sertraline, and paroxetine are approved for obsessive compulsive disorder (OCD) in adults. Clomipramine, fluoxetine, fluvoxamine, and sertraline have FDA approval for use in pediatric OCD. Bupropion, in contrast, is not approved for the treatment of any anxiety disorder.

Studies of antidepressants have yielded mixed results in substance use disorders, impulse-control disorders, and migraine. For example, SSRIs may be helpful in reducing alcohol consumption in some forms of alcohol misuse (type A or late onset alcoholism and heavy drinking or alcohol dependence with comorbid depression) but counterproductive in others (type B or early onset alcoholism) (251). Bupropion is indicated for the treatment of nicotine dependence, but has not been reported to be helpful in other substance use disorders (234). SSRIs have been reported to be both effective and ineffective in various impulse control disorders, such as trichotillomania, pathological gambling, compulsive shopping, and psychogenic excoriation (252,253). Mixed results have similarly been reported for antidepressants in migraine prevention, with most positive data supporting amitriptyline (254).

Mood Stabilizers

Lithium, valproate, carbamazepine, most second generation antipsychotics, and some first generation antipsychotics have all been shown to be effective in acute mania (60,66,68,166,255). Lithium, the atypical antipsychotics olanzapine and quetiapine, and the novel anticonvulsant lamotrigine have each been shown to be effective in acute bipolar depression (60,65,68,255). Lithium, valproate, olanzapine, and lamotrigine all have evidence of maintenance efficacy (60,68,255). However, lithium, valproate, and olanzapine appear to be more effective for preventing mania than depression, whereas lamotrigine appears to be more effective for preventing depression than mania (68).

    None of these medications have been evaluated in obesity. Indeed, the majority of these medications are associated with weight gain (27,32–34). Agents that are primarily weight neutral or associated with minimal weight gain are lamotrigine, the atypical antipsychotics aripiprazole and ziprasidone, and the typical antipsychotic molindone (27). To date, no pharmacologic agent has been identified that has clearly documented antimanic properties and is also associated with weight loss.

    Unfortunately, the effectiveness of these agents in binge eating behavior and eating disorders with binge eating, conditions that are related to bipolar disorders as well as to depressive disorders and obesity, has not been adequately studied. Lithium, valproate, and carbamazepine have all been reported to be effective in isolated cases of BN with comorbid bipolar disorder (187). Lithium was also reported effective in an open trial in women with BN (256). A subsequent placebo controlled trial in 91 female BN patients without bipolar disorder showed lithium (mean level 0.62 mEq/L) was not superior to placebo in decreasing binge eating episodes, except possibly in depressed patients (257). However, this study is difficult to interpret because nondepressed patients receiving placebo showed just as significant a reduction in binge eating as did nondepressed patients receiving lithium. A small ($n = 6$) controlled trial of carbamazepine in BN was negative, but also had methodological limitations (258). Possibly consistent with their weight gain profiles, atypical antipsychotics have been reported to induce binge eating behavior in persons with eating and psychotic disorders (259–261). Valproate has been reported to increase binge eating and weight gain in patients with BED and comorbid bipolar disorder (262).

Many of these agents have been reported to be effective in other conditions that co-occur with depressive and bipolar disorders. Thus, lithium, valproate, carbamazepine, olanzapine, and risperidone have been found to be effective in various conditions with impulsive features, such as intermittent explosive disorder, borderline personality disorder, and conduct disorder (136). Valproate and atypical antipsychotics may have anxiolytic properties, respectively, as monotherapy in panic disorder and as adjunctive agents in refractory OCD, PTSD, or GAD (136,263). Valproate has been shown superior to placebo in controlled trials in migraine prevention, for which it has an FDA indication (264).

The therapeutic profiles of available psychotropics are important to be cognizant of, because these agents may have utility in the psychiatric and general medical disorders that can co-occur in the obese patient with a mood disorder. Conversely, obesity may develop as a side effect in mood disorder patients from the use of agents associated with weight gain, including in patients receiving them for comorbid conditions.

Antiepileptics

Topiramate and zonisamide are novel antiepileptics reported clinically to have antimanic, antidepressant, and long-term mood stabilizing properties in patients with bipolar I and II disorders (197,265–269). Controlled studies of topiramate in acute bipolar mania in adults, however, did not demonstrate separation from placebo on mania ratings, although the drug was superior to placebo in a prematurely terminated study in adolescent mania (270,271). Topiramate was also comparable to bupropion in reducing depressive symptoms in a single-blind comparator trial in bipolar I depression (197). To date, there have been no double-blind, placebo-controlled studies of topiramate monotherapy in bipolar depression, unipolar major depression, or in the long-term maintenance treatment of bipolar or depressive disorders. Nor have there been any controlled studies of zonisamide in depressive or bipolar disorders. Thus, the complete thymoleptic profiles of these two novel anticonvulsants are presently unknown.

Topiramate and zonisamide were each associated with anorexia and weight loss in controlled studies in patients with epilepsy (272–274). This finding of weight loss led to positive double-blind, placebo-controlled studies of both drugs in patients with obesity (275–277). For topiramate, the weight loss was shown to be dose related and to plateau after 12–18 months of treatment. Topiramate has also been shown in double-blind, placebo-controlled trials to be effective in many of the conditions that co-occur with mood disorders, including BED, BN, alcohol dependence, and migraine (278–281). Moreover, topiramate was associated with weight loss in the controlled trials in these conditions, in the controlled bipolar mania trials, and in the single-blind bipolar depression trial. Open data suggest zonisamide may reduce binge eating and induce weight loss in patients with BED (282). Both topiramate and zonisamide have been used successfully to treat weight gain and obesity in patients with bipolar disorder receiving mood stabilizers and antipsychotics (265,283–286).The weight loss has sometimes been long term and associated with improvement in metabolic indices. Two open-label, prospective trials suggest that initiating treatment with the combination of topiramate with either risperidone or olanzapine may successfully stabilize mood in patients with bipolar disorder while preventing weight gain (284,285). Additionally, topiramate has been used to treat weight gain in patients with treatment-resistant major depression receiving antidepressants, in patients with anxiety disorders receiving SSRIs, and in patients with schizophrenia receiving antipsychotics (287–292). The mechanism(s) of the anorectic and weight loss effects of these drugs are unknown, but topiramate's may be related to its anti-glutamatergic action whereas zonisamide's has been hypothesized to be due to its dual effects on serotonin and dopamine (275,277,278).

Psychostimulants

Although no stimulant is approved by the FDA for the treatment of a mood disorder, these agents are relatively commonly used in patients with depressive and bipolar disorders for several reasons (293–296). First, their effectiveness in various depressive syndromes remains unclear. A review of 10 controlled studies published in 1989 suggested stimulants were not superior to placebo as monotherapy in the short-term treatment of outpatient major depression (294). However, many of these studies had methodological limitations, including unclear entry criteria and high placebo response rates. Second, mounting reports, including several double-blind, placebo-controlled studies, have found stimulants effective in treating depressive syndromes associated with general medical illness (295,296). Thus, *d*-amphetamine was shown superior to placebo in reducing anxious-depressive symptoms in obese patients; methylphenidate was found superior to placebo in older, depressed, medically ill patients; and *d*-amphetamine, methylphenidate, and pemoline were each found superior to placebo in reducing depressive symptoms and fatigue in ambulatory patients with human immunodeficiency virus disease (297–300). There have also been reports of the successful use of various stimulants to augment antidepressants in treatment-resistant and treatment-refractory mood disorder patients. For example, *d*-amphetamine has been used to potentiate MAOIs, TCAs, and SSRIs in patients with treatment-refractory major depression

(296,301,302). Similarly, modafinil, a novel alerting agent approved for the treatment of narcolepsy and obstructive sleep apnea, has been used as an adjunctive agent to treat residual fatigue, sleepiness, and hypersomnia in patients with major depressive disorder and bipolar disorder (303–307).

A third reason stimulants are frequently used in mood disorder patients is that the conditions for which they are approved, namely ADHD and (for modafinil) obstructive sleep apnea, often co-occur with mood disorders (122). Moreover, there are reports that some of these agents may be effective in other conditions that co-occur with mood disorders. Thus, methylphenidate has been reported to reduce binge eating and purging in BN, including in patients resistant to antidepressants (308–310).

Virtually all psychostimulants, with the possible exception of the novel agent modafinil, are associated with appetite suppression and weight loss (29). [Modafinil was associated with weight loss in one short-term study, but not in the clinical trials in patients with narcolepsy, even though narcolepsy may be associated with obesity (303,304,311,312)]. Some of these agents (phentermine, diethylpropion, mazindol, and phenylpropynolamine) have FDA approval for the short-term treatment of obesity (29–31). Although not approved for long-term use, phentermine's weight loss effects have been shown to persist for up to one year (313). The appetite suppressant and weight loss effects of these drugs have been attributed to their enhancement of brain catecholamine function, which includes promotion of dopamine and norepinephrine release and blockade of dopamine and norepinephrine reuptake.

Although not classified as a stimulant, atomoxetine is a highly selective norepinephrine reuptake inhibitor approved for use in ADHD that has been associated with anorexia and weight loss in children and adults (314,315). It has also been shown to reduce food consumption in animal models of feeding (316). Preliminary open data suggest atomoxetine may have antidepressant properties, but the drug has not yet been evaluated in obesity (317).

Dopamine Agonists

Dopamine agonists have received preliminary study in mood disorders and obesity. Regarding mood disorders, several of these drugs (amantadine, bromocriptine, cabergoline, pergolide, and pramipexole) have been reported in open studies to be effective when used adjunctively in patients with treatment-resistant depression (318–323). Pramipexole has been shown superior to placebo and comparable to fluoxetine as monotherapy in reducing depressive symptoms in an eight-week dose finding study of major depression ($N = 174$) (324). At 1.0 mg/day, pramipexole was superior to placebo; at 5.0 mg/day, the drug also appeared to be effective but the high drop out rate precluded statistical analysis. Pramipexole has also been shown superior to placebo in two small ($N = 22$ and 21) six-week studies as adjunctive therapy in bipolar depression (mean dose 1.7 mg/day in both studies) (325,326). In addition, amantadine has been shown to be more effective than placebo and pemoline in treating fatigue in patients with multiple sclerosis (327). Unfortunately, effects on weight were not reported in any of these studies.

Regarding obesity, bromocriptine (1.6–2.4 mg/day) was shown superior to placebo in reducing weight and improving glucose tolerance in an 18-week study in 17 obese patients (328). Bromocriptine was also shown to improve glycemic control and glucose tolerance in a placebo-controlled, 16-week study of 22 obese patients with type 2 diabetes who were prescribed a weight maintaining diet (329). Although no other dopamine agonists have been assessed in the treatment of obesity, open studies suggest amantadine may be helpful for weight gain due to atypical antipsychotics and mood stabilizers, including in patients with bipolar disorder (330,331). For example, Floris et al. (330) treated 12 patients (2 with bipolar disorder) with amatadine (mean dose = 175 mg/day) who had experienced a mean weight gain of 7 kg since beginning olanzapine therapy. Weight gain ceased almost immediately following addition of amantadine in all 12 patients. After six months, all but one of the patients lost weight, and mean weight loss was 3.5 kg.

Opiate Antagonists

Animal and human studies indicate that the endogenous opiod system is involved in the regulation of affective responses and eating behavior (332–334). Naltrexone is a competitive opioid receptor antagonist approved by the FDA for treating opiate and alcohol dependence that has been reported to also have short-term anorectic and weight loss properties in substance use disorder patients, healthy volunteers, and obese persons (333,334). Three small eight-week, placebo-controlled studies of naltrexone in obesity, however, have been negative (335–337). Dosages evaluated in these studies were 50 and l00, 200, and 300 mg/day, respectively. Similarly, placebo-controlled studies suggest naltrexone at doses of 50–150 mg/day is ineffective in binge eating associated with BN or BED (338,339). Case reports and open studies, though, suggest higher doses of the drug (200–400 mg/day) may be effective in some patients with BN and BED, including those refractory to antidepressants (340–342). In these patients, naltrexone was associated with therapeutic weight loss and improvement in metabolic parameters.

Despite evidence indicating that the opioid system is involved in the regulation of affect and the high comorbidity between mood and substance use disorders, opiate antagonists have not been studied in controlled trials in mood disorders. A preliminary double-blind, placebo-controlled study, however, found naltrexone (mean dose 187.5 mg) to be effective in pathological gambling (104,131,332,343). Extensive research has shown that pathological gambling is related to substance use, mood, and attention deficit hyperactivity disorders (344). In addition, problem gambling may be associated with binge eating and use of weight control efforts (345). Thus, naltrexone may be helpful for the obese mood disorder patient who has a co-occurring substance use or impulse control disorder, or treatment-resistant binge eating, especially if the binge eating has addictive or impulsive features.

ANTI-OBESITY DRUGS IN MOOD AND RELATED DISORDERS

As discussed earlier, the psychostimulants amphetamine and methylphenidate, which are effective in inducing weight loss but are no longer approved for obesity because of their questionable efficacy in weight-loss maintenance and their abuse potential, have been the most extensively studied centrally-active weight loss agents in depression (29,171,293–296). We were unable to find published controlled trials of other centrally acting antiobesity agents in mood disorders. However, preliminary data suggest that some of these agents may have antidepressant properties. The serotonergic agents fenfluramine and/or dexfenfluramme (which have been removed from the market for safety concerns) have been reported to improve depressed mood in obesity, as well as premenstrual depression, bipolar depression, seasonal affective disorder, and BN (297,346–349). Fenfluramine has also been shown to be superior to placebo in treating binge eating associated with both BN and BED, although in the latter study it was not associated with significant weight loss. Sibutramine and its metabolites have displayed antidepressant properties in animal models of depression (349–352). Although there are no published studies of sibutramine in patients with major depressive disorder, the drug has been shown superior to placebo in reducing depressed mood, along with binge eating behavior and body weight, in obese patients with BED (353).

Further supporting the possibility that these agents have antidepressant properties are reports that they have induced mania and manic symptoms. Thus, as noted earlier, various stimulants, fenfluramine, and sibutramine have each been associated with the induction of manic syndromes (35–37,39). These agents should therefore be used cautiously in patients with bipolar disorders.

There have been no controlled studies of peripherally acting antiobesity agents (e.g., gastrointestinal lipase inhibitors) in obese patients with mood disorders, though cases of patients with major depression and bipolar disorder successfully receiving orlistat for psychotropic-associated weight gain have been described (354–356). In one report, orlistat promoted varying degrees of weight loss (1–8.7% of body weight) over an eight-week period with minimal changes in psychotropic drug plasma levels (355). However, there is a case report of one patient with bipolar II disorder who developed depression after addition of orlistat to venlafaxine upon three successive occasions (357). There are also case reports of eating disorder patients abusing the drug (358–360). We observed an obese patient with BN who misused orlistat to compensate for her binge eating behavior in the midst of a major depressive episode (360). Thus, our group will use orlistat in obese patients with mood disorders, but we monitor mood symptoms very closely. Also, in obese patients with comorbid eating pathology (with or without mood disorders), we further monitor the patient's eating behavior and use of the drug. We tend to avoid using orlistat in patients with severe binge eating, any type of purging behavior, or poor insight into their pathological eating behaviors.

RESPONSE TO COMBINATION TREATMENT

Another important treatment similarity shared by obesity and mood disorders is that both conditions may respond to combination therapy. Thus, several drug–drug combinations have been reported to be effective in controlled trials for obesity, major depression, and bipolar disorder. These include fenfluramine with phentermine for obesity; antidepressants with lithium for major depression; mood stabilizers (lithium or valproate) with atypical antipsychotics (olanzapine, risperidone, and quetiapine) for bipolar I mania; and fluoxetine with olanzapine for bipolar I depression (29,68,181,361). (Unlike for obesity, however, mood disorders have been shown to respond better to these combination treatments than to single drug treatments in controlled trials.) In addition, obesity, major depression, and bipolar disorder have each been shown to respond better to pharmacotherapy in combination with psychological treatments than to pharmacotherapy alone in randomized controlled trials (362–369). Although not yet formally tested, such combination treatment approaches are likely to be especially important in the management of some obese patients with mood disorders.

ASSESSMENT OF THE PATIENT WITH OBESITY AND A MOOD DISORDER

Patients with comorbid obesity and a mood disorder may present with complaints related to their weight, their mood disorder, or another comorbid general medical or mental disorder as their primary reason for obtaining treatment. Thus, the patient presenting with overweight or obesity (especially severe obesity) should be evaluated for a mood disorder, whereas the patient presenting with signs and symptoms of a mood disorder should be evaluated for a weight disorder, including overweight and obesity as well as abdominal obesity and the metabolic syndrome. Not uncommonly in the comorbid patient, stabilizing a disorder that the patient is not requesting immediate treatment for (hypomania or major depression) may be clinically indicated in order to stabilize the disorder directly related to the patient's chief complaint (obesity). It is therefore crucial to assess the relative severity of both conditions in the comorbid patient, the distress and impairment both conditions are causing the patient, the presumed etiologic relationship among the conditions (if any) for that patient, and the patient's goals, treatment preferences, and resources for treatment.

A complete assessment for a lifetime mood disorder includes a psychiatric and medical history, family and social history, and mental status exam with a focus on current and lifetime mood, psychotic, anxiety, substance use, eating, and impulse control disorder signs and symptoms. Because bipolar disorder frequently presents as depression, comorbid Axis I disorders, Axis II personality disorders, behavioral dysregulation (including hypersexuality and antisocial behavior), or general medical disorders (e.g., migraine and other types of pain), it is important to carefully evaluate for a history of hypomania or mania, including subthreshold hypomanic symptoms, in patients with these presentations (370). Because patients often have difficulty identifying or recognizing hypomania, the use of screening instruments, such as the Mood Disorder Questionnaire (MDQ) or the Hypomania Symptom Checklist, and structured clinical interviews, such as the Structured Clinical Interview for DSM-IV (SCID), in combination with consultation of a significant other (with the patient's permission), will improve the identification of bipolarity, particularly "soft" or "occult" forms (371–373).

A complete assessment of obesity by a mental health professional should at minimum include determination of the patient's height, weight, and BMI; lifetime weight history; general medical history, including presence or absence of those conditions that are associated with obesity and mood disorders; and assessment of family weight and general medical problems (374). Other useful parameters to assess include waist circumference, vital signs and certain laboratory parameters, such as fasting glucose, lipid profile, and liver function tests. Ideally, in the treatment of a patient with obesity and mood disorder, there should be collaboration between the patient's mental health professional and his or her primary care provider.

OBESITY AND DEPRESSIVE DISORDERS

When treating an obese patient with a depressive disorder, management of the obesity and depression ideally should proceed concurrently. This entails keeping both conditions a focus of clinical concern with regular monitoring of depressive symptoms, weight, and appropriate medical variables (e.g., vital signs and metabolic indices) as treatment progresses.

However, the clinical situation may dictate that treatment of one condition should proceed before treatment of another. Thus, if the depression is mild and the patient's primary goal is to achieve weight loss through changing his or her diet and exercise habits, a standard behavior weight loss program might be safely initiated before treating the depression. Alternatively, if specialized treatment is available, cognitive behavior therapy (CBT) focusing on both weight loss and depressive symptoms would be another option. Inadequate adherence or progress with behavioral weight management or CBT should prompt consideration of pharmacotherapy of depressive symptoms—either with an antidepressant with a weight loss profile (bupropion, venlafaxine, or an SSRI) or an anti-obesity agent with potential antidepressant properties (sibutramine). Conversely, if a moderate to severe major depressive episode is present, or if depressive symptoms are associated with functional impairment, suicidal ideation, or psychotic features, the depression probably should be pharmacologically treated before a behavioral weight management program is initiated. Antidepressants that have weight loss properties or are weight neutral might be chosen as first-line agents. Topiramate or zonisamide might be considered as adjunctive therapy in patients inadequately responsive to antidepressant treatment or those who have associated affective instability, hyperphagia (especially if there is a compulsive component), or comorbid binge eating behavior, BED, BN, substance abuse, or migraine. Stimulants or dopamine agonists could be considered as adjunctive therapy in patients with residual fatigue, comorbid ADHD, binge eating, or significant general medical illness. Use of lithium augmentation and antidepressants associated with weight gain, such as TCAs, MAOIs, or mirtazapine, would be reserved for patients with treatment-resistant depression. Topiramate, zonisamide, stimulants, or dopamine agonists could also be added to the regimens of those patients who respond to such agents but who experience appetite stimulation or weight gain.

In patients whose mood has stabilized (in response to pharmacotherapy or psychotherapy) but who remain overweight or obese, additional pharmacotherapy (e.g., topiramate, zonisamide, orlistat, or naltrexone) or psychotherapy (e.g., behavioral weight management or CBT) could be added to treat obesity. Such patients with severe obesity could also be considered for bariatric surgery.

OBESITY AND BIPOLAR DISORDERS

In managing obese patients with a bipolar disorder, treatment of the bipolar disorder and obesity ideally should proceed concurrently if at all possible. Mood stabilization, however, is critical. Thymoleptic agents that have the optimal efficacy and appetite and weight profiles should be employed. Lithium, ziprasidone, and aripiprazole appear to be the antimanic agents associated with the least weight gain. Lamotrigine, which is effective in acute bipolar depression and as a maintenance treatment, is largely weight neutral and thus can be particularly helpful for the obese bipolar patient who is depressed and prone to switching with standard antidepressants. When utilizing pharmacotherapy for weight loss, agents that are potentially mood stabilizing or mood neutral (e.g., topiramate, zonisamide, and orlistat) might be used before those that are potentially mood destabilizing (e.g., sibutramine). As patients with bipolar disorder in general often require multiple medications for optimal response, obese patients with bipolar disorders are similarly likely to require combination pharmacotherapy. Various combinations of mood stabilizers, second generation antipsychotics, anticonvulsants, antidepressants, and/or anti-obesity agents may therefore be needed for optimal individualized response.

Psychotropic-associated weight gain in bipolar disorder can be managed with adjunctive treatment with psychotropics with appetite suppressant, weight loss, or anti-bingeing properties, and/or with centrally or peripherally acting-anti-obesity agents, depending on the patient's particular clinical situation. Thus, topiramate or zonisamide may be added when there is associated appetite stimulation, overeating, binge eating, mood instability, substance abuse, and/or migraine. Venlafaxine, SSRIs, bupropion, or sibutramine may be added when there are associated depressive, binge eating, or night eating symptoms, but should be avoided as long as there are manic, hypomanic, mixed, or cycling symptoms. Psychostimulants or dopamine agonists may be added for associated depressive and/or binge eating symptoms if the patient is already receiving an antidepressant, particularly if the patient has prominent fatigue or a medical disorder contributing to his or her depressive symptoms. Orlistat may be considered in patients who are overeating, but should be used cautiously in those who are binge eating, purging, or both.

In our experience, a substantial number of bipolar patients with overweight or obesity, especially those with soft spectrum disorders, refuse treatment with standard mood stabilizers because of the stigma associated with the diagnosis of bipolar disorder, the weight gain associated with standard mood stabilizers, or both. In such patients, as long as they are not acutely manic, we often begin treatment with topiramate or zonisamide as monotherapy, especially if the patient has comorbid binge eating. In our clinical experience, many of these patients will display weight loss and improvement in any comorbid binge eating. Although the response in associated mood symptoms is variable, the therapeutic alliance is often strengthened because of the weight loss and reduction in binge eating. This often leads to the patient's acceptance of adjunctive treatment with a standard mood stabilizer in the future if needed.

Extremely little is known about bariatric surgery for the stable bipolar patient with severe obesity. There is one case of the successful use of intravenous valproate for the treatment of manic symptoms that developed in a patient with schizoaffective disorder, bipolar type after bariatric surgery (375). The patient was eventually stabilized on oral valproate 5000 mg/day (with a serum concentration of 123 mg/mL) and clozapine 325 mg/day, suggesting he was absorbing at least the valproate.

CONCLUSION

Obesity and mood disorders are both serious public health problems that overlap to a clinically significant degree. Many psychotropic medications have adverse or therapeutic effects on appetite, weight, binge eating, and even primary obesity. Conversely, some anti-obesity agents may have effects on binge eating and mood.

Thus, for patients with obesity and mood disorders, first-line treatments would include psychotropics with maximal efficacy for their mood disorder that also possesses appetite suppressant, weight-loss, or anti-binge eating properties as well as optimal tolerability and safety. If such a drug is not available for a patient's particular psychopathology, drugs that are weight neutral followed by drugs that have lower weight-gaining liabilities could be chosen, provided that the drugs have comparable efficacy, tolerability, and safety. A thorough understanding of the relationships among obesity, mood disorders, the adverse and therapeutic effects of psychotropic drugs on appetite, binge eating, weight and metabolism, and the effects of anti-obesity agents on eating behavior, mood, and psychopathology should enable optimal medical treatment of the obese mood disorder patient's psychopathology while minimizing weight gain or, ideally, promoting weight loss and improving metabolic health.

REFERENCES

1. Black DW, Goldstein RB, Mason EE. Prevalence of mental disorders in 88 morbidly obese bariatric clinic patients. Am J Psychiatry 1992; 149:227–234.
2. Friedman MA, Brownell KD. Psychological correlates of obesity: moving to the next research generation. Psychol Bull 1995; 17:3–20.
3. Britz B, Siegfried W, Ziegler A, et al. Rates of psychiatric disorders in a clinical study group of adolescents with extreme obesity and in obese adolescents ascertained via a population based study. Int J Obes 2000; 24:1707–1714.
4. Carpenter KM, Hasin DS, Allison DB, et al. Relationships between obesity and DSM-IV major depressive disorder, suicide ideation, and suicide attempts: results from a general population study. Am J Public Health 2000; 90:251–257.
5. Faith MS, Matz, PE, Jorge MA. Obesity-depression associations in the population. J Psychosom Res 2002; 53:935–942.
6. Roberts RE, Deleger S, Strawbridge WJ, et al. Prospective association between obesity and depression: evidence from the Alameda County Study. Int J Obes Relat Metab Disord 2003; 27:514–521.
7. Stunkard AJ, Faith MS, Allison KC. Depression and obesity. Biol Psychiatry 2003; 54:330–337.
8. Onyike CU, Crum RM, Lee HB, et al. Is obesity associated with major depression? Results from the Third National Health and Nutrition Examination Survey. Am J Epidemiol 2003; 158:1139–1147.
9. Rosmond R. Obesity and depression: same disease, different names? Med Hypotheses 2004; 62:976–979.

10. McElroy SL, Kotwal R, Malhotra S, et al. Are mood disorders and obesity related? A review for the mental health professional. J Clin Psychiatry 2004; 65:634–651.
11. Sullivan M, Karlsson J, Sjörstöm L, et al. Swedish obese subjects (SOS)—an intervention study of obesity. Baseline evaluation of health and psychosocial functioning in the first 1743 subjects examined. Int J Obes Relat Metab Disord 1993; 17:503–512.
12. Goldstein LT, Goldsmith SJ, Anger K, et al. Psychiatric symptoms in clients presenting for commercial weight reduction treatment. Int J Eat Disord 1996; 20:191–197.
13. Cugini P, Cilli M, Salandri A, et al. Anxiety, depression, hunger and body composition: III. Their relationships in obese patients. Eat Weight Disord 1999; 4:115–120.
14. Csabi G, Tenyi T, Molnar D. Depressive symptoms among obese children. Eat Weight Disord 2000; 5:43–45.
15. Dixon JB, Dixon ME, O'Brien PE. Depression in association with severe obesity. Changes with weight loss. Arch Int Med 2003; 163:2058–2065.
16. Erermis S, Cefin N, Tamar M, et al. Is obesity a risk factor for psychopathology among adolescents? Pediatr Int 2004; 46:296–301.
17. Weissenburger J, Rush AJ, Giles DE, et al. Weight changes in depression. Psychiatry Res 1986; 17:275–283.
18. Frank E, Carpenter LL, Kupfer DJ. Sex differences in recurrent depression: are there any that are significant? Am J Psychiatry 1998; 145:41–45.
19. Stunkard AJ, Fernstrom MH, Price A, et al. Direction of weight change in recurrent depression. Consistency across episodes. Arch Gen Psychiatry 1990; 47:857–860.
20. Michelson D, Amsterdam JD, Quitkin FM, et al. Changes in weight during a 1-year trial of fluoxetine. Am J Psychiatry 1999; 156:1170–1176.
21. Elmslie JL, Silverstone JT, Mann JI, et al. Prevalence of overweight and obesity in bipolar patients. J Clin Psychiatry 2000; 61:179–184.
22. Pine DS, Goldstein RB, Wolk S, et al. The association between childhood depression and adulthood body mass index. Pediatrics 2001; 107:1049–1056.
23. McElroy SL, Frye MA, Suppes T, et al. Correlates of overweight and obesity in 644 patients with bipolar disorder. J Clin Psychiatry 2002; 63:207–213.
24. Fagiolini A, Frank E, Houck PR, et al. Prevalence of obesity and weight change during treatment in patients with bipolar I disorder. J Clin Psychiatry 2002; 63:528–533.
25. Fagiolini A, Kupfer DJ, Houck PR, et al. Obesity as a correlate of outcome in patients with bipolar I disorder. Am J Psychiatry 2003; 60:112–117.
26. Keck PE Jr, McElroy SL. Bipolar disorder, obesity, and pharmacotherapy-associated weight gain. J Clin Psychiatry 2003; 64:1426–1435.
27. Patten SB. "Diet pills" and major depression in the Canadian population. Can J Psychiatry 2001; 46:438–440.
28. Appolinario JC, Bueno JR, Coutinho W. Psychotropic drugs in the treatment of obesity: what promise? CNS Drugs 2004; 18:629–651.
29. Bray GA, Greenway FL. Current and potential drugs for treatment of obesity. Endocrine Reviews 1999; 20:805–875.

30. Yanovski SZ, Yanovski JA. Drug therapy. Obesity. N Engl J Med 2002; 346:591–602.
31. Bray GA, Bouchard C, eds. Handbook of Obesity. Clinical Applications. 2nd ed. New York: Marcel Dekker, 2004.
32. Ackerman S, Nolan LJ. Bodyweight gain induced by psychotropic drugs. Incidence, mechanisms and management. CNS Drugs 1998; 9:135–151.
33. Zimmermann U, Kraus T, Himmerich H, et al. Epidemiology, implications and mechanisms underlying drug-induced weight gain in psychiatric patients. J Psychiatr Res 2003; 37:193–220.
34. Arrone LJ, Segal KR. Weight gain in the treatment of mood disorders. J Clin Psychiatry 2003; 64(suppl 8):22–29.
35. Raison CL, Klein HM. Psychotic mania associated with fenfluramine and phentermine use. Am J Psychiatry 1997; 154:711.
36. Bowden CL, Dickson J, Jr. Mania from dexfenfluramine. J Clin Psychiatry 1997; 58:548–549.
37. Bagri S, Reddy G. Delirium with manic symptoms induced by diet pills [letter]. J Clin Psychiatry 1998; 59:83.
38. Zimmer JE, Gregory RJ. Bipolar depression associated with fenfluramine and phentermine. J Clin Psychiatry 1998; 59:383–384.
39. Cordeiro Q, Vallada H. Sibutramine-induced mania episode in a bipolar patient. Int J Neuropsychopharmacol 2002; 5:283–284.
40. Patten SB. Major depressive episodes and diet pills. Expert Opin Pharmacother 2002; 3:1405–1409.
41. Shannon PJ, Leonard D, Kidson MA. Fenfluramine and psychosis [letter]. Br Med J 1974; 3:576.
42. Devan GS. Phentermine and psychosis. Br J Psychiatry 1990; 156:442–443.
43. Preval H, Pakyvrek AM. Psychotic episode associated with dexfenfluramine. Am J Psychiatry 1997; 154:1624–1625.
44. Cleare AJ. Phentermine, psychosis, and family history [letter]. J Clin Psychopharmacol 1996; 16:470–471.
45. Taflinski T, Chojnacka J. Sibutramine-associated psychotic episode. Am J Psychiatry 2000; 157:2057–2058.
46. Björntorp P, Brodoff BN, eds. Obesity. Philadelphia: J.B. Lippincott, 1992.
47. Wadden TA, Van Itallie TB, eds. Treatment of the Seriously Obese Patient. New York: Guilford Press, 1992.
48. Allison DB, Pi-Sunyer FX, eds. Obesity Treatment Establishing Goals, Improving Outcomes, and Reviewing the Research Agenda. New York: Plenum Press1995.
49. National Task Force on the Prevention and Treatment of Obesity. Long-term pharmacotherapy in the management of obesity. JAMA 1996; 276: 1907–1915.
50. National Heart, Lung, and Blood Institute (NHLBI) and National Institute for Diabetes and Digestive and Kidney Diseases (NIDDKD) Clinical Guidelines on the Identification, Evaluation, and Treatment of Overweight and Obesity in Adults. The Evidence Report. National Institute of Health: Bethesda, MD, 1998. NIB Publication No. 98–4083. (Available at www.nhlbi.nih.gov/guidelines/obesity/ob-gdlns.htm.).

51. Douketis JD, Feightner JW, Attia J, et al. Periodic health examination, 1999 update: 1. Detection, prevention and treatment of obesity. Canadian Task Force on Preventive Health Care. CMAJ 1999; 160:513–525.
52. Fairburn CG, Brownell KD, eds. Eating Disorders and Obesity. A Comprehensive Handbook. 2nd ed. New York: Guilford Press, 2002.
53. Health Development Agency. The management of obesity and overweight. An analysis of reviews of diet, physical activity and behavioral approaches. Evidence briefing. United Kingdom, October, 2003.
54. Scottish Intercollegiate Guidelines Network. Management of obesity in children and young people. A national clinical guideline. Edinburgh: Royal College of Physicians, 2003.
55. McTigue KM, Harris R, Hemphill B, et al. Screening and interventions for obesity in adults: summary of the evidence for the U.S. Preventative Services Task Force. Ann Intern Med 2003; 139:933–949.
56. Kushner RF. Roadmaps for Clinical Practice: Case Studies in Disease Prevention and Health Promotion. In: Assessment and Management of Adult Obesity: A Primer for Physicians. Chicago: American Medical Association, 2003.
57. Thompson JK, ed. Handbook of Eating Disorders and Obesity. Hoboken, New Jersey: Wiley, 2004.
58. Avenell A, Broom J, Brown TJ, et al. Systematic review of the long-term effects and economic consequences of treatments for obesity and implications for health improvement. Health Technol Assess 2004; 8:1–182.
59. American Psychiatric Association. Practice guideline for the treatment of patients with major depressive disorder (revision). Am J Psychiatry 2000; 157(suppl):1–45.
60. American Psychiatric Association. Practice guideline for the treatment of patients with bipolar disorder (revision). Am J Psychiatry 2002; 159(suppl):1–50.
61. American Academy of Child and Adolescent Psychiatry: Practice parameters for the assessment and treatment of children and adolescents with depressive disorders. J Am Acad Child Adolesc Psychiatry 1998; 37(suppl):635–835.
62. American Academy of Child and Adolescent Psychiatry Official Action. Practice parameters for the assessment and treatment of children and adolescents with bipolar disorder. J Am Acad Child Adolesc Psychiatry 1997; 36:138–157.
63. Bauer M, Whybrow PC, Angst J, et al. World Federation of Societies of Biological Psychiatry (WFSBP) Guidelines for Biological Treatment of Unipolar Depressive Disorders, Part 1: acute and continuation treatment of major depressive disorder. World J Biol Psychiatry 2002; 3:5–43.
64. Bauer M, Whybrow PC, Angst J, et al. World Federation of Societies of Biological Psychiatry (WFSBP) Guidelines for Biological Treatment of Unipolar Depressive Disorders, Part 2: maintenance treatment of major depressive disorder and treatment of chronic depressive disorders and subthreshold depression. World J Biol Psychiatry 2002; 3:69–86.
65. Grunze H, Kasper S, Goodwin G, et al. World Federation of Societies of Biological Psychiatry (WFSBP) Guidelines for the Biological Treatment of

Bipolar Disorders, Part 1: treatment of bipolar depression. World J Biol Psychiatry 2002; 3:l15–124.

66. Grunze H, Kasper S, Goodwin G, et al. World Federation of Societies of Biological Psychiatry (WFSBP) Guidelines for the Biological Treatment of Bipolar Disorders, Part II: treatment of mania. World J Biol Psychiatry 2003; 4:5–13.

67. Boland PJ, Keller MB. Treatment of depression. In: Schatzberg AF, Nemeroff CB, eds. The American Psychiatric Publishing Textbook of Psychopharmacology. 3rd ed. Washington, DC: American Psychiatric Publishing, 2004:847–864.

68. Keck PE Jr, McElroy SL. Treatment of biolar disorder. In: Schatzberg AF, Nemeroff CB, eds. The American Psychiatric Publishing Textbook of Psychopharmacology. 3rd ed. Washington, DC: American Psychiatric Publishing, 2004:865–883.

69. Mustillo S, Worthman C, Erkanli A, et al. Obesity and psychiatric disorder: developmental trajectories. Pediatrics 2003; 111:851–859.

70. Kinder LS, Carnethon MR, Palaniappan LP, et al. Depression and the metabolic syndrome in young adults: findings from the Third National Health and Nutrition Examination Survey. Psychosom Med 2004; 66:316–322.

71. Muller-Oerlinghausen B, Passoth P-M, Poser W, et al. Impaired glucose tolerance in long-term lithium-treated patients. Int Pharmacopsychiat 1979; 14:350–362.

72. Shiori T, Kato T, Murashita J, et al. Changes in the frequency distribution pattern of body weight in patients with major depression. Acta Psychiatr Scand 1993; 88:356–360.

73. Thakore JH, Richards PJ, Reznek RH, et al. Increased abdominal fat deposition in patients with major depressive illness as measured by computed tomography. Biol Psychiatry 1997; 41:1140–1142.

74. Weber-Hamann B, Hentschel F, Kniest A, et al. Hypercortisolemic depression is associated with increased intra-abdominal fat. Psychosom Med 2002; 64:274–277.

75. Kendler KS, Eaves LJ, Walters EE, et al. The identification and validation of distinct depressive syndromes in a population-based sample of female twins. Arch Gen Psychiatry 1996; 53:391–399.

76. Pine DS, Cohen P, Brook J, et al. Psychiatric symptoms in adolescence as predictors of obesity in early adulthood: a longitudinal study. Am J Public Health 1997; 97:1303–1310.

77. Miller GE, Stetler CA, Carney RM, et al. Clinical depression and inflammatory risk markers for coronary heart disease. Am J Cardiol 2002; 90:1279–1283.

78. Lamertz CM, Jacobi C, Yassouridis A, et al. Are obese adolescents and adults at higher risk for mental disorder. A community survey. Obes Res 2002; 10:1152–1160.

79. Wyatt RJ, Henter ID, Mojtabai R, et al. Height, weight, and body mass index (BMI) in psychiatrically ill US Armed Forces personnel. Psychol Med 2003; 33:363–368.

80. Hasler G, Merikangas K, Eich D, et al. Psychopathology as a risk factor for being overweight. American Psychiatric Association 156th Annual Meeting New Research Abstracts, San Francisco, CA, May 17–22, 2003, NR 106, 39–40.

81. Richardson LP, Davis R, Poulton R, et al. A longitudinal evaluation of adolescent depression and adult obesity. Arch Psychiatr Adolesc Med 2003; 157:739–745.

82. Folsom AR, Kushi LH, Anderson KE, et al. Associations of general and abdominal obesity with multiple health outcomes in older women. The Iowa Women's Health Study. Arch Intern Med 2000; 160:2117–2128.

83. Bray GA, Bouchard C, eds. Handbook of Obesity. New York: Marcel Dekker, 2004.

84. Silverstein B. Gender difference in the prevalence of clinical depression: the role played by depression associated with somatic symptoms. Am J Psychiatry 1999; 156:480–482.

85. Gold PW, Chrousos GP. Organization of the stress system and its dysregulation in melancholic and atypical depression: high vs low CRH/NE states. Mole Psychiatry 2002; 7:254–275.

86. Angst J, Gamma A, Sellaro R, et al. Toward validation of atypical depression in the community: results of the Zurich cohort study. J Affect Disord 2002; 72:125–138.

87. Sullivan PF, Prescott CA, Kendler KS. The subtypes of major depression in a twin registry. J Affect Disord 2002; 68:273–284.

88. Posternak MA, Zimmerman M. Partial validation of the atypical features subtype of major depressive disorders. Arch Gen Psychiatry 2002; 59:70–76.

89. Flores BH, Musselman DL, De Battista C, et al. Biology of mood disorders. In: Schatzberg AF, Nemeroff CB, eds. The American Psychiatric Publishing Textbook of Psychopharmacology. 3rd ed. Washington, DC: American Psychiatric Publishing, 2004:717–763.

90. Faith MS, Johnson SL, Allison DB. Putting the *behavior* into the behavior genetics of obesity. Behav Genet 1997; 27:423–439.

91. Barsh GS, Farooqui S, O'Rahilly S. Genetics of body-weight regulation. Nature 2000; 404:644–651.

92. Bouchard C, Pérusse L, Rice T, et al. Genetics of human obesity. In: Bray GA, Bouchard C, eds. Handbook of Obesity. Etiology and Pathophysiology. 2nd. New York: Marcel Dekker, 2004:157–355.

93. Becker KG. The common variants/multiple disease hypothesis of common complex genetic disorders. Med Hypotheses 2004; 62:309–317.

94. Sullivan PF, Neale MC, Kendler KS. Genetic epidemiology of major depression: review and meta-analysis. Am J Psychiatry 2000; 157:1552–1562.

95. Kelsoe JR. Arguments for the genetic basis of the bipolar spectrum. J Affect Disord 2003; 73:183–197.

96. Lesch KP. Gene-environment interaction and the genetics of depression. J Psychiatry Neurosci 2004; 29:174–184.

97. Johnson JG, Cohen P, Kasen S, et al. Childhood adversities associated with risk for eating disorders or weight problems during adolescence or early adulthood. Am J Psychiatry 2002; 159:394–400.

98. Johnson JG, Cohen P, Kasen S, et al. Association of maladaptive parental behavior with psychiatric disorder among parents and their offspring. Arch Gen Psychiatry 2001; 58:453–460.

99. Batten SV, Asian M, Maciejewski PK, et al. Childhood maltreatment as a risk factor for adult cardiovascular disease and depression. J Clin Psychiatry 2004; 65:249–254.

100. Ozanne SE, Fernandez-Twinn D, Hales CN. Fetal growth and adult diseases. Semin Perinatol 2004; 28:81–87.

101. Must A, Spadano J, Coakley EH, et al. The disease burden associated with overweight and obesity. JAMA 1999; 282:1523–1529.

102. Bray GA. Risks of obesity. Endocrinol Metab Clin North Am 2003; 32:787–804.

103. Maser JD, Cloninger CR, eds. Comorbidity of Mood and Anxiety Disorders. Washington, DC: American Psychiatric Press, 1990.

104. Tohen M, ed. Comorbidity in Affective Disorders. New York, NY: Marcel Dekker, 1999.

105. Eaton WW. Epidemiologic evidence on the comorbidity of depression and diabetes. J Psychosom Res 2002; 53:903–906.

106. Musselman DL, Betan E, Larsen H, et al. Relationship of depression to diabetes types 1 and 2: epidemiology, biology, and treatment. Biol Psychiatry 2003; 54:317–329.

107. Keck PE Jr, Buse JB, Dagogo-Jack S, et al. Managing metabolic concerns in patients with severe mental illness. Minneapolis, MN: Postgraduate Medicine, McGraw-Hill, 2003.

108. Golden SH, Williams JE, Ford DE, et al. Depressive symptoms and the risk of type 2 diabetes: the atherosclerosis risk in communities study. Diabetes Care 2004; 27:429–435.

109. Jonas BS, Franks P, Ingram DD. Are symptoms of anxiety and depression risk factors for hypertension? Longitudinal evidence from the National Health and Nutrition Examination Survey I Epidemiologic Follow-Up Study. Arch Fam Med 1997; 6:43–49.

110. Bosworth HB, Bartash RM, Olsen MK, et al. The association of psychosocial factors and depression with hypertension among older adults. Int J Ger Psychiatry 2003; 18:l142–1148.

111. Musselman DL, Evans DL, Nemeroff CB. The relationship of depression to cardiovascular disease: epidemiology, biology, and treatment. Arch Gen Psychiatry 1998; 55:580–592.

112. Ford DE, Mead LA, Chang DP, et al. Depression is a risk factor for coronary artery disease in men: the precursors study. Arch Int Med 1998; 158: 1422–1426.

113. Ferketich AK, Schwartzbaum JA, Frid DJ, et al. Depression as an antecedent to heart disease among women and men in the NHANES I study. Arch Int Med 2000; 160:1261–1268.

114. Jonas BS, Mussolino ME. Symptoms of depression as a prospective risk factor for stroke. Psychosom Med 2000; 62:463–471.

115. Ohira T, Hiroyasu I, Satoh S, et al. Prospective study of depressive symptoms and risk of stroke among Japanese. Stroke 2001; 32:903–908.

116. Carney RM, Freedland KE, Miller GE, et al. Depression as a risk factor for cardiac mortality and morbidity. A review of potential mechanisms. J Psychosom Res 2002; 53:897–902.

117. Jones DJ, Bromberger JT, Sutton-Tyrrell K, et al. Lifetime history of depression and carotid atherosclerosis in middle-aged women. Arch Gen Psychiatry 2003; 60:153–160.
118. Lett HS, Blumenthal JA, Babyak MA, et al. Depression as a risk factor for coronary artery disease: evidence, mechanisms, and treatment. Psychosom Med 2004; 66:305–315.
119. Strike PC, Steptoe A. Psychosocial factors in the development of coronary artery disease. Prog Cardiovasc Dis 2004; 46:337–347.
120. Thomas AJ, Kalaria RN, O'Brien JT. Depression and vascular disease: what is the relationship? J Affect Disord 2004; 79:81–95.
121. Calabrese JR, Hirschfield RMA, Reed M, et al. Impact of bipolar disorder on a US community sample. J Clin Psychiatry 2003; 64:425–432.
122. Ohayon MM. The effects of breathing-related sleep disorders on mood disturbances in the general population. J Clin Psychiatry 2003; 64:1195–1200.
123. Ohayon MM, Schatzberg AF. Using chronic pain to predict depressive morbidity in the general population. Arch Gen Psychiatry 2003; 60:39–47.
124. Marcus DA. Obesity and the impact of chronic pain. Clin J Pain 2004; 20:186–191.
125. Hoyer EH, Mortensen PB, Olesen AV. Mortality and causes of death in a total national sample of patients with affective disorders admitted for the first time between 1973 and 1993. Br J Psychiatry 2000; 176:76–82.
126. Pennix BW, Beekman AT, Honig A, et al. Depression and cardiac mortality. Results from a community-based longitudinal study. Arch Gen Psych 2001; 58:221–227.
127. Ösby U, Brandt L, Correia N, et al. Excess mortality in bipolar and unipolar disorders in Sweden. Arch Gen Psychiatry 2001; 58:844–850.
128. Merikangas KR, Angst J, Isler H. Migraine and psychopathology. Results of the Zurich cohort study of young adults. Arch Gen Psychiatry 1990; 47:849–853.
129. Newport DJ, Nemeroff CB. Depression in the medically ill. In: Tohen M, ed. Comorbidity in Affective Disorders. New York: Marcel Dekker, 1999:57–104.
130. Sax KW, Strakowski SM. The co-occurrence of bipolar disorder with medical illness. In: Tohen M, ed. Comorbidity in Affective Disorders. New York: Marcel Dekker, 1999:1–25.
131. Kessler RC. Comorbidity of unipolar and bipolar depression with other psychiatric disorders in a general population survey. In: Tohen M, ed. Comorbidity in Affective Disorders. New York: Marcel Dekker, 1999:1–25.
132. McElroy SL, Altshuler LL, Suppes T, et al. Axis I psychiatric comorbidity and its relationship to historical illness variables in 288 patients with bipolar disorder. Am J Psychiatry 2001; 158:420–426.
133. Angst J, Sellaro R, Ries Merikangas K. Multimorbidity of psychiatric disorders as an indicator of clinical severity. Eur Arch Psychiatry Clin Neurosci 2002; 252:147–154.
134. Melartin TK, Rysälä HJ, Leskelä US, et al. Current comorbidity of psychiatric disorders among DSM-IV major depressive disorder patients in psychiatric care in the Vantaa Depression Study. J Clin Psychiatry 2002; 63:126–134.
135. Kessler RC, Berglund P, Dernier O, et al. The epidemiology of major depressive disorder. Results from the National Comorbidity Survey Replication (NCS-R). JAMA 2003; 289:3095–3105.

136. McElroy SL. Diagnosing and treating comorbid (complicated) bipolar disorder. J Clin Psychiatry 2004; 65(suppl 15):35–44.
137. Regier DA, Farmer ME, Rae DS, et al., Comorbidity of mental disorders with alcohol and other drug abuse. Results from Epidemiologic Catchment Area (ECA) Study. JAMA 1990; 264;2511–2518.
138. Chen Y-W, Who C, Dilsaver SC. Comorbidity of panic disorder in bipolar illness: evidence from the epidemiologic catchment area survey. Am J Psychiatry 1995; 152:280–282.
139. Chen Y-W, Dilsaver SC. Comorbidity for obsessive-compulsive disorder in bipolar and unipolar disorders. Psychiatry Res 1995; 59:57–64.
140. Kessler RC, Rubinow DR, Holmes C, et al. The epidemiology of DSM-III-R bipolar I disorder in a general population survey. Psychol Med 1997; 27:1079–1089.
141. Angst J. The emerging epidemiology of hypomania and bipolar II disorder. J Affect Disord 1998; 50:143–151.
142. Yanovski SZ, Nelson JE, Dubbert BK, et al. Association of binge eating disorder and psychiatric disorder in obese subjects. Am J Psychiatry 1993; 150:1472–1479.
143. Specker S, deZwaan M, Raymond N, et al. Psychopathology in subgroups of obese women with and without binge eating disorder. Comp Psychiatry 1994; 35:185–190.
144. Bulik CM, Sullivan PF, Kendler KS. Medical and psychiatric morbidity in obese women with and without binge eating. Int J Eat Dis 2002; 32:72–78.
145. Andrews G, Slade T, Issakidis C. Deconstructing current comorbidity: data from the Australian National Survey of Mental Health and Well-Being. Br J Psychiatry 2002; 181:306–314.
146. Frank E, Cyranowski JM, Rucci P, et al. Clinical significance of lifetime panic spectrum symptoms in the treatment of patients with bipolar I disorder. Arch Gen Psychiatry 2002; 59:905–911.
147. Fagiolini A, Kupfer DJ, Rucci P, et al. Suicide attempts and ideation in patients with bipolar I disorder. J Clin Psychiatry 2004; 65:509–514.
148. Blumenthal JA, Lett HS, Babyak MA, et al. Depression as a risk factor for mortality after coronary artery bypass surgery. Lancet 2003; 9:409–421.
149. Williams LS, Ghose SS, Swindle RW. Depression and other mental health diagnoses increase mortality risk after ischemic stroke. Am J Psychiatry 2004; 161:1090–1095.
150. DiMatteo MR, Lepper HS, Croghan TW. Depression is a risk factor for noncompliance with medical treatment. Arch Int Med 2000; 160:2101–2107.
151. Marcus MD, Wing RR, Guare J, et al. Lifetime prevalence of major depression and its effect on treatment outcome in obese type II diabetic patients. Diabetes Care 1992; 15:253–255.
152. Ciechanowski PS, Katon WJ, Russo JE. Depression and diabetes: impact of depressive symptoms on adherence, function, and costs. Arch Int Med 2000; 160:3278–3285.
153. Ciechanowski PS, Katon WJ, Russo JE, et al. The relationship of depressive symptoms to symptom reporting, self care and glucose control in diabetes. Gen Hosp Psychiatry 2003; 25:246–252.

154. Stunkard AJ, Rush J. Dieting and depression reexamined. A critical review of reports of untoward responses during weight reduction for obesity. Ann Int Med 1974; 81:526–533.
155. Wing RR, Epstein LH, Marcus MD, et al. Mood changes in behavioral weight loss programs. J Psychosom Res 1984; 28:189–196.
156. Smoller JW, Wadden TA, Stunkard AJ. Dieting and depression: a critical review. J Psychosom Res 1987; 31:429–440.
157. Herpetz S, KielmanR, Wolf AM, et al. Does obesity surgery improve psychosocial functioning? A systematic review. Int J Obes Relat Metab Disord 2003; 27:1300–1314.
158. Waters GS, Poiries WJ, Swanson MS, et al. Long-term studies of mental health after the Greenville gastric bypass operation for morbid obesity. Am J Surg 1991; 161:154–157.
159. Hsu LK, Benotti PN, Dwer J, et al. Nonsurgical factors that influence the outcome of bariatric surgery: a review. Psychosom Med 1998; 60:338–346.
160. Clark MM, Niaura R, King TK, et al. Depression, smoking, activity level, and health status: pretreatment predictors of attrition in obesity treatment. Addict Behav 1996; 21:509–513.
161. Linde JA, Jeffery RW, Levy RL, et al. Binge eating disorder, weight control self-efficacy and depression in overweight men and women. Int J Obes Relat Metab Disord 2004; 28:418–425.
162. Zeller M, Kirk S, Claytor R, et al. Predictors of attrition from a pediatric weight management program. J Pediatr 2004; 144:466–470.
163. Jenkins I, Djuric Z, Darga L, et al. Relationship of psychiatric diagnosis and weight loss maintenance in obese breast cancer survivors. Obes Res 2003; 11:1369–1375.
164. Klem ML, Wing RR, McGuire MT, et al. Psychological symptoms in individuals successful at long-term maintenance of weight loss. Health Psychol 1998; 17:336–345.
165. Phelan S, Hill JO, Lang W, et al. Recovery from relapse among successful weight maintainers. Am J Clin Nutr 2003; 78:1079–1084.
166. Schatzberg AF, Nemeroff CB, eds. The American Psychiatric Publishing Textbook of Psychopharmacology. Washington, DC: American Psychiatric Publishing, 2004.
167. Ghaemi SN, ed. Polypharmacy in Psychiatry. New York: Marcel Dekker, 2002.
168. Haddock CK, Poston WS, Dill PL, et al. Pharmacotherapy of obesity: a quantitative analysis of four decades of published randomized clinical trials. Int J Obes Relat Metab Disord 2002; 26:262–273.
169. Arterbum DE, Crane PK, Weenstra DL. The efficacy and safety of sibutramine for weight loss: a systematic review. Arch Int Med 2004; 164:994–1003.
170. O'Meara S, Riemsma R, Shirran L, et al. A systematic review of the clinical effectiveness of orlistat used for the management of obesity. Obes Rev 2004; 5:51–68.
171. Wilding J. Clinical evaluation of anti-obesity drugs. Curr Drug Targets 2004; 5:325–332.

172. Geddes JR, Carney SM, Davies C, et al. Relapse prevention with antidepressant drug treatment in depressive disorders: a systematic review. Lancet 2003; 361:653–661.
173. Stewart JW, Tricamo E, McGrath PJ, et al. Prophylactic efficacy of phenelzine and imipramine in chronic atypical depression: likelihood of recurrence on discontinuation after 6 months' remission. Am J Psychiatry 1997; 154: 31–36.
174. Kornstein SG, Schatzberg AF, Thase ME, et al. Gender differences in treatment response to sertraline and imipramine in chronic depression. Am J Psychiatry 2000; 157:1445–1452.
175. Wohlfarth T, Storosum JG, Elferink AJA, et al. Response to tricyclic antidepressants: independent of gender? Am J Psychiatry 2004; 161:370–372.
176. Keller MB, Ryan ND, Strober M, et al. Efficacy of paroxetine in the treatment of adolescent major depression: a randomized, controlled study. J Am Acad Child Adolesc Psychiatry 2001; 40:762–772.
177. Hazell P, O'Connell D, Heathcote D, et al. Tricyclic drugs for depression in children and adolescents. Cochrane Database Syst Rev 2002; (2):CD002317.
178. Rothschild AJ. Challenges in the treatment of depression with psychotic features. Biol Psychiatry 2003; 53:680–690.
179. Whittington CJ, Kendall T, Fonagy P, et al. Selective serotonin reuptake inhibitors in childhood depression: systematic review of published versus unpublished data. Lancet 2004; 363:1341–1345.
180. Brent DA. Antidepressants and pediatric depression—the risk of doing nothing. N Engl J Med 2004; 351:1598–1601.
181. Tohen M, Vieta E, Calabrese J, et al. Efficacy of olanzapine and olanzapine-fluoxetine combination in the treatment of bipolar I depression. Arch Gen Psychiatry 2003; 60:1079–1088.
182. Ghaemi SN, Hsu DJ, Soldani F, et al. Antidepressants in bipolar disorder: the case for caution. Bipolar Disord 2003; 5:421–433.
183. Altshuler LL, Suppes T, Black D, et al. Impact of antidepressant discontinuation after acute bipolar depression remission rates of depressive relapse at 1-year follow-up. Am J Psychiatry 2003; 160:1252–1262.
184. Ghaemi SN, Rosenquist KJ, Ko JY, et al. Antidepressant treatment in bipolar versus unipolar depression. Am J Psychiatry 2004; 161:163–165.
185. Gijsman HJ, Geddes JR, Rendell JM, et al. Antidepressants for bipolar depression: a systematic review of randomized, controlled trials. Am J Psychiatry 2004; 161:1537–1547.
186. Martin A, Young C, Leckman JF, et al. Age effects on antidepressant-induced manic conversion. Arch Pediatr Adolesc Med 2004; 158:773–780.
187. McElroy SL, Kotwal R, Keck PE Jr, et al. The comorbidity of bipolar and eating disorders: distinct or related disorders with shared dysregulations. J Affect Disord 2005; 86:107–127.
188. Fava M. Weight gain and antidepressants. J Clin Psychiatry 2000; 61(suppl 11):37–41.
189. Sussman N, Ginsberg DL, Bikoff J. Effects of nefazodone on body weight: a pooled analysis of selective serotonin reuptake inhibitor-and imipramine-controlled trials. J Clin Psychiatry 2001; 62:256–260.

190. McGuirk J, Silverstone T. The effect of the 5-HT re-uptake inhibitor fluoxetine on food intake and body weight in healthy male subjects. Int J Obes 1990; 14:361–372.
191. Harto NE, Spera KF, Branconnier RJ. Fluoxetine-induced reduction of body mass in patients with major depressive disorder. Psychopharmacol Bull 1988; 24:220–223.
192. Goldstein DJ, Hamilton SH, Masica DN, et al. Fluoxetine in medically stable, depressed geriatric patients: effects on weight. J Clin Psychopharmacol 1997; 17:365–369.
193. Edwards JG, Anderson I. Systemic review and guide to selection of selective serotonin reuptake inhibitors. Drugs 1999; 57:507–533.
194. Harto-Traux N, Stem WC, Miller LL, et al. Effects of bupropion on body weight. J Clin Psychiatry 1983; 44:183–186.
195. Settle EC, Stahl SM, Batey SR, et al. Safety profile of sustained-release bupropion in depression: results of three clinical trials. Clin Ther 1999; 21:454–463.
196. Croft H, Houser TL, Jamerson BD, et al. Effect on body weight of bupropion sustained-release in patients with major depression treated for 52 weeks. Clin Ther 2002; 24:662–672.
197. McIntyre RS, Mancini DA, McCann S, et al. Topiramate versus bupropion SR when added to mood stabilizer therapy for the depressive phase of bipolar disorder: a preliminary single-blind study. Bipolar Disord 2002; 4:207–213.
198. Rudolph RL, Fabre LF, Feighner JP, et al. A randomized, placebo-controlled, dose-response trial of venlafaxine hydrochloride in the treatment of major depression. J Clin Psychiatry 1998; 59:116–122.
199. Kraus T, Haack M, Schuld A, et al. Body weight, the tumor necrosis factor system and leptin production during treatment with mirtazepine or venlafaxine. Pharmacopsychiatry 2002; 35:220–225.
200. Malhotra S, King KH, Welge JA, et al. Venlafaxine treatment of binge eating disorder, associated with obesity: a series of 35 patients. J Clin Psychiatry 2002; 63:802–806.
201. Fava M, Judge R, Hoog SL, et al. Fluoxetine versus sertraline and paroxetine in major depressive disorder; changes in weight with long-term treatment. J Clin Psychiatry 2000; 61:863–867.
202. Bandelow B, Behnke K, Lenoir S, et al. Sertraline versus paroxetine in the treatment of panic disorder: an acute, double-blind noninferiority comparison. J Clin Psychiatry 2004; 65:405–413.
203. Curzon G, Gibson EL, Oluyomi AO. Appetite suppression by commonly used drugs depends on 5HT receptors but not on 5HT availability. Trend Pharmacol Sci 1998; 13:21–25.
204. Learned-Coughlin SM, Bergström M, Savitcheva I, et al. In vivo activity of bupropion at the human dopamine transporter as measured by positron emission tomography. 2003; 54:800–805.
205. Dong J, Blier P. Modification of norepinepherine and serotonin, but not dopamine, neuronal firing by bupropion treatment. Psychopharmacology 2001; 155:52–57.
206. Harvey AT, Rudolph RL, Preskom SH. Evidence of the dual mechanisms of action of venlafaxine. Arch Gen Psychiatry 2000; 57:503–509.

207. Levine LR, Enas GG, Thompson WL, et al. Use of fluoxetine, a selective serotonin reuptake inhibitor in the treatment of obesity: a dose response study. Int J Obes 1989; 13:635–645.
208. Marcus MD, Wing RR, Ewing L, et al. A double-blind, placebo-controlled trial of fluoxetine plus behavior modification in the treatment of obese binge-eaters and non-binge-eaters. Am J Psychiatry 1990; 147:876–881.
209. Darga LL, Carroll-Michals L, Botsford SJ, et al. Fluoxetine's effect on weight loss in obese subjects. Am J Clin Nutr 1991; 54:321–325.
210. Wise SD. Clinical studies with fluoxetine in obesity. Am J Clin Nutr 1992; 55(suppl 1):181S–184S.
211. Goldstein DJ, Rampey AH Jr, Enas GG, et al. Fluoxetine: a randomized clinical trial in the treatment of obesity. Intl J Obesity 1994; 18:129–135.
212. Sayler ME, Goldstein DJ, Roback PJ, et al. Evaluating success of weight-loss programs, with an application to fluoxetine weight-reduction clinical trial data. Int J Obes Relat Metab Disord 1994; 18:742–751.
213. Norris SL, Zhang X, Avenell A, et al. Efficacy of pharmacotherapy for weight loss in adults with type 2 diabetes mellitus: a meta-analysis. Arch Int Med 2004; 164:1395–1404.
214. Bitsch M, Skrumsager BK. Femoxetine in the treatment of obese patients in general practice. A randomized group comparative study with placebo. Int J Obes 1987; 11:183–190.
215. Szkudlarek J, Elsborg L. Treatment of severe obesity with a highly selective serotonin re-uptake inhibitor as a supplement to a low calorie diet. Int J Obes Relat Metab Disord 1993; 17:681–683.
216. Ljung T, Ahlberg AC, Holm G, et al. Treatment of abdominally obese men with a serotonin reuptake inhibitor: a pilot study. J Int Med 2001; 250: 219–224.
217. Abell CA, Farquhar DL, Galloway SM, et al. Placebo controlled double-blind trial of fluvoxamine maleate in the obese. J Psychosom Res 1986; 30:143–146.
218. deZwaan M, Nutzinger DO. Effect of fluvoxamine on total serum cholesterol levels during weight reduction. J Clin Psychiatry 1996; 57:346–348.
219. Ricca V, Mannucci E, DiBernardo M, et al. Sertraline enhances the effects of cognitive-behavioral treatment on weight reduction of obese patients. J Endocrinol Invest 1997; 20:727–733.
220. Wadden TA, Bartlett SJ, Foster GD, et al. Sertraline and prevention training following treatment by very low calorie diet: a controlled clinical trial. Obes Res 1995; 3:549–557.
221. Breum L, Bjerre V, Bak JF, et al. Long-term effects of fluoxetine on glycemic control in obese patients with non-insulin-dependent diabetes mellitus or glucose intolerance: influence on muscle receptor kinase activity. Metabolism 1995; 44:1570–1576.
222. Maheux P, Ducros F, Bourque J, et al. Fluoxetine improves insulin sensitivity in obese patients with non-insulin-dependent diabetes mellitus independently of weight loss. Int J Obes 1997; 21:97–102.
223. Bailey DL, LeMelledo JM. Effects of serotonin reuptake inhibitors on cholesterol levels in patients with panic disorder. J Clin Psychopharmacol 2003; 23:317–319.

224. Lara N, Baker GB, Archer SL, et al. Increased cholesterol levels during paroxetine administration in healthy men. J Clin Psychiatry 2003; 64:1455–1459.

225. Papakosras GI, Petersen T, Sonawalla SB, et al. Serum cholesterol in treatment-resistant depression. Neuropsychobiology 2003; 47:146–151.

226. Kopf D, Westphal S, Luley CW, et al. Lipid metabolism and insulin resistance in depressed patients: significance of weight, hypercortisolism, and antidepressant treatment. J Clin Psychopharmacol 2004; 24:527–531.

227. Huang T-L, Chen J-F. Lipid and lipoprotein levels in depressive disorders with melancholic feature or atypical feature and dysthymia. Psychiatry Clin Neurosci 2004; 58:295–299.

228. Poyurovsky M, Pashinian A, Gil-Ad I, et al. Olanzapine-induced weight gain in patients with first episode schizophrenia: a double-blind, placebo-controlled study of fluoxetine addition. Am J Psychiatry 2002; 159:1058–1060.

229. Barak Y, Lampl Y, Achirn A, et al. Fluoxetine induced weight loss: a pilot study in postpartum women. Isr J Psychiatry Relat Sci 1995; 32:51–54.

230. Achiron A, Barak Y, Noy S, et al. Fluoxetine treatment for weight reduction in steroid-induced obesity: a pilot study in myasthenia gravis patients. Eur Neuropsychopharmacol 1999; 9:111–113.

231. Gadde KM, Parker CB, Maner LG, et al. Bupropion for weight loss: an investigation of efficacy and tolerability in overweight and obese women. Obes Res 2001; 9:544–551.

232. Anderson JW, Greenway FL, Fujioka K, et al. Bupropion SR enhances weight loss: a 48-week double-blind, placebo-controlled trial. Obes Res 2002; 10:633–641.

233. Jain AK, Kaplan RA, Gadde KM, et al. Bupropion SR vs placebo for weight loss in obese patients with depressive symptoms. Obes Res 2002; 1049–1056.

234. Hays JT, Ebbert JO. Bupropion sustained release for treatment of tobacco dependence. Mayo Clin Proc 2003; 78:1020–1024.

235. Poyurovsky M, Isaacs I, Fuchs C, et al. Attentuation of olanzapine-induced weight gain with reboxetine in patients with schizophrenia: a double-blind, placebo-controlled study. Am J Psychiatry 2003; 160:297–302.

236. Bodkin JA, Lasser RA, Wines JD Jr, et al. Combining serotonin reuptake inhibitors and bupropion in partial responders to antidepressant monotherapy. J Clin Psychiatry 1997; 58:137–145.

237. Nelson JC. Augmentation strategies with serotonergic-noradrenergic combinations. J Clin psychiatry 1998; 59:65–68.

238. Lam RW, Hossie H, Solomons K, et al. Citalopram and bupropion-SR: combining versus switching in patients with treatment-resistant major depression. J Clin Psychiatry 2004; 65:337–340.

239. Nelson JC, Mazure CM, Jatlow PI, et al. Combining norepinephrine and serotonin reuptake inhibition mechanisms for treatment of depression: a double-blind, randomized study. Biol Psychiatry 2004; 55:296–300.

240. Gill D, Hatcher S. Antidepressants for depression in medical illness. Cochrane Database Syst Rev 2000; (4):CD001312.

241. Cheer SM, Goa KL. Fluoxetine. A review of its therapeutic potential in the treatment of depression associated with physical illness. Drugs 2001; 61:81–110.

242. Glassman AH, O'Connor CM, Califf RM, et al. Sertraline Antidepressant Heart Attack Randomized Trial (SADHEART) Group. Sertraline treatment of major depression in patients with acute MI or unstable angina. JAMA 288:701–709.
243. Fortner MR, Brown K, Varia IM, et al. Effect of bupropion SR on the quality of life in elderly depressed patients with comorbid medical disorders. Prim Care Companion J Clin Psychiatry 1999; 1:174–179.
244. Jorge RE, Robinson RG, Amdt S, et al. Mortality and post stroke depression: a placebo-controlled trial of antidepressants. Am J Psychiatry 2003; 160:1823–1829.
245. Sauer WH, Berlin JA, Kimmel SE. Effect of antidepressants and their relative affinity for the serotonin transporter on the risk of myocardial infarction. Circulation 2003; 108:32–36.
246. Hudson JI, Pope HG Jr, Carter WP. Pharmacologic therapy of bulimia nervosa. In: Goldstein DJ, ed. The Management of Eating Disorders and Obesity. Totowa, NJ: Humana Press, 1999:19–32.
247. Bacaltchuk J, Hay P. Antidepressants versus placebo for people with bulimia nervosa. Cochrane Database Syst Rev 2003;CD003391.
248. Romano SJ, Halmi KA, Sarkar NP, et al. A placebo-controlled study of fluoxetine in continued treatment of bulimia nervosa after successful acute fluoxetine treatment. Am J Psychiatry 2002; 159:96–102.
249. Carter WP, Hudson JL, Lalonde JK, et al. Pharmacologic treatment of binge eating disorder. Int Eat Disord 2003; 34(suppl):S74–S88.
250. Stein DJ, Hollander E, eds. Textbook of Anxiety Disorders. Washington, DC: American Psychiatric Publishing, 2002.
251. Pettinati HM, Kranzler HR, Madaras. The status of serotonin-selective pharmacotherapy in the treatment of alcohol dependence. In: Galanter M, ed. Recent Developments in Alcoholism. Vol 16. Research on Alcoholism Treatment: New York, Kluwer Academic, 2003:247–262.
252. McElroy SL, Arnold LA. Impulse Control Disorders. In: Gabbard GO, ed. Treatment of Psychiatric Disorders. 3rd ed. Washington, DC: American Psychiatric Press, 2001:2435–2471.
253. Hollander E, Stein DJ, eds. Clinical Manual of Impulse Control Disorders. Washington, D.C, American Psychiatric Publishing, 2005.
254. Silberstein SD, Lipton RB, Dalessio DJ, eds. Wolff's Headache and Other Head pain, 7th ed. New York, Oxford University Press, 2001.
255. Bauer MS, Mitchner L. What is a "mood stabilizer"? An evidence-based response. Am J Psychiatry 2004; 161:3–18.
256. Hsu LKG. Treatment of bulimia with lithium. Am J Psychiatry 1984; 141:1260–1262.
257. Hsu LKG, Clement L, Santhouse R, et al. Treatment of bulimia nervosa with lithium carbonate. A controlled study. J Nerv Men Dis 1991; 179:351–355.
258. Kaplan AS, Garfinkel PE, Darby PL, et al. Carbamazepine in the treatment of bulimia. Am J Psychiatry 1983; 140:1225–1226.
259. Brewerton TD, Shannon M. Possible clozapine exacerbation of bulimia nervosa. Am J Psychiatry 1992; 149:1408–1409.

260. Crockford DN, Fisher G, Barker P. Risperidone, weight gain, and bulimia nervosa. Can J Psychiatry 1997; 42:326–327.
261. Thiesen FM, Linden A, König IR, et al. Spectrum of binge eating symptomatology in patients treated with clozapine and olanzapine. J Neural Transm 2003; 110:111–121.
262. Shapira NA, Goldsmith TD, McElroy SL. Treatment of binge-eating disorder with topiramate: a clinical case series. J Clin Psychiatry 2000; 61:368–372.
263. McIntyre R, Katzman M. The role of atypical antipsychotics in bipolar depression and anxiety disorders. Bipolar Disord 2003; 5(suppl 2):20–35.
264. Freitag FG. Divalproex in the treatment of migraine. Psychopharmacol Bull 2004; 37(suppl 2):98–115.
265. McElroy SL, Suppes T, Keck PE Jr, et al. Open-label adjunctive topiramate in the treatment of bipolar disorders. Biol Psychiatry 2000; 47:1025–1033.
266. McElroy SL, Keck PE Jr. Topiramate. In: Schatzberg AF, Nemeroff CB, eds. American Psychiatric Publishing Textbook of Psychopharmacology, 3rd ed. Arlington, VA: American Psychiatric Publishing, 2004:627–636.
267. Kanba S, Yagi G, Kamijima K, et al. The first open study of zonisamide, a novel anticonvulsant, shows efficacy in mania. Prog Neuropsychopharmacol Biol Psychiatry 1994; 18:707–715.
268. McElroy SL, Suppes T, Keck PE Jr, et al. Open-label adjunctive zonisamide in the treatment of bipolar disorders: a prospective trial. J Clin Psychiatry 2005; 66:617–624.
269. Baldassano CF, Ghaemi SN, Chang A, et al. Acute treatment of bipolar depression with adjunctive zonisamide: a retrospective chart review. Bipolar Disord 2004; 6:432–434.
270. Powers PS, Sachs GS, Kushner SF, et al. Topiramate in adults with acute bipolar I mania: pooled results. American Psychiatric Association 157th Annual Meeting, New York, May 1–6, 2004.
271. DelBello MP, Findling RL, Kushner S, et al. A pilot controlled trial of topiramate for mania in children and adolescents with bipolar disorder. J Am Acad Child Adoles Psychiatry 2005; 44:539–547.
272. Reife R, Pledger G, Wu SC. Topiramate as add-on therapy: pooled analysis of randomized controlled trials in adults. Epilepsia 2000; 41(suppl 1):566–571.
273. Ben-Menachem E, Axelsen M, Johanson EH, et al. Predictors of weight loss in adults with topiramate treated epilepsy. Obes Res 2003; 11:556–562.
274. Leppik IE. Zonisamide, a novel antiepileptic agent. Today's Therapeutic Trends 1999; 17:181–195.
275. Bray GA, Hollander P, Klein S, et al. for the U.S. Topiramate Research Group. A 6-month randomized, placebo-controlled, dose-ranging trial of topiramate for weight loss in obesity. Obes Res 2003; 11:722–733.
276. Wilding J, Gaal LV, Rissanen A, et al. A randomized double-blind placebo-controlled study of the long-term efficacy and safety of topiramate in the treatment of obese subjects. Int J Obes Relat Metab Disord 2004; 28:1399–1410.
277. Gadde KM, Francicy DM, Wagner HR II, et al. Zonisamide for weight loss in obese adults. A randomized, controlled trial. JAMA 2003; 289:1820–1825.

278. McElroy SL, Arnold LM, Shapira NA, et al. Topiramate in the treatment of binge eating disorder associated with obesity: a randomized, placebo-controlled trial. Am J Psychiatry 2003; 160:255–261.

279. Hoopes SP, Reimherr FW, Hedges DW, et al. Treatment of bulimia nervosa with topiramate in a randomized, double-blind, placebo-controlled trial, part 1: improvement in binge and purge measures. J Clin Psychiatry 2003; 64: 1335–1341.

280. Johnson BA, Ait-Daoud N, Bowden CL, et al. Oral topiramate for treatment of alcohol dependence: a randomized controlled trial. Lancet 2003; 361:1677–1685.

281. Brandes JL, Saper JR, Diamond M, et al. Topiramate for migraine prevention: a randomized controlled trial. JAMA 2004; 291:965–973.

282. McElroy SL, Kotwal R, Hudson JI, et al. Zonisamide in the treatment of binge-eating disorder: an open-label, prospective trial. J Clin Psychiatry 2004; 65:50–56.

283. Chengappa KNR, Levine J, Rathore D, et al. Long-term effects of topiramate on bipolar mood instability, weight change and glycemic control: a case series. Eur Psychiatry 2001; 16:186–190.

284. Vieta E, Goikolea JM, Olivares JM, et al. 1-year follow-up of patients treated with risperidone and topiramate for a manic episode. J Clin Psychiatry 2003; 64:834–839.

285. Vieta E, Sanchez-Moreno J, Goikolea JM, et al. Effect on weight and outcome of long-term olanzapine and topiramate combination treatment in bipolar disorder. J Clin Psychopharmacol 2004; 24:374–378.

286. Woods TM, Eichner SF, Franks AS. Weight gain mitigation with topiramate in mood disorders. Ann Pharmacother 2004; 38:887–891.

287. Gordon A, Price LH. Mood stabilization and weight loss with topiramate. Am J Psychiatry 1999; 156:968–969.

288. Teter CJ, Early JJ, Gibbs CM. Treatment of affective disorder and obesity with topiramate. Ann Pharmacother 2000; 34:1262–1265.

289. Dursun SM, Devarajan S. Accelerated weight loss after treating refractory depression with fluoxetine plus topiramate: possible mechanisms of action? [Letter] Can J Psychiatry 2001; 45:287–288.

290. Carpenter LL, Leon Z, Yasmin S, et al. Do obese depressed patients respond to topiramate? A retrospective chart review. J Affect Disord 2002; 69:251–255.

291. Van Ameringen M, Mancini C, Pipe B, et al. Topiramate treatment for SSRI-induced weight gain in anxiety disorders. J Clin Psychiatry 2002; 63:981–984.

292. Dursun SM, Devarajan S. Clozapine weight gain, plus topiramate weight loss. Can J Psychiatry 2000; 45:198.

293. Chiarello RJ, Cole JO. The use of psychostimulants in general psychiatry. A reconsideration. Arch Gen Psychiatry 1987; 44:286–295.

294. Satel SL, Nelson JC. Stimulants in the treatment of depression: a critical overview. J Clin Psychiatry 1989; 50:241–249.

295. Masand PS, Tesar GE. Use of stimulants in the medically ill. Psychiatr Clin North Am 1996; 18:515–547.

296. Fawcett J, Busch KA. Stimulants in psychiatry. In: Schatzberg AF, Nemeroff CB, eds. Textbook of Psychopharmacology. 2nd ed. Washington, DC: American Psychiatric Press, 1998:503–522.

297. Rickels K, Hesbacher P, Fisher E, et al. Emotional symptomatology in obese patients treated with fenfluramine and dextroamphetamine. Psychol Med 1976; 6:623–630.
298. Wallace AE, Kofoed LL, West AN. Double-blind, placebo-controlled trial of methylphenidate in older, depressed, medically ill patients. Am J Psychiatry 1995; 152:929–931.
299. Wagner GJ, Rabkin R. Effects of dextroamphetamine on depression and fatigue in men with HIV: a double-blind, placebo-controlled trial. J Clin Psychiatry 2000; 61:436–440.
300. Breitbart W, Rosenfeld B, Kaim M, et al. A randomized,double-blind, placebo-controlled trial of psychosimulants for the treatment of fatigue in ambulatory patients with human immunodeficiency virus disease. Arch Int Med 2001; 161:411–420.
301. Fawcett J, Kravitz HM, Zajecka JM, et al. CNS stimulant potentation of monoamine oxidase inhibitors in treatment-refractory depression. J Clin Psychopharmacol 1991; 11:127–132.
302. Nierenberg AA, Dougherty D, Rosenbaun JF. Dopaminergic agents and stimulants as antidepressant augmentation strategies. J Clin Psychiatry 1988; 59(suppl 5):60–63.
303. U.S. Modafinil in Narcolepsy Multicenter Study Group. Randomized trial of modafinil as a treatment for the excessive daytime somnolence of narcolepsy. Neurology 2000; 54:1166–1175.
304. Moldofsky H, Broughton RJ, Hill ID. A randomized trial of the long-term, continued efficacy and safety of modafinil in narcolepsy. Sleep Med 2000; 1:109–116.
305. Dinges DF, Weaver TE. Effects of modafinil on sustained attention performance and quality of life in OSA patients with residual sleepiness while being treated with CPAP. Sleep Med 2003; 4:393–402.
306. DeBattista C, Doghramji K, Menza MA, et al. Adjunct modafinil for the short term treatment of fatigue and sleepiness in patients with major depressive disorder: a preliminary double-blind, placebo-controlled study. J Clin Psychiatry 2003; 64:1057–1064.
307. Fernandes PP, Petty F. Modafinil for remitted bipolar depression with hypersomnia. Ann Pharmacother 2003; 37:1807–1809.
308. Schweickert LA, Strober M, Moskowitz A. Efficacy of methyphenidate in bulimia nervosa comorbid with attention deficit disorder: a case report. Int J Eating Disord 1997; 21:299–301.
309. Sokol MS, Gray NS, Goldstein A, et al. Methylphenidate treatment in bulimia nervosa associated with Cluster B Personality Disorder. Int J Eat Disord 1999; 25:233–237.
310. Drimmer EJ. Stimulant treatment of bulimia nervosa with and without attention-deficit disorder: three case reports. Nutrition 2003; 19:76–77.
311. Makris AP, Rush CR, Frederich PC, et al. Wake-promoting agents with different mechanisms of action: comparison of effects of modafinil and amphetamine on food intake and cardiovascular activity. Appetite 2004; 42:185–195.
312. Kok SW, Overeem S, Visscher TLS, et al. Hypocretin deficiency in narcoleptic humans is associated with abdominal obesity. Obes Res 2003; 11:1147–1154.

313. Glazer G. Long-term pharmacotherapy of obesity 2000: a review of efficacy and safety. Arch Int Med 2001; 161:1814–1824.
314. Wernicke JF, Kratochvil CJ. Safety profile of atomoxetine in the treatment of children and adolescents with ADHD. J Clin Psychiatry 2002; 63(suppl 12):50–55.
315. Michelson D, Adler L, Spencer T, et al. Atomoxetine in adults with ADHD: two randomized, placebo-controlled studies. Biol Psychiatry 2003; 53:112–120.
316. Gehlert DR, Dreshfield L, Tinsley F, et al. The selective norepinephrine reuptake inhibitor, LY368975, reduces food consumption in animal models of feeding. J Pharmacol Exp Ther 1998; 287:122–127.
317. Chouinard G, Annable L, Bradwein J, et al. An early phase II clinical trial with followup of tomoxetine (LY139603) in the treatment of newly admitted depressed patients. Psychopharmacol Bull 2003; 21:73–76.
318. Huber TJ, Dietrich DE, Emrich HM. Possible use of amantadine in depression. Pharmacopsychiatry 1999; 32:47–55.
319. Stryjer R, Strous RD, Shaked G, et al. Amantadine as augmentation therapy in the management of treatment-resistant depression. Int Clin Psychopharmacol 2003; 18:93–96.
320. Sitland-Marken PA, Wells BG, Froemming JH, et al. Psychiatric applications of bromocriptine therapy. J Clin Psychiatry 1990; 51:68–82.
321. Takahashi H, Yoshida K, Higuchi H, et al. Addition of a dopamine agonist, cabergoline, to a serotonin-noradrenalin reuptake inhibitor, milnacipran as a therapeutic option in the treatment of refractory depression: two case reports. Clin Neuropharmacol 2003; 26:230–232.
322. Izumi T, Inove T, Kitagawa N, et al. Open pergolide treatment of tricyclic and heterocyclic antidepressant-resistant depression. J Affect Disord 2000; 61: 127–132.
323. Lattanzi L, Dell'Osso L, Cassano P, et al. Pramipexole in treatment-resistant depression: a 16-week naturalistic study. Bipolar Disord 2002; 4:307–314.
324. Corrigan MH, Denahan AQ, Wright CE, et al. Comparison of pramipexole, fluoxetine, and placebo in patients with major depression. Depress Anxiety 2000; 11:58–65.
325. Goldberg JF, Burdick KE, Endick CJ. Preliminary randomized, double-blind, placebo-controlled trial of pramipexole added to mood stabilizers for treatment-resistant bipolar depression. Am J Psychiatry 2004; 161:564–566.
326. Zarate CA Jr, Payne JL, Singh J, et al. Pramipexole for bipolar II depression: a placebo-controlled proof of concept study. Biol Psychiatry 2004; 56:54–60.
327. Krupp LB, Coyle PK, Doscher C, et al. Fatigue therapy in multiple sclerosis: results of a double-blind, randomized, parallel trial of amantadine, pemoline, and placebo. Neurology 1995; 45:1956–1961.
328. Cincotta AH, Meieer AH. Bromocriptine (Ergoset) reduces body weight and improves glucose tolerance in obese subjects. Diabetes Care 1996; 19: 667–670.
329. Pijl H, Ohashi S, Matsuda M, et al. Bromocriptine: a novel approach to the treatment of type 2 diabetes. Diabetes Care 2000; 23:1154–1161.
330. Floris M, Lejeune J, Deberdt W. Effect of amantadine on weight gain during olanzapine treatment. Eur Neuropsychopharmacol 2001; 11:181–182.

331. Gracious BL, Krysiak TE, Youngstrom EA. Amantadine treatment of psychotropic-induced weight gain in children and adolescents: case series. J Child Adolesc Psychopharmacol 2002; 12:249–257.
332. Zubieta JK, Ketter TA, Bueller JA, et al. Regulation of human affective responses by anterior cingulated and limbic μ-opioid neurotransmission. Arch Gen Psychiatry 2003; 60:1145–1153.
333. deZwaan M, Mitchell JE. Opiate antagonists and eating behavior in humans: a review. J Clin Pharmacol 1992; 32:1061–1072.
334. Yeomans MR, Gray RW. Opioid peptides and the control of human ingestive behavior. Neurosci Biobeh Rev 2002; 26:713–728.
335. Malcom R, O'Neil PM, Sexauer JD, et al. A controlled trial of naltrexone in obese humans. Intl J Obes 1985; 9:347–353.
336. Atkinson RL, Berke LK, Drake CR, et al. Effects of long term therapy with, naltrexone on body weight in obesity. Clin Pharmacol Ther 1985; 38: 419–422.
337. Mitchell JE, Morley JE, Levine AS, et al. High dose naltrexone therapy and dietary counseling for obesity. Biol Psychiatry 1987; 22:35–42.
338. Mitchell GE, Christenson G, Jennings J, et al. A placebo-controlled, double-blind crossover study of naltrexone hydrochloride in outpatients with normal weight bulimia. J Clin Psychopharmacol 1989; 9:94–97.
339. Alger SA, Schwalberg MD, Bigaouette JM, et al. Effect of a tricyclic antidepressant and opiate antagonist on binge eating behavior in normoweight bulimic and obese, binge-eating subjects. Am J Clin Nutr 1991; 53:865–871.
340. Jonas JM, Gold MS. The use of opiate antagonists in treating bulimia: a study of low dose versus high dose naltrexone. Psychiatry Res 1988; 24:195–199.
341. Marrazzi MA, Markham KM, Kinzie J, et al. Binge eating disorder: response to naltrexone. Int J Obes Relat Metab Disord 1995; 19:143–145.
342. Raingeard I, Courtet P, Renard E, et al. Naltrexone improves blood glucose control in type 1 diabetic women with severe and chronic eating disorders. Diab Care 2004; 27:847–848.
343. Kim SW, Grant JE, Adson DE, et al. Double-blind naltrexone and placebo comparison study in the treatment of pathological gambling. Biol Psychiatry 2001; 49:914–921.
344. Sood ED, Pallanti S, Hollander E. Diagnosis and treatment of pathological gambling. Curr Psychiatry Rep 2003; 5:9–15.
345. Engwall D, Hunter R, Steinberg M. Gambling and other risk behaviors on university campuses. J Am Coll Health 2004; 52:245–255.
346. Brezezinski AA, Wurtman JJ, Wurtman RJ, et al. Dexfenfluramine suppresses the increased calorie and carbohydrate intake and improves the mood of women with premenstrual depression. Obstet Gynecol 1990; 76:296–301.
347. Murphy DL, Slater S, de la Vega CE, et al. The serotonergic neurotransmitter system in the affective disorders-a preliminary evaluation of the antidepressant and antimanic effects of fenfluramine. In: Deniker P, Radonco-Thomas C, Villeneuve A, eds. Neuropsychopharmacology. New York: Pergamon Press, 1978:675–682.
348. O'Rourke D, Wurtman JJ, Wurtman RJ, et al. Treatment of seasonal depression with d-fenfluramine. J Clin Psychiatry 1989; 50:343–347.

349. Blouin AG, Blouin JH, Perez EL, et al. Treatment of bulimia with fenfluramine and desipramine. J Clin Psychopharmacol 1988; 8:261–269.
350. Stunkard A, Berkowitz R, Tanrikut C, et al. d-Fenfluramine treatment of binge eating disorder. Am J Psychiatry 1996; 153:1455–1459.
351. Buckett WR, Thomas PL, Luscombe GP. The pharmacology of sibutramine hydrochloride (BTS 54 524), a new antidepressant which induces rapid noradrenergic down-regulation. Prog Neuro Psychopharmacol Biol Psychiatry 1988; 12:575–584.
352. Glick SD, Haskew RE, Maisonneuve IM, et al. Enantioselective behavioral effects of sibutramine metabolites. Eur J Pharmacol 2000; 397:93–102.
353. Appolinario JC, Bacaltchuk J, Sichieri R, et al. A randomized, double-blind, placebo-controlled study of sibutramine in the treatment of binge-eating disorder. Arch Gen Psychiatry 2003; 60:1109–1116.
354. Anghelescu I, Klawe C, Benkert O. Orlistat in the treatment of psychopharmacologically induced weight gain. J Clin Psychopharmacol 2000; 20:716–717.
355. Hilger E, Quiner S, Ginzel I, et al. The effect of orlistat on plasma levels of psychotropic drugs in patients with long-term psychopharmacotherapy. J Clin Psychopharmacol 2002; 22:68–70.
356. Schwartz TL, Jindal S, Simionescu M, et al. Effectiveness of orlistat versus diet and exercise for weight gain associated with antidepressant use: a pilot study. J Clin Psychopharmacol. 2004; 24:555–556.
357. Benazzi F. Depression induced by orlistat (xenical). Can J Psychiatry 2000; 45:87.
358. Fernandez-Aranda F, Amor A, Jimenez-Murcia S, et al. Bulimia nervosa and misuse of orlistat: two case reports. Int J Eat Disord 2001; 30:458–461.
359. Cochrane C, Malcolm R. Case report of abuse of orlistat. Eat Behav 2002; 3:167–169.
360. Malhotra S, McElroy SL. Orlistat misuse in bulimia nervosa. Am J Psychiatry 2002; 3:492–493.
361. Bauer M, Adli M, Baethge C, et al. Lithium augmentation therapy in refractory depression: clinical evidence and neurobiological mechanisms. Can J Psychiatry 2003; 48:440–448.
362. Wadden TA, Berkowitz RI, Sarwer DB, et al. Benefits of lifestyle modification in the pharmacologic treatment of obesity: a randomized trial. Arch Int Med 2001; 161:218–227.
363. Phelan S, Wadden TA. Combining behavioral and pharmacological treatments for oesity. Obes Res 2002; 10:560–574.
364. Keller MB, McCullough JP, Klein DN, et al. A comparison of nefazodone, the cognitive-behavioral analysis system of psychotherapy, and their combination for the treatment of chronic depression. N Engl J Med 2000; 342:1462–1470.
365. Hegerl V, Plattner A, Moller HJ. Should combined pharmaco-and psychotherapy be offered to depressed patients? Eur Arch Psychiatry Clin Neurosci 2004; 254:99–107.
366. Pampallona S, Bollini P, Tibaldi G, et al. Combined pharmacotherapy and psychological treatment for depression. A systematic review. Arch Gen Psychiatry 2004; 61:714–719.

367. Miklowitz DJ, George EL, Richards JA, et al. A randomized study of family focused psychoeducation and pharmacotherapy in the outpatient management of bipolar disorder. Arch Gen Psychiatry 2003; 60:904–912.
368. Colom F, Vieta E, Martinez-Aran A, et al. A randomized trial on the efficacy of group psychoeducation in the prophylaxis of recurrences in bipolar patients whose disease is in remission. Arch Gen Psychiatry 2003; 60:402–407.
369. Lam DH, Watkins ER, Hayward P, et al. A randomized controlled study of cognitive therapy for relapse prevention for bipolar affective disorder: outcome of the first year. Arch Gen Psychiatry 2003; 60:145–152.
370. Angst J, Gamma A, Benazzi F, et al. Toward a redefinition of subthreshold bipolarity: epidemiology and proposed criteria for bipolar II, minor bipolar disorders and hypomaaia. J Affect Disord 2003; 73:133–146.
371. Hirshfeld RMA, Williams JBW, Sptizer RL, et al. Development and validation of a screening instrument for bipolar spectrum disorder: the Mood Disorder Questionnaire. Am J Psychiatry 2000; 157:1873–1875.
372. Benazzi F. Toward better probing for hypomania of bipolar II disorder by using Angst's checklist. Int J Meth Psychiatr Res 2004; 13:1–9.
373. First MB, Spitzer RL, Gibbon M, et al. Structured Clinical Interview for the DSM-IV-TR Axis I Disorders Research Version Patient Edition (SCID I/P). New York, Biometrics Research Department, New York State Psychiatric Institute, 2001.
374. Yanovski SZ. A practical approach to treatment of the obese patient. Arch Fam Med 1993; 2:309–316.
375. Kaltsounis J, De Leon OA. Intravenous valproate treatment of severe manic symptoms after gastric bypass surgery: a case report. Psychosomatics 2000; 41:454–456.

17

Medical Management of Obesity and Binge Eating

Scott Crow

Department of Psychiatry, University of Minnesota,
Minneapolis, Minnesota, U.S.A.

Kerry Wangen

Department of Psychiatry, University of California–Irvine,
Orange, California, U.S.A.

Pharmacotherapy is an important aspect of treatment for individuals with obesity and binge eating. The extant literature regarding controlled trials of medications for the treatment of obesity and binge eating disorder (BED) has been reviewed in chapter 10. In this chapter, we lay the rationale for using pharmacologic approaches in the treatment of persons with obesity and binge eating, and make recommendations about treatment approaches.

Why consider medication management for the treatment of this illness? This is a reasonable question to ask. The majority of studies in this area (reflecting the rest of the eating disorders field) have involved psychotherapy treatments, and a number of manualized psychotherapies have shown good results in the treatment of BED. Similarly, behavioral weight loss therapy has also been shown to provide some benefit—not only for weight loss, but for binge eating. However, psychotherapeutic and behavioral weight loss approaches have substantial limitations, which necessitate the consideration of medication treatments. First, psychotherapeutic treatments are not widely available. Most psychotherapeutic treatments that have been studied for BED and those which are frequently advocated by experts in this field are highly specialized, manualized therapies of relatively short duration which appear to be rarely provided and difficult to find; this has clearly been proven true for bulimia nervosa, but is almost certainly true for BED as well (1). Treatments such as cognitive behavioral therapy or interpersonal therapy may be available in major metropolitan areas that contain an eating disorder specialty center, but they are certainly not widely available otherwise. Second, limitation of the existing psychotherapies for BED is that for the most part they result in little, if any, weight loss (2). This is problematic because both patients and their referring physicians are seeking weight loss in addition to control of binge eating behavior. Third, as has been described elsewhere, there is a high degree of comorbidity between binge eating and BED and other forms of psychopathology (3). Some of these common forms of psychopathology (particularly mild-to-moderate depression and anxiety) might be amenable to interventions such as cognitive behavioral therapy, but other relatively frequent forms may not respond to these psychotherapies, particularly severe depression, bipolar disorder, and substance abuse. Furthermore, even if specialized psychotherapies provide some benefit for the comorbid psychopathology, behavioral weight loss treatments would not. On the other hand, a number of pharmacologic agents discussed below have well-demonstrated efficacy in the treatment of various types of comorbid psychopathology. For all these reasons, the clinician may well consider pharmacotherapy.

APPROACH TO THE PATIENT WITH BINGE EATING DISORDER

The approach to pharmacologic treatment of BED is similar to that typically used in the treatment of other psychiatric illness, with some exceptions. First among these is the paramount importance of making treatment goals explicit. For example, when a patient presents for treatment of depression, both patient and treating physician are in agreement about the goal of pharmacotherapy: the relief of target depressive symptoms. On the other hand, in the treatment of BED, there are at least two common goals: relief of binge eating symptoms and weight loss. It is our clinical impression that not only is weight loss an extremely common goal, but that for many patients, weight loss is the preferred goal of treatment, over and above cessation of binge eating. Likewise, if the referring professional is a primary care physician or medical subspecialist, weight loss goals may be particularly important in achieving metabolic benefits.

As discussed in chapter 10, a number of agents have demonstrated efficacy for decreasing binge eating symptoms, in selected instances, and also weight loss. The selection of appropriate agents depends to a substantial degree on the overall clinical situation, as described later.

Obese Patients with Binge Eating, Without Other Prominent Psychopathology

The broadest range of potential options exists for those with binge eating and obesity who are without other psychopathology in need of pharmacotherapy. For this group, all the "psychiatric" and "weight loss" medications described in chapters 12 and 13 may play a role. A critical decision point in choosing between these types of medications involves assessing the urgency of associated weight loss (either in the eyes of the patient or his/her medical provider). When weight loss is a prominent goal, appetite suppressant medications such as sibutramine, phentermine, or perhaps topiramate may be an optimal starting point for treatment. With the treatment of obesity, a critical part of initiating treatment is clarifying the rate at which weight loss can be expected for patients. In our experience, this can be even more important in the treatment of BED because patients often assume that the cessation of binge eating will itself resolve in marked weight loss; clinically, this rarely true.

Obese Individuals with Binge Eating and Other Psychopathology

Comorbid psychopathology is extremely common in BED, even in community samples not seeking treatment, and is still higher in those seeking treatment. Thus, it will be quite routine to address binge eating in the context of other psychiatric problems. Fortunately, as reviewed in chapter 10, a number of medications with demonstrated efficacy for binge eating were first developed and have been widely studied for the treatment of many of these common comorbidities, so at times pharmacologic treatments in this setting can target multiple symptom domains. Pertinent areas are described below.

MOOD AND ANXIETY DISORDERS

Many of the psychotropic agents previously studied in BED generally have well recognized antidepressant and anxiolytic effects. Major depression, dysthymia, and various anxiety disorders frequently co-occur with BED. When BED and either a depressive or an anxiety disorder are present, a rational approach involves the selection of a drug known to have both anti-binge eating and antidepressant and/or anxiolytic effects. Practically speaking, this leaves the clinician with the choice of several serotonin selective reuptake inhibitors (SSRIs) (e.g., fluoxetine, sertraline, fluvoxamine, citalopram, or escitalopram) or the tricyclic (TCA) antidepressant desipramine (DMI). For most clinicians, DMI would be a rare choice due to diminishing familiarity with this and the other TCAs, as well as a higher side effect burden, including a somewhat elevated (though much lower with DMI than with other TCAs) risk of weight gain. Appropriate dosing of the SSRIs for BED is not clearly defined. Higher doses of fluoxetine (i.e., 60 mg/day) are widely viewed as the pharmacologic standard of treatment for bulimia nervosa and many experts would strive to achieve similarly high doses for BED. It seems reasonable to think that such high doses may be more effective in treating BED, but data to clearly answer this question are lacking.

One important consideration in the use of these antidepressant and anxiolytic drugs in the treatment of BED is the issue of weight loss. As noted above, weight loss is an extremely common treatment goal for patients, yet a major frustration in previous treatment trials for BED is that psychotropic agents that have shown good efficacy for binge eating have generally shown little if any positive impact on weight. It seems prudent, then, to try to combine psychotropic treatment with a well-designed behavioral weight loss program, although the efficacy of such combination treatment in patients with BED has not yet been shown. Also, whether patients will comply with such interventions over lengthy periods of time is somewhat questionable.

PSYCHOTIC AND BIPOLAR DISORDERS

The treatment of bipolar disorder has particularly seen marked change over the last decade with the identification of multiple new effective mood stabilizers and the introduction of a whole new generation of antipsychotics with much broader spectrums of action, both in terms of targeted symptoms and in terms of the number of individuals for whom these drugs show efficacy. Even though the numbers of patients affected with BED and comorbid bipolar or psychotic disorders may be relatively small compared with depressive disorders, these conditions may co-occur more than once expected (4,5). Moreover, many of the new agents used to treat bipolar and psychotic disorders have marked effects on body weight and on eating behavior. The mechanisms by which these drugs affect weight are likely diverse and may include diminished resting metabolic rate, increased food intake, change in macronutrient choice, and for some individuals "carbohydrate craving" and perhaps frank binge eating behavior (5). Such effects may inadvertently have an adverse impact on individuals who have binge eating.

There is good evidence to suggest that primary care physicians rarely inquire about binge eating and it seems rather unlikely that psychiatrists do so with much higher frequency (6). It has been common to suggest that changes in eating behavior or weight induced by these psychotropic drugs should be treated by routine behavioral weight loss interventions, but existing evidence suggests that these interventions are neither particularly well suited nor effective for such individuals (7). Therefore, scrupulous avoidance of weight gain in this population is critical. The selection of agents with limited risk for weight gain such as ziprasidone, aripiprazole, or perhaps risperidone may be preferable to agents with high rates of weight gain, particularly olanzapine or clozapine.

DURATION OF TREATMENT FOR BINGE EATING

The course of binge eating is somewhat unclear. On one hand, individuals seeking treatment in controlled trials in the U.S. have a typical duration of illness of roughly two decades, indicating that this is a highly stable chronic condition (2). On the other hand, studies of persons with BED from the community have suggested that the symptoms are somewhat less stable (8,9). Adding to this confusion is the fact that most controlled trials of pharmacotherapy for BED have had a duration of only a few months, which is almost certainly less than the optimal length of treatment for this condition. Finally, community-based effectiveness studies of pharmacologic (or other) treatment for BED of some sort needed to definitively answer this question do not exist. Thus, one is left attempting to generalize from pharmacologic treatment studies for weight loss, bulimia nervosa, and perhaps for major depression.

One clear source of information on treatment duration evolves from the body of literature reviewed in chapter 10 regarding pharmacologic treatment for obesity. There is increasing acceptance of the concept that long-term pharmacologic treatment is needed in order to achieve long-term positive benefits for obesity, and that one would expect a cessation of treatment benefit for most patients when pharmacologic treatment ceases. For weight-related aspects of BED treatment, this almost certainly holds true. On the other hand, achieving the goal of binge eating cessation may not require such truly long-term treatment; in fact, the literature on bulimia nervosa treatment suggests that treatments longer than a few months are needed but that chronic or lifelong treatment is typically not necessary. In studies that have compared the clinical course of bulimia nervosa with BED, BED participants have generally been more prone toward symptom remission than those with BN, so perhaps somewhat shorter term treatment may be reasonable for BED (9). Finally, many treatments employed for BED would also be selected (as reviewed above) for their antidepressant and/or anxiolytic effects. Here, again, there is much more consensus about the need for longer and at times lifelong treatment.

How then to summarize this literature? For BED not complicated by comorbid psychopathology where the major target is cessation of binge eating, a medication trial of approximately one year followed by taper and careful observation seems reasonable. For individuals with BED where treatment of obesity is an important additional focus, longer term pharmacotherapy will probably provide the best clinical result; in this case, duration of pharmacologic treatment would proceed very much as it typically would in the treatment of uncomplicated obesity. Finally, when comorbid psychopathology is an additional major treatment goal, the need for pharmacologic treatment for the comorbid mood or anxiety disorder may long exceed the duration of the eating disorder symptoms. If one has selected an agent with both anti-binge eating and antidepressant (or anxiolytic) effects, those treatments may be required long beyond the effective resolution of the binge eating symptoms.

REFERENCES

1. Crow SJ, Mussell MP, Peterson CB, Mitchell JE, Knopke A. Adequacy of prior treatment in patients with bulimia nervosa. Int J Eat Disord 1999; 25(1):39–44.
2. Wonderlich SA, de Zwaan M, Mitchell JE, Peterson CB, Crow SJ. Psychological and dietary treatments for binge eating disorder: conceptual implications. Int J Eat Disord 2003; 24(suppl):S58–S73.
3. Mussell M, Mitchell J, deZwaan M, Crosby R, Crow S. Clinical characteristics associated with binge eating in obese females: A descriptive study. Int J Obesity 1996; 20(4):324–331.
4. Kruger S, Shugar G, Cooke RG. Comorbidity of binge eating disorder and the partial binge eating syndrome with bipolar disorder. Int J Eat Disord 1996; 19:45–52.
5. Thiesen FM, Linden A, König IR, Martin M, Remschmidt H, Hebebrand J. Spectrum of binge eating symptomatology in patients treated with clozapine and olanzapine. J Neural Transm 2003; 110:111–121.
6. Crow SJ, Peterson CB, Levine AS, Thuras P, Mitchell JE. A survey of obesity treatment practices among primary care providers. Int J Eat Disord 2004; 35: 348–353.
7. Ball MP, Coons VB, Buchanan RW. A program for treating olanzapine-related weight gain. Psychiatr Serv 2001; 52:967–969.
8. Fitchter MM, Quadflieg N, Gnutzmann A. Binge eating disorder: Treatment outcome over a 6-year course. J Psychosom Res 1998; 44:385–405.
9. Fairbum CG, Cooper Z, Doll HA, Norman P, O'Connor M. The natural course of bulimia nervosa and binge eating disorder in young women. Arch Gen Psychiatry 2000; 57:659–665.

18

Weight Loss Surgery for the Treatment of Morbid Obesity

Reena Bhargava, Calvin Selwyn, and Keith S. Gersin
*Division of GI and Endocrine Surgery, Department of Bariatric Surgery,
University of Cincinnati School of Medicine, Cincinnati, Ohio, U.S.A.*

INTRODUCTION

Obesity is a multifactorial disease process influenced by genetics, culture, economics, and psychological issues (1). There are various degrees of obesity ranging from overweight to morbidly obese (Table 1). The notion that obesity represents a failure of individual willpower is unscientific and prejudicial. Identification of effective obesity treatment modalities continues to challenge clinicians, researchers, and industry. Results from the American National Health and Nutrition Examination Survey demonstrate that approximately 65% of Americans aged 20 years of age or older are overweight [body mass index (BMI) > 25] and 31% are obese or morbidly obese (2). Among American children and adolescents, 21% to 24% are overweight and 10% to 11% are obese or morbidly obese (3). The costs of obesity are enormous as between 2% and 8% of health care expenditures are for obesity-related diseases (4). In 1990, there were 300,000 deaths annually attributable to obesity. This number has increased to 320,000–400,000 obesity related deaths in 2004 (5,6). Obesity now ranks above tobacco use as an adverse health indicator and is second only to cigarette smoking as a cause of preventable death in the United States (6).

Current modalities for the treatment of morbid obesity include dietary modification, exercise, pharmacologic intervention, and surgery. Surgical

Table 1 Obesity Classification. Weight Loss Surgery Is Offered to Those with a BMI of ≥40 or ≥35 if Comorbidities Are Present

	Obesity class	BMI (kg/m^2)
Underweight		<18.5
Normal		18.5–24.9
Overweight		25.0–29.9
Obesity	I	30.0–34.9
	II	35.0–35.9
Extreme obesity	III	≥40.0

Abbreviation: BMI, body mass index.

intervention has been offered to those patients who are refractory to non-surgical methods of weight loss and who have a BMI ≥ 40 (Fig. 1) or ≥35 if comorbidities are present. In 1991, the National Institutes of Health consensus conference concluded that changes in behavior, diet, pharmacologic intervention, and education have proven relatively ineffective as long-term weight loss treatments, and that surgery is currently the most effective and durable weight loss method (6). The American Society for Bariatric Surgery (ASBS) estimates that more than 144,000 patients will have bariatric surgery in 2004—an increase from 2002 when 67,000 patients underwent gastric bypass for treatment of morbid obesity (7).

HISTORY

Obesity surgery stems from surgical weight loss identified in patients who underwent gastric and small bowel resections for treatment of diseases other than morbid obesity. Weight loss procedures have been performed based on malabsorptive techniques, restrictive techniques, and a combination of

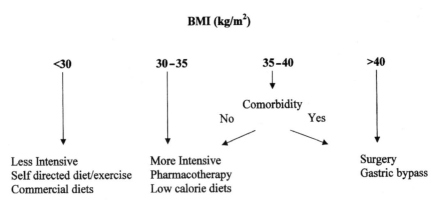

Figure 1 Treatments for obesity based on BMI. *Abbreviation*: BMI, body mass index.

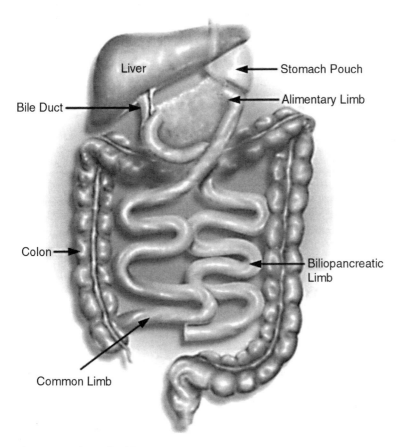

Figure 2 Jejuno–ileal bypass.

both. Early attempts at weight loss procedures based on properties of malabsorption did so via shortening the length of the digestive tract through which food was absorbed (8,9). The jejuno–ileal bypass was effective in achieving weight loss from the bypass of significant lengths of small bowel (Fig. 2). Although effective in achieving weight loss, several complications of malabsorption ensued, including socially limiting diarrhea, vitamin and protein deficiencies, arthritis, renal failure, liver failure, and death (7,10). These early malabsorptive operations should no longer be performed for surgical weight loss. If recognized, they should be reversed or converted to acceptable weight loss procedures (7,10).

In the 1960s gastric bypass surgery was pioneered by Dr. Edward Mason at the University of Iowa, emerging from observations of sustained weight loss after gastric ulcer surgery and stomach resection (7). This procedure offered both components of weight loss surgery that have been

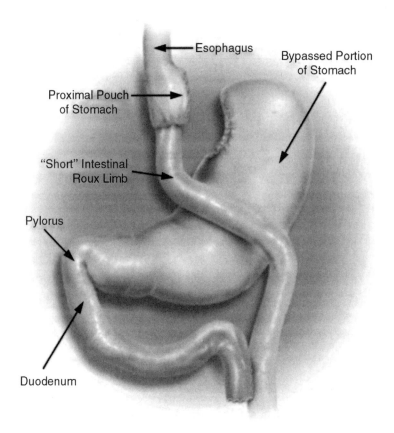

Figure 3   Roux-en-Y gastric bypass.

previously used singularly: malabsorption and restriction. The complications from this Roux-en-Y gastric bypass (RNYGB) were less than those
reported from the earlier performed jejuno–ileal bypass and specifically
did not include the severe malabsorptive side effects (Fig. 3) (7,11).

In 1982 vertical banded gastroplasty (VBG) was introduced (Fig. 4)
(12). VBG is a restrictive procedure limiting caloric intake by reducing food
volume. The benefit of purely restrictive procedures is that, unlike their
malabsorptive counterparts, there is a decreased likelihood of nutritional
deficiencies, since nutrient absorption is unaffected by the restrictive component of the surgery. Although effective in achieving weight loss, patients are
counseled to avoid ingesting high calorie liquids because doing so may lead
to weight loss failures. Indeed, VBG has fallen out of favor due to inferior
long-term weight loss as compared with RNYGB (13).

The first laparoscopic RNYGB was reported by Wittgrove et al. (14)
in 1994. The advent of minimally invasive surgical techniques has helped

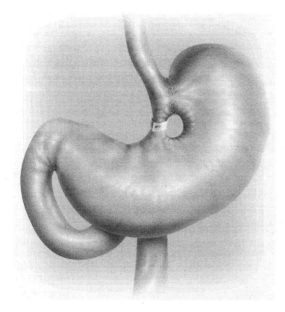

Figure 4 Vertical banded gastroplasty.

place laparoscopic surgery at the forefront of bariatric surgery. Complex procedures, once performed with large incisions, are now being performed laparoscopically with equal safety and efficacy (15). Moreover, patients may benefit from minimally invasive RNYGB due to decreased postoperative pain, a decrease in the frequency of iatrogenic splenectomies, fewer wound complications, shorter hospital lengths of stay, and an overall decrease in mortality (Table 2) (15–17).

Laparoscopic adjustable banding was approved for use by the United States Food and Drug Administration in 1991 (18). Analogous to VBG, this is a restrictive procedure which involves placement of an inflatable silastic cuff around the upper portion of the stomach (Fig. 5). The inflatable band is adjusted on an outpatient basis via saline injection through a subcutaneously accessed port. Patients are advised that weight loss may be less than that reported with RNYGB (47.5% vs. 61.6%. respectively) (19). Complications of band erosion and slippage have been reduced with improved techniques in band placement (20).

SURGICAL CRITERIA

Bariatric surgery, despite the dramatic effects on appearance, is not a cosmetic procedure and should not be performed for this indication. Indications for surgical weight loss are for the improvement or resolution

Table 2 A Comparison of Randomized and Cohort Studies for Laparoscopic Versus Open RNYGB

Parameter	Author				
	Lujan/Spain	Nguyen/US	Schauer	Biertho	DeMaria
Study type	Randomized	Randomized	Cohort	Cohort	Cohort
Approach	Lap/Open	Lap/Open	Lap	Lap	Lap
Operative time	186 vs. 202[a]	225 vs. 195[a]	260	–	198
Conversion	5%	2.5%	1.1%	2.0%	2.8%
Early morbidity	23% vs. 29%	7.6% vs. 9.2%	3.3%	4.2%	7.1%[c]
Late morbidity	11% vs. 24%[a]	18.9% vs. 15.2%	18.9%	8.1%	16.4%[c]
LOS (menu)	5.2 vs. 7.9[a]	4.0 vs. 8.4[a]	3.6	3.0[b]	4.0
BMT range	36–80 kg/m^2	40–60 kg/m^2	35–68 kg/m^2	27–77 kg/m^2	40–71 kg/m^2

Mean operative time in minutes; LOS, in days.
[a]Significant difference ($p < 0.05$) between laparoscopic and open.
[b]Median LOS.
[c]Extrapolated from separated morbidity data.
Abbreviation: RNYGB, Roux-en-Y gastric bypass.
Source: From Ref. 27.

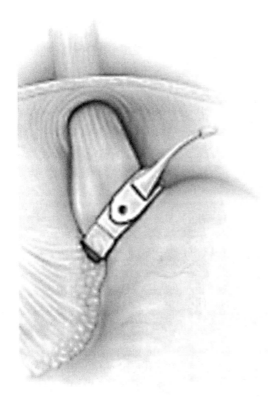

Figure 5 Laparoscopic adjustable banding.

of comorbid adverse health conditions present in many morbidly obese people. The term "morbid obesity" was developed to describe the significant morbidity associated with severe obesity including diabetes, sleep apnea, venous stasis, heart failure, deep venous thrombosis, pulmonary emboli, hypertension, degenerative arthritis, gallstones, hernias, and an increased incidence of ovarian, breast, prostate, and colon cancer (21). Candidates for bariatric surgery have a BMI of ≥35 in the presence of comorbidities or a BMI of ≥40 in the absence of comorbidities (7). Individuals with a BMI less than 35 are counseled on nonsurgical methods of weight loss such as pharmacologic intervention, dietary modification, exercise, and psychotherapy.

SURGICAL RISKS

The risk of maintaining oneself in a morbidly obese state needs to be weighed against the risks of bariatric surgery which is a major operation whether performed laparoscopically or open. Those individuals who are

Table 3 Comparison of Major Complications After Laparoscopic Versus Open RNYGB Complications

Complications	Laparoscopic GBP ($n = 79$)	Open GBP ($n = 76$)	p value
Gastrointestinal			
Anastomotic leak	1	1	
Gastric pouch outlet obstruction	0	1	
Hypopharyngeal perforation	1	0	
Jejunojejunostomy obstruction	3	0	
Pulmonary			
Pulmonary embolism	0	1	
Respiratory failure	0	1	
Gastrointestinal bleeding	1	0	
Wound infection	0	2	
Retained laparotomy sponge	0	1	
Total	6 (7.6%)	7 (9.2%)	.78[a]

[a]Fisher exact tests.
Abbreviation: RNYGB, Roux-en-Y gastric bypass; GBP, gastric bypass.
Source: From Ref. 26.

at increased risk for any elective surgical procedure are not candidates for weight loss surgery and may include those with prohibitive cardiorespiratory disease. Risks are stratified into those occurring early (within 24–48 hours) and those occurring late (after 48 hours). Early risks include gastric leaks, bleeding, and pulmonary emboli, whereas later risks include infection, anastomotic stricture, and obstructions (Table 3). The overall morbidity resulting from bariatric surgery is 9.6% to 10% and the resultant mortality has been reported as 0.1% to 1.5% (4,19,22,23). Improved outcomes are realized in the setting of experienced bariatric surgeons in conjunction with a qualified bariatric team composed of surgeons, dieticians, exercise physiologists, and mental health professionals (24,25).

CONCLUSION

Bariatric surgery is one of several options for morbidly obese individuals seeking weight loss. Current data suggests marked improvement in co-morbidities from resultant weight loss. Although improved cosmesis may result of surgical weight loss, it should not be the criteria for which surgery is performed. Appropriate patient education includes dietary counseling, support group counseling, and preoperative psychological evaluation, exercise, and pulmonary evaluation, as well as lifelong surgical follow-up. A well-educated patient and established bariatric team is imperative for successful outcomes. The decision to undergo weight loss surgery should be made after consideration of all weight loss options and should involve patients, families, and clinicians.

REFERENCES

1. Obesity and Genetics: A public health perspective (February 2002) Center for Disease Control and Prevention.
2. (NHANES) National Health & Nutrition Examination survey 1990–2000.
3. Trioano RP, Flegel KM. Overweight children and adolescents: description, epidemiology and demographics. Pediatrics 1998; 101:497–504.
4. Gastrointestinal Surgery for Severe Obesity. NDH Consens Statement 1991 March 25–27; 9(1):1–20.
5. Allison DB, Fontaine KR, Manson JE, Stevens J, Vanltallie TB. Annual deaths attributable to obesity in the United States. JAMA 1999; 282(16):1530–1538.
6. Prevalence of Overweight and Obesity Among Adults: United States, 1999–2002: National Center for Health Statistics, CDC.
7. MacGregor A, MD, CME director, ASBS, 2000.
8. Buchwald H, Williams SE. Bariatric surgery worldwide 2003. Obes Surg 2004; 14(9):1157–1164.
9. Buchwarld H, Buchwald JN. Evolution of operative procedures for the management of morbid obesity 1950–2000.
10. Griffen WO Jr, Bivins BA, Bell RM. The decline and fall of the jejunoileal bypass. Surg Gynecol Obstet 1983; 157(4):301–308.
11. Hocking MP, Davis GL, Franzini DA, Woodward ER. Long-term consequences after jejunoileal bypass for morbid obesity. Dig Dis Sci 1998; 43(11): 2493–2499.
12. Mason EE. Vertical banded gastroplasty for obesity. Arch Surg 1982; 117(5): 701–706.
13. Sugerman HJ, Kellum JM Jr, DeMaria EJ, Reines HD. Conversion of failed or complicated vertical banded gastroplasty to gastric bypass in morbid obesity. Am J Surg 1996; 171(2):263–269.
14. Higa KD, Boone KB, Ho T, Davies OG. Laparoscopic Roux-en-Y gastric bypass for morbid obesity. Arch Surg 2000; 135:1029–1033.
15. Wittgrove AC, Clark GW, Schubert KR. Laparoscopic gastric bypass, Roux-en-Y: Technique and result in 75 patients with 3–30 months follow-up. Obes Surg 1996; 6(6):500–504.
16. Podnos YD, Jimenez JC, Wilson SE, Stevens CM, Nguyen NT. Complications after laparoscopic gastric bypass: a review of 346 cases. Arch Surg 2003; 138(9): 95–61.
17. Fried M, Peskova M, Kasalicky M. The role of laparoscopy in the treatment of morbid obesity. Obes Surg 1998; 8(5):520–523.
18. Ren CJ, Weiner M, Allen JW. Favorable early results of gastric banding for morbid obesity: the American experience. Surg Endosc 2004; 18(3):543–546. Epub 2004 Feb 02.
19. Buchwald H, Avidor Y, Braunwald E, Jensen MD, Pories W, Fahrbach Schoelles K. Bariatric surgery: a systematic review and meta-analysis. JAMA 2004; 292(14):1724–1737.

20. Nehoda H, Hourmont K, Sauper T, et al. Laparoscopic gastric banding in older patients. Arch Sug 2001; 136:1171–1176.
21. Lara MD, Kothari SN, Sugerman HJ. Surgical management of obesity: a review of the evidence relative to the health benefits and risks. Treat Endocrinol 2005; 4(1):55–64.
22. Livingston EH. Procedure incidence and in-hospital complication rates of bariatric surgery in the United States. Am J Surg 2004; 188(2):105–110.
23. Fernandez AZ Jr, Demaria EJ, Thicansky DS, et al. Multivariate analysis of risk factors for death following gastric bypass for treatment of morbid obesity. Ann Surg 2004; 239(5):698–702; discussion 702–703.
24. Nguyen NT, Moore C, Stevens CM, Chalifoux S, Mavandadi S, Wilson S. The practice of bariatric surgery at academic medical centers. J Gastrointest Surg 2004; 8(7):856–860; discussion 860.
25. Wadden TA, Sarwer DB, Womble LG, Foster GD, McGuckin BG, Schimmel A. Psychosocial aspects of obesity and obesity surgery. Surg Clin North Am 2001; 81(5):1001–1024.
26. Nguyen NT, Goldman C, Rosenquist CJ, et al. Laparoscopic versus open gastric bypass: A randomized study of outcomes, quality of life, and costs. Ann Surg 2001; 234(3):279–291.
27. Brolin RE. Laparoscopic versus open gastric bypass to treat morbid obesity. Ann Surg 2004; 239(4):438–440.

19

The Role of Bariatric Surgery in the Obese Patient with Psychopathology

James E. Mitchell, Tricia Cook Myers,
and Lorraine Swan-Kremeier

*Neuropsychiatric Research Institute, University of North Dakota
School of Medicine and Health Sciences Department of Clinical Neuroscience,
University of Erlangen, Erlangen, Germany*

Martina de Zwaan

*Department of Psychosomatic Medicine,
University of Erlangen, Erlangen, Germany*

INTRODUCTION

As has been widely recognized in the media in recent years, overweight and obesity have become increasingly important public health concerns, and currently the majority of adults in the United States are overweight or obese (1,2). This problem is not confined to the United States, as it is clear that obesity is a growing public health problem around the world. While the reasons for this are complex and while adult body weight is to a certain extent heritable, the crucial variables in this change appear to be the increasing availability of highly palatable energy-dense food and the lack of exercise. Basically, the increase in the amount of energy intake has not been balanced by an increase in physical activity. Therefore, this imbalance in the "energy in/energy out" equation has resulted in this marked increase in problems with weight (3–6).

As obesity becomes more common, and as the modest efficacy of behavioral and pharmacological approaches available to us has been repeatedly demonstrated, bariatric surgery has increasingly been used as a means of treatment for obesity. Such procedures were performed rarely prior to 20 years ago, but the number of procedures has escalated dramatically and probably will continue to do so, owing not only to the increasing rate of obesity but also to the increasing safety and efficacy of the bariatric surgery approaches now available (7). As the utilization of bariatric surgery increases, the number of individuals who present for bariatric surgery who have psychiatric conditions will likewise increase, and given the marked demands placed on bariatric surgery recipients to modify their behavior and lifestyle, there have been growing concerns about the ability of some individuals, given their psychopathology, to adapt to such changes. The purpose of this chapter is to address the question of the role of bariatric surgery in obese patients with psychopathology. We will attempt to do this by covering six areas:

1. What are the psychopathological contraindications to the use of the bariatric surgery?
2. How should bariatric surgery candidates be screened for psychopathology?
3. What are the rates of psychopathology among bariatric surgery candidates?
4. What is the impact of bariatric surgery on psychopathology rates at follow-up?
5. What is the impact of presurgery psychopathology on outcome of bariatric surgery?
6. How can comorbid psychopathology be treated to insure a better response and long-term outcome following bariatric surgery procedures?

PSYCHOPATHOLOGY CONTRAINDICATIONS

The psychopathological contraindications to bariatric surgery remain controversial (8). Part of this is attributable to the fact that as procedures have been performed on a wider variety of patients it has become apparent that many patients with significant comorbid psychopathology or other cognitive abnormalities often do quite well with the surgery given the proper support and encouragement. Nonetheless, most bariatric surgery programs would agree that the following constitutes a list of probable contraindications:

1. *Dementia.* Patients with dementing illness, most of whom are elderly, should not be considered as candidates for bariatric surgery procedures in most situations. There are several reasons for

this. First, it would be difficult for such individuals to truly give informed consent. Second, even the least invasive procedures, such as the LapBand, require significant modifications in dietary behavior and are accompanied by significant unavoidable pain and discomfort. For these reasons, it seems unethical to perform such procedures on these patients. In addition, demented patients' capacity to cooperate with proper aftercare is clearly marginal at best. Also, many patients with dementia are at risk for problems such as aspiration pneumonia, which may be more of a problem postoperatively given the changes in intake patterns necessitated by the surgery. The issue of bariatric surgery in patients with dementia rarely arises, however, since most demented patients have problems achieving adequate energy intake rather than being over-weight. These guidelines, though, would apply to dementia from a variety of causes, including dementing-like syndromes in patients post-head trauma.

2. *A developmental disability.* Individuals with significant cognitive limitation, particularly those with severe mental retardation, clearly are not candidates for bariatric surgery for some of the reasons that are outlined earlier. What the exact cutoff should be in terms of intelligence is unclear. Some patients with marginal intelligence appear to be able to give informed consent and adapt adequately to post-bariatric surgery demands. There have been case reports of individuals with Prader Willi Syndrome (PWS) having undergone bariatric surgery, given the hazards of the extreme obesity associated with this condition (9). Bariatric surgery appears to be an option to consider for the management of obesity in PWS, particularly in patients with higher IQs. Therefore, mental retardation is not an absolute contraindication to bariatric surgery, but dependent on the practical ability of the patient to give informed consent and to cooperate with aftercare.

3. *Psychoses.* Generally patients with persistent psychotic disorders that are unremitting, such as those with chronic schizophrenia, would not be considered candidates for bariatric surgery, again, given the demands of aftercare and the changes that are necessitated in eating behavior. However, following the introduction of atypical antipsychotics, which allow some patients with schizophrenia to function at a much higher social level than was possible previously, a chronic psychotic disorder should probably no longer be regarded as an absolute contraindication.

Indeed, we know that obesity is very common among patients with schizophrenia, and as mentioned, some will function very well on stable doses of atypical antipsychotics and appear to be able to give informed consent and cooperate with aftercare.

Thus, this is an area that appears now to be a relative contraindication, which needs a careful evaluation in each case.

Individuals who have illnesses that present intermittently with psychotic features, such as psychotic depression, bipolar disorder, or other periodic but transient psychoses, certainly can be considered for these procedures if their illness is in remission. However, this raises interesting problems concerning medication regimens around the time of surgery, the possible precipitation of psychoses postoperatively (which is a period of great stress), and the need for careful psychiatric monitoring and input in the pre- and postsurgical management of these patients.

4. *Active substance abuse/dependence.* Most centers would say that patients who are actively abusing alcohol or drugs would not be candidates for bariatric surgery. Again, there are several reasons for this. First is the possibility of an untoward outcome, given the possibility of withdrawal symptoms or the emergence of frank delirium tremens in alcohol dependent patients in the postoperative period, which would markedly increase both the morbidity and mortality associated with the procedure. There obviously are also concerns about these individuals' ability to cooperate with proper aftercare and to make the necessary dietary changes. A third concern is their longevity, in that such patients are seen as a risk for a variety of untoward medical complications without surgery and these complications may be enhanced through exposure to general anesthesia, major surgery, and the demands for major lifestyle changes. However, it is clear that some patients who have had active substance abuse problems have undergone bariatric surgery successfully and probably many patients who have had such problems actively deny them at the time of evaluation so as not to discourage the surgeon from accepting them as a surgical candidate (10). A criterion of a period of at least six months of abstinence might be required as a useful period to demonstrate sobriety and ability to not use substances and to be able to cooperate with aftercare.

5. *Adolescents and children.* Although age less than 18 years was long considered a contraindication, older adolescents are increasingly being considered for bariatric surgery, particularly for the more easily reversible interventions such as gastric banding (11–14).

6. *Other problems.* The last category basically includes anyone who for any reasons is not able to give informed consent and/or cooperate in the aftercare necessary postoperatively. Possible categories here would include patients with severe intractable seizure disorders, patients with severe somatoform disorders who would be at high risk for major adjustment problems and medical complaints postoperatively, and individuals with severe treatment

resistant obsessive–compulsive disorder, whose ritualistic behavior and obsessionality may make it impossible for them to be actively involved in their own aftercare. Another possibility would be individuals with severe personality disorders such as borderline personality characterized by self-injurious behavior. To operate on such patients might result in unpredictable psychological decompensation and also expose the surgical team to the risk of a variety of adverse complications that are best avoided.

SCREENING BARIATRIC SURGERY CANDIDATES FOR PSYCHOPATHOLOGY

Practices vary widely across bariatric surgery programs in terms of what is required or expected in terms of psychological assessment. Options vary from no requirements to a series of self-report questions asked as part of standard intake, either in written form or as part of the interview, through an in-depth psychosocial assessment by a mental health professional skilled in working with bariatric surgery patients, including psychological testing. At times, the depth of the evaluation will depend on insurance requirements rather than on any particular bias on behalf of the bariatric surgery group. For example, a number of third party payers in the United States require that a psychosocial assessment be done by a mental health practitioner before patients can undergo bariatric surgery procedures. In some clinics this is routine practice, regardless of third party payer requirements. In other clinics, it is optional depending on the observations that the members of the surgical team have made of the patient, or to the patients' responses on self-report measures or interview. Upon reflection, it is interesting that third party payers would require a psychosocial assessment for bariatric procedures when they indeed do not require such assessments for patients receiving any other type of surgery. However, many surgeries are not elective, as are bariatric surgery procedures. Nonetheless, the requirement for psychosocial assessment by some insurance companies may reflect a long held bias that these are particularly "dangerous" procedures for patients with significant psychopathology.

Nevertheless, given that rates of psychopathology are high in the general population and may be elevated in the severely obese, and given that bariatric surgery does impact significantly long term on a variety of behaviors necessitating marked changes in individuals' routines and eating behaviors, it would seem that a psychosocial evaluation is highly desirable and occasionally critical. The question then becomes how best to obtain this evaluation in the most cost effective manner. Before turning to specific data gathering techniques, it is important to remember one variable that characterizes patients undergoing a psychosocial assessment when they are a candidate for bariatric surgery: most are very desirous of having the procedure, and are very alert to the possibility that certain things they might say might dissuade the surgeon, the third party payor, or the health care team from approving them for the procedure. Therefore, if they have had or currently have certain psychiatric problems there will be a tendency for the patient to either downplay their severity or not to mention them at all. This has been shown previously in research, where patients retrospectively, after they have had the surgery, will admit to having had psychiatric problems that they initially had denied prior to the surgery (10). Because of this, any information obtained from the patient must be considered carefully in terms of its importance.

PSYCHIATRIC INTERVIEW

The psychosocial assessment is designed to obtain detailed information about any comorbid psychiatric problems, as well as information about weight history, previous weight loss attempts, social support, and other environmental circumstances which might impact outcome. Usually, the patient will be seeing the clinician as a requirement of the bariatric surgery team and will be somewhat guarded and concerned about the implications of the interview. Therefore, it is best at the beginning to lay out what will transpire, and what sorts of problems might lead the interviewer to recommend that the candidate not undergo the procedure, or at least have it postponed until some sort of psychological intervention can be introduced, and to indicate what information will and will not be shared with the team. In particular, it is important to state that if the patient has active problems with alcohol or substance abuse, or has been having certain psychotic symptoms, that this would make it difficult for them to adhere to the required changes after the surgery. Therefore, it would be in their best interest to share such information with the interviewer so that a treatment plan could be outlined. Generally, a forthright statement of these problems at the beginning will result in more reliable data gathering than attempting to "sneak up" on the patient through questioning.

A second data gathering strategy that can be useful is the use of a self-report standardized database which the patient can complete prior to being seen for evaluation. Such databases include detailed questioning about current or previous psychosocial problems. Examples include the "Eating Disorder Questionnaire" developed by our group and the "Weight and Lifestyle Inventory" developed by Wadden and Foster (15,16). Patients can be mailed such forms and asked to complete them in advance and bring them to the clinic appointment, providing the clinician with considerable background information before the interview. Obtaining data in this way assures that the clinician can focus the interview on particular points of concern.

A number of clinics find it useful to include certain standardized psychometric instruments as part of the evaluation process to provide further information about psychosocial issues. These may include the following:

1. *Questionnaire on eating and weight patterns-revised (QEWP-R)* (17). This is a 28-item scale designed to assess the presence or absence of binge eating and binge eating disorder (BED).
2. *Social functioning-36 (SF-36)* (18). This instrument measures eight areas of social functioning; it is one of the most widely used quality of life measures. Areas assessed include physical functioning, role physical, bodily pain, general health, vitality, social functioning, role emotional, and mental health.
3. *Beck depression inventory (BDI)* (19). This is an extensively used and well validated 21-item self report measure of depression.
4. *Impact of weight on quality of life-lite (IWQOL-Lite)* (20). This is a quality of life measure designed specifically for obese individuals, and has excellent psychometric properties. The scale has five domains (work, public distress, self-esteem, sexual life, and physical function) as well as a total score.

Although rarely employed in usual clinical practices, in depth information about comorbid psychopathology can be obtained by using structured interviews to assess for DSM diagnoses including the structured clinical interview for DSM-IV Axis I (SCID-I) and the Structured Clinical Interview for DSM-IV Axis II (SCID-II).

RATES OF PSYCHOPATHOLOGY

Obese individuals seeking bariatric surgery are at substantial risk for psychopathology. Whether obesity leads to psychopathology (such as depression or anxiety), perhaps through discrimination and isolation, or psychopathology leads to obesity (such as BED causing weight gain), is not always entirely known. However, recent evidence suggests that most obesity cannot be directly attributed to psychological symptoms. Nonetheless, knowledge of psychiatric status provides valuable information in terms of the variables that may be associated with poorer surgical outcome and increased rates of complications.

Studies of psychopathology in individuals seeking bariatric surgery have differed in their rigor and methodology, yielding different findings and making it difficult to compare results. Some have employed semistructured interviews while others have relied on clinical interviews. Self-report questionnaires have also been used. These research studies have shown that 27–42% of patients evaluated for bariatric surgery meet DSM criteria for one or more axis I disorders (21,22). Mood, anxiety, and eating disorders are the most common and will be discussed in more detail further. In addition, the frequency of personality disorders will also be reviewed.

Mood Disorders

Research in recent years supports the notion that many symptoms of depression seen in the obese are the result of societal views and discrimination of the obese as well as the physical and medical' complications of being overweight (23). It also seems clear that the presence of BED, female gender, and larger body mass index (BMI) increase the likelihood of depression and anxiety (23). Women with a BMI ≥ 30 have been shown to be 37% more likely to have had a major depressive episode within a year of assessment than were normal or overweight females (24). Additionally, Hafner et al. (25) found that morbidly obese individuals had somewhat higher levels of anxiety and depression than their normal weight peers.

Comparisons of the rates of depression and anxiety in pre-bariatric surgery patients in contrast to rates in the general population have shown mixed results, highlighting the importance of appropriate control group selection. Although more than a quarter of individuals seeking surgical intervention for their weight report a lifetime history of major depressive disorder, a much smaller percentage of presurgery patients endorse current symptomatology (26,27).

Binge Eating Disorder

BED is a widely studied eating disorder (a form of EDNOS) that is listed in the DSM-1V appendix as a diagnosis for further study (28). Individuals with BED report a loss of control while eating a large amount of food in a short period of time. They also experience marked distress and endorse three or more of the following symptoms: (*i*) eating until uncomfortably full, (*ii*) eating rapidly, (*iii*) eating large quantities when not hungry, (*iv*) eating alone due to embarrassment, and (*v*) feeling disgusted, depressed, or guilty after overeating.

The prevalence of BED in individuals seeking weight loss surgery ranges from 1% to 46% (29–35). In addition, up to 73% of preoperative patients engage in regular "grazing," or endorse other significant eating disturbances (36). For example, in one study, approximately 10% of bariatric patients met criteria for night eating syndrome before surgery (27). Yet rates of bulimia nervosa are reported to be very low (10,29). Prior to surgery, bariatric patients report less restraint and more disinhibition and hunger than do conventional weight loss controls on the three factor eating questionnaire (TFEQ) (37). In addition, patients with binge eating are more likely to be distressed and meet criteria for other DSM disorders than are non-binge eaters.

Personality Disorders

There is evidence that almost a quarter of individuals seeking bariatric surgery meet DSM criteria for at least one axis II disorder (38–42). For example, Larsen reported that 22% of 90 patients about to undergo bariatric surgery met criteria for a personality disorder (39). In another study, 20% of patients met criteria for one or more personality disorders, the most common being dependent personality disorder (9%), personality disorder NOS (6%), schizoid personality disorder (4%), and borderline personality disorder (3%) (27). Other studies have shown that passive dependent traits are more common in obese individuals seeking bariatric surgery than in normal weight controls (39).

PSYCHOPATHOLOGY RATES AT FOLLOW-UP

Herpertz et al. (34) performed a thorough review of the literature on the impact of bariatric surgery on psychosocial outcome. All 40 studies included in the review had a minimal follow-up period of at least one year. Eight of the 40 studies looked specifically at rates of psychopathology. All employed a prospective and nonrandomized design. The review showed that in general weight loss surgery lead to a decline in the prevalence of DSM axis I disorders but did not alter the course of axis II disorders. Regarding BED, the specific surgical procedure impacted outcome but, overall, there appeared to be an improvement in BED criteria post-bariatric surgery of any kind. Specific categories are addressed in more detail further.

Mood and Anxiety Disorders

Research studies that have assessed both pre- and postsurgical psychopathology show that prevalence rates of depression and anxiety after surgery are significantly lower than rates before surgery (34). Specifically, depressive symptomatology as measured by the BDI decreases markedly, and the decrease is correlated with the amount of lost weight at long-term follow-up (43,44).

Likewise, scores on the anxiety and global severity scales of the SCL-90 R are reduced following surgery, especially for those who lost the most weight (45). There are also notable improvements in generalized anxiety disorder and phobias after surgery (39,46). Although one study suggested that suicide rates were higher post-bariatric surgery than in a community sample, it is impossible to determine if there were any legitimate changes in suicide rates or gestures, given attrition rates during follow-up across studies (44). In addition, BMI matched controls rather than community members may be a better comparison group (34).

Not surprisingly, the more weight lost, the greater the decrease in symptoms of depression and anxiety, regardless if conventional or surgical means are used (34,38). However, in contrast to nonsurgical means of weight reduction (i.e., very low caloric diets, behavior modification, exercise, and drugs), bariatric surgery is less likely to result in psychiatric disturbance. Not only are rates of depression and preoccupations with food significantly less, but also patients endorse greater self-confidence and well-being and improved quality of life following bariatric surgery in comparison with more conservative methods of weight control (47,48).

Of concern, however, is the finding that patients who have noted improvements in mood and anxiety post-bariatric surgery may experience a return of these symptoms two to three years after the surgery, at the same time that they may experience weight regain, indicating the possible need for supportive or other interventions during this time (32,33,49).

Binge Eating Disorder

Significant reductions in binge eating usually occur after obesity surgery in patients with BED. In the longest follow-up to date, Mitchell et al. (10) assessed gastric bypass patients 13–15 years postsurgery. They found that while 49% of patients met BED criteria prior to the surgery, only 6.4% met full criteria at follow-up. Twelve percent of patients at follow-up met all BED criteria with the exception of eating "a large amount of food." There were also significant decreases on the M-FED (an interview designed to collect longitudinal data) (50) in dissatisfaction with weight and shape, impact of weight and shape on self-perception, and fear of gaining weight.

Although bariatric surgery is associated with improvements in binge eating, there may be a tendency for some patients to experience an increase in disinhibition and hunger and a decrease in restraint about two years postsurgery, with resulting weight gain (33,44,48). However, evidence of the recurrence of binge eating has been mixed, with some studies reporting that patients are able to maintain normalized eating up to three years postsurgery (31).

Different surgical interventions alter anatomy in various ways and may therefore differentially impact eating behavior. Some surgeries merely limit the amount of intake (e.g., LapBand) while others also incorporate malabsorption (e.g., gastric bypass). Following restrictive surgery such as gastroplasty or gastric banding, patients report a decrease in binge eating but an increased occurrence of vomiting (40,42).

Patients usually experience involuntary vomiting during the first few postoperative weeks. During that period, they frequently discover that they can vomit with ease after eating. The modified anatomical situation in the upper GI tract supports the development of a new eating pathology. In some patients, surgeons even recommend that they induce vomiting to decrease discomfort rather than experience lengthy nausea and vomiting. Overtime, some patients purposely overeat knowing it might result in *spontaneous* vomiting which then will prevent weight gain. Others *self-induce* vomiting as a response to fullness and epigastric discomfort or as a counter-measure to the consumption of a forbidden food. In both instances, the behavior could be labeled as "semi-purposeful." It is unclear if and to what extent postoperative vomiting represents purging behavior.

Powers et al. (42) reported that 5.5 years after restrictive surgery, 79% of the patients were vomiting at least occasionally and 33% were vomiting weekly. Mitchell et al. (10) reported that 13–15 years after gastric bypass, 68.8% of the patients reported continued problems with vomiting. In this study, the authors found an unexpectedly low level of distress caused by regular vomiting (10). It is unclear, however, if the vomiting in these patients occurred entirely, involuntarily, or if it was some kind of "purging mechanism." In addition, it might be difficult to elicit the extent to which the patients accept vomiting in order to not regain weight or to lose more weight. They might not be honest about it or not fully aware about it themselves. Even if the vomiting occurs spontaneously, some patients might welcome the effect that this might have on their weight or shape. Such thoughts might serve as a cognitive reinforcer for further vomiting.

Outcome after gastric bypass, which incorporates malabsorption, is essentially the same as gastroplasty or gastric banding procedures (10,51). Biliopancereatic diversion, while offering similar improvements in binge eating, does not seem to lead to increased rates of vomiting (30,51–53).

In short, it is difficult to distinguish between what should be considered normal eating and pathological eating after bariatric surgery, since all eating behavior will be different from that presurgery and from the eating behavior of the normal population. Patients are forced to adopt an eating style that is characterized by restraint, restriction of food varieties, and ritualistic behavior around how food is eaten (e.g., with frequent intake of small amounts of foods and extensive chewing before swallowing). Indeed, post-bariatric surgery eating behavior resembles that of patients with more classic eating disorders (i.e., anorexia nervosa and bulimia nervosa) in many ways.

Personality Disorders

Personality disorders are not markedly altered by bariatric surgery, which makes sense given that these conditions are ususally persistent and pervasive (34). For example, Larsen (39) found that the frequency of axis II diagnoses was not significantly impacted by weight loss surgery. Although not widely supported by other studies, there is some evidence that personality traits, as measured by the Millon Clincial Multiaxial Inventory (MCMI), can be altered in a positive manner post-bariatric surgery (54). In this study, the investigators found a significant decrease on the schizoid, avoidant, and passive-aggressive subscales. At the same time, patients displayed increases on the histrionic and narcissistic subscales, which the authors hypothesized to be due to improved socialization. Similar results were obtained in two studies by Chandarana et al. (55,56). Another study used the Dutch Shortened MMPI and the Dutch Personality Inventory, and showed significant improvements in social inadequacy and shyness (57). These results may not necessarily reflect a change in personality per se, but rather that postsurgical weight loss, patients feel more comfortable in social situations.

IMPACT OF PSYCHOPATHOLOGY ON OUTCOME

Building upon the aforementioned prevalence rates of psychopathology in bariatric surgery patients, research has begun to investigate the impact of psychiatric comorbidity on surgical outcome. Measuring outcome in this population is complicated not only by variations in surgical procedures, but also by the multifaceted impact of bariatric surgery on patients' functioning. There are a variety of ways in which outcome can be measured. The most common measure has been weight loss; however, changes in other conditions, including medical complications, psychiatric status, psychosocial functioning, eating patterns, and quality of life are also important in understanding the outcome of bariatric surgery. It is likely that these areas are highly intercorrelated and that outcome is multidimensional (58). What follows is a review of research investigating the impact of psychopathology on bariatric surgery outcome.

Psychiatric Comorbidity

Recent research has attempted to investigate the impact of psychiatric comorbidity on weight loss following bariatric surgery. Most of these investigations have concluded that presurgical psychiatric status does not negatively impact bariatric surgery outcome when weight loss is used as the outcome measure (21,26,40,41,46,52). However, a review of the findings reveals great variability in independent variables and surgical procedures, making definitive conclusions impossible.

Schrader et al. (59) investigated whether psychosocial factors, including psychiatric history, contributed to weight loss following gastroplasty, gastric bypass, or gastrogastrostomy. Patients participated in a presurgical semistructured interview and weight measurements at 6, 12, 24, and 36 months. The presence of a psychiatric history did not predict weight loss or noncompliance following surgery in this study; however, psychiatric history was not clearly defined. Hafner et al. (25) hypothesized that presurgical psychopathology would predict less successful weight loss following "gastric restriction surgery." The results did not support their hypothesis; the presence of depression, anxiety, phobias, obsessions, somatization, aggression, assertiveness, or marital dissatisfaction did not predict less weight loss. Hsu et al. (60) similarly found that psychiatric status previous to and/or following vertical banded gastroplasty (VBG) did not affect weight loss.

One study did suggest that more severe psychological problems, as measured by the Minnesota Multiphasic Personality Inventory (MMPI), were correlated with poorer weight loss in a sample of women who underwent VBG. The authors concluded, however, that "there was no direct or linear relationship between severity of psychological disturbance and surgical outcome" (58). Rather, types of psychopathology, including emotional lability, self injurious behaviors, impaired interpersonal functioning, suspiciousness, self-defeating behaviors, and familial psychiatric history were associated with poorer weight loss.

In sum, when weight loss is used as the outcome measure, studies suggest that presurgical psychiatric comorbidity does not negatively impact bariatric surgery outcome. However, when other measures of outcome are considered, it is apparent that the presence of psychopathology does impact patients' postsurgical experience and functioning in important ways. Studies have investigated the impact of psychopathology on such outcomes, including medical complications, worsening psychiatric status, and eating behavior (37,59,61–63).

Valley and Grace (61) found that a history of psychiatric hospitalizations, MMPI scale elevations, negative life events, and lack of social support failed to predict weight loss in a sample of patients undergoing horizontal reinforced gastroplasty. A history of psychiatric hospitalizations and lack of social support, however, predicted increased medical complications and decreased satisfaction with surgical outcome. The authors concluded that the severity of psychopathology was correlated with the presence and severity of medical complications and hypothesized that these patients may have used food as a source of coping with negative emotionality presurgically. This in turn resulted in poor compliance with dietary recommendations and subsequent medical complications.

Another study found that increased psychopathology correlated with increased improvements in psychological functioning (as measured by reductions in MMPI scale score elevations) and also with postoperative medical and psychological complications (59). Powers et al. (37) found that a presurgical diagnosis of depression or anxiety was associated with postsurgical problems including medical complications, eating disturbances, psychosexual adjustment difficulties, and impaired social functioning. These investigations highlight the importance of thorough presurgical psychiatric assessment and the need for the consideration of the multifaceted nature of bariatric surgery outcome.

Eating Specific Comorbidity

The presence of eating disorders as a specific form of psychopathology has also been the subject of investigation in bariatric surgery outcome studies. Although there are case reports describing patients developing anorexia nervosa and bulimia nervosa after bariatric surgery, research has primarily focused on investigating the impact of BED and related eating patterns, including night eating syndrome and grazing, on the outcome of bariatric surgery (42,64–66).

As noted, the rates of BED in the bariatric surgery population are significant. Including subthreshold binge eating, grazing, and night eating only increase the prevalence rates of disturbed overeating behavior among these patients. When strict diagnostic criteria related to consuming an objectively large amount of food is considered, bariatric surgery appears to be a "cure" for BED. Kalarchian et al. (29) reported that binge eating was eliminated for all of 22 patients classified presurgically as binge eaters at four-month follow-up. This is explained by the fact that patients are no longer able to physically consume an objectively large amount of food. However, some patients with a history of binge eating continued to experience a sense of loss of control characteristic of binge eating after bariatric surgery. Similarly, Powers et al. (38) reported elimination of binge eating in all subjects with presurgical BED; however, it would appear that binge eating was again defined by consuming objectively large amounts of food. Given the mechanical limitations resulting from bariatric surgery, outcome measures for binge eating in this population will need to be modified, especially the criterion for eating an objectively large amount of food, when determining the presence of binge eating and its impact on outcome.

Whether or not presurgical eating disorders (e.g., BED) or disordered eating patterns (e.g., grazing and night eating) impact surgical outcome therefore depends in part upon the surgical procedure as well as the outcome measure being used. Several studies have attempted to discern whether a history of BED is associated with poor weight loss outcome (10,38,60,65,66). Mitchell et al. (10) found that patients who redeveloped binge eating behaviors, excluding the requirement of consuming a large amount of food, following gastric bypass demonstrated a greater likelihood of weight regain. Kalarchian et al. (67) found that almost half of subjects in their study experienced a sense of loss of control while eating, and that binge eating was associated with greater weight regain and elevated scores on measures of eating pathology. Taken together, this research suggests that presurgical binge eating may place patients at higher risk for the reemergence of eating problems and greater weight regain in the long term. In contrast to the results of these studies, Powers et al. (38) did not find an association between presurgical binge eating or night eating and weight loss or weight regain. Others found that presurgical binge eating predicted a higher vomiting frequency after gastric banding with a higher complication rate (e.g., neostoma stenosis) (40).

Research investigating psychopathology in bariatric surgery patients highlights the high prevalence of psychiatric comorbidity in this population. Although great variability in patient populations, outcome measures, follow-up periods, and surgical methodologies used make it difficult to draw definitive conclusions, it is apparent that psychiatric and eating related comorbidity impact surgical outcome, particularly medical complications, weight loss, and weight maintenance. Further investigation into comorbid psychopathology, eating behavior, psychosocial functioning, and quality of life presurgically and longitudinally is needed to guide developments in patient selection as well as appropriate interventions for patients at risk of poor outcome.

TREATMENT OF COMORBID PSYCHOPATHOLOGY

Although few in number, investigations have been conducted examining the impact of psychosocial interventions aimed at enhancing outcome, including nonspecific psychotherapy, preoperative weight loss programs, behavioral therapy, brief strategic therapy, and cognitive behavioral interventions for bariatric surgery patients (68–74). Although highly variable in sample size and selection, surgical procedures, interventions, and outcome measures, research has shown some promising results.

Support Groups

The provision of support groups as a component of bariatric surgery services is increasingly common. It has been suggested that emotional support is necessary for a successful surgical outcome (75). Marcus and Elkins (75) put forth a model for supportive group therapy which addresses issues pertinent to gastric bypass patients presurgically, the first six months following surgery, and beyond. Their model includes emphasis on self-responsibility, relapse prevention, and group process. Their work has found that patients who are intelligent, motivated, psychologically open, and who are more distressed by obesity and changes subsequent to surgery are most likely to benefit. There is also some evidence that suggests that attendance at support groups may enhance weight loss.

Psychoeducation Programs

Psychoeducation regarding surgical procedures, potential complications, and necessary dietary and lifestyle changes is routinely provided. Horchner and Tuinebreijer (76) studied the impact of presurgical psychoeducation on postoperative pain, vomiting, and analgesic use in a sample of patients undergoing VBG. Patients received verbal, written, and audiovisual materials. Although the differences were not statistically significant, patients receiving this structured psychoeducation program seemed to experience less postoperative pain and vomiting and shorter hospital stays.

Behavioral Weight Loss Interventions

Investigations have been conducted into the safety and efficacy of preoperative weight loss programs and their impact on bariatric surgery outcome. Martin et al. (69) found that although preoperative weight loss did not determine psychiatric complications or wound healing, it seemed to reduce length of hospital stay. Another study found that although presurgical weight loss interventions may not impact postsurgical weight loss, it may reduce the occurrence of eating disturbances such as excessive sweet eating (70).

Psychotherapeutic Interventions

Traditional psychotherapy interventions have also been the subject of investigation in bariatric surgery patients. Tucker et al. (71) investigated the impact of behavioral interventions on the adjustment to postsurgical eating and lifestyle changes following gastric bypass surgery. Although patients receiving behavioral treatment did not differ in weight loss, daily caloric intake, or frequency of vomiting or pain, they did demonstrate higher levels of psychosocial functioning and greater physical activity. Brief strategic therapy has also shown promising results, particularly for patients with a history of BED and sweet eating (72).

Given the well established efficacy of cognitive behavioral therapy for many of the axis I disorders prevalent in bariatric surgery patients (i.e., depression, anxiety, and BED), cognitive behavioral interventions appear particularly well suited for these patients. In view of the significant changes in eating patterns required postsurgically, behavioral strategies for adopting new eating patterns and eliminating those that could interfere with weight loss and contribute to weight regain, such as sweet eating, grazing, and subjective binge eating, could significantly enhance outcome. In light of the presence of psychosocial comorbidity, interventions targeting cognitive restructuring, impulse control, body image, stress management, problem solving, and interpersonal functioning would also be appropriate. Relapse prevention techniques would likely be effective given the risk for reemergence of eating pathology for some patients and weight regain in the long term for most.

Kalarchian and Marcus (73) have outlined the multiple functions of cognitive behavioral interventions during the preoperative, postoperative, and longer-term adjustment phases for the bariatric surgery patient. In addition, Saunders (74) has developed a structured intervention program utilizing cognitive behavioral interventions, particularly targeting patients with binge eating symptoms. Interventions were particularly beneficial in increasing awareness of problematic eating patterns and developing adaptive coping skills and alternatives to self-nurturing.

SUMMARY

As overweight and obesity increase in prevalence, additional patients with psychopathology will be presenting for evaluation for bariatric surgery. Some conditions appear to be contraindications, including dementia, chronic psychoses, mental retardation, and active substance abuse/dependence. Patients can be screened by using standardized databases, self-report forms, and interviews. Certain forms of psychopathology, particularly mood and anxiety disorders and BED, are common among surgical candidates. While many of these problems often improve with postsurgical weight loss, such a comorbidity may result in adjustment problems after surgery, and BED, if recurrent, may lead to weight regain over the long term. Certain psychosocial interventions, currently under development, may improve the outcome of such patients.

REFERENCES

1. Binkley JE, Eales J, Jekanowski M. The relation between dietary change and rising US obesity. Int J Obes Relat Metab Disord 2000; 24:1032–1039.
2. Drewnowski A. Nutrition transition and global dietary trends. Nutrition 2000; 16:486–487.
3. French SA, Story M, Jeffery RW. Environmental influences on eating and physical activity. Annu Rev Public Health 2001; 22:309–335.
4. National Heart, Lung, and Blood Institute (NHLBI). Clinical guidelines on the identification, evaluation, and treatment of overweight and obesity in adults: The evidence report. Obes Res 2000; Bethesda, MD: National Institute of Health.
5. Schoeller DA. Limitations in the assessment of dietary energy intake by self-report. Metabolism 1995; 44:18–22.
6. Bray GA. Risks of obesity. Endocrinol Metab Clin North Am 2003; 32:787–804.
7. Craig BM, Tseng DS. Cost-effectiveness of gastric bypass for severe obesity. Am J Med 2002; 113:491–498.
8. Segal A, Libanori HT, Azevedo A. Bariatric surgery in a patient with possible psychiatric contraindications. Obes Surg 2002; 12:598–601.
9. Kobayashi J, Kodama M, Yamazaki K, et al. Gastric bypass in a man with Prader-Willi syndrome and morbid obesity. Obes Surg 2003; 13:803–805.
10. Mitchell JE, Lancaster KL, Burgard MA, et al. Long-term follow-up of patients' status after gastric bypass. Obes Surg 2001; 11:464–468.
11. Soper RT, Mason EE, Printen KJ, Zellweger H. Gastric bypass for morbid obesity in children and adolescents. J Pediatr Surg 1975; 10(1):51–58.
12. Abu-Abeid S, Gavert N, Klausner JM, Szold A. Bariatric surgery in adolescence. J Pediatr Surg 2003; 38:1379–1382.
13. Sugerman HJ, Sugerman EL, DeMaria EJ, et al. Bariatric surgery for severely obese adolescents. J Gastrointest Surg 2003; 7:102–107.
14. Breaux CW. Obesity surgery in children. Obes Surg 1995; 5:279–284.
15. Mitchell JE, Hatsukami D, Eckert ED, Pyle R. Eating disorders questionnaire. Psychopharmacol Bull 1985; 21:1025–1043.

16. Wadden TA, Foster GD, Letizia KA. Response of obese binge eaters to treatment by behavior therapy combined with very low calorie diet. J Consult Clin Psychol 1992; 60:808–811.
17. Spitzer RL, Devlin M, Walsh TB, et al. Binge eating disorder: a multi-site field trial of the diagnostic criteria. Int J Eat Disord 1992; 11:191–203.
18. Ware JE, Kosinski M, Keller SD. SF-36 Physical and Mental Summary Scales: A User's Manual. Boston, MA: The Health Institute, 1994.
19. Beck AT, Ward CH, Mendelson M, et al. An inventory for measuring depression. Arch Gen Psychiatry 1961; 4:561–571.
20. Kolotkin RL, Crosby RD, Kosloski KD, Williams GR. Development of a brief measure to assess quality of life in obesity. Obes Res 2001; 9:102–111.
21. Gentry K, Halverson JD, Heisler S. Psychological assessment of morbidly obese patients undergoing gastric bypass: a comparison of preoperative and postoperative adjustment. Surgery 1984; 95:215–220.
22. Gertler R, Ramsey-Stewart G. Preoperative psychiatric assessment of patients presenting for gastric bariatric surgery (surgical control of morbid obesity). Aust N Z J Surg 1986; 56:157–161.
23. Wadden TA, Sarwe DB, Womble LG, Foster GD, McGuckin BG, Schimmel A. Psychosocial aspects of obesity and obesity surgery. Surg Clin North Am 2001; 81:1001–1024.
24. Carpenter KM, Hasin DS, Allison DB, et al. Relationships between obesity and DSM-IV major depressive disorder, suicide ideation, and suicide attempts: results from a general population study. Am J Public Health 2000; 90:251–257.
25. Hafner RJ, Watts JM, Rogers J. Psychological status of morbidly obese women before gastric restriction surgery. J Psychosomatic Res 1987; 31:607–612.
26. Halmi KA, Long M, Stunkard AJ, Mason E. Psychiatric diagnosis of morbidly obese gastric bypass patients. Am J Psychiatry 1980; 137:470–472.
27. Powers PS, Boyd F, Blair CR, Stevens B, Rosemurgy A. Psychiatric issues in bariatric surgery. Obes Surg 1992; 2:315–325.
28. American Psychiatric Association. Diagnostic and Statistical Manual of Mental Disorders, 4th ed. Washington, DC: American Psychiatric Association, 1994.
29. Kalarchian MA, Wison GT, Brolin RE, Bradley L. Effects of bariatric surgery on binge eating and related psychopathology. Eating and Weight Disord 1999; 4:1–5.
30. Adami GF, Gandolfo P, Bauer B, Scopinaro N. Binge eating in massively obese patients undergoing bariatric surgery. Int J Eat Disord 1995; 17:45–50.
31. Adami GF, Meneghelli A, Bressani A, Scopinaro N. Body image in obese patients before and after stable weight reduction following bariatric surgery. J Psychosom Res 1999; 46:275–281.
32. Hsu LKG, Sullivan SP, Benotti PN. Eating disturbances and outcome of gastric bypass surgery: a pilot study. Int J Eat Disord 1997; 21:385–390.
33. Hsu LK, Benotti PN, Dwer J, et al. Nonsurgical factors that influence the outcome of bariatric surgery: a review. Psychosom Med 1998; 60:338–346.
34. Herpertz S, Kielmann R, Wolf AM, Langkafel M, Senf W, Hebebrand J. Does obesity surgery improve psychosocial functioning? A systematic review. Int J Obes 2003; 27:1–15.

35. de Zwaan M, Mitchell JE, Howell LM, Monson N, Swan-Kremeier L, Crosby RD. Characteristics of morbidly obese patients before gastric bypass surgery. Compr Psychiatry 2003; 44:428–434.
36. Saunders R, Johnson L, Teschner J. Prevalence of eating disorders among bariatric surgery patients. Int J Eat Disord 1998; 6:309–317.
37. Stunkard AJ, Messick S. The three-factor eating questionnaire to measure dietary restraint, disinhibition and hunger. J Psychosom Res 1985; 29:71–83.
38. Karlsson J, Sjostrom L, Sullivan M. Swedish obese subjects (SOS)—an intervention study of obesity. Two-year follow-up of health-related quality of life (HRQL) and eating behavior after gastric surgery for severe obesity. Int J Obes Rel Metab Disord 1998; 22:113–126.
39. Larsen F. Psychosocial function before and after gastric banding surgery for morbid obesity. A prospective psychiatric study. Acta Psychiatr Scand Suppl 1990; 359:1–57.
40. Powers P, Rosemurgy A, Boyd, F, Perez A. Outcome of gastric restriction procedures: weight, psychiatric diagnoses, and satisfaction. Obes Surg 1997; 7:471–477.
41. Powers PS, Rosemurgy AS, Coovert DL, Boyd FR. Psychosocial sequelae of bariatric surgery: a pilot study. Psychosomatics 1988; 29:283–288.
42. Powers PS, Perez A, Boyd F, Rosemurgy A. Eating pathology before and after bariatric surgery: a prospective study. Int J Eat Disord 1999; 25:293– 300.
43. Larsen F, Torgersen S. Personality changes after gastric banding surgery for morbid obesity. A prospective study. J Psychosom Res 1989; 33:323–334.
44. Larsen JK, Geenen R, van Ramsorst B, et al. Psychosocial functioning before and after laparoscopic adjustable gastric banding: a cross sectional study. Obes Surg 2003; 13:629–636.
45. Guisado JA, Vaz FJ, Lopez-lbor JJ, Lopez-lbor MI, del Rio J, Rubio MA. Gastric surgery and restraint from food as triggering factors of eating disorders in morbid obesity. Int J Eat Disord 2002; 31:97–100.
46. Hafner RJ, Rogers J, Watts JM. Psychological status before and after gastric restriction as predictors of weight loss in the morbidly obese. J Psychosom Res 1990; 34:295–302.
47. Sullivan M, Karlsson J, Sjostrom L, Taft C. Why quality of life measures should be used in the treatment of patients with obesity. In: Bjorntrop P, ed. International Textbook of Obesity. London: John Wiley and Sons, 2001.
48. Andersen T, Backer OG, Stokholm KH, Quaade F. Randomized trial of diet and gastroplasty compared with diet alone in morbid obesity. N Engl J Med 1984; 310:352–356.
49. Pories WJ, MacDonald KG. The surgical treatment of morbid obesity. Curr Opin Gen Surg 1993; 1:195–202.
50. Agras WS, Crow SJ, Halmi KA, Mitchell JE, Wilson GT, Kraemer HC. Outcome predictors for the cognitive behavior treatment of bulimia nervosa: data from a multisite study. Am J Psychiatry 2000; 157:1302–1308.
51. Halmi KA, Mason E, Falk JR, Stunkard A. Appetitive behavior after gastric bypass for obesity. Int J Obes Rel Metab Disord 1981; 5:457–464.
52. Rowston WM, McCluskey SE, Gazet J-C, Lacey JH, Franks G, Lynch D. Eating behavior, physical symptoms and psychological factors associated with

weight reduction following the Scopinaro operation as modified by Gazet. Obes Surg 1992; 2:355–360.

53. Adami GF, Gandolfo P, Meneghelli A, Scopinaro N. Binge eating in obesity: a longitudinal study following biliopancreatic diversion. Int J Eat Disord 1996; 20:405–413.

54. Millon T. Millon Clinical Miltiaxial Invenotry Manual. 3rd ed. Minneapolis, Minnesota: Interpretive Scoring Systems, 1983.

55. Chandarana P, Holliday R, Conlon P, Deslippe T. Psychosocial considerations in gastric stapling surgery. J Psychosom Res 1988; 32:85–92.

56. Chandarana PC, Conlon P, Holliday RL, Deslippe T, Field VA. A prospective study of psychosocial aspects of gastric stapling surgery. Psychiat J Univ Ott 1990; 15:32–35.

57. Van Germert WG, Severeijns RM, Greve JWM, Groenman N, Soeters PB. Psychological functioning of morbidly obese patients after surgical treatment. Int J Obes 1998; 22:393–398.

58. Barrash J, Rodriguez E, Scott DH, Mason EE, Sines JO. The utility of MMPI subtypes for the prediction of weight loss after bariatric surgery. Int J Obes 1987; 11:115–128.

59. Schrader G, Stefanovic S, Gibbs A, Elmslie R, Higgins B, Slavotinek A. Do psychosocial factors predict weight loss following gastric surgery for obesity? Aust N Z J Psychiatry 1990; 24:496–499.

60. Hsu LKG, Betancourt S, Sullivan SP. Eating disturbances before and after vertical banded gastroplasty: a pilot study. Int J Eat Disord 1996; 19:23–34.

61. Valley V, Grace DM. Psychosocial risk factors in gastric surgery for obesity: identifying guidelines for screening. Int J Obes 1987; 11:105–113.

62. Clark MM, Balsiger BM, Sletten CD, et al. Psychosocial factors and 2-year outcome following bariatric surgery for weight loss. Obes Surg 2003; 13:739–745.

63. Saltzstein EC, Gutmann MC. Gastric bypass for morbid obesity: preoperative and post-operative psychological evaluation of patients. Arch Surg 1980; 115:21–28.

64. Atchison M, Wade T, Higgins B, Slavotinek T. Anorexia nervosa following gastric reduction surgery for obesity. Int J Eat Disord 1998; 23:111–116.

65. Rand CSW, Macgregor AMC, Hankins GC. Eating behavior after gastric bypass surgery for obesity. South Med J 1987; 80:961–964.

66. Thompson JK, Weinsier RL, Jacobs B. Self-induced vomiting and subclinical bulimia following gastroplasty surgery for morbid obesity: a case description and report of a multi-component cognitive-behavioral treatment strategy. Int J Eat Disord 1985; 4:609–615.

67. Kalarchian MA, Marcus MD, Wilson GT, Labouvie EW, Brolin RE, LaMarca LB. Binge eating among gastric bypass patients at long-term follow-up. Obes Surg 2002; 12:270–275.

68. Kinzl J, Trefalt E, Fiala M, Biebl W. Psychotherapeutic treatment of morbidly obese patients after gastric banding. Obes Surg 2002; 12:292–294.

69. Martin L, Tijiauw-Ling T, Holmes R, Becker D, Horn J, Bixler E. Can morbidly obese patients safely lose weight preoperatively? Am J Surg 1995; 169: 245–253.

70. van de Weijgert E, Ruseler C, Elte J. Long-term follow-up after gastric surgery for morbid obesity: preoperative weight loss improves the long-term control of morbid obesity after vertical banded gastroplasty. Obes Surg 1999; 9:426–432.
71. Tucker J, Samo J, Rand C, Woodward E. Behavioral interventions to promote adaptive eating behavior and lifestyle changes following surgery for obesity: results of a two-year outcome evaluation. Int J Eat Disord 1991; 10:689–698.
72. Caniato D, Skorjanec B. The role of brief strategic therapy on the outcome of gastric banding. Obes Surg 2002; 12:666–671.
73. Kalarchian M, Marcus M. [in press]. Management of the bariatric surgery patient: is there a role for the cognitive behavior therapist? Cog Behav Practice 2003; 10:112–119.
74. Saunders R. Compulsive eating and gastric bypass surgery: what does hunger have to do with it? Obes Surg 2001; 11:757–761.
75. Marcus JD, Eikins GR. Development of a model for a structured support group for patients following bariatric surgery. Obes Surg 2004; 14:103–106.
76. Horchner R, Tuinebreijer W. Preoperative preparatory program has no effect on morbidly obese patients undergoing a LapBand operation. Obes Surg 1999; 9:250–257.

Index

Weight gain
  antidepressants induce, 278, 309
  antipsychotic medications induce, 25,
      243, 318–324
  atypical neuroleptics induce, 156
  drug-induced, 6
  medication associated, mechanisms
      of, 324–330
  oral-contraceptives induce, 15
  psychiatric medications induced, 175
Weight gain post smoking cessation,
      agents for reducing
  nicotine gum, 130
  nicotine inhaler, 133
  nicotine nasal spray, 132
  nicotine patch, 131
Weight history, 219
Weight loss, 222, 262, 263, 272, 277
  behavioral treatment in, 236
  induced, 71, 97, 387
  maintenance, 389

[Weight loss]
  medications for, 263
    categories of, 334
Weight loss, short-term, 230. *See also*
      VLCD
Weight maintenance, 241, 242
Weight management, in psychiatric
      populations, 331–333
Weight regain, 262
Weight-reducing diets, 331
Wellbutrin, 361
WHR. *See* Waist-to-hip ratio

Xenical, 359

Zonisamide, drug inducing weight loss,
      277, 278, 363, 385

About the Editors

SUSAN L. McELROY is Professor of Psychiatry and Neuroscience and Director of the Psychopharmacology Research Program, University of Cincinnati College of Medicine, Ohio. Dr. McElroy received the M.D. degree from Cornell University Medical School, Ithaca, New York. She completed a residency in internal medicine at Columbia Presbyterian Hospital, New York, New York, and a residency in Psychiatry at McLean Hospital, Belmont, Massachusetts.

DAVID B. ALLISON is Professor of Biostatistics, Head of the Section on Statistical Genetics, and Director of the Clinical Nutrition Research Center, University of Alabama at Birmingham. Dr. Allison received the Ph.D. degree from Hofstra University, Hempstead, New York, and completed a post-doctoral fellowship at the Johns Hopkins University School of Medicine, Baltimore, Maryland, and a second post-doctoral fellowship at the National Institutes of Health (NIH)-funded New York Obesity Research Center at St. Luke's/Roosevelt Hospital Center.

GEORGE A. BRAY is Boyd Professor, Pennington Biomedical Research Center, Louisiana State University System, Baton Rouge. He is an internationally recognized authority on obesity and the various medical conditions associated with obesity. Dr. Bray received the A.B. degree from Brown University, Providence, Rhode Island, and the M.D. degree from Harvard Medical School, Boston, Massachusetts.